REHABILITATION OF THE SPINE

A PRACTITIONER'S MANUAL

REHABILITATION OF THE SPINE

A PRACTITIONER'S MANUAL

Editor

CRAIG LIEBENSON, DC
Los Angeles, California

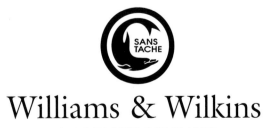

Williams & Wilkins
A WAVERLY COMPANY

BALTIMORE • PHILADELPHIA • LONDON • PARIS • BANGKOK
HONG KONG • MUNICH • SYDNEY • TOKYO • WROCLAW

1996

Editor: John P. Butler
Managing Editor: Linda S. Napora
Production Manager: Laurie Forsyth
Copy Editor: Cathy Nancarrow
Designer: Susan Blaker
Typesetter: Graphic World
Printer: Maple Press
Binder: Maple Press

Rose Tree Corporate Center
1400 North Providence Road
Building II, Suite 5025
Media, Pennsylvania 19063-2043   USA

Accurate indications, adverse reactions, and dosage schedules for drugs are provided in this book, but it is possible that they may change. The reader is urged to review the package information data of the manufacturers of the medications mentioned.

Printed in the United States of America

Library of Congress Cataloging-in-Publication Data

Rehabilitation of the spine : a practioner's manual / editor, Craig
  Liebenson.
          p.   cm.
    Includes index.
    ISBN 0-683-05032-X
    1. Backache—Chiropractic treatment.   2. Backache—Physical
therapy.   I. Liebenson, Craig.
    [DNLM: 1. Back Pain—rehabilitation.   WE 720 R345 1996]
  RZ265.S64R44   1996
  617.3′7506—dc20
  DNLM/DLC
  for Library of Congress   95-12867
                                                              CIP

The Publishers have made every effort to trace the copyright holders for borrowed material. If they have inadvertently overlooked any, they will be pleased to make the necessary arrangements at the first opportunity

96 97 98 99
2 3 4 5 6 7 8 9 10

Reprints of chapters may be purchased from Williams & Wilkins in quantities of 100 or more. Call Isabella Wise in the Special Sales Department, (800) 358-3583.

Foreword

Backache is a 20th century medical disaster. All our knowledge, resources and efforts have certainly not solved the problem. There is some suspicion that we may actually have made matters worse.

We now have investigations and therapies to deal confidently and quite effectively with serious spinal diseases and major neurologic problems. The real problem is non-specific low back pain: the everyday bodily symptom that affects most of us at some time in our adult lives. Traditional medical management for back pain is rest, based on orthopedic principles and teaching. But there is little scientific evidence for rest, and all the epidemiologic evidence is that this approach has failed. Prolonged rest is not only bad for backs, it is disastrous for patients. Musculoskeletal nutrition and health depend on movement and use.

Over the past decade there has been growing evidence that back pain is best treated by active rehabilitation. It is now time to rethink our whole approach to low back pain and disability. We must consider and deal with the physical problem in the patient's back but we must also look at how that individual deals with the pain and how it affects his or her life. The aim of health care is to relieve pain as much as we can, but backache is often a recurrent problem, and we must also help patients get on with their lives even if they still have some symptoms.

Dr. Liebenson and his colleagues are to be congratulated for this presentation of the modern approach to spinal problems. They take the best scientific evidence available, integrate it with chiropractic, and apply it to routine clinical practice. This book is a very practical contribution to the revolution that is now taking place in the care of patients with low back pain.

GORDON WADDELL, MD, FRC
Western Infirmary
Glascow, Scotland

Foreword

Modern chiropractic has a rich and colorful heritage. As a profession, it has tenaciously held to the value of manual treatment for disorders of structure and function, specifically the merit of high velocity, low amplitude manipulation or adjustment of the spine. A survey of the field of alternatives show few other treatment options as promising for spine-related disorders. Over the past several years, scientific studies have justified that commitment with findings favoring patient benefit through pain control and functional improvement by inclusion of manipulation/adjustment in the treatment plan. Multiple evidence and consensus based guidelines commissioned or conducted by the RAND Corporation; United States, Canadian and British governments have recommended manipulation for activity intolerance from low back, leg, neck and headache pain. Such symptoms, and their treatment, have ranged across a wide spectrum of pathoanatomical diagnoses.

Regional data suggests that up to 40% of patients with spine pain in the United States consult Chiropractors for their initial treatment. As a result, unprecedented opportunity exists to implement a vision of leadership in conservative management of these conditions. Despite the advances in our understanding of the appropriate uses of spinal manipulative/adjustment for effective results under controlled circumstances, the story for the patient and health care provider is not so simple. Each patient brings a constellation of factors into the doctor-patient interaction. They include severity, duration and number of prior episodes of the complaint; comorbid conditions; underlying physical condition; patient attitude; cultural and socioeconomic influences; and psychosocial functioning status. The successful outcome of clinical intervention will depend on the balance of these factors, random confounding complications that arise during treatment and the clinical effectiveness of the treatment plan.

Multidisciplinary cooperation between the various health care disciplines that deal with spine disorders has been accelerating over the past decade. Legitimate clinical collaboration, including joint ventures, have begun. Vertical integration of the services as "clinics without walls" or in centers for "one-stop shopping" offer significant advantages for the delivery of high quality health care at reduced cost. Indeed, successful therapies can be expedited and unsuccessful treatments identified more quickly through concerted team effort that focuses on patient outcomes.

As information has accumulated that supports the use of SMT for spine related disorders, a collateral body of evidence has developed that calls into question the continued use of any form of passive treatment for chronic cases. Manipulation or adjustment is, by definition, a passive treatment. That is, one where the patient concedes responsibility for their condition to the efforts of the provider and for which they take minimal personal responsibility. Persistent utilization of passive care promotes chronicity and physician dependence. These patients require different treatment that supports the therapeutic gains obtained from the passive care while tranferring responsibility for sustaining them back to the patient.

Dr. Liebenson, as editor of this work, has overseen the collection of a family of international experts whose multidisciplinary skills are dedicated to optimizing patient outcome. The approach that is detailed affords the reader a chance to understand the realistic and practical applications of pathophysiology and pathomechanics of injury. Application of these principles balances the need of the pateint to return to pre-injury activity as quickly as possible while permitting sufficient time for healing and rebuilding of the tissues. The methods arm the provider with relevant tools to assess progress and advance the patient's recovery with reasonable dispatch.

The doctor, using the considerations of this text, may thus avoid slavish adherence to time frames of treatment based on animal studies of tissue repair, as proposed by some, using the injury model to guide clinical decision making. Animal studies, no doubt, are important sources of information on the mechanisms of repair and the time required to reach various levels of tissue strength from controlled and predetermined extents of injury. After the first few days, however, they have little application directly to the clinical experience as there is rare opportunity to know the same detail of microscopic tissue injury within our patients. For the information on patient response, we must rely on clinical data that is generalizable and means of assessment specific to the patient and his/her circumstances.

Dr. Liebenson and his broad team of contributors are to be commended for assembling the elements necessary for a chiropractor wishing to focus in the field of rehabilitation. Likewise, their vision for integrated care will help position the chiropractor for stronger participation in the health care delivery systems of the future.

JOHN J. TRIANO, DC, MA
Texas Back Institute

Preface

Rehabilitation of the locomotor system is fast becoming the standard of care for neuromusculoskeletal disorders. The "sports medicine" model has been applied to the back and termed functional restoration. *Rehabilitation of the Spine: A Practitioner's Manual* has been designed to integrate the fields of chiropractic, myofascial therapy, and exercise into a cost-effective approach for spinal disorders. Learning how to transition from the passive care-based therapies to the active care approaches is at the heart of rehabilitation of the locomotor system. But, it is much more than that, too.

Today, quality care means that each patient is offered the specific type of care that he or she needs. Advice, manipulation, and exercise are valuable tools that this book integrates into a new paradigm of care. Appropriate measurement of outcomes is also part of the modern approach. Although expensive, functional capacity testing equipment has flourished in medicolegal and multidisciplinary clinics in the last decade; alternative low cost, reliable, valid approaches are presented here. In addition to active care and outcomes measurement, the third pillar of a rehabilitation practice is the identification of psychosocial factors that may predispose a patient to disability or chronic pain. These "illness behaviors" should be identified early in care to avoid treatment dependency and patient dissatisfaction.

This manual has many individual sections covering the basic skills of rehabilitation. For instance, functional assessment, manual resistance techniques, stabilization exercises, and patient education are each presented with dozens of photographs and figures showing the "how to" for each skill. These skills are in turn integrated with the introductory chapters on standards of care and the functional pathology of the motor system so that application in practice "Monday morning" can be achieved. Chapter 18 offers protocols bringing together the various elements learned and can serve as an instant reference in your practice.

Rehabilitation of the Spine is a practical guidebook for identification of rehabilitation candidates and solutions. Hopefully, restoring function in the locomotor system will become the standard for managing our patients with complex neuromusculoskeletal disorders.

CRAIG LIEBENSON
Los Angeles, California

Acknowledgments

I have had the good fortune to have had my chiropractic education complemented by introduction to a broader paradigm of care involving the muscular system through studying with Leon Chaitow, Janet Travell, and Richard Hamilton. Further study with the great Czech neurologists and manual medicine practitioners, Karel Lewit and Vladimir Janda, laid the groundwork for integrating rehabilitation with manipulative therapy. In particular, they have contributed to our approach and comprehensive analysis of the locomotor system, which enables clinicians to see how various functional pathologies, such as stiff joints, tight muscles, and weak muscles are all part of a chain of events amenable to a specific prescription of manipulation and rehabilitation. Another great teacher, Dennis Morgan, introduced to chiropractic, some of the most creative training methods for making active care possible in just about any patient with spinal pain.

Many conversations with one of the grandfathers of spinal surgery and pioneers of taking a functional view of spinal problems, William Kirkaldy-Willis, has helped sharpen my view of the locomotor system. I also owe much to Joseph Howe, whose expertise in musculoskeletal radiology and wondrously open mind have helped keep me determined to finish this project. I have regularly been challenged by David Simons, the indefatigable champion of myofascial pain syndromes. The Los Angeles College of Chiropractic (LACC), in particular Alan Adams, Rita Pierce, and Reed Phillips, have all contributed greatly to this work through their support of programs at LACC, designed to not only bring together those working at the cutting edge but to expand the chiropractic practice to include rehabilitation.

I could not have accomplished this task without the tremendous support of Nehmet Saab, head librarian at LACC. My editors, Linda Napora and Laurie Forsyth, have also been a regular source of support and encouragement driving me on to the finish line.

Contributors

GEORGE E. BECKER, M.D.
Medical Staff
Department of Orthopaedic Surgery and Psychiatry
California-Pacific Medical Center
San Francisco, California

JEAN P. BOUCHER, Ph.D.
Professor
Department of Kinanthropology
University of Quebec at Montreal
Montreal, Quebec, Canada

PIERRE-MARIE GAGEY, M.D.
President, Association Francaise de Posturologie
Manager, Institut Medical de Posturologie
Paris, France

RENÉ GENTAZ, M.D.
Association Francaise de Posturologie
Paris, France

PAUL D. HOOPER, D.C.
Chair, Department of Principles and Practice
Los Angeles College of Chiropractic
Whittier, California

JERRY HYMAN, D.C.
Los Angeles, California

GARY JACOB, D.C.
Santa Monica, California

VLADIMIR JANDA, M.D.
Chief, Department of Rehabilitation Medicine
Postgraduate Institute of Medicine
University Hospital
Srobarova, Prague, Czechoslovakia

WILLIAM H. KIRKALDY-WILLIS, M.D.
Emeritus Professor
Orthopaedic Department
Royal University Hospital
University of Saskatchewan
Saskatoon, Saskatchewan, Canada

KAREL LEWIT, MUDr.
Neurological Clinic
Medical Faculty
Charles University
Prague-Vinohrady, Czech Republic

CRAIG LIEBENSON, D.C.
Los Angeles, California

LEONARD N. MATHESON, Ph.D.
Director
Employment and Rehabilitation Institute of California
Santa Ana, California

ROBIN MCKENZIE, F.N.Z.S.P., D.I.P., M.T.
The McKenzie Institute International
Waikanae, New Zealand

VERT MOONEY, M.D.
Medical Director, UCSD Spine and Joint Conditioning Center
Professor of Orthopaedic Surgery
University of California, San Diego
San Diego, California

JEFF OSLANCE, D.C.
San Diego, California

M. VÁVROVÁ, P.T.
Prague, Czech Republic

LUDMILA F. VASILYEVA, M.D.
Associate Professor
The Novokuznetsk Advanced Doctor's Training Institute
The Department of Conventional Medicine
Novokuznetsk, Russia

HOWARD VERNON, D.C., F.C.C.S.
Associate Dean
Director of the Center for The Study of Spinal Health
Canadian Memorial Chiropractic
Toronto, Ontario, Canada

ROBERT G. WATKINS, M.D.
Kerlan, Jobe Orthopaedic Clinic
Inglewood, Calfornia

Contents

I

BASIC PRINCIPLES

1 GUIDELINES FOR COST-EFFECTIVE MANAGEMENT OF SPINAL PAIN

CRAIG LIEBENSON

MISDIAGNOSIS AND MISMANAGEMENT OF THE PROBLEM

Emerging evidence indicates the problem of low back pain has been mismanaged on a grand scale. From over-prescription of bed rest to overuse of surgical intervention and advanced imaging techniques, the costs related to low back pain are uncontained. The U.S. government recently issued federal guidelines on acute low back pain aimed at promoting a quality care model.[1] Reassurance, activity modification, manipulation, over-the-counter medications, and exercise were recommended as the key elements of such a model.[1]

Epidemic

From 60 to 80% of the general population suffer lower back pain at some time in their lives.[1–6] Most of these individuals recover within 6 weeks, but 5 to 15% are unresponsive to treatment and have continued disability[7–10] (Fig. 1.1). The minority of patients who do not recover within 3 months account for up 75 to 90% of the total expenses related to this health care problem,[11–17] which exceed $60 billion per year in the United States.[17] The 7.4% of patients who are out of work for 6 months account for 75.6% of the total cost[18] (Fig. 1.2). The majority of these costs (60%) are attributable to indemnity, with only 40% related to treatment[11,15] (Table 1.1).

Among those patients whose symptoms resolve, recurrences are common. In some studies, recurrence rates were as low as 22 to 36%.[19–21] Berquist-Ullman and Larsson found that 62% of patients with acute back pain suffered at least one recurrence during 1 year of follow-up.[10] A long-term study revealed that 45% of patients had at least one significant recurrence within 4 years.[22]

The incidence rate, cost of chronicity and disability, and high recurrence rate add up to a problem of epidemic proportions. In his Volvo award winning paper, Waddell stated, "Conventional medical treatment for low-back pain has failed, and the role of medicine in the present epidemic must be critically examined."[23] The cause of this epidemic involves a number of factors. The reasons for this failure of treatment and potential solutions are presented in Table 1.2.

Overemphasis on a Structural Diagnosis

After Mixter and Barr's discovery that compression of a nerve root by a herniated disk could cause sciatica, the medical profession has believed strongly in the pathoanatomic basis for back and leg pain.[24,25] Structural evidence of a disk hernia is present in more than 90% of patients with appropriate symptoms.[26–29] Unfortunately, even when using such advanced imaging techniques as myelography, CT scanning, or magnetic resonance imaging, the same positive findings are also present in 28 to 50% of normal, asymptomatic individuals.[26–30] Thus, imaging tests have high sensitivity (few false negatives) but low specificity (high false-positive rate) for identifying disk problems. Even when the diagnosis of disk hernia is relevant, such pathologic change tends to resolve without surgical intervention. Bush et al. reported, "A high proportion of intervertebral disc herniations have the potential to resolve spontaneously. Even if patients have marked reduction of straight leg raising, positive neurologic signs, and a substantial intervertebral disc herniation (as opposed to a bulge), there is potential for making a natural recovery, not least due to resolution of the intervertebral disc herniation."[31]

Other structural pathologic changes have also been overrated as causes of back pain. Little correlation exists between radiologic signs of degeneration and clinical symptoms.[32–38] Nachemson said, "Even when strict radiographic criteria are adhered to, 'disk degeneration' is demonstrated with equal incidence in subjects with or without pain."[39] In a study of cadaveric specimens, Videman et al. found no correlation between structural pathologic findings and a history of low back pain.[40] Spondylolisthesis is an exception; patients with this abnormality have an increased incidence of episodes of low back pain.[38] Segmental instability and isolated disk resorption are other diagnoses that cannot be validated as causative factors of low back pain.[39]

An interesting situation exists with respect to two popular diagnoses—the facet and sacroiliac syndromes. Although it is known that these structures are pain sensitive, it is notoriously difficult to confirm the diagnosis of either condition.[41,42] Schwarzer et al. used a combination of screening and confirmatory anaesthetic zygapophyseal joint blocks along with typical examination procedures (i.e., extension with rotation) and could not correlate injection response with any single

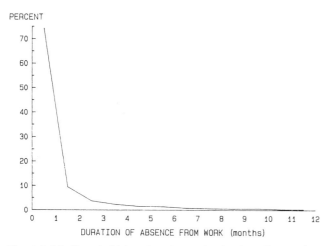

Fig. 1.1. Likelihood of injured workers returning to active employment as work absence increases. Quebec, 1981. (From Spitzer WO, Le Blanc FE, Dupuis M, et al: Scientific approach to the assessment and management of activity-related spinal disorders: A monograph for clinicians. Report of the Quebec Task Force on Spinal Disorders. Spine 12 (Suppl 7):S1, 1987.)

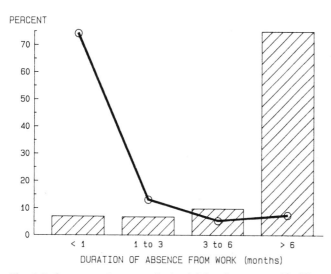

Fig. 1.2. Compensation costs for back injury in groups with different durations of absence from work. Quebec, 1981. (From Spitzer WO, Le Blanc FE, Dupuis M, et al: Scientific approach to the assessment and management of activity-related spinal disorders: A monograph for clinicians. Report of the Quebec Task Force on Spinal Disorders. Spine 12 (Suppl 7):S1, 1987.)

set of clinical features (history or examination).[43] In contrast, a study involving chronic neck pain patients who had suffered whiplash revealed that double anesthetic blocks could identify painful joints in 40 to 68% of patients.[44] In another study involving the use of diagnostic blocks, investigators reported that between 13 and 30% of patients with chronic low back pain experienced pain generated from the sacroiliac joint.[45]

Most patients with low back pain do not have structural pathologic conditions that can be clearly determined as the cause of their symptoms.[46] For this reason, most such cases are classified with the label "nonspecific back pain." According to Frymoyer, "Most commonly, diagnosis is speculative and unconfirmed by objective testing."[47] The Quebec Task force states that "before we become mesmerized with the developing diagnostic technology, such techniques must be adjudicated rigidly as to their cost/benefit, risk/benefit, and cost/effectiveness ratios."[18] Perhaps with diagnostic blocks paving the way, other less expensive tests may be found to compare favorably to this potentially important "gold standard."

Overprescription of Bed Rest

Because of the failure to pinpoint the specific pain generators in low back pain, bed rest and analgesics have become the typical treatment. The self-limiting course of most low back pain episodes has given justification to this practice of symptomatic treatment. As it turns out, this seemingly benign prescription of prolonged bed rest has been shown to be one of the most costly errors in musculoskeletal care. Allan and Waddell said, "Tragically, despite the best of intentions to relieve pain, our whole approach to backache has been associated with increasing low back disability. Despite a wide range of treatments, or perhaps because none of the them provide a lasting cure, our whole strategy of management has been negative, based on rest. We have actually prescribed low back disability!"[25] The Quebec report stated, "Bed rest is not necessary for low back pain without significant radiation. When prescribed, it should last no longer than 2 days.

Table 1.1. Percentage of Costs by Type of Treatment and Compensation

Back Pain Costs	Percent	Percent
Medical costs		33
Physician's fees	11	
Hospital costs	11	
Diagnostic tests	4	
Physical therapy	3	
Drugs	2	
Appliances	2	
Disability		67
Temporary	22	
Permanent	45	
Total costs		100

Adapted with permission from Pope MH, Frymoyer JW, Andersson G (eds): Occupational Low Back Pain. New York, Praeger, 1984, p 107.

Table 1.2. The Low Back Pain Epidemic

The Problem	The Solution
Overemphasis on structural diagnosis	ID deconditioning syndrome
Overprescription of bed rest	Early, aggressive conservative therapy
Overuse of surgery	Active care for subacute cases
Ignoring abnormal illness behavior	Early ID of disability predictors

Prolonged bed rest may be counterproductive."[18] Deyo and colleagues performed a controlled clinical trial comparing 2 days against 2 weeks of bed rest. They concluded that not only was 2 days of bed rest as effective as 2 weeks, but also the negative effects of prolonged immobilization were also limited.[48]

Overuse of Surgery

The overuse of surgery has been perhaps the single most damaging medical intervention for back pain sufferers. Bigos and Battie said, "Surgery seems helpful for at most 2% of patients with back problems, and its inappropriate use can have a great impact on increasing the chance of chronic back pain disability."[46] In his Volvo award paper, Waddell said, "Such dramatic surgical successes unfortunately only apply to approximately 1% of patients with low back disorders. Our failure involves the remaining 99% . . . for whom the problem has become progressively worse."[23] Saal and Saal supervised care for a group of patients referred by neurologists for surgery. They attempted rehabilitation for these patients and made the following observations: "Surgery should be reserved for those patients for whom function cannot be satisfactorily improved by a physical rehabilitation program . . . Failure of passive nonoperative treatment is not sufficient for the decision to operate."[49]

In 1970, Hakelius performed a study that revealed that the majority of sciatica patients responded to conservative care.[50] In 1983, Weber reported that, even in properly selected patients, there is no difference in outcome between surgically and conservatively treated patients at 2 years.[51] Saal and Saal and their colleagues discovered, "The premise that operative patients fare better in the first year is contrary to our results."[49] In 1992, Bush stated that, "86% of patients with clinical sciatica and radiologic evidence of nerve root entrapment were treated successfully by aggressive conservative management."[31]

The notion that surgery is necessary in a patient with a large disk extrusion is not supported in the literature. According to Saal and Saal, "The presence of disk extrusion does not adversely effect the outcome of nonoperative treatment and should not be used as overwhelming evidence that surgery is necessary."[49] Bush et al. found that, "Indeed, the intervertebral disc pathomorphology that might seem best suited to surgical resection is in fact that which shows the most significant incidence of natural regression . . . These results confirm that if the pain can be controlled, nature can be allowed to run its course with the partial or complete resolution of the mechanical factor . . . . Lumbar herniated nucleus pulposus can be treated non-operatively with a high degree of success."[31]

Surgery clearly has its place in the treatment of lumbar spine disorders. Conservative care practitioners must be able to select the patients who satisfy the criteria for surgical intervention. These criteria are more strict than previously believed. Bush said, "In some cases, symptoms may have been

more promptly relieved by surgery, but this has a significant morbidity and rarely mortality. Surgery is not invariably successful."[31] Allen and Waddell, using the strongest possible language, blame their colleagues, "The rapid and enthusiastic expansion of disc surgery soon exposed its limitations and failures. It was accused of leaving more tragic human wreckage in its wake than any other operation in history."[25] Frymoyer describes a particularly difficult patient group on which to perform surgery: "One place where treatment has an adverse effect is surgical management of patients with compensation."[47] Schneider and Kahanovitz echoed these same remarks, noting that even in patients who had an apparently successful operation for sciatica, if their problem is compensable, they are still at significant risk for recurrence and disability.[52]

Overemphasis on a Psychogenic Diagnosis

According to Dworkin,[53] "Pain report often occurs in the absence of pathophysiology or any discernible peripheral somatic changes. This finding implies the need to reexamine our limited understanding of pain, rather than leaping to the conclusion that such pains must be psychogenic." LaRocca commented on this problem in his Presidential Address to the Cervical Spine Research Society Annual Meeting in December of 1991: "An assumption is made that there is a pathological entity operating in the spine to produce pain which, if eliminated or controlled, should result in pain relief in every instance . . . The clinician, having spent his resources, is conditioned to resolve the matter by deciding that a psychological explanation is the only alternative . . . The error here is the automatic leap to psychology. It assumes that all organic factors have been considered, when in reality the clinician's appreciation of the complexity of such factors is often severely limited."[54] According to Merskey, "Slater and Glithero[55] showed that 60% of patients diagnosed by distinguished neurologists as having hysteria did suffer from, or develop, relevant physical disease that might account for their symptoms . . ."[56] Merskey goes on to conclude that most regional pain syndromes are not psychogenic in origin and are often mislabeled as such.[57–59]

This is not to say that pain behavior does not accompany pain sensation. Dworkin says, "Finally, there is no inconsistency in accepting the likelihood that chronic pain patients experience distress in the form of depression, anxiety, and multiple nonspecific physical symptoms, without having recourse to the diagnosis or classification of their pain condition as psychogenic."[53] Pain behavior is common and should be recognized and addressed. Although acute pain is directly related to painful stimuli, nociception, and tissue injury, chronic pain is attributable only in part to physical events.[59–63] Chronic illness behavior and disability are only partially related to nociceptive influences.[61,64–66] Psychosocial illness behavior, including depression, inactivity, and pain avoidance, are the rule with chronic pain sufferers.[67–71]

Because most patients do not have a diagnosable structural cause of their symptoms, a functional disorder should be assumed. Pain in the locomotor system should be viewed as a sign of impaired function. Nonspecific or idiopathic back pain most likely has to do with muscle or joint dysfunction with resultant soft tissue irritation and pain generation. Treatments designed for injury states or disk lesions inevitably fail, thus causing depression, despair, and illness behavior.[72–76]

Abnormal illness behavior was defined by Pilowsky[77] as a patient's inappropriate or maladaptive response to a physical complaint (Table 1.3). This situation typically occurs when no organic cause for a patient's back pain can be identified. Descartes' view of pain as a warning signal of impending harm has led to the advice to "let pain be your guide," which is helpful in acute situations when nociceptive factors predominate. In chronic cases, however, behavior should be encouraged that focuses on functional reactivation and not on pain avoidance. In fact, it is necessary for chronic pain patients to focus on increasing their activities in spite of their pain.

QUALITY CARE: COST CONTAINMENT STRATEGIES FOR MANAGING SPINAL PAIN

Feuerstein[78] has modeled how rehabilitation deals with assessment and multidisciplinary management of medical status (internal, neurologic, musculoskeletal), physical capabilities (functional capacity, work capacity), work demands (biomechanical, psychophysical), and psychosocial/behavioral resources (coping skills, job satisfaction, family situation).

A quality care approach begins with primary prevention and the aggressive treatment of any acute pain episodes. Manipulation is a proven cost saver in this regard.[1] Overutilization of expensive imaging techniques to make a structural diagnosis should be avoided.[1,18] Strict criteria for prescribing bed rest or surgery should be maintained. After studying a group of patients with operable disk lesions, Bush et al. commented that "Even if patients have marked reduction of straight leg raising, positive neurologic signs, and a substantial intervertebral disc herniation (as opposed to a bulge), . . . if the pain can be controlled, nature can be allowed to run its course with the partial or complete resolution of the mechanical factor."[31]

Patients with subacute pain should be educated about the benign nature of pain and the dangers of deconditioning, and be encouraged about the benefits and safety of becoming more active. Functional restoration programs concentrating on quantification of functional deficits, exercise, education, and psychologic intervention have proven their success with chronically disabled low-back pain sufferers or recurrent pain patients (Table 1.4).

Primary Prevention

Because first-time back pain patients are likely to suffer recurrences, successful primary prevention would be of great value in reducing this epidemic disorder. Unfortunately, little scientific literature addresses this topic. Those engaged in repetitive lifting or prolonged sitting occupations may be at higher risk, but few studies have evaluated whether treatment can lower these risks. Two of the best studies performed to date involve nurses and nurse's aides.[79,80] Gundewell et al. showed that exercises can impart a preventive benefit, and Videman et al. showed that skill training can reduce future injuries.[79,80] Skill training, ergonomic modifications, and improved fitness are all probable ways to prevent first-time occurrences of back pain.

Primary Conservative Care

A pro-active disability management program aggressively treats acute pain episodes with conservative care. The Quebec report stated that, "Management strategies should be directed at maximizing the number of workers returning to work before 1 month and minimizing the number whose spinal disorder keeps them idle for longer than 6 months."[18] Most traditionally minded physicians are still ignorant of the dangers of bed rest and immobilization.[1] They are too passive in their approach to lower back pain. Troup said, "The first attack is the ideal time for active and perhaps aggressive treatment. But if it is tacitly assumed that the vast majority of patients recover from back pain whether or not they are treated, then the opportunity may be missed."[81] The natural history of lower back pain is toward resolution in 80% of patients within 6 weeks. The 20% who are resistant to this generally favorable natural history, however, have a 50% chance of becoming permanently disabled if their symptoms persist for 6 months (Fig. 1.3).

Linton and co-workers demonstrated that early aggressive treatment (patient education, exercise instruction, physical therapy) was superior to traditional treatment approaches (rest and analgesics without physical therapy for 3 months), "Properly administered Early Active Intervention may therefore decrease sick leave and prevent chronic problems, thus saving considerable resources."[82] This study is particularly powerful in that the risk of developing chronic pain was eight

Table 1.3. Abnormal Illness Behavior

Symptom magnification syndrome
Pain-avoidance behavior
Psychologic distress
Catastrophizing as a coping strategy
Anxiety
Treatment dependency

Table 1.4. Quality Care for Low Back Pain

Primary prevention
Primary conservative care for acute episodes
Secondary functional restoration for subacute and recurrent cases
Tertiary multidisciplinary functional restoration for chronic, disabled
  patients

PROBABILITY OF RETURNING TO WORK

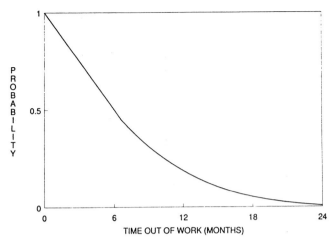

Fig. 1.3. The probability of recovering from low back pain. (From Frymoyer JW: Epidemiology of spinal disorders. In Mayer TG, Mooney V, Gatchel RJ (eds): Contemporary Conservative Care for Painful Spinal Disorders. Philadelphia, Lea & Febiger, 1991.)

times lower in the Early Active Intervention group than in the traditional group. Many doctors consulting in managed care situations today wrongly conclude that care should be minimized for back pain sufferers because most will get better regardless of care.

MANIPULATIVE THERAPY RESULTS IN LESS DISABILITY AND INCREASED PATIENT SATISFACTION

Manipulative therapy has clearly established its cost effectiveness in patients with acute and subacute low back pain.[1,83–85] Jarvis and colleagues found, in comparing medical versus chiropractic treatment for identical diagnoses, that "cost for care was significantly more for medical claims, and compensation costs were 10-fold less for chiropractic claims."[86] Authors of a recent meta-analysis looked at studies comparing spinal manipulation to other conservative treatments for acute low back pain and found significantly better rates of recovery for those individuals treated with manipulation.[83] In fact, they concluded that manipulative therapy has demonstrated a 34% better rate of recovery at the 3-week mark than other conservative therapies.[83]

Patient satisfaction is a critical aspect to reducing disability and treatment costs. Chiropractics (which offers over 90% of the spinal manipulations) has shown higher levels of patient satisfaction than family practitioner visits for back pain.[87–89] This level of satisfaction may be attributable in part to the thorough explanations that chiropractors give their patients regarding the nature of their symptoms (facet, myofascial, disk, etc.).[89]

Shekelle noted that the expert Rand panel recommendations for spinal manipulation included about 12 manip-

ulations over a 1-month period.[84] Certain studies excluded from the meta-analysis were those such as Meade's, which included other therapies, the effects of which could not be disentangled from those of manipulation.[84,85] The study by Meade and co-workers was one of a select few that suggested manipulation was beneficial for chronic low back pain.[85] Triano et al reported recently that in patients with low back pain over 7 weeks, an average of 10.5 treatments with chiropractic manipulation resulted in improved function and significantly reduced pain.[90] Erhard and Delitto demonstrated that patients receiving manipulation and exercise outperformed those receiving exercise alone.[91]

EARLY RETURN TO WORK IS A KEY

Aggressive care gives the best chance for early return to work. Litigation neurosis is easy for disabled workers to acquire. Promoting bed rest and prolonged inactivity only increases the likelihood of prolonged disability. Treatments that mobilize the patient and attempt to return them to work quickly are advantageous. Communication between doctor and employer is essential because certain job modifications may be necessary to ensure worker safety on return to work. Deyo and associates said, "Our data support a recent trend toward earlier mobilization of patients with back pain . . . . early return to work may help to prevent the emergence of chronic back pain syndromes, with their enormous human and monetary costs."[48] Cats-Baril and Frymoyer also said, "It would seem that people who are able to work through the acute phase of a low back pain episode or those who go back to work even if the pain has not disappeared after a period of rest are unlikely to become disabled . . . . keeping people at work is very effective therapy."[92] Waddell succinctly stated that, "Prolonged time away from work in itself makes recovery and return to work progressively less likely."[23]

Secondary Functional Restoration

Prolonged passive care in an attempt to ameliorate the suffering of back pain patients can lead to patient dependency. In the acute stages of an injury, such care is necessary; however, when the chemical signs of inflammation are missing, a more active, patient participatory type of care is required. Oland and Tveiten said, ". . . resources from the health services should be used in the subacute stage to enhance diagnosis, treatment, and rehabilitation and to inform the public of the benign, self-limiting course of low-back pain and the positive effect of physical training."[93]

Secondary functional restoration care that focuses on specific functional goals and patient education should be the mode of care for subacute or recurrent pain patients. Comprehensive rehabilitation involves functional capacity testing, physical training, education about biomechanics and ergonomics, and identification of psychosocial predictors of disability (Table 1.5).

Table 1.5. Functional Restoration

Functional capacity evaluation
Rehabilitation of the motor system
Patient education
Identification of psychosocial factors (disability predictors)

FUNCTIONAL CAPACITY EVALUATION

Functional reactivation requires assessment of the functional status of the patient's motor system. Evaluation of posture and movement or static and dynamic function is essential and should include assessment of joint mobility, muscle strength, coordination, endurance, and flexibility. Postural analysis and job or activity skills should also be assessed.

An objective functional capacity evaluation can be performed inexpensively and helps the doctor understand exactly what areas need improvement. Many of the functional tests also provide ideal outcome assessment measurements, which provide the patient with visual feedback of their baseline functional capacity and lets them see their progress over time. It is also crucial for communication with third-party payers or for documentation in medicolegal cases. "Low-tech" tests have proven reliability.[94] Such tests correlate better with disability than do dynametric tests.[95] Overuse of technically advanced tests can lead to increased expense, and therefore such methods should be used only if necessary.

ACTIVE CARE VS. PASSIVE CARE

In a comparative study of passive physical therapy versus rehabilitation, Mitchell and Carmen found, "Active exercise to provide mobility, muscle strengthening, and work conditioning has shown superior results . . . substantial savings have been realized in the number of days absent from work and savings in the dollars expended for compensation benefits. There was an initial increase in health care costs resulting from the intensity of the treatment, but these costs were more than offset by savings in wage loss cost."[96] Lindstrom et al. compared a group of patients treated with exercises and education to a control group that received more traditional treatment. They documented earlier return to work and decreased re-injury in the rehabilitation group.[97]

The notion that active exercise can be harmful in an individual with back pain is incorrect. Guided exercise by a properly trained rehabilitation specialist is the optimal treatment program for the subacute population. A key is exercising to a pre-established quota rather than to a pain limit.[74,97] Waddell stated, "There is no evidence that activity is harmful and, contrary to common belief, it does not necessarily even aggravate the pain."[23] Saal and Saal treated a group of patients that had back and leg pain and were referred for surgery. They concluded, "All patients had undergone an aggressive physical rehabilitation program consisting of back school and stabilization exercise training . . . 92% return to work rate."[49] Active rehabilitation is essential for all patients, including those for whom surgery is being considered. Again, Saal and Saal said the failure of passive nonoperative treatment is not sufficient support of the decision to operate.[49]

In one notable study concerning the treatment of uncomplicated, acute back pain patients, Faas et al. reported that exercise was no better than usual care by a general practitioner.[98] One obvious criticism of this study is that exercises were given on a "generic" basis rather than being customized to the needs of each patient. This investigation can be contrasted with eight other controlled studies, all of which showed substantial benefit from exercise that lasted for at least 6 months to 2 years.[97,99–104] In a well-controlled study looking at exercise in failed back surgery patients, Timm found that "low-tech" exercises (stabilization and McKenzie) gave a greater benefit than "high-tech" exercises (Cybex).[104]

Mooney said, "Prolonged rest and passive physical therapy modalities no longer have a place in the treatment of the chronic problem."[105] According to Waddell, "The main theme of management must change from rest to rehabilitation and restoration of function."[23]

PATIENT EDUCATION FOR DISABILITY PREVENTION

Patient education, especially regarding skill training and ergonomics as well as self-care methods, has shown promise in reducing the costs associated with disabling lower back pain.[106–110] Berquist-Ullman and Larsson showed that, when compared to a control group, patients with acute lower back pain who received a 4-hour back school returned to work sooner and had few recurrences in the following year.[10] A recent study concluded, "Differences between back school participants and a comparison group indicated significantly fewer injuries among the back school participants in the 6-month post-intervention period."[99] Participants had one half as many re-injuries as nonparticipants. They also demonstrated significant reductions in lost work time costs. Although these results are impressive, some studies have questioned the long-term results of back schools.[111–113]

IDENTIFICATION OF PSYCHOSOCIAL FACTORS (DISABILITY PREDICTORS)

It is the responsibility of the rehabilitation specialist to be on the lookout for early signs of a disability prone patient. According to Frymoyer, "if a patient is identified early in the course of the low back pain episode to have a high risk for disability, early, aggressive rehabilitative efforts may be more successful and cost effective than permitting the patient to have a longer period of disability with its resultant economic, social and medical consequences."[47]

The problem of chronicity or "delayed recovery" occurs when disability is disproportionate to impairment.[114] Many researchers believe psychologic characteristics may be more important than biomechanical ones.[68–70,74,75] Frymoyer said, "There is increasing evidence from the general field of disability, and specifically low back disability, that a 'disability prone profile' can be identified and used to predict potential disability before the condition becomes truly chronic."[47] Job dissatisfaction is one of the only proven predictors of disabling back pain.[115] According to Cats-Baril and Frymoyer,[116] other predictors of low back disability include work status and job satisfaction; injury being viewed as compensable; past hospitalization; and the patient's educational level.

Recent studies indicate that it may be possible to identify acute back pain patients with psychologic predispositions to becoming chronically disabled.[117,118] In the Minnesota Multiphasic Personality Inventory (MMPI), responses indicating increased catastrophizing as a pain-coping strategy as well as emotional distress appear to be promising discriminators.[117–122] Depression, anxiety, hypochondriasis, and hysteria are related to poor surgical outcome.[72,116] The "bio-psychosocial" model has been proposed by Waddell to address the disability problem in patients with low back pain[23] (Table 1.6).

Tertiary Multidisciplinary Functional Restoration

Tertiary treatment of the chronic, disabled patient with *multidisciplinary functional restoration* has demonstrated its cost effectiveness. A combination of technically advanced functional capacity evaluation, exercise training, and psychosocial intervention are essential to the program's success. With a functional restoration approach, Mayer et al. allowed 87% of chronically disabled people to return to work compared to only 41% of a comparison group.[123] Hazard et al. reported that 81% of the treatment group returned to work compared to only 21% of the control group.[124] When Sachs et al. used less psychologic intervention, 73% returned to work compared with 38% in the control group. This approach was less costly than that used by Mayer or Hazard and their colleagues.[125] Oland and Tveiten attempted a modified program in Europe, but they had difficulty achieving similar results.[93] Alaranta et al. compared a multidisciplinary functional restoration program to a primarily passive care approach and documented improved function, pain, and disability levels.[126] In contrast to most other multidisciplinary approaches, their approach involved the use of low cost, "low-tech" functional capacity measures.

Multidisciplinary functional restoration includes the components described in Table 1.7.

Table 1.6. Biopsychosocial Approach to Low Back Disability

Restore function
Promote return to work
Decrease pain
Reduce distress
Reduce abnormal illness behavior

CONCLUSION

With consensus-based guidelines emerging as the best chance to cut costs associated with diagnosis and treatment of low back pain, it is incumbent on us to be aware of the direction in which new findings lead. Quality care will result in better patient satisfaction and reduced costs. Manipulation and exercise both appear to be of value if our beliefs are based on the scientific literature. Future studies will hopefully flush out which patients respond better to what type of care and what are appropriate timelines for transferring from passive to active care.

Table 1.7. Multidisciplinary Functional Restoration

Quantifiable, functional capacity evaluation
Physical reconditioning of the impaired "weak link"
Work hardening
Behavioral disability management
Ongoing outcome assessment using objective criteria

REFERENCES

1. Bigos S, Bowyer O, Braen G, et al: Acute Low Back Problems in Adults. Clinical Practice Guideline. Rockville, MD, U.S. Department of Health and Human Services, Public Health Service, Agency for Health Care Policy and Research, 1994.
2. Hult L: The Munkfors investigation. Acta Orthop Scand Suppl 16, 1954.
3. Frymoyer JW, Pope MH, Costanza MC, et al: Epidemiologic studies of low-back pain. Spine 5:419, 1980.
4. Svensson HO, Andersson GBJ: Low back pain in forty to forty-seven year old men. I. Frequency of occurrence and impact on medical services. Scand J Rehabil Med 14:47, 1982.
5. Valkenburg HA, Haanen HCM: The epidemiology of low back pain. Clin Orthop 179:9, 1983.
6. Biering-Sorensen F: A prospective study of low back pain in a general population. I. Occurrence, recurrence and aetiology. Scand J Rehabil Med 15:71, 1983.
7. Benn RT, Wood PH: Pain in the back: An attempt to estimate the size of the problem. Rheumatol Rehabil 14:121, 1975.
8. Horal J: The clinical appearance of low back pain disorders in the city of Gothenburg, Sweden. Acta Orthop Scand Suppl 18:1, 1969.
9. Rowe ML: Low back pain in industry. J Occup Med 11:161, 1969.
10. Berquist-Ullman M, Larsson U: Acute low back pain in industry. Acta Orthop Scand Suppl 170:1, 1977.
11. Webster BS, Snook SH: The cost of 1989 workers' compensation low back pain claims. Spine 19:1111, 1994.
12. Snook SH: Low back pain in industry. In White AA, Gordon SL (eds): Symposium on Idiopathic Low Back Pain. St Louis, CV Mosby, 1982.
13. Spengler DM, Bigos SJ, Martin NA, et al: Back injuries in industry: A retrospective study. I. Overview and cost analysis. Spine 11:241, 1986.
14. Frymoyer JW, Pope MH, Clements JH, et al: Risk factors in low-back pain: An epidemiological study. J Bone Joint Surg [Am] 65:213, 1983.
15. Andersson GBJ, Pope MH, Frymoyer JW: Epidemiology. In Pope MH, Frymoyer JW, Andersson G (eds): Occupational Low Back Pain. New York, Praeger, 1984, pp 101–114.
16. Morris A: Identifying workers at risk to back injury is not guesswork. Occup Health Saf 55:16, 1985.
17. Frymoyer JW: Epidemiology. In Frymoyer JW, Gordon SL (eds): Symposium on New Perspectives on Low Back Pain. Park Ridge, American Academy of Orthopaedic Surgeons, 1989, pp 19–33.

18. Spitzer WO, Le Blanc FE, Dupuis M, et al: Scientific approach to the assessment and management of activity-related spinal disorders: A monograph for clinicians. Report of the Quebec Task Force on Spinal Disorders. Spine 12(Suppl 7):S1, 1987.

19. Rossignol M, Suissa S, Abenheim L: Working disability due to occupational back pain: Three-year follow-up of 2,300 compensated workers in Quebec. J Occup Med 30:502, 1988.

20. Abenheim L, Suissa S, Rossignol M: Risk of recurrence of occupational back pain over a three year follow up. Br J Ind Med 45:829, 1988.

21. Frymoyer JW, Rosen JC, Clements J, et al: Psychologic factors in low-back-pain disability. Clin Orthop 195:178, 1985.

22. Dillane JB, Fry J, Kalton G: Acute back syndrome-a study from general practice. Br Med J 2:82, 1966.

23. Waddell G: A new clinical model for the treatment of low-back pain. Spine 12:634, 1987.

24. Mixter WJ, Barr JS: Rupture of the intervertebral disc with involvement of the spinal canal. N Engl J Med 211:210, 1934.

25. Allan DB, Waddell G: An historical perspective on low back pain and disability. Acta Orthop Scand Suppl 60:1, 1989.

26. Wiesel SE, Tsourmans N, Feffer HL, et al: A study of computer-assisted tomography. I. The incidence of positive CAT scans in an asymptomatic group of patients. Spine 9:549, 1984.

27. Rothman RH, et al: A study of computer-assisted tomography. Spine 9:548, 1984.

28. Hitselberger WE, Witten RM: Abnormal myelograms in asymptomatic patients. J Neurosurg 28:204, 1968.

29. Boden SD, Davis DO, Dina TS, et al: Abnormal magnetic-resonance scans of the lumbar spine in asymptomatic subjects. J Bone Joint Surg [Am] 72:403, 1990.

30. Jensel MC, Brant-Zawadzki MN, Obuchowski N, et al: Magnetic resonance imaging of the lumbar spine in people without back pain. N Engl J Med 2:69, 1994.

31. Bush K, Cowan N, Katz DE, et al: The natural history of sciatica associated with disc pathology: A prospective study with clinical and independent radiologic follow-up. Spine 17:1205, 1992.

32. Frymoyer JW, Newberg A, Pope MH, et al: Spine radiographs in patients with low-back pain: An epidemiological study in men. J Bone Joint Surg [Am] 66:1048, 1984.

33. Fullenlove TM, Williams AJ: Comparative roentgen findings in symptomatic and asymptomatic backs. JAMA 168:572, 1957.

34. LaRocca H, Macnab IA: Value of pre-employment radiographic assessment of the lumbar spine. Can Med Assoc J 101:383, 1969.

35. Magora A, Schwartz A: Relation between the low back pain syndrome and x-ray findings. Scand J Rehabil Med 8:115, 1976.

36. Splithoff CA: Lumbosacral junction: Roentographic comparison of patients with and without back ache. JAMA 152:1610, 1953.

37. Torgeson WR, Dotler WE: Comparative roentgenographic study of the asymptomatic and symptomatic lumbar spine. J Bone Joint Surg [Am] 58:850, 1976.

38. Dabbs VM, Dabbs LG: Correlation between disk height narrowing and low-back pain. Spine 15:1366, 1990.

39. Nachemson AL: Newest knowledge of low back pain. Clin Orthop 279:8, 1992.

40. Videman T, Nurminen M, Troup JDG: Lumbar spinal pathology in cadaveric material in relation to history of back pain, occupation, and physical loading. Spine 15:728, 1990.

41. Butler D, Trafinmow JH, Andersson GBJ, et al: Disks degenerate before facets. Spine 15:111, 1990.

42. Jackson RP: The facet syndrome—Myth or reality? Clin Orthop 279:110, 1992.

43. Schwarzer AC, April CN, Derby R, et al: Clinical features of patients with pain stemming from the lumbar zygapophyseal joints. Spine 19:1132, 1994.

44. Barnsley L, Lord SM, Wallis BJ, et al: The prevalence of chronic cervical zygapophyseal joint pain after whiplash. Spine 20:20, 1995.

45. Schwarzer AC, April CN, Bogduk N: The sacroiliac joint in chronic low back pain. Spine 20:31, 1995.

46. Bigos, S, Battie MC: Back disability prevention. Clin Orthop 221:121, 1987.

47. Frymoyer JW: Predicting disability from low back pain. Clin Orth 279:103, 1992.

48. Deyo RA, Diehl AK, Rosenthal M: How many days of bed rest for acute low back pain?. N Engl J Med 315:1064, 1986.

49. Saal JA, Saal JS: Nonoperative treatment of herniated lumbar intervertebral disc with radiculopathy. Spine 14:431, 1989.

50. Hakelius A: Prognosis in sciatica. Acta Orthop Scand Suppl 129:1, 1970.

51. Weber H: Lumbar disc herniation: A controlled prospective study with ten years of observation. Spine 8:131, 1983.

52. Schneider PL, Kahanovitz N: Clinical testing in chronic low back pain. Surg Rounds Orthop 4:19, 1990.

53. Dworkin SF: Perspectives on psychogenic versus biogenic factors in orofacial and other pain states. APS Journal 3:172, 1992.

54. LaRocca H: A taxonomy of chronic pain syndromes. 1991 Presidential Address, Cervical Spine Research Society Annual Meeting, December 5, 1991. Spine 10:S344, 1992.

55. Slater E, Glithero E: A follow-up of patients diagnosed as suffering from "hysteria." J Psychosom Res 9:9, 1965.

56. Merskey H: Limitations of pain behavior. APS Journal 2:101, 1992.

57. Merskey H: Regional pain is rarely hysterical. Arch Neurol 45:915, 1988.

58. Merskey H: The importance of hysteria. Br J Psychiatry 149:23, 1986.

59. International Association for the Study of Pain: Pain terms: A list with definitions and notes on usage. Pain 6:249, 1979.

60. Loeser JD, Fordyce WE: Chronic pain. In Carr JE, Dendgerink HA (eds): Behavioral Science in the Practice of Medicine. New York, Elsevier, 1983.

61. Philips HC, Jahanshahi M: The components of pain behavior report. Behav Res Ther 24:117, 1986.

62. Zarkowska E, Philips HC: Recent onset vs. persistent pain: Evidence for a distinction. Pain 25:365, 1987.

63. Waddell G: A new clinical model for the treatment of low back pain. In Weinstein JN, Wiesel SW (eds): The Lumbar Spine: The International Society for the Study of the Lumbar Spine. Philadelphia, WB Saunders, 1990, pp 38–56.

64. Linton SJ: The relationship between activity and chronic pain. Pain 21:289, 1985.

65. Fordyce WE, McMahon R, Rainwater G, et al: Pain complaint-exercise performance relationship in chronic pain. Pain 10:311, 1981.

66. Nachemson A: Work for all, for those with low back pain as well. Clin Orthop 179:77, 1983.

67. Bortz WM: The disuse syndrome. West J Med 141:691, 1984.

68. Engel GL: Psychogenic pain and the pain prone patient. Am J Med 26:899, 1959.

69. Naliboff BD, Cohen MJ, Swanson GA, et al: Comprehensive assessment of chronic low back pain patients and controls: Physical abilities, level of activities, psychological adjustment and pain perception. Pain 23:121, 1985.

70. Szasz TS: The painful person. Lancet 88:18, 1968.

71. Waddell G, Main CJ, Morris EW, et al: Chronic low back pain, psychological distress and illness behavior. Spine 9:209, 1984.

72. Wiltse LL, Rocchio PF: Preoperative psychological tests as predictors of success of chemonucleolysis in the treatment of the low back syndrome. J Bone Joint Surg [Am] 57:478, 1975.

73. Fordyce WE, Brochway JA, Bergman JA, et al: Acute back pain: A control-group comparison of behavioral vs. traditional management methods. J Behav Med 9:127, 1986.

74. Fordyce WE, Fowler RS, Lehmann JF, et al: Operant conditioning in the treatment of chronic pain. Arch Phys Med Rehabil 54:399, 1973.

75. Sternbach RA, Timmermans G: Personality changes associated with reduction of pain. Pain 1:177, 1975.

76. Waddell G, Morris EW, DiPaoloa M, et al: A concept of illness tested as an improved basis for surgical decisions in low back disorders. Spine 11:712, 1986.

77. Pilowsky I: A general classification of abnormal illness behavior. Br J Med Psychol 51:131, 1979.

78. Feuerstein M: A multidisciplinary approach to the prevention, evaluation, and management of work disability. J Occup Rehab 1:11, 1991.

79. Gundewell B, Liljeqvist M, Hansson T: Primary prevention of back symptoms and absence from work. Spine 18:587, 1993.

80. Videman T, Ranhala H, Asp S, et al: Patient-handling skill, back injuries and back pain. An intervention study in nursing. Spine 2:148, 1989.

81. Troup JDG: The perception of musculoskeletal pain and incapacity for work: Prevention and early treatment. Physiotherapy 74:435, 1988.

82. Linton SJ, Hellsing AL, Andersson D: A controlled study of the effects of an early intervention on acute musculoskeletal pain problems. Pain 54:353, 1993.

83. Shekelle PG, Adams AH, Chassin MR, et al: Spinal manipulation for low-back pain. Ann Intern Med 117:590, 1992.

84. Shekelle PG: Spine update: Spinal manipulation. Spine 19:858, 1994.

85. Meade TW, Dyer S, Browne W, et al: Low back pain of mechanical origin: Randomized comparison of chiropractic and hospital outpatient treatment. Br Med J 300:1431, 1990.

86. Jarvis V, Phillips RB, Morris EK: Cost per case comparison of back injury claims of chiropractic versus medical management for conditions with identical diagnostic codes. J Occup Med 33:847, 1991.

87. Cherkin DC, MacCornack FA: Patient evaluations of low back pain care from family physicians and chiropractors. West J Med 51:355, 1989.

88. Cherkin DC: Family physicians and chiropractors: What's best for the patient? J Fam Pract 35:505, 1992.

89. Curtis P, Bove G: Family physicians, chiropractors, and back pain. J Fam Pract 35:551, 1992.

90. Triano J, McGregor M, Hondras M, et al: Manipulative therapy versus education programs in chronic low back pain. Spine 20:948, 1995.

91. Erhard RE, Delitto A: Relative effectiveness of an extension program and a combined program of manipulation and flexion and extension exercises in patients with acute low back syndrome. Phys Ther 74:1093, 1994.

92. Cats-Baril WL, Frymoyer JW: Identifying patients at risk of becoming disabled because of low-back pain. Spine 16:607, 1991.

93. Oland G, Tveiten GT: A trial of modern rehabilitation for chronic low-back pain and disability. Spine 16:457, 1991.

94. Alaranta H, Hurri H, Heliovaara M, et al: Non-dynametric trunk performance tests: Reliability and normative data. Scand J Rehab Med 26:211, 1994.

95. Rissanen A, Alaranta H, Sainio P, et al: Isokinetic and non-dynametric tests in low-back pain patients related to pain and disability index. Spine 19:1963, 1994.

96. Mitchell RI, Carmen GM: Results of a multicenter trial using an intensive active exercise program for the treatment of acute soft tissue and back injuries. Spine 15:514, 1990.

97. Lindstrom A, Ohlund C, Eek C, et al: Activation of subacute low back patients. Phys Ther 4:279, 1992.

98. Faas A, Chavannes AW, van Eijk J Th M, et al: A randomized, placebo-controlled trial of exercise therapy in patients with acute low back pain. Spine 18:1388, 1993.

99. Catchlove R, Cohen K: Effects of a directive return to work approach in the tratment of workmens' compensation patients with chronic pain. Pain 14:181, 1992.

100. Fordyce WE, Brockway JA, Bergman JA, et al: Acute back pain: A control group comparison of behavioural vs. traditional management methods. J Behav Med 9:127, 1986.

101. Mayer TG, Gatchel RJ, Kishino ND, et al: Objective assessment of spine function following industrial injury: A prospective study with comparison group and one-year follow-up. Spine 10:482, 1985.

102. Linton SJ, Bradley LA, Jensen I, et al: The secondary prevention of low back pain: A controlled study with follow-up. Pain 36:197, 1989.

103. Kellet KM, Kellett DA, Nordholm LA: Effects of an exercise program on sick leave due to back pain. Phys Ther 71:283, 1991.

104. Timm KE: A randomized-control study of active and passive treatments for chronic low back pain following L5 laminectomy. J Occup Sports Phys Ther 20:276, 1994.

105. Mooney V: Where is the pain coming from?. Spine 12:754, 1987.

106. Brown KC, Sirles AT, Hilyer JC, et al: Cost-effectiveness of a back school intervention for municipal employees. Spine 17:1224, 1992.

107. Moffett JAK, Chase SM, Portek I, et al: A controlled, prospective study to evaluate the effectiveness of a back school in the relief of chronic low back pain. Spine 11:120, 1986.

108. Versloot JM, Schilstra AJ, Tolen FJ, et al: Back school in industry. A prospective longitudinal controlled study (3 years). ISSLS Meeting, Miami, FL, April 13–17, 1988.

109. Nordin M, Frankel V, Spengler DM: A preventive back care program for industry. Presented at the International Lumbar Spine Meeting, Paris, May 1981.

110. Berwick DM, Budman S, Feldstein M: No clinical effect of back schools in an HMO. Spine 14:8, 1989.

111. Lankhorst GJ, van de Stadt RJ, Vogelaar TW, et al: The effect of the Swedish back school in chronic idiopathic low back pain. Scand J Rehabil Med 15:141, 1983.

112. Lindquist S, Lundberg B, Wikmark R, et al: Information and regimen on low back pain. Scand J Rehabil Med 16:113, 1984.

113. Genaidy AM: A training programme to improve human physical capability for manual handling jobs. Ergonomics 34:1, 1991.

114. Derebery VJ, Tullis W: Delayed recovery in the patient with a work compensable injury. J Occup Med 25:829, 1983.

115. Bigos SJ, Battie MC, Spengler DM, et al: A prospective study of work perceptions and psychosocial factors affecting the report of back injury. Spine 16:1, 1991.

116. Cats-Baril WL, Frymoyer JW: Identifying patients at risk of becoming disabled because of low-back pain. Spine 16:605, 1991.

117. Waddell G, Newton M, Henderson I, et al: A fear-avoidance beliefs questionnaire and the role of fear-avoidance beliefs in chronic low back pain and disability. Pain 52:157,168, 1993.

118. Iezzi A, Adams HE, Stokes GS, et al: An identification of low back pain groups using biobehavioral variables. J Occup Rehab 2:19, 1992.

119. Reesor KA, Craig KD: Medically incongruent chronic back pain: Physical limitations, suffering and ineffective coping. Pain 32:34, 1988.

120. Turk DC, Rudy TE: Toward an empirically derived taxonomy of chronic back pain patients: Integration of psychological assessment data. J Consult Clin Psychol 56:233, 1988.

121. Feuerstein M, Thebarge RW: Perceptions of disability and occupational stress as discriminators of work disability in patients with chronic pain. J Occup Rehab 1:185, 1991.

122. Wifling FG, Klonoff H, Kokan P: Psychological, demographic and orthopaedic factors associated with prediction of outcome of spinal fusion. Clin Orthop 90:153, 1973.

123. Mayer TG, Gatchel RJ, Mayer H, et al: A prospective two-year study of functional restoration in industrial low back injury. JAMA 258:1763, 1987.

124. Hazard RG, Fenwick JW, Kalisch SM, et al: Functional restoration with behavioral support. Spine 14:157, 1989.

125. Sachs BL, David JF, Olimpio D, et al: Spinal rehabilitation by work tolerance based on objective physical capacity assessment of dysfunction. Spine 15:1325, 1990.

126. Alaranta H, Rytokoski U, Rissanan A, et al: Intensive physical and psychosocial training program for patients with chronic low back pain. Spine 19:1339, 1994.

2 Integrating Rehabilitation into Chiropractic Practice (Blending Active and Passive Care)

CRAIG LIEBENSON

Rehabilitation and chiropractic (manual medicine) are perfect partners in the delivery of high quality neuromusculoskeletal health care. Disorders of the locomotor system often resolve spontaneously, but high recurrence rates dictate a more proactive approach. Manipulation and exercise are the two methods that have become the standard of care, especially in the costly arena involving low back pain. New treatments must prove their value against these "gold standards." Combining passive and active care is a new art that requires certain fundamental skills, which are outlined in this chapter.

FUNCTIONAL PATHOLOGY OF THE MOTOR SYSTEM

Clinically significant structural abnormalities, such as disk syndromes, are present in less than 20% of patients with low back pain. In the absence of trauma or relevant pathoanatomic change, the primary goals of care should be restoration of function and prevention of disability, including the chief functions of the locomotor system; strength, endurance, flexibility, coordination, and balance. Patients should be educated about the negative effects of immobilization and deconditioning and the safety/benefits of early mobilization and controlled activity. Rehabilitation is guided by evaluation of the functional capacity and work demands of the individual. This evaluation also provides ideal outcome measures of quality care.

Deconditioning Syndrome

Rehabilitation attempts to address physical, and if necessary psychologic, deconditioning that accompanies most persistent pain syndromes. Muscular disuse leads to weakness, incoordination, atrophy, and loss of flexibility. Joint immobilization leads to bone demineralization, capsular adhesions, and decreased ligamentous stress tolerance (including annular weakness). Cardiovascular fitness is diminished. Deconditioning affects not only peripheral anatomic structures, but also afferent systems, such as proprioception involved in balance as well as central neuromotor control of movement and posture.

Although a specific pain generator often is difficult to pin down, the deconditioning syndrome can be identified in most patients with chronic or recurrent back pain by the presence of immobility, muscle weakness, and pain-avoidance behavior. It encompasses many of the typical physical and psychologic signs associated with back pain patients. The various interconnections between these clinical signs are shown in Figure 2.1.

The overemphasis on treatment of conjectured structural pathologic change (disk, facet, etc.) has resulted in a failure to identify or focus on intrinsic functional losses, psychosocial factors, and extrinsic environmental stressors (work demands). This failure to recognize the limited reach of clinical diagnosis has especially plagued the medical community, whose overconfidence in the diagnosis of disk syndromes has promoted an overly passive approach involving rest and medication. The overemphasis of this nonmanagement philosophy is typically grounded in the belief that the natural history of most back pain episodes leads to resolution. Unfortunately, by encouraging inactivity, this approach results in immobilization of tissues and leads to deconditioning of the musculoskeletal system. Deyo encourages maintaining function as the mainstay of treatment when a specific diagnosis is elusive.[1]

Chiropractors or myofascial specialists who concentrate exclusively on passive intervention (i.e., spinal adjustments, trigger point therapy) to treat a specific pain generator (joint or soft tissue) are also placing patients at risk for deconditioning. *Unless the patient is educated to control environmental stressors and trained to recondition functional deficits, pain recurrences and treatment dependency will be the rule rather than the exception.*

NEGATIVE EFFECTS OF IMMOBILIZATION

Prolonged immobilization results in compromise of the musculotendinous, ligamentous-articular, osseous, cardiovascular, and central nervous systems[2-51] (Figs. 2.2 and 2.3; Table 2.1).

Prolonged immobilization after an injury can lead to scar tissue formation and lowered fatigue tolerance of injured tissues. Soft tissue healing has three phases: inflammation, repair, and remodeling. Some form of local tissue immobilization is usually advisable during the inflammatory phase, which usually peaks around the third day after injury. Toward the end of the inflammatory phase, fibroblasts are found in increasing numbers in the injured area. These fibroblasts contribute to scar formation. In a study of calf contusions in rats, Lehto and colleagues found that connective tissue scar formation will persist and become fibrotic rather than be

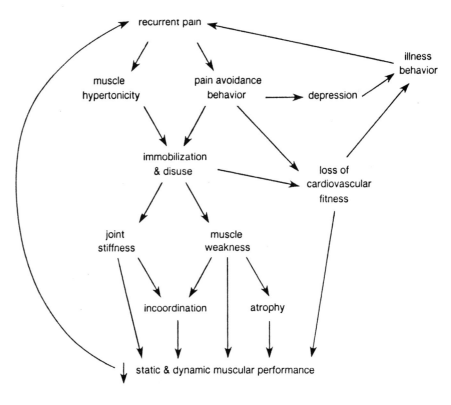

Fig. 2.1. Pathophysiology of deconditioning syndrome. (Adapted with permission from Liebenson C: Pathogenesis of chronic back pain. J Manipulative Physiol Ther 15:303, 1992.)

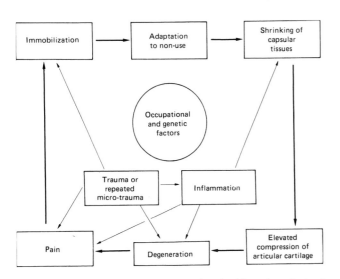

Fig. 2.2. Biochemical changes associated with reduced physical activity. (From Troup JDG, Videman T: Inactivity and the aetiopathogenesis of musculoskeletal disorders. Clin Biomech 4:175, 1989.)

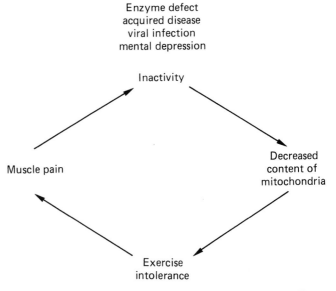

Fig. 2.3. Effects of musculoskeletal immobilization. (From Troup JDG, Videman T: Inactivity and the aetiopathogenesis of musculoskeletal disorders. Clin Biomech 4:175, 1989.)

absorbed if the acute inflammatory reaction is allowed to persist.[45] These authors suggest early, aggressive management of injuries to limit enlargement of the injured area.[45]

During the repair phase, passive and active motion of the tissues positively affects the injured tissues. Classic work on knee cartilage by Salter and co-workers showed that after 3 weeks of immobilization, intra-articular adhesions complicate the repair phase of soft tissue healing.[12] Either intermittent active motion or continuous passive motion prevented such adhesion formation.[12]

The remodeling phase involves lysis of adhesions and reorientation of collagen fibers along the lines of imposed stress. Again, prolonged immobilization is a negative factor in proper healing. In studies of rhesus monkeys, Noyes studied the effects of 8 weeks of immobilization on ligament stiffness and failure rate.[3] Ligament stiffness was reduced to 69% of

Table 2.1. Negative Effects of Immobilization

Joints
    Shrinks joint capsules[2,3]
    Increases compressive loading[4]
    Leads to joint contracture[5,6]
    Increases synthesis rate of glycosaminoglycans[7–9]
    Increase in periarticular fibrosis[10–12]
    Irreversible changes after 8 weeks immobilization[13,14]
Ligament
    Lowers failure or yield point[2,3,6,15–17]
    Decreased thickness of collagen fibers[18–20]
Disk biochemistry
    Decreases oxygen[21]
    Decreases glucose[21]
    Decreases sulfate[21]
    Increases lactate concentration[22]
    Decreases proteoglycan content[22]
Bone
    Decreases bone density[23–31]
    Eburnation[4]
Muscle
    Decreased thickening of collagen fibers[18,32]
    Decreased oxidative potential[33–35]
    Decreased muscle mass[22,36–39]
    Decreased sarcomeres[40]
    Decreased cross-sectional area[41–43]
    Decreased mitochondrial content[44]
    Increased connective tissue fibrosis[45]
    Type 1 muscle atrophy[42,46,47]
    Type 2 muscle atrophy[48,49]
    20% loss of muscle strength per week[50]
Cardiopulmonary
    Increased maximal heart rate[51]
    Decreased VO_2 max[51]
    Decreased plasma volume[51]

(From Liebenson C: Pathogenesis of chronic back pain. J Manipulative Physiol Ther 15:303, 1992.)

normal after 8 weeks. After 5 months of reconditioning, stiffness was reduced to only 7% of normal levels.[3] Five months of reconditioning improved the tissue failure rate to 80% of normal, and after 12 months of reconditioning, the rate was completely normal.[3]

FUNCTIONAL DEFICITS ARE PROSPECTIVELY CORRELATED WITH LOW BACK PAIN

Patients typically become inactive when they experience pain, and this inactivity promotes deconditioning. With deconditioning comes greater susceptibility to typical postural or occupational repetitive strains. A chronic cycle of recurring pain is easily established unless function is restored. If pain relief is the only goal of treatment, and functional restoration is ignored, painful recurrences are more likely. Sports medicine specialist Stanley Herring says, "signs and symptoms of injury abate, but these functional deficits persist. . . . adaptive patterns develop secondary to the remaining functional deficits."[50] Focusing on function helps patients to develop control over their symptoms and to prevent recurrences.

In many retrospective studies, investigators have documented that various functional changes in musculoskeletal performance are associated with episodes of back pain, although they cannot determine if these changes are a cause or a result of the pain. Prospective studies come closer to identifying etiologic factors. The goal of such research is to identify what factors are causally linked to low back pain episodes in a predictive manner. The following studies are all prospective.

Many researchers have found that muscle strength is prospectively correlated with future incidences of disabling back pain. Chaffin first demonstrated in 1973 a correlation between decreased muscular strength and increased incidence of low back pain.[52,53] Cady et al. found decreased isometric lifting strength and endurance in firemen who later developed first time episodes of low back pain.[54] Rowe found decreased abdominal muscle strength in 50% of those who later developed symptoms.[55]

Losses in muscle strength have also been found to correlate with the increased likelihood of recurrences in an individual once they have suffered a disabling back injury. Biering-Sorenson found that individuals with the greatest number of recurrences of lower back pain had decreased isometric trunk muscle strength in flexion and extension.[56] Troup et al. reported that decreased dynamic trunk flexion strength is a good predictor of recurrences or persistence of lower back pain.[57]

In one study, physically fit nurse's aides had shorter recovery periods after injury than those who were less fit.[58] Gundewall et al. demonstrated that nurses and nurse's aides who spent 20 minutes per day for 13 months exercising their backs had fewer injuries than those who did not exercise.[59] These two groups were divided randomly and the exercises included trunk extension strength and endurance as well as pushing and pulling. Videman et al. found that back injuries could be reduced by increasing the patient handling skill of nurses.[60]

The correlation between losses in normal flexibility and the likelihood of developing a disabling episode of back pain is not as clear,[61] although decreases in normal flexibility do relate to a higher than normal rate of recurrence.[57,61] Troup and co-workers found a decrease in sagittal flexibility, especially in extension, in those persons who later developed symptoms.[57]

Deyo and Bass reported that decreased physical activity, along with smoking and weight factors, were predictive of future episodes of lower back pain.[62] The American Academy of Orthopedic Surgeons stated that "functional deficits become the dominant physical impairment associated with disability in the patient with chronic back problems."[63] Table 2.2 summarizes the functional losses prospectively correlated with episodes of back pain.

Biomechanical Factors

Musculoskeletal structures (ligaments, joints, disks, muscles, etc.) are constantly subjected to biomechanical forces such as tension, torsion, compression, or shear. When functional capacity is less than work or activity demands, microfailure

Table 2.2. Intrinsic Functional Losses Correlated Prospectively with Back Pain Episodes

Muscle strength[52,53]
Isometric lifting strength/endurance[54]
Abdominal strength[55,57]
Isometric flexion/extension strength[56]
Physical fitness[54,58]
Job skill[60]
Extension mobility[57]
Physical activity[59,62]

(fatigue) and eventual injury are the result (Fig. 2.4). The stress/ strain curve explains the mechanics of the relationship between external load (stress) and tissue deformation (strain). The applied or elongating force is termed stress. The amount or percent of elongation is the strain. Stress is measured in newtons and strain in percent (%) elongation.

Loading of biologic tissues produces a characteristic stress/strain curve demonstrating the amount of stress (loading) required to produce a set amount of strain (percent elongation or deformation)[64] (Fig. 2.5). The initial concave portion of the curve is the "toe" region, which corresponds to the initial tissue distraction involving a structural change from a crimped, wavy fibril organization to a more straightened, parallel arrangement.[2] In the toe region, little force or energy is required to take the slack out of the tissue, but the tissue quickly becomes stiffer, resisting further elongation. If greater forces are present, tissue deformation occurs with accompanying microfailure. Only 4% deformation is necessary to cause microfailure.[64]

After prolonged or repeated loading—sometimes, just 15 minutes—tissue *creep* will occur, resulting from the "gradual rearrangement of collagen fibers, proteoglycans and water in the ligaments or capsule being stressed."[64] Once a tissue is stressed, it tends to have difficulty returning to its initial length. The energy lost after prolonged or repetitive loading is called *hysteresis,* and is represented by the difference between the new and old stress/strain curves (Fig. 2.6). Hysterisis only occurs when loading exceeds the point at which all crimp is removed from the tissues (4% elongation). According to Bogduk and Twomey, "the further a structure is stressed beyond its toe phase, the more bonds are broken and the greater the hysteresis and set."[64]

Mild strains can cause microdamage, and if repeated, they frequently result in tissue deformation.[64] According to Bogduk and Twomey, "what proportion of collagen fibers need to fail before macroscopic failure of a ligament or capsule is not known . . . "[64] At a certain point after loading has led to tissue fatigue and microinjury, tissues begin to fail and frank rupture of structural elements occurs. Under conditions of exposure to prolonged cycles of repetitive stress, less external load is required to cause tissue failure. Bogduk and Twomey conclude that hysteresis makes fatigued tissues more vulnerable to injury, "after prolonged strain, ligaments, capsules and intervertebral discs of the lumbar spine may creep, and they may be liable to injury if sudden forces are unex-

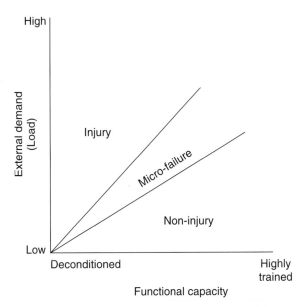

Fig. 2.4. Relationship between external demand and functional capacity.

STRESS

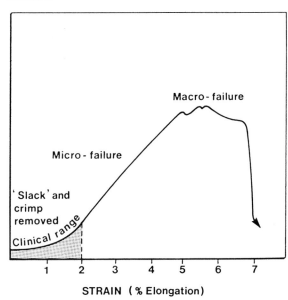

Fig. 2.5. Stress-strain curve for a ligament. (From Bogduk N, Twomey LT: Clinical Anatomy of the Lumbar Spine. 2nd Ed. Melbourne, Churchill Livingstone, 1991.)

pectedly applied during their vulnerable, recovery phase."[64] According to Andersson, "It is generally believed that repetitive loading causes failure because of fatigue of the various tissues."[65] Brinckmann and Pope conclude, " . . . under repetitive loading, the yield stress of these materials and the strength of structures built from these materials is reduced with respect to the stress or strength observed under a single load cycle"[66] (Fig. 2.7). *Reducing exposure to high levels of load—such as trunk flexion with either compression or rotation—is one of the most important tenets of prevention of low*

STRESS

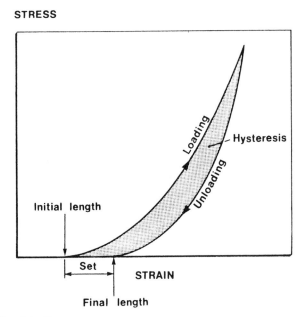

Fig. 2.6. Stress-strain curve illustrating hysteresis. When unloaded, a structure regains shape at a rate different to that at which it deformed. Any difference between the initial and final shape is the "set." (From Bogduk N, Twomey LT: *Clinical Anatomy of the Lumbar Spine.* 2nd Ed. Melbourne, Churchill Livingstone, 1991.)

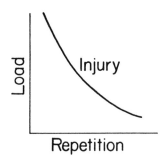

Fig. 2.7. A fatigue curve illustrates the importance of repetition and load to fatigue failure. (From Andersson GBJ: Occupational biomechanics. In Weinstein JN, Wiesel SW (eds): *The Lumbar Spine.* Philadelphia, WB Saunders, 1990.)

back pain. Similarly, frequent microbreaks, taken as often as every 20 minutes, can help reduce the chance of injury after exposure to repetitive overloading. Frequent microbreaks can prevent the instability that arises after tissue creep has occurred. Such breaks can prevent repetitive strain injuries noted after prolonged static loading such as from sitting or repetitive overuse from sports or occupational activities.

The more impaired the soft tissue, the less stress required to reach the soft tissue fatigue or failure point. *Immobilized tissues are more vulnerable than normal tissues to similar amounts of mechanical stress (Fig. 2.8).*[1] *Preventing the negative effects of immobilization is one of the primary goals of rehabilitation for musculoskeletal complaints.*

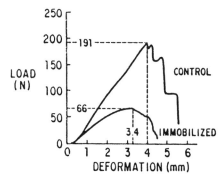

Fig. 2.8. The strength of rested tissue deteriorates dramatically compared to normal tissue. In this medial collateral ligament of a rabbit knee that rested for 9 weeks, two thirds of the strength has been lost. (From Mooney V: The subacute patient: To operate or not to operate. In Mayer TG, Mooney V, Gatchel RJ (eds): *Contemporary Conservative Care for Painful Spinal Disorders.* Baltimore, Williams & Wilkins, 1991.)

Neurophysiologic Factors

As the active component of our locomotor system, muscles are often called on consciously or by reflex to protect other tissues under stress. Compensatory adaptations (facilitative and inhibitory) typically follow any strain, whether or not it is painful. What may begin as a segmental, reflex muscular adaptation to pain may become "programmed" in the form of a new movement pattern stored in the central nervous system. Injury, inflammation, joint nociceptive activity, sensitization of dorsal horn neurones, or pain perception can all trigger muscular reactions. These adaptations are an essential part of the deconditioning syndrome.

IS THERE A PAIN CYCLE?

The existence of a pain-spasm-pain cycle has been a well-accepted concept of physical therapy and chiropractics. As a criteria for therapeutic decision making, it is one of the most influential "a priori" assumptions of many practitioners, especially among those who use extensive passive techniques and/or soft tissue manipulation. Its validity is unproven, however, and currently, it is often ignored. The literature does show that prolonged or intense pain can lead to both psychologic (abnormal illness behavior) and neurologic (dorsal horn sensitization) consequences. Either or both of these behavioral and physiologic dysfunctions are at the heart of the transition from an acute to a chronic pain syndrome. Significant external loading that exceeds intrinsic functional capacity leads to tissue fatigue and altered biomechanics. To maintain spinal stability following biomechanical changes, such as can occur after creep and hysteresis, type I and type II afferents are stimulated to maintain accurate proprioception (Table 2.3). The initial firing from the joint mechanoreceptors, muscle spindle afferents, and Golgi tendon organ afferents allows adaptation to occur so the fatiguing tissues can avoid failure. Because these receptors are adaptive, they do not continue to discharge if the biomechanical changes are

Table 2.3 Nerve Types and Functions

FAST MYELINATED LARGE		SLOW UNMYELINATED SMALL	
Low Threshold/Adaptive		High Threshold/ Nonadapting	
I	II	III	IV
A alpha	A beta and gamma	A delta	C
Golgi tendon, primary muscle spindle, efferents to skeletal muscle	Secondary muscle spindle, gamma efferent to intrafusal muscle spindle	Acute pain	Chronic pain, postganglionic autonomic, dorsal root afferents

present for a long period of time. As a result, repetitive strains eventually exhaust the adaptive capacity of the body's defenses and lead to painful injury.

Once tissue failure occurs, inflammation, mediated by bradykinin, substance P, and prostaglandin E2, lead to stimulation of nonadaptive, types III and IV nociceptive afferents. Various changes in the muscular system occur automatically when injury occurs. *For instance, muscle inhibition follows acute low back pain or knee injury/inflammation.*[67,68] *Additionally, increased neuromuscular tone also results from strong nociceptive stimulation.*[69–71] Protective mechanisms—normal illness behavior—to immobilize an injured area are usually appropriate in the acute stage. If they become memorized as a "pain-motor program," however, they can lead to a chronic state. *Abnormal illness behavior, such as excessive or prolonged stress, fear, or anxiety, will affect the neuromuscular system behaviorally via conditioning and physiologically from the limbic center, thus providing an ideal terrain for chronic pain.*

Testing with evoked potentials of patients with chronic back pain revealed lower pain thresholds and higher than normal evoked responses at thresholds than are noted in normal subjects.[72] Magnetoencephalographic study with sub, supra, and standard intracutaneous electric shock stimuli in chronic back sufferers also revealed a higher than normal pain-evoked magnetic field.[73] It was concluded that this heightened response was attributable to central nervous system hyperresponsiveness in the primary somatosensory cortex.

Acute pain involves biomechanical insult (i.e., injury, repetitive strain), biochemical mediation (inflammation), facilitation of algesic pathways, and finally neuromuscular adaptation. If repetitive biomechanical insult is not avoided; abnormal illness behavior is present; or deconditioning occurs, resulting in inadequate neuromuscular adaptation, then chronic pain with central nervous system involvement (corticalization) can be expected.

To prevent the transition from acute to chronic pain, three things should occur once the initial acute, inflammatory phase has passed: (1) patient education about how to identify

and limit external sources of biomechanical overload; (2) early identification of psychosocial factors of abnormal illness behavior; and (3) identification and rehabilitation of the functional pathology of the motor system (i.e., deconditioning syndrome). This third aspect involves looking for specific joint and muscle dysfunctions so that patient reactivation can be promoted and deconditioning prevented. Figure 2.9 shows how chronic pain can arise from deconditioning syndrome.

Pain is derived from the Latin term "poena" meaning penalty or punishment. Unfortunately, pain does not always serve as a good early-warning system, but often arises only after damage is done. Pain alone is just a symptom—the conscious perception of nociceptive activity. *If pain relief is the only goal of care, then deconditioning and various functional pathologies will remain as precursors to future biomechanical failures. Functional restoration in addition to pain relief are appropriate goals because prevention of recurrent or chronic pain is the ultimate goal of a cost containment-oriented approach.* In as much as we can identify specific functional pathologies that are causally linked—trigger points or overactive muscles, weak muscles or abnormal movement patterns, and joint dysfunction—we can then not only provide symptomatic (pain) relief, but also restore function. Even in the absence of uncovering a clear chain of functional pathologic changes, identifying deficits in functional capacity can drive the reactivation of the patient by remediating pain avoidance behavior.

MUSCULAR PAIN, TENSION, AND INHIBITION

Muscles are often ignored while joints or disks receive the majority of recognition as potential pain generators. For

THE PAIN CYCLE:

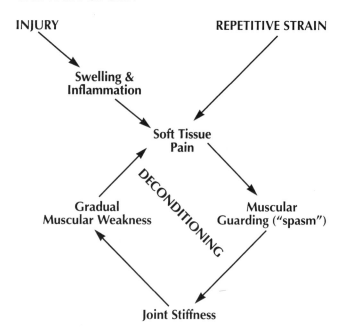

Fig. 2.9. The pain cycle.

years, skeptics have enjoyed pointing out the unproven nature of such clinically popular concepts as myofascial trigger points. Reviewing the literature on muscle pain, however, reveals the error of this omission.

Traumatic injuries overload the structural components of muscles and lead to frank tissue disruption and failure. Under these circumstances, increased muscle pain is predominantly a result of neurochemical events. Traumatized muscles release various chemicals capable of activating nociceptive pain generators.[74] These chemicals can also activate nociceptive pathways via potassium, bradykinin, or histamine extravasation.

Increased muscle tone or "spasm" has been widely used as a descriptor for patients with palpable stiffness in their soft tissues. Unfortunately, viscoelastic connective tissue and neuromuscular factors are rarely differentiated. Additionally, terms such as increased muscle tone, muscle tension, tightness, stiffness, shortening, hypertonicity, spasm, fibrosis, and others are used loosely and without adequate definition. Scientific work in this field has been lacking, but researchers are beginning to redress this situation.[74,75]

Although it is admittedly unproven, muscle tension is widely believed to go hand in hand with pain. Muscles as the active components of the locomotor system are responsible for both reflex and centrally mediated adaptations to repetitive strain, injury, or pain.

The significance and validity of palpable increases of soft tissue tension or stiffness have been called into question by, among other things, the poor reproducibility of electromyography (EMG) and the poor reliability of palpation. Nonetheless, as Paillard explains, muscle tone is a key aspect of motor control: "Muscle tone, once widely used as a basic semiological dimension of clinical neurology, is now almost totally ignored by neurophysiology. It certainly deserves new considerations as a potent contextual dimension of motor performance."[76]

The organ of muscle tone is thought to be the muscle spindle, which sets the sensitivity of the muscle to stretch. Boyd refers to the muscle spindle as ". . . a marvel of control engineering, incorporating many of the features of an engineering 'servo-control' system."[77] In theory, muscle tone is greatly influenced by the amount of gamma activity present: the greater the background gamma activity, the larger the intrafusal spindle response to any given change in muscle length (Fig. 2.10). The gamma system is under the control of descending impulses from the extrapyramidal motor pathways. These higher cortical centers (i.e., the limbic lobe) are more active under conditions of emotional stress.

Many examples of increased soft tissue tension are unequivocal, such as cases of acute lumbar strain, torticollis, acute appendicitis, peritonitis, and whiplash. To what degree such neuromuscular changes are attributable to reflex, central, or other mechanisms is unclear. It is also unproven to what extent the muscle spindle or gamma system participates. Increased EMG activity in muscles has been shown, as in the case of the loss of the lumbar flexion relaxation response, in

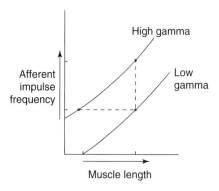

Fig. 2.10. Influence of muscle length on spindle impulse frequency at two different levels of gamma motoneuron activity. (From Korr IM: Proprioceptors and somatic dysfunction. J Am Osteopath Assoc 74:638, 1975.)

patients with low back disability.[78] In addition, sustained EMG activity has been found in the nidus of trigger points.[79] It has also been noted that when pressure is applied to an active trigger point, EMG activity increases in muscles in the referred pain zone.[80]

Static overstrain, such as from prolonged sitting or slumping, has often been suggested as a high risk activity for individuals with a back problem. Sustained contractions of only 4% of the maximum voluntary contraction possible have been shown to lead to negative effects.[65,81] Metabolites are produced that stimulate groups III and IV afferents and increase gamma motor neuron activity. It has also been shown that increased interstitial potassium concentrations sensitize the groups III and IV muscle afferents,[82] resulting in an increase in the sensitivity to stretch of muscles with convergent afferent input[83] (Figs. 2.11 and 2.12).

Study of muscle fibers has shown that conditions of constant load affect the ability of a muscle to achieve efficient relaxation.[74] As a result, tension and pressure build up in the muscle.[74] The more the muscle contracts, the greater the energy expenditure. Local ischemia is another key factor involved in increased muscle tone. Under conditions of ischemia, groups III and IV muscle afferents become more sensitive to stretch[84] (Fig. 2.13).

Ischemia itself is not painful; however, if a muscle contracts under ischemic conditions, pain develops within 1 minute.[85] Bradykinin is released during ischemia and is therefore thought to be associated with ischemia-produced pain.[74] Under eccentric muscular conditions, mild overload may swell muscle fibers without inflammation.[86] Heavy eccentric exercise leads to swelling and necrotic inflammation.[87]

Joint receptors, if stimulated, cause both facilitation and inhibition of muscles. Low intensity stimulation of joint afferents in the knee have been shown to influence the sensitivity to stretch of muscles around the knee.[69,87–90] Also, reflex inhibition of muscles has been noted when joints and ligaments are arthritic or swollen;[67,91,92] vastus medialis inhibition is the most famous example.[91] Muscle fatigability resulting from in-

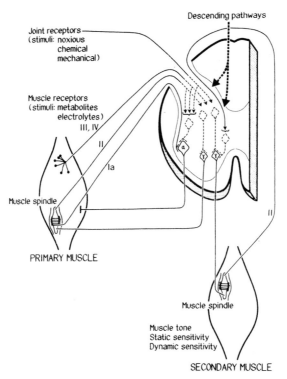

Fig. 2.11. Pathophysiologic model for mechanisms possibly involved in the genesis and spread of muscular tension in occupational muscle pain and chronic musculoskeletal pain syndromes. (From Johansson H, Sokja P: Pathophysiological mechanisms involved in genesis and spread of muscular tension in occupational muscle pain and in chronic musculoskeletal pain syndromes. A hypothesis. Med Hypotheses 35:196, 1991.)

Fig. 2.12. Increase in muscle tone with chronic irritation of the small nociceptor afferents from skeletal muscles. (From Dvorak J: Neurological and biomechanical aspects of back pain. In Buerger AA, Greenman PE (eds): Empirical Approaches to the Validation of Spinal Manipulation. Springfield, Charles C Thomas, 1985.)

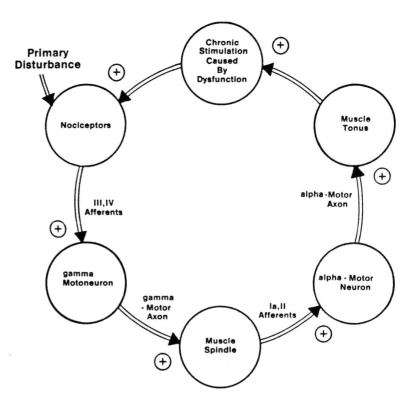

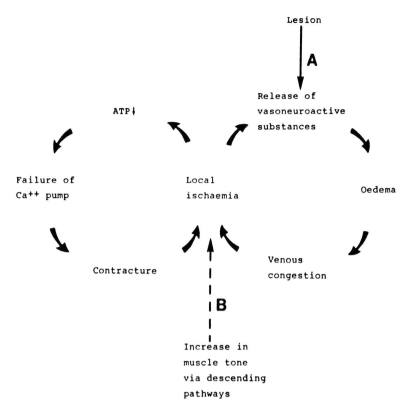

Fig. 2.13. Local vicious cycles in damaged muscle as a possible peripheral mechanism for chronic muscle pain. The right-hand cycle is assumed to be started by a tissue lesion that releases vasoneuroactive substances (path A). The central factor of the cycles is ischemia, which can be produced by venous congestion, local contracture, and tonic activation of muscles by descending motor pathways (path B). (From Mense S: Nociception from skeletal muscle in relation to clinical muscle pain. Pain 54:241, 1993.)

hibition of certain muscles required for a task is a likely contributor to overload injury or pain.[93,94]

Hides et al. documented unilateral wasting of the multifidus muscle in patients with acute low back pain.[68] With real-time sonography, they measured cross-sectional area (CSA) of the muscle and determined that the wasting was isolated to one vertebral segment. The wasting occurred rapidly in a localized area and was thus not considered to be the result of disuse atrophy. The authors were able to correlate the area of wasting with a dysfunctional segment identified on clinical manual examination (i.e., motion palpation). In patients with chronic back pain, CT scanning demonstrated generalized atrophy but a relative increase in the CSA on the symptomatic side.[95] Such a relative increase in the CSA could be explained by the findings of increased paraspinal muscle activity[96] and histologic evidence of type I fiber hypertrophy on the symptomatic side and type II fiber atrophy bilaterally in persons with chronic back pain.[97]

Bullock-Saxton et al. described gluteus maximus and medius inhibition during gait, and their subsequent facilitation after a brief course of propriosensory retraining.[98] Janda also reported reciprocal inhibition of the abdominal muscles as a result of stiff, overactive erector spinae muscles.[99] He showed that the abdominals became spontaneously stronger following inhibition and stretching of the erector spinae. Headley successfully demonstrated inhibition of the lower trapezius muscle during shoulder flexion or abduction when active trigger points in the upper trapezius are present.[94] Simons also reported inhibition of the deltoid muscle during shoulder flexion when infraspinatus trigger points are present.[80]

The initial muscular reaction to pain and injury has traditionally been assumed to be increased tension and stiffness. Data in the literature indicate inhibition is at least as significant. Tissue immobilization occurs secondarily, which leads to joint stiffness and disuse muscle atrophy. Such changes become a habit, mediated by central motor regulatory pathways as a new "pain-motor program" forms.

The combination of trigger points, muscle inhibition, and joint dysfunction are key peripheral components of the functional pathology of the motor system. If sustained over a period of time, these components may outlive the elimination of what caused them in the first place. This fact is of concern in cases of cumulative trauma (repetitive strain) disorders and prevention of recurrences after acute injury.

JOINT DYSFUNCTION AND PAIN

According to Schaible and Grubb, "The major sensation that is ascribed to the joint is pain."[100] The joint is involved in pain, proprioceptive, reflex muscular, reflex sympathetic, and other neurobiologic events. These events are depicted in Figure 2.14. Although joint afferents participate in movement and position sense, proprioception is primarily a muscle sense.[100,101]

Hypersensitivity (increased or abnormal pain response) of joints to movement is a key factor in the development of the deconditioning syndrome. Groups III and IV afferents can develop "long-lasting 'sensitization' to mechanical stimuli after the onset of joint inflammation. . . . many of them have been found to exhibit ongoing discharges when the joint is kept in its resting position."[100] Mechano-insensitive afferents are also

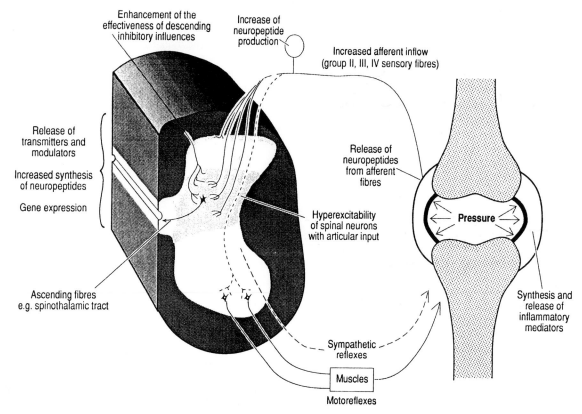

Fig. 2.14. Overview of neuronal events in the course of an inflammation in the joint. (From Schaible HG, Grubb BD: Afferent and spinal mechanisms of joint pain. Pain 55:5, 1993.)

present. These "silent nociceptors" also can become pain producers when sensitized by inflammation.[100]

Joints as a source of pain are all too frequently ignored. In a study of 318 consecutive patients with intractable neck pain, examined by provocation diskography and/or zygapophyseal joint blocks, 26% of the patients had symptoms associated with a joint, whereas 53% had symptoms related to a disk.[102] In a similar study, 56 patients with neck pain and no signs of nerve root involvement of at least 6 months duration were examined. The results showed 23% had a symptomatic joint, 20% had a symptomatic disk, and 41% had symptoms related to both a disk and a facet joint.[103]

Referred pain is often ascribed to nerve root irritation, but joints are also a likely source. Activated joint afferents are capable of giving rise to referred pain. Cat spinal cord neurons with knee input had convergent input from muscles in the thigh and lower leg and the skin.[100] Cutaneous receptive fields were found as distant as in the foot.

Johansson et al. reviewed the motor reflex effects of joint afferent excitation.[69] Under non-noxious stimuli, joint afferents excite significant amounts of reflex gamma motoneuron activity,[69] which probably assists in the regulation of stiffness. Long-lasting noxious stimulation results in activation of the flexion reflex (Fig. 2.15). Joints are also supplied with efferent sympathetic nerve fibers, which are capable of consistent reflex discharges.[100]

As mentioned previously, joint inflammation can give rise to reflex inhibition of muscles.[67,91,92] The knee was the model

in these studies, but spinal joint dysfunction has been correlated with muscle wasting in patients with acute low back pain as well.[68]

SUBLUXATION, REFERRED PAIN, AND NEUROPATHIC PAIN

The chiropractic "subluxation" involves biomechanical alterations such as viscoelastic stiffness in addition to neurophysiologically mediated dorsal horn sensitization. Such sensitization has a neuroanatomic basis in primary afferents and secondary dorsal horn neurons. Because of neuroplasticity, a reduced pain threshold from primary afferents coupled with an exaggerated pain response leads to hyperalgesia and referred pain. Today's pain scientists call this sensation "neuropathic pain." Previous research was led by osteopaths who termed this neuromechanical phenomena the "facilitated segment." Patterson says of the facilitated segment that " . . . because of abnormal afferent or efferent sensory inputs to a particular area of the spinal cord, that area is kept in a state of constant increased excitation. This facilitation allows normally ineffectual or subliminal stimuli to become effective in producing efferent output from the facilitated segment . . ."[104] (Fig. 2.16)

As long ago as 1883, Sturge suggested that an injury could trigger a change in the central nervous system such that normal inputs would evoke an exaggerated response.[105] In 1893, MacKenzie proposed that referred pain could result after sensory impulses from injured tissue have created

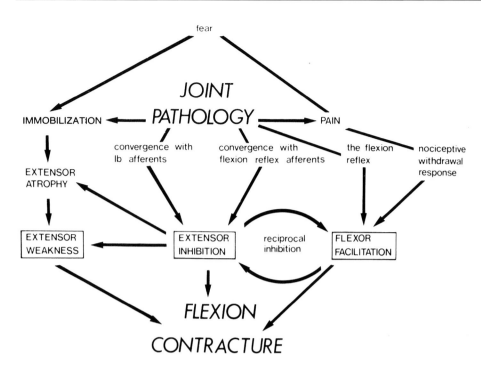

Fig. 2.15. Suggested network of factors contributing to fixed flexion of a damaged joint. (From Young A, Stokes M, Iles JF: Effects of joint pathology on muscles. Clin Orthop 219:21, 1987.)

an "irritable focus" in specific spinal cord segments.[106] Perl et al.[107] and Kenshalo and co-workers[108] made the initial experiments that showed that noxious sensory stimuli produced heightened sensitivity of dorsal horn neurons to future stimuli.

A new concept called "neuropathic pain" is being put forward to explain the common clinical presentation of persistent pain, hypersensitivity, and poor motor control in the absence of a patho-anatomic or neurologic explanation. Because of the poor correlation between presenting symptoms and objective physical signs, the pain experienced by these patients is commonly mislabeled psychogenic. According to Merskey, "There is increasing evidence that signs and symptoms that were taken to be proof of hysteria—or of behavioral disorder—such as a failure of complaints to observe anatomical boundaries, may have a physical basis."[109,110] "Regional pain syndromes and regional loss of sensitivity can have a pathophysiological origin related to expansion of receptor fields through the responses to peripheral injury of spinal cord neurons."[109,110] According to Nachemson, "various pools of nerve cells in the dorsal columns can be hypersensitized and thus can signal a painful condition even though there is very little peripheral input."[111]

The implications of this research in validating the complaints of millions of pain sufferers is remarkable. *The subluxation hypothesis backed steadfastly by the chiropractic profession appears to be on the verge of scientific validation—in a modified form—by an independent group of neurophysiologists studying pain mechanisms and behavior.* That this group of scientists make no mention of chiropractic and only occasionally refer to the physical medicine theories of myofascial pain by Travell and Rinzler and of zygapophyseal pain by Bogduk and Twomey is intriguing.[64,109,112] What is

most exciting is that they are attacking the notion that pain patients with few objective signs have psychogenic pain.

Neuropathic pain is considered common in causalgia, reflex sympathetic dystrophy, post-herpetic neuralgia, stroke, syringomyelia, syringobulbia, multiple sclerosis, and spinal cord injury. Neuropathic pain can also result from a repetitive strain initiating strong afferent nociceptive barrage to dorsal horn neurons, eventually leading to sensitization of those neurons because of central nervous system plasticity. *As a result of sensitization of secondary dorsal horn neurons or a decreased threshold for primary peripheral afferents—including normally pain-insensitive groups I and II afferents, input from normal mechanoreceptor afferents can be interpreted as nociceptive.*[113] Sensitization results in allodynia, deep hyperalgesia, poor motor control, and an expansion of the receptor field.

Neuropathic pain is related to:

Allodynia–Lowering of pain threshold (even to non–noxious stimuli) and pain that arises from activation of sensory channels not ordinarily involved in pain (e.g., low threshold mechanoreceptors [LTM]).
Test: Sensitivity to non–noxious stimuli as in light palpation or percussion of noninjured tissues and pain with physiologic joint movement.
Hyperalgesia–Increase in response to suprathreshold (i.e., noxious) stimuli. Mechanical hyperalgesia is pain during movements in the working range or pain on gentle pressure. Closely related to persistent pain.
Test: Positive jump sign (patient withdrawal) with soft tissue palpation of noninjured tissue. Withdrawal with passive overpressure at the end of the physiologic range of joint movement.
Cutaneous Hypoesthesia–Decreased sensation or sensitivity.
Test: Decreased sensation to pin prick.

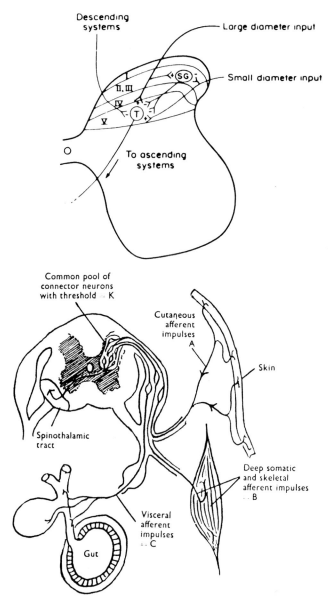

Fig. 2.16. Physiologic mechanism of the "irritable focus" in the grey matter of the spinal cord. (From Grieve GP: Simulated visceral disease. In Grieve GP (ed): Modern Manual Therapy of the Verteberal Column. Edinburgh, Churchill Livingstone, Edinburgh, 1986.)

Poor Motor Control–Incoordination or poor balance.
Test: Incoordinated movement patterns or gait; positive Rhomberg or Hautant test.
Referred Pain or Secondary Hyperalgesia–Spread of pain or hyperalgesia to uninjured or normal tissue in a dermatomal or nondermatomal distribution.
Test: Trigger point evaluation, pain mapping.
Sympathetic Symptoms–Vasomotor effects.
Test: Moisture, thermal changes in tissues.

Neuropathic symptoms have been shown to be related in part to convergent input in the dorsal horn from skin and/or deep somatic (visceral and nonvisceral) struc-

tures. Stimulation of viscera does not always produce pain, but visceral afferents projecting into the dorsal horn do typically converge with skin and/or deep somatic structures.[114–117]

Convergence and central neural plasticity provide the neuroanatomic basis for pain referral. It has been reported that many afferent units, when noxiously stimulated, elicit pain in two distinct receptive fields (RF).[118] Branching of the afferent fiber near its termination point is the likely anatomic explanation. According to Mense, this convergence would, "reduce the spatial resolution of the nociceptive system and thus could contribute to the diffuse nature of deep pain."[72] It has been shown that dorsal horn neurons are able to change the size, number, and sensitivity of their RF under the influence of noxious stimuli.[119,120]

When noxious stimuli are applied experimentally, referred pain into new RF typically takes a few minutes to occur.[72] Neuroplasticity seems to be operating as new central nervous connections are formed after peripheral injury. It has been shown that visceral pain, such as from a coronary infarct, can be referred to a muscle like the pectoralis major.[112] The muscular target for referred pain may also show signs of hyperalgesia.[121]

The presence of nondermatomal referred pain and hyperalgesia implies that central changes independent of convergence are operative.[122] An example is the situation in which referred pain spreads to the site of an old injury. An angina attack has been shown to refer pain directly to an old vertebral fracture.[123] It has also been demonstrated that 1 week after dental surgery, pin prick of the nasal mucosa can produce referred pain to the treated teeth.[124] Distant referral of pain to a nondermatomal area can also occur, such as in cardiac pain referring to the ear.[125] It has also been shown that a decrease in the flexion withdrawal reflex threshold is present in women after gynecologic surgery.[71]

What is Sensitization? Sensitization is a change in the stimulus-response profile of dorsal horn neurons so that they respond to mechanoreceptive afferents as if they were nociceptors.[126–128] Willis explains that a nociceptive barrage leads to central sensitization of dorsal horn neurons:[126] "If these nociceptive neurons have **convergent** input from mechanoreceptors, their responses to both innocuous and noxious mechanical stimuli will then be increased. . . . Sensitization then causes formerly subthreshold responses to reach threshold and trigger discharges."[126] According to Mayer and colleagues, "Overwhelming evidence supports the conclusion that a change in the central processing of input from low-threshold mechanoreceptors is responsible for secondary hyperalgesia to light touch."[128] Silent nociceptors that are mechano-insensitive also can become mechanosensitive once sensitized.[100] Table 2.4 lists the neural changes associated with sensitization and Figure 2.17 depicts the pathophysiology of sensitization.

How Do Mechanoreceptor Afferents Cause Pain? The Neurochemistry of Neuropathic Pain. The pathophysiology of neuropathic pain involves peripheral and central neural

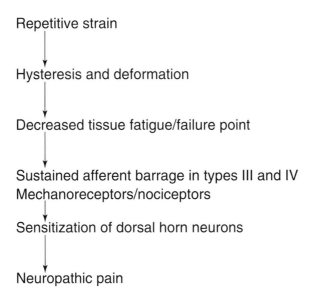

Fig. 2.17. The pathophysiology of sensitization.

events. Sustained activity in types III and IV (small diameter) primary afferents leads to a release of excitatory amino acids (glutamate) and neuropeptides (substance P) in the dorsal horn. Increased concentration of these neurochemical mediators lowers the firing threshold for primary sensory afferents.[126,127] In the presence of certain neurotransmitters, secondary dorsal horn neurons may become hyper-responsive because of excitatory amino acids acting at N-methyl-D-aspartate (NMDA) receptor sites and activating dorsal horn nociceptive neurons.[126,127] Secondary neuron hyper-responsiveness after repeated stimulation is called "wind-up" and is often short term. Inhibitory amino acids such as GABA are present to dampen this exaggerated response, but, over time, segmental inhibition is deactivated by the flood of excitatory amino acids.[129,130] Long-lasting changes appear to be the result of oncogene activation by strong nociceptive input.[126] Oncogenes such as c-fos enter the nucleus of the neuron and regulate other gene activity. According to Willis, "The implications of this chain of events are still unclear, but a potential result could be long-term changes in the responsiveness of nociceptive neurons."[126]

Pathoanatomic Changes in Neuropathic Pain. Peripheral nerves can sprout after peripheral nerve injury so that low threshold mechanoreceptors can extend to terminate within the superficial dorsal horn and make direct connection with nociceptors.[130,131] According to Dubner, peripheral nerve damage leads to an expansion of the low threshold portion of wide dynamic range (WDR) neurons because of a loss of sur-

rounding inhibition.[130] Increased excitability leads to excitotoxicity.[128,131,132] The most sensitive neurons are small local circuit inhibitory neurons.[130] Morphologic changes have been demonstrated in the rat dorsal horn after partial nerve injury.[130,133]

CORTICALIZATION OF PAIN AND CENTRAL MOTOR REGULATION

The locomotor system has peripheral (sensory and motor) and central (programming) components. The peripheral components (somatosensory, vestibular, visual) provide input and feedback (afferent) as well as carry out the instructions (efferent) of the central motor regulatory centers (cortex, cerebellum, basal ganglia, etc.) (Figs. 2.18 and 2.19). Prolonged or intense noxious, sensory stimulation can lead to dorsal horn sensitization, reorganization of somatotopic maps, limbic dysfunction, and "reprogramming" of movement patterns.

Abnormal illness behavior in response to subacute pain encourages chronicity. Poor sleep habits, high levels of emotional stress, and excessive fear or anxiety may stem from a limbic dysfunction. This condition negatively affects the musculoskeletal system by promoting physical and psychologic deconditioning. Magnetoencephalographic and evoked potential studies in patients with chronic low back pain have demonstrated central nervous system hyper-responsiveness in the primary somatosensory cortex.[72,73] Magnetoencephalography has revealed a somatotopic cortical map reorganization in patients who underwent reconstructive surgery.[134] That the central nervous system is involved in painful musculoskeletal disorders is no longer a question.

In response to chronic pain, new movement patterns are adopted that attempt to reduce noxious stimuli; these are often termed "pain-motor programs." Movement patterns repeated

Table 2.4. Results of Sensitization[112]

Increased spontaneous activity of types III and IV primary afferents
Prolonged after discharges of afferents to repeated stimulation
Decreased threshold to afferent input
Expanded receptive fields of dorsal horn neurons

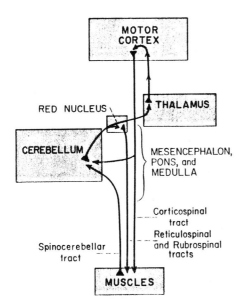

Fig. 2.18. Pathways for cerebellar control of voluntary movements. (From Guyton AC: Basic Neuroscience. Philadelphia, WB Saunders, 1987.)

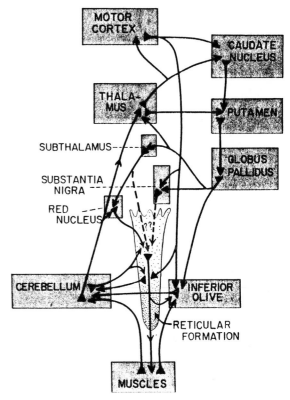

Fig. 2.19. Pathways for cerebellar "error" control of involuntary movements. (From Guyton A: Basic Neuroscience, Philadelphia, WB Saunders, 1987.)

often enough are learned by the cerebellum. This new central programming is called an "engram." In regard to this programming, Paillard says, "The existence in all animals of a consolidated repertoire of motor capacities, either inherited or secondarily acquired, is now an incontrovertible fact of contemporary neurophysiology."[76] Treatment of chronic conditions will likely fail if only peripheral targets (i.e., muscles, joints, etc.) are addressed. *Successful care for the chronic patient will likely involve treatments aimed at the peripheral pain generators, central motor regulation, and psychosocial factors.*

Clinical Features

MUSCULAR IMBALANCE

When muscles react to protect the body from harm or to reduce pain, certain muscles become overactive while others are inhibited. As a result, joint stress is altered and greater muscle fatigue results. For such protective reactions, the postural or antigravity muscles are activated most easily. Conversely, muscles with a primarily dynamic or phasic function tend to be inhibited when physical stress is present. Janda and co-workers, who studied these typical muscle reactions in both neurologic and orthopedic patients, call this common clinical phenomena "muscle imbalance."[135–137]

Janda and colleagues explained that the basis for most muscle imbalances comes from our predictable response to stressful environmental demands (constrained postures, repetitive tasks, gravity stress, inactivity). They identified that the postural muscles tend toward overuse and eventual shortening, whereas the phasic muscles tend toward disuse and weakness[134–137] (Table 2.5). These muscles are often grouped as paired antagonists and appear to be affected by

Sherrington's Law of Reciprocal Inhibition (Fig. 2.20). *Thus, if a postural muscle such as the iliopsoas becomes shortened from overuse, not only will it mechanically limit the range of motion of its antagonist the gluteus maximus, but also it will neurologically inhibit its action as well.* This combination of biomechanical and neurophysiologic influences is a strong stimulus to the creation and maintenance of muscular imbalances.

Electromyographic (EMG) data (Fig. 2.21) show that a tight erector spinae muscle will be active during its reverse action, trunk flexion, and thus inhibits the action of the ago-

Table 2.5. Postural and Phasic Muscles[135]

Postural (Tend to hyperactivity)	Phasic (Tend to hypoactivity)
Triceps surae	Tibialis anterior
Hamstrings	Gluteus maximus
Adductors	Gluteus medius
Rectus femoris	Rectus abdominus
Tensor fascia latae (TFL)	Lower/middle trapezius
Psoas	Scaleni/longus colli
Erector spinae	Deltoids
Quadratus lumborum (QL)	Digastrics
Pectoralis	
Upper trapezius	
Sternocleidomastoid (SCM)	
Suboccipital	
Masticatories	

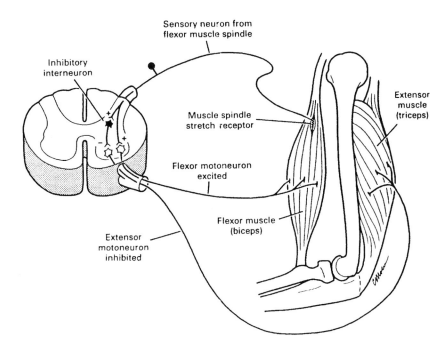

Fig. 2.20. Reciprocal inhibition of motor neurons to the opposing muscle. Impulses from the contracted muscle excite motor units in the same muscle (facilitory synaptic influence designated with a plus sign) and inhibit, through an interneuron, motor units in the opposing muscle (inhibitory synaptic influence designated with a minus sign). (From Lehmkuhl LD, Smith LK: Brunnstrom's Clinical Kinesiology. Philadelphia, FA Davis, 1983.)

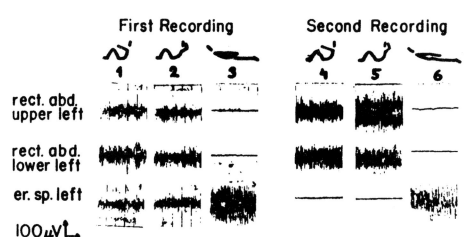

Fig. 2.21. Electromyographic activity before and after stretching tight muscles. (From Janda V: Muscles, central nervous motor regulation and back problems. In Korr IM (ed): Neurobiologic Mechanisms in Manipulative Therapy. New York, Plenum, 1978.)

nist, the abdominals. After the erector spinae muscle has been stretched, not only does it relax during trunk flexion, but also a significant, spontaneous facilitation effect is seen in the abdominal muscles. Figure 2.22 shows the typical lower crossed syndrome, which frequently develops as a result of muscular imbalance in the lumbopelvic region.

The postural or antigravity muscles maintain erect standing in gait. The majority of normal gait is spent on one leg; therefore, special emphasis is placed on the muscles involved in one leg standing. Sedentary life in modern society results in overuse of postural muscles, thus encouraging tightness to develop. Simultaneously, the phasic or dynamic muscles tend to become weak from disuse. Postural and phasic muscles are made up of mixed fiber types; however, "slow-twitch" fibers (type I) are predominant in postural muscles and "fast-twitch" (type II) fibers are predominant in phasic muscles. Table 2.6 describes the characteristics of these different types.

An intermediate muscle type is FR—"fast-twitch fatigue resistant." This type resists fatigue but also has fast contraction and relaxation speeds. The FR type has both aerobic and anaerobic metabolic capacity. Like type I units at rest, a high metabolic price is paid for maintaining this fiber type.

Muscle types can be converted with training.[138,139] With regular electrical stimulation, phasic muscle fibers can begin to have altered contractile characteristics within 2 weeks.[139] By 6 weeks of training, histochemical appearance is altered, and within 5 months, the muscle behaves entirely like a postural muscle. Keeping rats under hypergravity can turn fast-twitch into slow-twitch fibers.[138] Endurance training can also alter muscle fiber characteristics. When stimulation or training is withdrawn, however, the muscle gradually regains its former properties.[138]

A growing body of evidence shows that muscle imbalances (muscle atrophy and hypertrophy) are present in

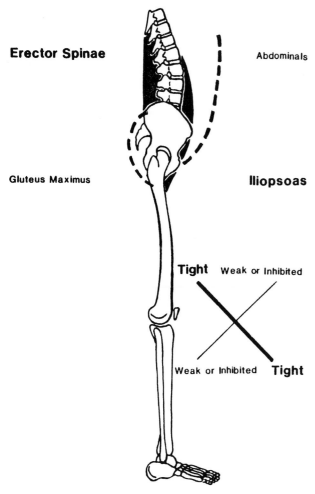

Erector Spinae

Abdominals

Gluteus Maximus

Iliopsoas

Tight Weak or Inhibited

Weak or Inhibited **Tight**

Fig. 2.22. The lower crossed syndrome. (From Jull G, Janda V: Muscles and Motor Control in Low Back Pain. In Twomey LT, Taylor JR (eds): Physical Therapy for the Low Back, Clinics in Physical Therapy, New York, Churchill Livingstone, 1987.)

patients with acute and chronic low back pain. *Hides et al. found unilateral, segmental wasting of the multifidus in acute back pain patients.[68] This change occurred rapidly and thus was not considered to be a disuse atrophy. Stokes et al. found generalized atrophy in patients with chronic back pain, but a relative increase in the CSA was noted on the symptomatic side.[95] Type I fiber hypertrophy on the symptomatic side and type II fiber atrophy bilaterally have been documented in chronic back pain patients.[97]*

Muscles housing trigger points have been shown to have dramatically different levels of EMG activity within the same functional muscle unit. Hubbard and Berkoff showed EMG hyperexcitability in the nidus of the trigger point in a taut band that had a characteristic pattern of reproducible referred pain.[79] Case studies have also revealed that trigger points in one muscle are related to inhibition of another functionally related muscle.[78,98] In particular, Simons showed that the deltoid muscle can be inhibited when there are infraspinatus trigger points.[80] Headley has shown that lower trapezius inhibition is related to trigger points in the upper trapezius.[94]

Muscle imbalances alter the performance of related movements. Repeated performance of abnormal movements leads inevitably to further strain, which can perpetuate muscular imbalances and joint dysfunction. In the work place, the combination of muscle imbalance and performing repetitive tasks in constrained postures has contributed to an epidemic of overuse syndromes.

Muscles that become overactive or tight are often said to be in "spasm." Loose application of the term spasm leads to inappropriate treatment selection. Clinical decision making would be better served if muscle tension or stiffness is viewed as being related to either viscoelastic, connective tissue, and/or neuromuscular factors. Trigger points, acute torticollis, appendicitis, lumbar strain with antalgic posture, and loss of the flexion-relaxation response in disabling lumbar pain syndromes are examples of increased neuromuscular tension.[76,77] Elevated EMG activity typically is present in such situations. Connective tissue changes in a muscle or its fascia, such as adhesion or scar formation, usually arise gradually after trauma when the acute, inflammatory phase is prolonged.[45] Improper healing allows fibroblast proliferation and eventual scar formation.[45] Viscoelastic changes without increased neuromuscular tension also occur in the gradual muscle shortening seen with aging and sedentariness.

A central source of increased neuromuscular tension is theorized to be dysfunction of the limbic system.[140] This condition is thought to be related to abnormal illness behavior—sleep disorder, depression, anxiety, fear—and is accompanied by *generalized* soft tissue tenderness. Sarno used the descriptive term "tension myositis," whereas others commonly refer to this neuromuscular tension as fibromyalgia.[141] Fibromyalgia patients tested with laser evoked potentials have been documented to have hyperalgesia.[142]

According to Janda, the most typical types of functional muscle weakness are as follows. *Tightness weakness* develops when a muscle is chronically shortened and eventually loses strength (i.e., psoas).[143] *Stretch weakness* occurs if a

Table 2.6. Characteristics of Muscle Types[119,120]

Characteristics	Type S "Slow-Twitch"	Type FF "Fast-Twitch Fatigable"
	Type I	*Type II*
Fatigability	Resistant	Easy
Metabolism	Oxidative	Anaerobic
Energy	Mitochondria/ATP	Glycogen
Capillary network	Extensive	Minimal
Metabolic preference	Constant muscle length	Muscle shortening
Speed of contraction, relaxation and force generation	Slow	Fast
Metabolism at rest	High	Low
Function	Posture "antigravity"	Phasic "fight or flight"

muscle is perpetually placed in a lengthened position so that the muscle spindles become desensitized to stretch (i.e., gluteus maximus).[143] *Arthrogenic weakness* occurs when nociceptive afferent barrage from a joint or ligament causes a reflex inhibition.[143] Examples are the vastus medialis after injury of the anterior cruciate ligament or meniscus or gluteus maximus weakness when a sacroiliac dysfunction is present.[143] Finally, *trigger point weakness* occurs when a muscle cannot fully activate all its contractile fibers because of the presence of a trigger point.[143]

Common types of muscular dysfunction, like trigger points, are best understood in the context of muscular imbalance. A short, tight postural muscle may house trigger points because of its increased metabolic demands and tension, which can produce ischemia and irritating metabolites. Also, an inhibited phasic muscle may form trigger points as a result of its greater than normal fatigability and thus susceptibility to overload and mechanical failure.

Table 2.7. Consequences of Muscular Imbalance

Altered joint mechanics/uneven distribution of pressure
Limited range of motion and compensatory hypermobility
Change in proprioceptive input
Impaired reciprocal inhibition
Altered programming of movement patterns

(From Janda V: Lecture, Los Angeles College of Chiropractic, Rehabilitation Certification Course, 1993.)

The general effects of muscular imbalance are listed in Table 2.7. Muscular imbalance is typically identified by postural analysis (two and one leg stance), gait analysis, muscle length tests, and evaluation of key movement patterns. *Postural analysis* (Fig. 2.23) seeks to identify structural asymmetries (i.e., oblique pelvis, winged scapula), pelvic position (i.e., anterior pelvic tilt, rotated pelvis), hypertrophied muscles (i.e., thoracolumbar erector spinae, upper trapezius), and atrophied muscles (i.e., gluteus maximus, lumbosacral

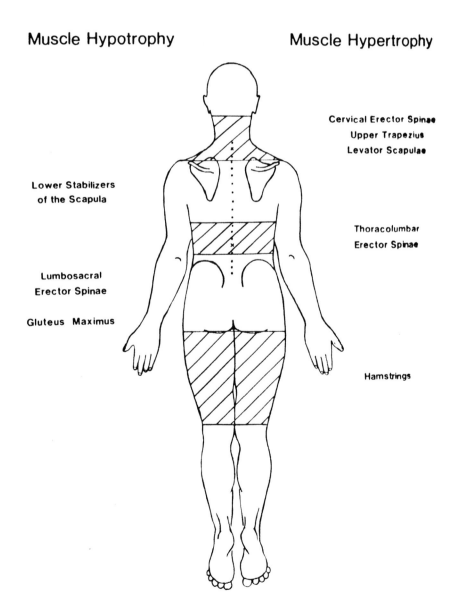

Muscle Hypotrophy

Muscle Hypertrophy

Lower Stabilizers
of the Scapula

Lumbosacral
Erector Spinae

Gluteus Maximus

Cervical Erector Spinae
Upper Trapezius
Levator Scapulae

Thoracolumbar
Erector Spinae

Hamstrings

Fig. 2.23. Depiction of the layer syndrome. (From Jull G, Janda V: Muscles and Motor Control in Low Back Pain. In Twomey LT, Taylor JR (eds): Physical Therapy for the Low Back, Clinics in Physical Therapy, New York, Churchill Livingstone, 1987.)

erector spinae). Postural analysis in one leg standing observes presence of gluteus medius weakness, pelvic obliquity, and other muscular compensations. *Gait analysis* mostly addresses hip mobility (decreased hip hyperextension), increased pelvic side shift (weakness of gluteus medius), compensatory hyperlordosis, and lack of pelvic motion attributable to a sacroiliac lesion. *Muscle length tests* are specific tests to identify the amount of muscle shortening present. Six basic, stereotypic *movement patterns* are tested to evaluate the muscle activation sequence or coordination during performance of key hip, trunk, scapulothoracic, scapulohumeral, and cervical movements.

CORRELATING MUSCULAR AND JOINT DYSFUNCTION

The most common pain generators are likely to be those structures housing the most nociceptors (articular surfaces, joint capsules, ligaments). Regardless of what is the exact pain generator, the entire motor system will react and compensate. Long after strained soft tissues have been injured, adaptive patterns will persist.

Muscles are the medium through which central motor commands or reflex spinal activity compensate for any disturbance. Certain muscles typically react when specific joints are injured or are dysfunctional. This relationship can work in either direction in that impairment in a muscle or joint will eventually lead to some compensatory change in its functional partner. Clearly, if a muscle is shortened or overactive, increased pressure and strain develop in the joint capsule and tendoperiosteal junction. Also, a muscle that is inhibited and weak is associated with poorer stability for the related joints, with compensatory fixations or even hypermobility resulting.

As described previously, Johansson et al. correlated non–noxious joint afferent activity with increased reflex gamma motoneuron activity.[69] They hypothesized that long-lasting noxious stimulation may activate the flexion withdrawal reflex.[69] Similar reflex discharges from the joints mediated by efferent sympathetic fibers were described by Schaible and Grubb.[100] Joint inflammation in the knee can lead to reflex muscle inhibition.[67,91,92] Hides et al. correlated segmental, reflex muscle atrophy in the low back with acute low back pain in patients in whom specific lumbar joint dysfunction was manually diagnosed.[68] Bullock-Saxton et al. showed a correlation between poor ankle joint stability and inhibition of the gluteus maximus and medius during walking.[98]

By understanding the relationship between specific muscles and joints, therapeutic shortcuts can often be uncovered. Finding a chain reaction between muscular imbalance, an altered movement pattern, and specific joint dysfunctions enables the clinician to find the key factors in the development of functional pathology, and thus catalyzes the therapeutic program. Lewit identified specific joint dysfunctions that are linked to individual dysfunctional muscles (Table 2.8).[144,145]

ALTERED MOVEMENT PATTERNS

The presence of pain, muscular imbalance, trigger points, or joint dysfunction alters the ability of the patient to perform

Table 2.8. Muscle and Joint Functional Chains[144]

Joint	Muscle
C0/1	Suboccipitals, SCM,* upper trapezius, (masticatories, submandibular)
C1/2	SCM, levator scapulae, upper trapezius
C2/3	SCM, levator scapulae, upper trapezius
C3/6	Upper trapezius, cervical erector spinae, (supinator, wrist extensor, biceps)
C6/T3	SCM, upper or middle trapezius, scaleni (subscapularis)
T3/T10	Pectoralis, thoracic erector spinae, serratus anterior (subscapularis)
T10/L2	Quadratus lumborum, psoas, abdominals, thoracolumbar erector spinae
L2/L3	Gluteus medius
L3/L4	Rectus femoris, lumbar erector spinae, adductors
L4/L5	Piriformis, hamstrings, lumbar erector spinae, adductors
L5/S1	Iliacus, hamstrings, lumbar erector spinae, adductors
SI	Gluteus maximus, piriformis, iliacus, hamstrings, adductors, contralateral gluteus medius
Coccyx	Levator ani, gluteus maximus, piriformis (iliacus)
Hip	Adductors

*SCM, sternocleidomastoid.

certain, stereotypic movement patterns. The negative relationship between various individual functional pathologic changes and the abnormal performance of basic movement patterns is self-perpetuating. Altered or faulty movement patterns themselves place new strains on the locomotor system and lead to the spread of a local problem beyond a single region.

Such movement patterns were first recognized clinically by Janda, who noticed that the classic muscle testing of Kendall and Kendall did not differentiate between normal recruitment of related muscles and "trick" patterns of substitution during a specific action. So-called "trick" movements are uneconomical and place unusual strain on the joints. They involve muscles in inefficient or incoordinated ways, which thus are prone to fatigue. On the classic test for prone hip extension, it is difficult to identify overactivity of the lumbar erector spinae or hamstrings as substitutes for an inhibited gluteus maximus. All that is noted is the overall strength or quantity of output, not how it is accomplished—its *quality.* Janda's tests are far more sensitive and allow the clinician to identify these clinically pertinent muscle imbalances and faulty movement patterns by seeing abnormal substitution during muscle testing protocols.

When a movement pattern is altered, the activation sequence or firing order of different muscles involved in a specific movement is disturbed. The prime mover may be slow to activate while synergists or stabilizers substitute and become overactive. New joint stresses will then be encountered. Sometimes, the timing sequence is normal but the overall range may be limited because of joint stiffness or antagonist muscle shortening.

A classic example of muscular imbalance causing an impaired movement pattern is when tight hip flexors are combined with weakness in the gluteus maximus, causing an inefficient or incoordinated hip extension movement pattern. The gluteus maximus may be inhibited and activate poorly

Table 2.9. Muscular Imbalance and Altered Movement Patterns

Weak Agonist	Overactive Antagonist	Overactive Synergist	Movement Pattern
Gluteus maximus	Psoas, rectus femoris	Erector spinae, hamstrings	Hip extension
Gluteus medius	Adductors	QL, TFL, piriformis*	Hip abduction
Abdominals	Erector spinae	Psoas	Trunk flexion
Serratus anterior	Pectoralis major/minor	Upper trapezius, levator scapulae, rhomboids	Trunk lowering from a push-up (scapular fixation)
Deep neck flexors	Suboccipitals	SCM*	Neck flexion
Lower and middle trapezius		Upper trapezius, levator scapulae, rhomboids	Shoulder abduction or flexion (scapular fixation)
Diaphragm		Scalenes, pectoralis major	Respiration

*QL, quadratus lumborum; TFL, tensor fascia latae; SCM, sternocleidomastoid.

during the movement, leading to overactivity of the stabilizers in the lumbar spine, the erector spinae muscles. Although such an altered pattern may have formed as a result of hip flexor compensation to a low back strain, hyperpronation problem, leg length inequality, etc., it eventually perpetuates instability by overstressing the lumbar joints on its own. In this case, the following functional pathologic abnormalities will be interconnected: shortening of the psoas, inhibition/weakness/trigger points of the gluteus maximus, overactivity/trigger points of the lumbar erector spinae, lumbar spine joint dysfunction, and altered coordination/endurance of hip extension, particularly during gait.

Testing individual muscles for strength without concern for the speed of activation or relaxation or the activation sequence of agonist, synergists, and stabilizers is an error. According to Korr, "The brain thinks in terms of whole motions, not individual muscles."[146] Muscles may have anatomic individuality, but they function interdependently, to create smooth, well-orchestrated movements.

Examples of typical pairs of overactive and weak muscles and the related altered movement patterns are listed in Table 2.9. These patterns are used as a screening evaluation to correlate joint overstress, trigger points, tight muscles, and inhibited or weak muscles. Other key functional demands such as squatting, lunging, reaching, etc. can also be assessed for muscle imbalances, incoordination, and other dysfunctions. *The purpose of identifying altered movement patterns and muscle imbalances is to discover what to stretch, strengthen, and adjust in patients with deconditioning syndrome. This information allows us to search for the clinical shortcuts afforded by understanding the connection between altered biomechanics and neurophysiology of patients with pathologic function of the motor system.*

Treatment of altered movement patterns is described in Table 2.10.

Pain motor programs, poor postural habits, or altered movement patterns are memorized just as is normal gait, skiing, or virtuoso musicianship. Inefficient or uneconomical movement patterns, once learned, will perpetuate the muscular imbalance and joint dysfunction that may have caused them. Treatment aimed at peripheral functional pathologic alterations, such as tight muscles, trigger points, or joint dysfunction, often fails if altered movement patterns are not iden-

tified and the individual is not re-educated. This need to relearn is an important reason why pain often outlasts the elimination of its cause.

Janda advanced the concept that the control of movement by the central nervous system can be re-educated. This theory was tested in a study in which propriosensory stimulation exercises were given to individuals in an attempt to improve the speed of recruitment of the gluteus maximus and gluteus medius muscles during gait.[98] Individuals performed balance exercises for 15 minutes per day for 1 week. These exercises led to significant increases in the speed of activation of the gait muscles. Such propriosensory retraining improved gluteal activity "automatically and subconsciously, and not as a voluntary muscle contraction."[98]

REHABILITATION OF THE MOTOR SYSTEM

Rehabilitation includes functional capacity evaluation, rehabilitative care, patient education, and psychosocial factors. It is ideally suited for managed care practices because it involves quantification of functional progress of the patient, outcomes assessment, proven cost-containment methods, and self-care.

Rehabilitation vs. Conservative Treatment

Rehabilitation is different from acute, conservative care. Conservative care is ideal for acute disorders. It focuses on stabilization of the injured part, pain control, and promotion of soft tissue healing. Rehabilitation is concerned with restoring musculoskeletal function in patients with subacute, chronic, and recurrent conditions. Rehabilitation attempts to prevent or manage disability through functional restoration, work hardening, and psychosocial intervention.

In the first issue of the Journal of Occupational Rehabilitation, Feuerstein described the changing paradigm of musculoskeletal care: "Active rehabilitation efforts using a sports

Table 2.10. Treatment for Altered Movement Patterns

Relax/stretch overactive/tight muscles
Mobilize/adjust stiff joints
Facilitate/strengthen weak muscles
Re-educate movement patterns on reflex, subcortical basis

medicine model directed at rapid safe return to work coupled with ergonomic intervention have replaced much of the traditional passive, i.e., modality-driven, approaches to rehabilitation of musculoskeletal injuries."[147]

The key difference between rehabilitation and traditional conservative care is the primary emphasis on function rather than pain relief. Patients are educated that pain perception will decrease as physical functioning improves. This focus transforms the patient from a passive, dependent recipient of care to an active participant engaged in the process of rehabilitation (Table 2.11), and the doctor's role becomes that of helper rather than healer.

Rehabilitation involves lifestyle changes and behavioral re-education (functional restoration), and thus is part of a biopsychosocial approach. The patient's suffering and illness are more important than a specific disease process. *Historically, this approach was appropriate for physically exceptional (athletes) and physically impaired (handicapped) individuals. Today, it is necessary for most pain patients. The indications for rehabilitation include the subacute stage of injury, chronic pain, disability, or recurrent pain. The purpose of rehabilitation is to treat or prevent deconditioning syndrome and abnormal illness behavior.*

Blending Active and Passive Care in Practice

To be a rehabilitation specialist, a health care provider must *identify "red flags," shift from passive to active care, understand the emerging guidelines for care, perform outcomes assessment and functional testing, and identify psychosocial factors relating to abnormal illness behavior.* It is important to rule out morphology, infection, carcinoma, and visceral, metabolic, rheumatologic, or neurologic diseases (red flags) before attempting rehabilitation.[148] Such patients should be referred to the appropriate specialists. Acute disk problems and traumatic injuries require following specialized conservative care protocols, but these patients eventually will become candidates for rehabilitation.

Current guidelines dictate that exercise and active care are crucial to the management of subacute, recurrent, and chronic conditions. Bed rest, medication, passive methods, injections, surgery, and manipulation all have their proper place in treatment planning. *Being able to define an appropriate rehabilitation goal depends on knowing how to judge functional status and work demands.* If an individual has a high work demand, greater functional status will need to be achieved. Injured workers should be viewed as "occupational athletes" facing high levels of stress/strain in their work place for

which they need to be properly trained. It is essential to address deconditioning and teach a worker how to reduce mechanical stress while simultaneously training them to improve their functional status.

Individuals with abnormal illness behavior are more likely to become disabled or to develop chronic pain syndromes. Quick shifting from passive (conservative) to active (rehabilitative) care can prevent much disability. Referral for multidisciplinary functional restoration, involving psychologic support and biobehavioral re-education may also be indicated.

Although treatment decisions are often made on the basis of a diagnosis, patients with spinal pain resist accurate labeling. Painful spinal syndromes are considered mechanical disorders most of the time, but many experts view the psychologic or social factors to be predominant. Pain-sensitive structures abound in the spinal region, and perhaps because of the overlap between sites of referred pain from muscles, joints, ligaments, fascia, nerves, etc., a diagnosis often is given on the basis of the physician's pathophysiologic philosophy rather than on any provable hypothesis (i.e., degenerative disk, sacroiliac or myofascial syndromes). Unfortunately, a certain pathoanatomic diagnosis can only be determined approximately 20% of the time,[111,149,150] including conditions ranging from disk syndromes and stenosis to the much rarer spinal trauma, rheumatologic disorders, and infectious or neoplastic diseases of the spine.

The obvious limitation of the Quebec Task Force classification is that it suggests that 80% of all back pain cases require no individualization of care. Attempts to subclassify the nonspecific pain group are under way, and progress has been reported by Delitto et al.[151] These authors have shown prescriptive validity for an approach that identifies extension and sacroiliac mobilization subclassifications.[151] Diagnostic anesthetic block tests have also been used to identify sacroiliac joint pathology as an etiologic factor in 10 to 30% of chronic low back pain patients.[152] Similar methods have demonstrated that greater than 50% of chronic neck pain after whiplash injury involves the cervical zygapophyseal joints.[153] Unfortunately, no physical examination tests correlate with the diagnostic block techniques.

Passive and active care are both important in case management, passive care being more important initially and active care later on. Table 2.12 describes the stages of treatment and their goals, and some specific interventions during these stages are outlined in Table 2.13. We must mention, however, some important exceptions. For instance, McKenzie methods may be used, even in acute cases. When these methods are

Table 2.11. Primary Goals of Rehabilitation and Conservative Care

	Pain Relief	Promote Tissue Healing	Functional Restoration	Passive Patient	Active Patient
Rehabilitation	−	−	+	−	+
Conservative care	+	+	−	+	−

(Adapted from Liebenson C: Rehabilitation of the chronic back pain patient. California Chiropractic Journal, July 1991.)

Table 2.12. Goals of Treatment

Acute Intervention	Remobilization	Rehabilitation and Reconditioning	Lifestyle Adaptations
Reduce inflammation No pain at rest Minimal pain with unstressed daily activities Decrease muscle "spasm"	Increase pain-free mobility Minimize deconditioning Promote tissue repair/regeneration	Increase muscle strength/endurance Improve coordination Increase flexibility Increase aerobic capacity Promote tissue remodeling	Improve ergonomic factors Education about biomechanics Address psychosocial factors

PAIN RELIEF & PROMOTION OF SOFT TISSUE HEALING

FUNCTIONAL RESTORATION

(Adapted from Triano J: Standards of care: Manipulative procedures. In White AH, Anderson R (eds): Conservative Care of Low Back Pain. Baltimore, Williams and Wilkins, 1991, pp 159–168.)

Table 2.13. Treatment Strategies

Acute Intervention	Remobilization	Rehabilitation and Reconditioning	Prevention and Lifestyle Factors
Rest/ice Supports/braces Gentle stretching Physical therapy Anti-inflammatories	Chiropractic adjustments Soft tissue manipulation Physical therapy Postural correction Functional exercise	Functional strengthening Stretching Cardiovascular fitness Balance and coordination	Stress management Ergonomics "work station" Biomechanics "lifting/bending" Diet/nutrition

ACTIVE CARE

PASSIVE CARE

successful, they are able to impart enormous cost savings. Similarly, a trial of manipulative therapy for a chronic sufferer who has not previously had such care is also indicated.

Rehabilitation of the motor system involves restoring normal joint mobility; inhibiting overactive musculature (including trigger points); improving muscular flexibility, coordination, strength, and endurance; stretching retracted soft tissues; propriosensory re-education; cardiovascular training; and postural re-education. Passive and active care are both required to achieve these goals (Table 2.14). Physical training alone would fail to address specific joint dysfunctions or movement incoordination. Chiropractic adjustments alone would fail to address muscle imbalances or faulty movement patterns. *Assessment should identify the various links in the chain of functional pathologic processes.* Often the problem is in the patient's posture or work activities. Regardless of what other influences exist, rehabilitating the motor system requires that we see the interrelationship between the functional parts and between the patient and his or her environment.

This approach is empiric in that one identifies functional deficits and seeks those interventions that can have the most

positive impact on improving functional integrity. Restoring function by reversing the deconditioning syndrome is the primary goal, as opposed to merely treating symptoms. Highly technical muscle function testing and training apparatuses are not necessary to achieve this end. *Practitioners in small, private practices who assess and treat functional pathologic problems while training and educating the patient in how to*

Table 2.14. Integrating Passive and Active Care in Rehabilitation

Goal: Improved posture and motor control on a reflex, semiautomatic basis
Increase mobility/flexibility
   Joint mobilization/adjustment
   Muscle relaxation/stretch
Improve coordination, strength, endurance
   Muscle facilitation
   "Spinal stabilization" or functional exercise training
   Propriosensory retraining
   Cardiovascular training
Postural re-education

Table 2.15. Factors that May Predict a Longer Recovery (from the Mercy Guideline)

History of more than 4 episodes
Longer than 1 week of symptoms before seeing a doctor
Severe pain
Pre-existing structural pathology or skeletal anomaly (i.e., spondy-lolisthesis) directly related to new injury or condition

(From Haldeman S, Chapman-Smith D, Petersen DM: Frequency and duration of care. In Guidelines for Chiropractic Quality Assurance and Practice Parameters. Gaithersburg, Aspen, 1993, pp. 115–130.)

prevent reoccurrences represent the cost-effective front line against today's soaring costs for caring for individuals with low back pain.

Case Management and Standards of Care
PROGNOSIS

The natural history of uncomplicated spinal disorders is toward resolution within 6 weeks.[148,150] More time may be necessary for moderate to severe traumatic injuries, prolapsed disks with nerve compression, or if certain complicating factors are present (Tables 2.15 and 2.16). Intervention for uncomplicated cases is considered successful if the patient is asymptomatic within 6 weeks. Traumatic injuries may require more time, depending on the severity of the injury. Disk problems may also require more time because of the poor healing potential of the avascular annulus fibrosis (particularly in smokers). The goal of modern care of the spine is to minimize the incidence of chronic pain and disability by focusing on restoration of function as soon as possible. Nordin comments, " . . . there is a very small window of time in low back pain care; we must act quickly within 4–6 weeks to bring patients into an active reconditioning program if we expect to return them to productive lives and prevent recurrence."[154]

Table 2.16. Risk Factors for Chronicity

History/Consultation
  Previous history of low back pain
  Total work loss in past 12 months
  Heavy smoking
  Personal problems—alcohol, marital, financial
  Adversarial medicolegal problems
  Low education attainment*
  Heavy physical occupation*
Questionnaires/Pain Drawings or Scales
  Radiating leg pain
  Low job satisfaction
  Psychologic distress and depressive symptoms—BMG
Examination
  Reduced straight leg raising
  Signs of nerve root involvement
  Reduced trunk strength and endurance (dynametric, nondynametric)
  Poor physical fitness (aerobic capacity)
  Disproportionate illness behavior (Waddell's signs)

*Only slightly increases the risk of chronicity, but significantly increases the difficulty of rehabilitation.
(Adapted from CSAG Clinical Standards Advisory Group Report on Back Pain. London, HMSO, 1994; 1–89.)

Patients have traditionally been categorized as having acute, subacute, chronic, or recurrent disease, depending on the stage of soft tissue healing or time course of their recovery.[155–157] The acute, inflammatory phase of soft tissue healing lasts between 24 and 72 hours. The subacute phase, in which repair and regeneration occur, lasts from 24 hours to 6 weeks. The final phase involves remodeling, which proceeds from the third week to 12 months after injury. These phases of soft tissue healing make sense for patients suffering traumatic injuries, but for individuals experiencing pain syndromes related to cumulative microtrauma, such a framework is not appropriate. *Because of the presence of abnormal illness behavior disproportionate to impairment or structural pathologic findings, the chronic stage is often entered as soon as 7 weeks after pain onset.*[150] According to Waddell, cases involving back pain should be regarded as acute, recurrent, or chronic.[158]

The individual suffering an episode of pain after injury or trauma should be better in 7 to 16 weeks.[159] The acute phase may last 1 week or until the patient has no pain at rest and he or she can perform unstressed daily activities.[159] Up to 3 to 7 days of "relative rest" and immobilization may be necessary. Prolonged immobilization must be avoided, however, because of its deleterious effects (see "Negative Effects of Immobilization"). The subacute phase should last 6 to 8 weeks if it is a minor to moderate injury.[159] This phase may last 8 to 16 weeks if the injury is moderate to severe.[159] For soft tissue injuries, any patient still experiencing symptoms at the 16-week mark should be considered in the chronic phase.[160] Soft tissue healing is complete at this point, except for the most severe injuries.

The popular medical practice of assigning the label "nonspecific or idiopathic back pain" is likely to lead to decreased patient satisfaction.[161] Some practical patient classifications should be sought that can be used to direct the choice of therapeutic intervention.[151] Most patients have a gradual or nontraumatic onset with nonradicular symptoms. Repetitive strain is the most likely etiology for the first time or recurrent symptoms. If there is no nerve root involvement, such pain episodes should be expected to resolve within the same time frame as allowed for mild to moderate injuries (6 to 8 weeks).[148,150] The presence of complicating factors as listed in Table 2.15 may legitimize additional care. *Justifying a longer recovery time because of the stages of soft tissue healing is an inappropriate application of an acute injury model to patients suffering from cumulative trauma or repetitive strain.*[150,159]

The patient with radicular symptoms (symptoms distal to the knee or elbow) and evidence of nerve root compression (i.e., nerve tension signs) is a specific example of a complicated case, the natural history of which involves greater than 6 weeks before resolution can be expected. This prognosis is due to a strong correlation between clinical symptoms and structural pathologic findings. Nonetheless, even patients with large disk prolapses can be expected to recover without surgery.[111,148,150,162,163] Treatment in such cases might follow a similar time frame as for moderate to severe injuries.

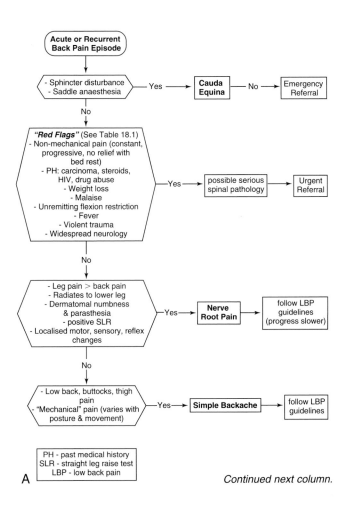

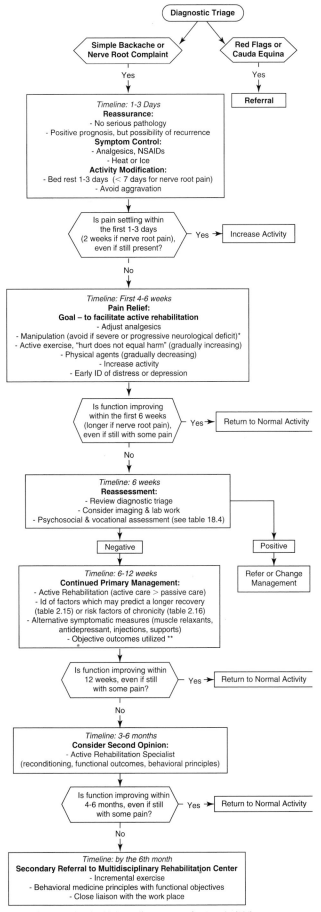

Fig. 2.24. (A) Diagnostic triage algorithm. (B) Treatment guidelines algorithm.

A

Acute or Recurrent Back Pain Episode

- Sphincter disturbance
- Saddle anaesthesia → Yes → **Cauda Equina** → No → Emergency Referral

No

"Red Flags" (See Table 18.1)
- Non-mechanical pain (constant, progressive, no relief with bed rest)
- PH: carcinoma, steroids, HIV, drug abuse
- Weight loss
- Malaise
- Unremitting flexion restriction
- Fever
- Violent trauma
- Widespread neurology

→ Yes → possible serious spinal pathology → Urgent Referral

No

- Leg pain > back pain
- Radiates to lower leg
- Dermatomal numbness & parasthesia
- positive SLR
- Localised motor, sensory, reflex changes

→ Yes → **Nerve Root Pain** → follow LBP guidelines (progress slower)

No

- Low back, buttocks, thigh pain
- "Mechanical" pain (varies with posture & movement)

→ Yes → **Simple Backache** → follow LBP guidelines

PH - past medical history
SLR - straight leg raise test
LBP - low back pain

Continued next column.

B

Diagnostic Triage

Simple Backache or Nerve Root Complaint — Yes

Red Flags or Cauda Equina — Yes → Referral

Timeline: 1-3 Days
Reassurance:
- No serious pathology
- Positive prognosis, but possibility of recurrence
Symptom Control:
- Analgesics, NSAIDs
- Heat or Ice
Activity Modification:
- Bed rest 1-3 days (< 7 days for nerve root pain)
- Avoid aggravation

Is pain settling within the first 1-3 days (2 weeks if nerve root pain), even if still present? → Yes → Increase Activity

No

Timeline: First 4-6 weeks
Pain Relief:
Goal – to facilitate active rehabilitation
- Adjust analgesics
- Manipulation (avoid if severe or progressive neurological deficit)*
- Active exercise, "hurt does not equal harm" (gradually increasing)
- Physical agents (gradually decreasing)
- Increase activity
- Early ID of distress or depression

Is function improving within the first 6 weeks (longer if nerve root pain), even if still with some pain → Yes → Return to Normal Activity

No

Timeline: 6 weeks
Reassessment:
- Review diagnostic triage
- Consider imaging & lab work
- Psychosocial & vocational assessment (see table 18.4)

Negative   Positive → Refer or Change Management

Timeline: 6-12 weeks
Continued Primary Management:
- Active Rehabilitation (active care > passive care)
- Id of factors which may predict a longer recovery (table 2.15) or risk factors of chronicity (table 2.16)
- Alternative symptomatic measures (muscle relaxants, antidepressant, injections, supports)
- Objective outcomes utilized **

Is function improving within 12 weeks, even if still with some pain? → Yes → Return to Normal Activity

No

Timeline: 3-6 months
Consider Second Opinion:
- Active Rehabilitation Specialist (reconditioning, functional outcomes, behavioral principles)

Is function improving within 4-6 months, even if still with some pain? → Yes → Return to Normal Activity

No

Timeline: by the 6th month
Secondary Referral to Multidisciplinary Rehabilitation Center
- Incremental exercise
- Behavioral medicine principles with functional objectives
- Close liaison with the work place

* Type of manipulation should change if no progress after 2 weeks (184).

** Treatment beyond 6 weeks must be tracked by acceptable, outcome assessment measurements. Failure to show significant progress by the 8th week of an uncomplicated case or the 16th week of a complicated case or nerve root complaint should result in

Table 2.17 summarizes the prognosis for the various general types of cases. The algorithm in Figure 2.24 is useful for understanding the indications for bed rest, manipulation, active care, and multidisciplinary functional restoration.

Certain patients can be identified early as being "disability prone."[164] A certain profile of the chronic pain or disability-prone patient has emerged that can be used to predict a poor response to care[164,165] (Table 2.18). These factors are not structural or functional (organic), but are psychosocial (nonorganic).[157,164] Such psychologic factors as poor pain coping strategies, excessive anxiety, depression, and symptom magnification are significant.[166–168] Social or economic factors like job dissatisfaction, pending litigation, low income level, and low education level are also important.[164,165,169] Waddell and colleagues studied the relationship between pain, impairment, and disability in patients with inappropriate signs of symptoms of illness behavior.[170] An individual who is unwilling to move from being a pain avoider to becoming a pain manager is such a patient. Excessive dependency on medication or passive forms of therapy, along with an unwillingness to develop internal control over symptoms by learning self-treatment skills, are clear signs of a potential chronic pain patient.

The treatment plan for spinal disorders focuses on aggressive, conservative care for promotion of soft tissue healing after an injury. When pain is a result of a repetitive strain, conservative care may be appropriate for pain relief, but treatment goals must quickly change to rehabilitation or restoration of function. Intervention involving manipulative therapy has demonstrated a clear advantage over other methods (reduced disability) in the initial care of the patients with pain.[171] Early, active intervention; preventative education; and rehabilitation approaches have all shown their positive impact on

Table 2.17. Prognosis for Musculoskeletal Pain Syndromes[159]

	Syndromes		
	Acute	Subacute	Chronic
Mild-moderate injury	2–3 days	6–8 weeks	—
Moderate-severe injury	<1 week	8–16 weeks	4–12 months
Repetitive strain	2–3 days	6–8 weeks	—
Nerve root compression	<1 week	8–16 weeks	4–12 months

Table 2.18. Profile of the Disability Prone Patient

Symptom magnification
Pain avoidance behavior
Psychologic distress
Job dissatisfaction
Anxiety
Treatment dependency
Catastrophizing as a coping strategy
Pending litigation

Table 2.19. Guidelines for Management of Uncomplicated Soft Tissue Musculoskeletal Pain Syndromes

1. Bed rest should not exceed 2 days and passive methods 6 to 8 weeks.
2. Treatment frequency is 2 to 5X/week for the first 2 weeks (passive care with manipulative therapy appropriate).
3. From week 3 to weeks 6 to 8, treatment frequency should be decreasing.
4. Functional capacity evaluation is recommended when patient is subacute (week 2 to 4) and mandatory at 6 to 8 weeks.
5. Progressive exercise prescription and self-care advice recommended within 1 to 2 weeks and mandatory at 6 to 8 weeks.
6. Evaluation by a rehabilitation specialist may be appropriate at 6 to 8 weeks.
7. Advanced imaging techniques are appropriate only when neurologic function is deteriorating or progressive exercise therapy has failed.
8. Evaluation by a pain behavioral specialist may be appropriate at 6 months.

reducing future recurrences and preventing the emergence of chronic pain syndromes.[59,60,172,173] Bush showed that aggressive conservative care is highly successful for the management of severe disk protrusions with nerve root compression.[163] Multidisciplinary, functional restoration programs have repeatedly demonstrated their success in returning the chronically disabled back pain sufferer to work.[160,174–176] Other studies have shown that failure of passive therapy approaches does not imply that active rehabilitation efforts will fail.[177,178]

Pain relief and prevention of recurrences are the primary aims of care. Restoring function is the means by which these ends are achieved. *In most uncomplicated cases involving subacute or recurrent pain, treatment aimed at pain relief and functional restoration takes between 2 and 6 weeks. Initial treatment frequency (three times per week for 2 weeks) is often sufficient to identify the key functional pathologic problems that will enable the health care provider to individualize a self-treatment strategy. Continued care with decreasing frequency for approximately another 4 weeks is usually appropriate.* Additional care is often required in cases of moderate to severe trauma, disk prolapse with nerve root compression, or chronic pain, or when significant complicating factors or abnormal illness behavior are present. The disability-prone patient often requires interdisciplinary referral. Table 2.19 provides an overview of these guidelines, which are also discussed in Chapter 21.

REPORT OF FINDINGS

Although it is sometimes considered speculative to assert that a specific tissue is the primary pain generator, it is not necessary to burden the patient with the diagnosis of nonspecific back pain.[161] Kirkaldy-Willis discussed the cardinal signs of different sources of nonspecific pain, such as facet, sacroiliac, and myofascial.[162] Cherkin and MacCornack noted that offering an explanation to patients and clearly outlining goals for care leads to greater patient satisfaction.[179,180] Bogduk and Simons summarized the key elements for diagnosing myofascial sources of pain from articular sources (see Chapter 18).[181]

After the patient has been given the working diagnosis, it is important to explain that although most people get better within 6 weeks, recurrences are the rule rather than the exception.[56] For this reason, it is prudent to spend some time teaching patients how to reduce further strain on their back and how to increase their intrinsic capacity to handle external demands. If a patient is "disability prone," psychosocial as well as biomechanical issues will need to be addressed. Referral to a psychologist specializing in biobehavioral education may be necessary.

Simple charts can be used (refer to Fig. 2.4) to educate the patient about the importance of reducing external demand and/or increasing functional capacity to prevent re-injury. The more external stress, the greater the chance of injury. Such extrinsic sources could include prolonged sitting, improper lifting technique, or repetitive manual handling activities. *The simplest way to avoid future problems is to reduce the external stress. In as much as this change is not always possible, intrinsic functional capacity can be increased.* Various intrinsic factors such as muscular imbalances of strength or flexibility, postural faults (i.e., slumped posture), structural asymmetry (i.e., short leg), impaired coordination or balance, or poor cardiovascular fitness also predispose to recurrent pain episodes. The dangers of even low level repetitive strains should be made clear (refer to Fig. 2.7). Instruction should stress taking frequent "microbreaks" from either prolonged static loading (i.e., desk work) or repetitive activities (i.e., manual material handling).

Whatever the pain complaint, proper management hinges on reducing strain so as to promote healing and to prevent recurrences. In the acute stage, especially with disk syndromes or trauma, reducing load on the injured structures is called "relative rest." This measure, along with chiropractic, physical therapy, and exercise, may be used to reduce tissue swelling or irritability and to promote a good environment for healing of soft tissue injuries.

Patients can be educated about the dangers of recurrences as pain subsides and the need to increase intrinsic back fitness and decrease exposure to harmful, extrinsic sources of back strain. Comparing the patient's treatment to that of an athlete will help to motivate the patient toward seeking more than just symptomatic relief. Tables 2.12 and 2.13, along with Figure 2.9, can be used to show the patient how the sports medicine paradigm of rehabilitation is the best method for achieving optimal results. For example, an injured patient learns that healing starts with inflammation. The goal of treatment is to decrease swelling and pain. The strategies used include rest, ice, supports, etc. A patient with subacute injury learns that their tissues are going through repair and various passive methods along with exercise are necessary to *relax and mobilize* their healing tissues and simultaneously prevent scar tissue and deconditioning. Next, this patient learns that they must *strengthen and stabilize* their "weak link" or injured tissues to prevent recurrences.

A patient who suffers pain without trauma learns that once serious medical causes are ruled out, treatment will focus on functional restoration. Ways to reduce exposure to harmful external stress and how to increase functional capacity are the focus of care. Rather than adhering to the philosophy of "no pain-no gain," the patient is taught how to "handle" pain. The difference between "hurt and harm" is explained. Stretching exercises may hurt slightly because stiff structures are being stretched, but strengthening exercises should be painless in their symptomatic areas. They may feel a "burn" in the muscle being trained, but they should not experience pain in their symptomatic area.

Manipulation and other therapies may be used to address key trigger points or joint dysfunctions with the goal of relaxing and mobilizing tense or stiff tissues (see Chapter 11). Then, patients learn about strengthening and stabilizing the "weak link" by training the "big" muscles (quadriceps, gluteal, abdominals) to do most of the work and to avoid overstraining the "smaller" postural muscles and deeper spinal structures. This training may lead to some postexercise soreness, but this discomfort should involve areas quite distinct from their primary area of complaint (see Chapter 14). While training these "big" muscles, the patient is taught to perceive their "safe" spinal posture. With repetition, they learn to control their posture better, by developing improved kinesthetic awareness, and to use the "big" muscles to perform most of the work, which takes strain off all the structures of the spine (disk, ligament, joint, etc.). Ultimately, their improved motor control should become automatic, requiring no conscious effort.

So long as the patient's case is uncomplicated, recovery can be expected within 6 weeks. If factors are present that complicate the case, these should be explained to the patient. Such a patient should be apprised of their poorer prognosis. It can be mentioned that approximately 15% of patients with low back pain develop chronic pain syndromes, and at least 33% of all patients suffer recurrences at some time. Complicated cases require pro-active management to defuse these "ticking time bombs." It is better to inform such patients of their risk for chronicity than to allow them to build up anger and resentment when they are frustrated by their unsatisfactory progress. A brief course of manipulative therapy, followed by aggressive rehabilitation efforts with an active care focus, are essential for these patients. If this sequence is unsuccessful, a biobehavioral approach incorporating multidisciplinary support is necessary.

REPORT TO THIRD PARTY PAYOR

It is important to be able to communicate the rationale for rehabilitation to the group responsible for financial reimbursement. With musculoskeletal injury or pain, changes will occur in the areas of strength, mobility/flexibility, balance, coordination, and cardiovascular fitness.[50] These functional losses are a result of immobilization and adaptation and are termed "deconditioning."[158] *To protect your right to reimbursement for services rendered that adhere to standards of care, follow these steps: (1) Document the presence of any complicating factors in the patient's history and examination; (2) Use outcomes assessment tools to document any functional changes or subjective improvement; (3) Differentiate clearly between passive and active care treatment approaches; and (4) Quote published guidelines (Quebec, Mercy, AHCPR and CSAG) to demonstrate the appropriateness and place of manipulation and exercise (active care).*[148,150,182]

It might be helpful to explain the phases of care and appropriate treatment selection for each phase. After a *mild to moderate injury,* the goals of initial treatment are to reduce inflammation/swelling, control pain, and rest the injured soft tissues. This acute stage of care typically lasts only 2 to 3 days. Treatment is inclusive of rest/ice, supports/braces, gentle stretching, physical therapy techniques, chiropractic joint manipulation, and nutritional supplements. Progress is measured by using specific, quantifiable outcomes assessment tools. Outcomes assessed include mobility and pain intensity (Visual Analog Scale).

Once inflammation has subsided, the patient enters the repair or regeneration phase of soft tissue healing. This phase usually lasts from 72 hours to 6 weeks. In this subacute stage, the goal of treatment is to promote the repair/regeneration process and remobilize the patient. This goal is accomplished by mobilizing the soft tissues. Treatment is inclusive of chiropractic joint manipulation, soft tissue manipulation, physical therapy techniques postural exercises, and individualized exercises for muscular imbalances. Progress is measured by improved mobility, decreased pain, and increased ability to perform normal activities of daily living (i.e., Oswestry Survey).

In cases *involving moderate to severe injury,* the acute stage may last up to 1 week and the subacute stage up to 16 weeks. A chronic phase follows in which the goal of treatment is to promote remodeling of the soft tissues and rehabilitate any lost musculoskeletal function. Remodeling after a moderate to severe injury can last up to 12 months. Treatment is inclusive of muscle stretching, strengthening, cardiovascular fitness, coordination exercises, and decreasing application of physical therapy techniques and chiropractic joint manipulation. The goal is rehabilitation of the patient to their preinjury level of functioning. Measurement of specific outcomes becomes essential to prevent patients from developing chronic pain syndromes. Outcomes evaluated include mobility, activities of daily living, and muscle strength.

For patients who suffer pain without any acute trauma, a *repetitive strain* is the likely explanation. Repetitive "microtrauma" from prolonged overuse and/or constrained postures leads to gradual deconditioning of the strained soft tissues. This deconditioning weakens the various musculoskeletal structures to the extent that painful injury can result without any trauma. Such pain can occur without the inflammation or swelling associated with an acute injury. The treatment is similar to that for mild to moderate acute injuries.

Another type of case is that involving the *patient with chronic pain.* This patient has completed all soft tissue healing, and often has abnormal illness behavior disproportionate to impairment or pathologic evidence. The goal of treatment is rehabilitation with an emphasis on functional restoration rather than on pain relief alone. Psychologic intervention to increase coping skills and to reduce fear is necessary in combination with a physical reactivation program.

Patients with uncomplicated cases and not suffering unstable injuries or chronic pain syndromes should be fully rehabilitated within 6 to 8 weeks. A severe whiplash, grades II or III knee ligament injury, or disk herniation with radiculitis are examples of unstable conditions that usually require treatment well beyond 6 to 8 weeks. Complicated cases may require more treatment time because of the presence of chronic pain with its associated physical and psychologic deconditioning.

By demonstrating to the third party payor what type of patient is being treated; the standard of care of treatment for that patient type; and progress being achieved through objective, quantifiable outcome measures, the clinician should be able to justify reasonable extensions of care for a complicated case (Table 2.20). When functional outcomes do not improve with care, then continued care is not justified and referral becomes appropriate.

INCREASING PATIENT ADHERENCE, COMPLIANCE, AND MOTIVATION

Converting a pain patient from a passive recipient of care to an active partner in their own rehabilitation involves behavioral psychology;[150,183] specifically, making the shift from being a pain avoider to a pain manager (Fig. 2.25). A key to this process is convincing the patient that their pain is not a stop light warning them away from all activity. Reassuring an individual that we do not advocate a no pain – no gain approach, and instead teaching them how to differentiate between hurt and harm, helps them become reactivated. Chronic pain requires a different coping strategy than is used for acute pain.[183,184] Increased activity is the goal, because greater stiff-

Table 2.20. Quantification of Symptomatic and Functional Progress

Date	SLR (degree)	VAS (low back) (%)	Trunk Flexion and Extension ROM	Oswestry (%)
2/9/94	30	85	20/60 and 5/25	78
2/16/94	60	50	40/60 and 15/25	54
3/1/94	75	26	50/60 and 20/25	30
3/16/94	85	1.3	60/60 and 22/25	04

*SLR, straight leg raise; VAS, visual analog scale; ROM, range of motion.

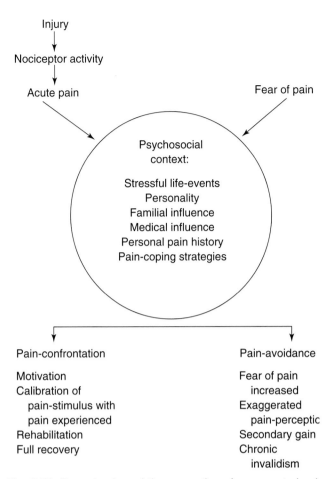

Injury

↓

Nociceptor activity

↓

Acute pain   Fear of pain

Psychosocial
context:

Stressful life-events
Personality
Familial influence
Medical influence
Personal pain history
Pain-coping strategies

Pain-confrontation   Pain-avoidance

Motivation   Fear of pain
Calibration of   increased
    pain-stimulus with   Exaggerated
    pain experienced   pain-perceptic
Rehabilitation   Secondary gain
Full recovery   Chronic
                                        invalidism

Fig. 2.25. Fear of pain and the generation of exaggerated pain perception. (From JDG Troup: The perception of musculoskeletal pain and incapacity for work; prevention and early treatment. Physiotherapy 74:435, 1988.)

ness and weakness will otherwise develop, which will only complete a vicious cycle causing more pain, not less. Once a pain avoider is identified, additional time spent with patient education is essential.

The primary goal of patient care is to reduce any disability. Often, patients have sacrificed different features of their lifestyle as a result of pain. An Oswesry survey can quantify this level of adjustment. Such things as decreased sitting tolerance can be identified in the history. The patient may say, "I can't go to the movies anymore." Individuals may have given up or compromised certain activities such as tennis or golf. If a patient says they always feel pain after 9 holes of golf, a goal may be to be able to play a full round. Sexual activity may also be a problem. Whatever lifestyle changes they have made as a result of their pain should be uncovered in the history. Then, the restoration of these activities becomes a mutually agreeable goal of rehabilitation. Establishing functional restoration as a goal, along with pain relief, is essential to achieving a positive outcome.

To achieve lasting pain relief, the patient is educated that their musculoskeletal function can and should be improved. If their muscles are too tight or weak, then it is ex-

plained that this tightness or weakness is what leads to irritation and pain with activity. They must learn that rehabilitation or restoration of function will prevent pain from arising in the first place, and although such rehabilitation may be more painful in the short term, improving function is the key to long–term pain relief. Always seeking temporary pain relief will do nothing to prevent the problem from starting again.

Patients can be reassured that most of their exercises will be relatively pain–free. Everything that can be done to relax and mobilize their tissues will be done before attempting to strengthen them. The ultimate goal is increased kinesthetic awareness and improved stability. Exercise will focus on strengthening the "big muscles" that are neighbors to the painful spinal or postural areas. The no pain-no gain philosophy does not apply to chronic pain rehabilitation. Exercises are performed until the point of muscle fatigue only so long as proper coordination is maintained. The only pain should be in the muscle being worked (a "burn"). If a symptomatic area (spinal muscles) is activated during the exercise, the movement is stopped. When we can achieve an intensity of training that leads to postexercise soreness in deconditioned tissues without exacerbating the original symptoms, we are well on our way to a successful outcome.

Objectification of function is a key tool in motivating patients. Helping patients focus on function rather than on pain is an important first step. Then, baseline levels of functional impairment, pain distribution and intensity, and level of disability should be quantified. These quantifiable baselines can be used to track the patient's progress objectively. Treatment should be guided by the results of the objective, functional capacity evaluation. Progress can be monitored at regular intervals (every 2 to 4 weeks) to give the patient accurate feedback on how they are improving. Seeing an increase in their walking and sitting tolerance as well as in the number of trunk curls serves as positive reinforcement. Pre- and post-treatment checks of painful maneuvers or measurable functional deficits (i.e., strength, flexibility) is an excellent way to motivate patients.

Rehabilitation seeks to reduce functional impairment. It does not focus on the symptoms. Quantification of functional capacity and patient education about well behaviors are the keys. Manipulation to restore function to key muscles and joints is essential to initiate patient reactivation. Finally, physical training that focuses on stabilizing the lumbopelvic region and trunk is the final step in rehabilitation of the motor system.

REFERENCES

1. Deyo RA: Measuring functional outcomes in therapeutic trials for chronic disease. Controlled Clin Trials 5:223, 1984.
2. Binkley J, Peat M: The effect of immobilization on the ultrastructure and mechanical properties of the rat medial collateral ligament. Clin Orthop 203:301, 1986.
3. Noyes F: Functional properties of knee ligaments and alterations induced by immobilization. Clin Orthop 123:210, 1977.
4. Videman T: Experimental models of osteoarthritis: The role of immobilization. Clin Biomech 2:223, 1987.

5. Akeson WH, Woo SLY, Amiel D, et al: Biomechanical and biochemical changes in the periarticular connective tissue during contracture development in the immobilized rabbit knee. Connect Tissue Res 2:315, 1974.

6. Woo SLY, Mathews JV, Akeson WH, et al: Connective tissue response to immobility: Correlative study of biomechanical and biochemical measurements of normal and immobilized rabbit knees. Arthritis Rheum 18:257, 1975.

7. Videman T, Michelsson JE, Rauhamaki R, et al: Changes in 35S–sulphate uptake in different tissues in the knee and hip regions of rabbits during immobilization, remobilization and the development of osteoarthritis. Acta Orthop Scand 47:290, 1976.

8. Eronen I, Videman T, Frimon C, et al: Glycosaminoglycan metabolism in experimental osteoarthrosis caused by immobilization. Acta Orthop Scand 49:329, 1978.

9. Videman T, Eronen I, Friman C: Glycosaminoglycan metabolism in experimental osteoarthritis caused by immobilization. Acta Orthop Scand 52:11, 1981.

10. Lloyd–Roberts GC: The role of capsular changes in osteoarthritis of the hip joint. J Bone Joint Surg [Br] 35:627, 1953.

11. Akeson WH, Amiel D, Mechanic GL, et al: Collagen cross-linking alterations in joint contractures: Changes in the reducible cross-links in periarticular connective tissue collagen after nine weeks of immobilization. Connect Tissue Res 5:15, 1977.

12. Salter R, Simmonds DR, Malcolm BW, et al: The biological effect of continuous passive motion on the healing of full-thickness defects in articular cartilage. J Bone Joint Surg [Am] 62:1232, 1980.

13. Finsterbush A, Friedman B: Reversibility of joint changes produced by immobilization in rabbits. Clin Orthop 111:290, 1975.

14. Paulos LE, Payne FC, Rosenberg TD: Rehabilitation after anterior cruciate ligament surgery. In Jackson D, Dre D (eds): The Anterior Cruciate Deficient Knee. St Louis: CV Mosby, 1987, pp 291–314.

15. Binkley J: Overview of ligament and tendon structure and mechanics: Implications for clinical practice. Physiother Can 41:24, 1989.

16. Wood SLY: Mechanical properties of tendons and ligaments. and nonlinear viscoelastic properties. Biorheology 19:385, 1982.

17. Noyes FR, Torvik PJ, Hyde WB, et al: Biomechanics of ligament failure. II. An analysis of immobilization, exercise, and reconditioning effects in primates. J Bone Joint Surg [Am] 1974.

18. Tipton CM, Vailas AC, Matthes RD: Experimental studies on the influences of physical activity on ligaments, tendons and joints: A brief review. In Astrand P-O, Grimby G (eds): Physical Activity in Health and Disease. Acta Medica Scandinavica Symposium Series no 2. Stockholm, Almqvist & Wiksell International, 1986, pp 157–168.

19. Tipton CM, James SL, Mergner W, et al: Influence of exercise on strength of medial collateral knee ligaments of dogs. Am J Physiol 218:894, 1970.

20. Tipton CM, Tcheng T, Mergner W: Ligamentous strength measurements from hypophysectomized rats. Am J Physiol 221:1144, 1971.

21. Holm S, Nachemson A: Nutritional changes in the canine intervertebral disc after spinal fusion. Clin Orthop 169:243, 1982.

22. Eyre D, Benya P, Buckwalter J, et al: Intervertebral Disc: Basic Science Perspectives. In Frymoyer JW, Gordon SL (eds): New Perspectives on Low Back Pain. Park Ridge, American Academy of Orthopaedic Surgeons, 1989, p 167.

23. Hansson TH, Roos BO, Nachemson A: Development of osteopenia in the fourth lumbar vertebra during prolonged bed rest after operation for scoliosis. Acta Orthop Scand 46:621, 1975.

24. Greenleaf JE: Physiological responses to prolonged bed rest and fluid immersion in humans. J Appl Physiol 57:619, 1984.

25. Smidt EL, Raab DM: Osteoporosis and physical activity. In Astrand P-O, Grimby G (eds): Physical Activity in Health and Disease. Acta Medica Scandinavica Symposium Series no 2. Stockholm, Almqvist & Wiksell International, 1986, pp 149–156.

26. Saville PD, Whyte MP: Muscle and bone hypertrophy. Clin Orthop 65:81, 1969.

27. Whedon GD, Shorr E: Metabolic studies in paralytic acute anterior poliomyelitis. J Clin Invest 36:941, 1957.

28. Walton JN, Warrick CK: Osseous changes in myopathy. Br J Radiol 27:1, 1954.

29. Abramson AS: Bone disturbances in injuries to the spinal cord and cauda equina. J Bone Joint Surg [Am] 30:982, 1948.

30. Gillespie JA: The nature of bone changes associated with nerve injuries and disuse. J Bone Joint Surg [Br] 36:464, 1954.

31. Geiser M, Trueta J: Muscle action, bone rarefaction and bone formation. J Bone Joint Surg [Br] 40:282, 1958.

32. Nakagawa Y, Totsuka M, Sato T, et al: Effect of disuse of the ultrastructure of the achilles tendon in rats. Eur J Appl Physiol 59:239, 1989.

33. Saltin B, Gollnick PD: Skeletal muscle adaptability: Significance for metabolism and performance. In Peachey LD, Adrian RH, Geiger SR (eds): Handbook of Physiology: Section 10. Skeletal Muscle. Bethesda, American Physiological Society, 1983, pp 555–631.

34. Henriksson J, Reitman JS: Time course of changes in human skeletal muscle succinate dehydrogenase and cytochrome oxidase activities and maximal oxygen uptake with physical activity and inactivity. Acta Physiol Scand 99:91, 1977.

35. Saltin B, Blomqvist G, Michell JH, et al: Response to exercise after bed rest and after training. Circulation 38(Suppl 7):1, 1968.

36. Flynn DE, Max SR: Effect of suspension hypokinesia/hypodynamia on rat skeletal muscle. Aviat Space Environ Med 56:1065, 1985.

37. Desplenches D, Mayet MH, Sempore B, et al: Structural and functional responses to prolonged hindlimb suspension in rat muscles. J Appl Physiol 63:558, 1987.

38. Hauschka ED, Roy RR, Edgerton VR: Size and metabolic properties of single muscle fibers in rat soleus after hindlimb suspension. J Appl Physiol 62:2338, 1987.

39. Thomason DB, Herrick RE, Baldwin KM: Activity influences on soleus muscle myosin during rodent hindlimb suspension. J Appl Physiol 63:138, 1987.

40. Goldspink G: Alterations in myofibril size and structure during growth, exercise, and changes in environmental temperature. In Peachey LD, Adrian RH, Geiger SR (eds): Handbook of Physiology: Section 10. Skeletal Muscle. Bethesda, American Physiological Society, 1983, pp 539–554.

41. Sargeant AJ, Davies CT, Edwards RH, et al: Functional and structural changes after disuse of human muscle. Clin Sci 52:337, 1977.

42. Gibson JNA, Smith K, Rennie MJ: Prevention of disuse muscle atrophy by means of electrical stimulation: Maintenance of protein synthesis. Lancet 8614:767, 1988.

43. Serra G, Tugnoli V, Eleopra R, et al: Neurophysiological evaluation of the muscular hypotrophy after immobilization. Electromyogr Clin Neurophysiol 29:29, 1989.

44. Wagenmakers AJM, Coakley JH, Edwards RTH: The metabolic consequences of reduced habitual activities in patients with muscle pain and disease. Ergonomics 31:1519, 1988.

45. Lehto M, Jarvinen M, Nelimarkka O: Scar formation after skeletal muscle injury. Arch Orthop Trauma Surg 104:366, 1986.

46. Ericksson H, Haggmark T: Comparison of isometric muscle training and electrical stimulation supplementing isometric muscle training in the recovery after major knee ligament surgery. Am J Sports Med 7:169, 1979.

47. Haggmark T, Ericksson E: Cylinder or mobile cast brace after knee ligament surgery: A clinical analysis and morphologic and enzymatic studies of changes in the quadriceps muscle. Am J Sports Med 7:48, 1979.

48. Banker BZ, Engel AG: Basic reactions of muscle. In Engel AG, Banker BZ (eds): Myology. Vol. 2. New York, McGraw-Hill, 1986, pp 845–907.

49. Engle AG, Banker BZ: Ultrastructural changes in diseased muscle. In Engel AG, Banker BZ (eds): Myology. Vol. 2. New York, McGraw-Hill, 1986, pp 909–1043.

50. Herring SA: Rehabilitation of muscle injuries. Med Sci Sports Exerc 22:453, 1990.

51. Katz DR, Kumar VN: Effects of prolonged bed rest on cardiopulmonary conditioning. Orthop Rev 11:89, 1982.

52. Chaffin DB, Park KS: A longitudinal study of low–back pain as associated with occupational weight lifting factors. Am Ind Hyg Assoc J 34:513, 1973.

53. Chaffin DB, Herrin GD, Keyserling WM: Preemployment strength testing: An updated position. J Occup Med 20:403, 1978.

54. Cady LD, Bischoff LP, O'Connel ER, et al: Strength and fitness and subsequent back injuries in firefighters. J Occup Med 21:269, 1979

55. Rowe ML: Low back pain in industry. J Occup Med 11:161, 1969.

56. Biering-Sorensen F: Physical measurements as risk indicators for low-back trouble over a one-year period. Spine 9: 106, 1984.

57. Troup JDG, Martin JW, Lloyd DCEF: Back pain in industry: A prospective study. Spine 6:61, 1981.

58. Dehlin O, Berg S, Andersson GBJ, et al: Effect of physical training and ergonomic counseling on the psychological perception of work and on the subjective assessment of low-back insufficiency. Scand J Rehabil Med 13:1, 1981.

59. Gundewell B, Liljeqvist M, Hansson T: Primary prevention of back symptoms and absence from work. Spine 18:587, 1993.

60. Videman T, Rauhala S, Asp K, et al: Patient-handling skill, back injuries, and back pain. Spine 14:148, 1989.

61. Battie MC, Bigos SJ, Fisher LD, et al: The role of spinal flexibility in back pain complaints within industry: A prospective study. Spine 15:768, 1990.

62. Deyo RA, Bass JE: Lifestyle and low back pain: The influence of smoking, exercise and obesity. Clin Res 35:577A, 1987.

63. Frymoyer JW: Epidemiology. In Frymoyer JW, Gordon SL (eds): Symposium on New Perspectives on Low Back Pain. Park Ridge, American Academy of Orthopaedic Surgeons, 1989, pp 19–33.

64. Bogduk N, Twomey LT: Clinical Anatomy of the Lumbar Spine. 2nd Ed. Churchill Livingstone, Melbourne, 1991.

65. Andersson GBJ: Occupational biomechanics. In Weinstein JN, Wiesel SW (eds): The Lumbar Spine: the International Society for the Study of the Lumbar Spine. Philadelphia, WB Saunders, 1990, p 213.

66. Brinckmann P, Pope MH: Effects of repeated loads and vibration. In Weinstein JN, Wiesel SW (eds): the Lumbar Spine: the International Society for the Study of the Lumbar Spine. Philadelphia, WB Saunders, 1990, p 172.

67. DeAndrade JR, Grant C, Dixon ASJ: Joint distension and reflex muscle inhibition in the knee. J Bone Joint Surg 47:313, 1965.

68. Hides JA, Stokes MJ, Saide M, et al: Evidence of lumbar multifidus muscles wasting ipsilateral to symptoms in patients with acute/subacute low back pain. Spine 19:165, 1994.

69. Johansson H, Sjolander P, Sojka P: Receptors in the knee joint ligaments and their role in the biomechanics of the joint. Crit Rev Biomed Eng 18:341, 1991.

70. Woolf CJ: Long term alterations in the excitability of the flexion reflex produced by peripheral tissue injury in the chronic decerebrate rat. Pain 18:325, 1984.

71. Dahl JB, Erichsen CJ, Fuglsang–Frederiksen A, et al: Pain sensation and nociceptive reflex excitability in surgical patients and human volunteers. Br J Anaesth 69:117, 1992.

72. Flor H, Birbaumer N, Furst M, et al: Evidence of enhanced peripheral and central responses of painful stimulation in states of chronic pain. Psychophysiology 30:S9, 1993.

73. Flor H, Birbaumer N, Braun C, et al: Chronic pain enhances the magnitude of the magnetic field evoked by painful stimulation. In Deecke L, Baumgartner C, Stroink G, et al (eds): Recent Advances in Biomagnetism. 9th International Conference on Biomagnetism, Vienna, 1993, pp. 72–73.

74. Mense S: Nociception from skeletal muscle in relation to clinical muscle pain. Pain 54:241, 1993.

75. Walsh EG: Muscles, Masses and Motion. The Physiology of Normality, Hypotonicity, Spasticity, and Rigidity. Oxford, MacKeith Press, Blackwell Scientific Publication Ltd, 1992.

76. Paillard J: Posture and locomotion: Old problems and new concepts. In Amblard B, Berthoz A, Clarac F (eds): Posture and Gait: Development, Adaptation and Modulation. Amsterdam, Elsevier Science Publishers, 1988, pp V–XII.

77. Boyd IA: The isolated mammalian muscle spindle. In Evarts EV, Wise SP, Bousfield D (eds): The Motor System in Neurobiology. Amsterdam, Elsevier, 1985.

78. Triano J, Schultz AB: Correlation of objective measure of trunk motion and muscle function with low-back disability ratings. Spine 12:561, 1987.

79. Hubbard DR, Berkoff GM: Myofascial trigger points show spontaneous needle EMG activity. Spine 18:1803, 1993.

80. Simons DG: Referred phenomena of myofascial trigger points. In Vecchiet L, Albe–Fessard D, Lindlom U: New Trends in Referred Pain and Hyperalgesia. Amsterdam, Elsevier, 1993.

81. Sato H, Ohashi J, Iwanaga K, et al: Endurance time and fatigue in static contractions. J Hum Ergol (Tokyo) 3:147, 1984.

82. Rybicki KJ, Waldrop TG, Kaufman MP: Increasing gracilis muscle interstitial potassium concentrations stimulate groups III and IV afferents. J Appl Physiol 58:936, 1985.

83. Johansson H, Sokja P: Pathophysiological mechanisms involved in genesis and spread of muscular tension in occupational muscle pain and in chronic musculoskeletal pain syndromes. A hypothesis. Med Hypotheses 35:196, 1991.

84. Kaufman MP, Longhurst JC, Rybicki KJ, et al: Effects of static muscular contraction on impulse activity of groups III and IV afferents in cats. J Appl Physiol 55:105, 1983.

85. Lewis T: Pain. Macmillan, London, 1942.

86. Friden J, Sfakianos PN, Hargens AR et al: Residual muscular swelling after repetitive eccentric contractions. J Orthop Res 6:493, 1988.

87. Stauber WT, Clarkson PM, Fritz VK et al: Extracellular matrix disruption and pain after eccentric muscle action. J Appl Physiol 69:868, 1990.

88. Johansson H, Sjolander P, Sojka P: Fusimotor reflexes in triceps surae muscle elicited by natural and electrical stimulation of joint afferents. Neuro-orthop 6:67, 1988.

89. Johansson H, Sjolander P, Sojka P, et al: Reflex actions on the gamma-muscle spindle systems acting at the knee joint elicited by the stretch of the posterior cruciate ligament. Neuro-orthop 8:9, 1989

90. Johansson H, Lorentzon R, Sjolander P, et al: The anterior cruciate ligament. A sensor acting on the y-muscle-spindle systems of muscles around the knee joint. Neuro-orthop 9:1, 1990.

91. Brucini M, Duranti R, Galleti R, et al: Pain thresholds and electromyographic features of periarticular muscles in patients with osteoarthritis of the knee. Pain 10:57, 1981.

92. Spencer JD, Hayes KC, Alexander IJ: Knee joint effusion and quadriceps reflex inhibition in man. Arch Phys Med Rehabil 65:171, 1984.

93. Stokes M, Edwards R, Cooper R: Effect of low frequency fatigue on human muscle strength and fatigability during subsequent stimulated activity. Eur J Appl Physiol 59:278, 1989.

94. Headley BJ: Muscle inhibition. Physical Therapy Forum, November 1, 1993, pp 24–26.

95. Stokes MJ, Cooper RG, Jayson MIV: Selective changes in multifidus dimensions in patients with chronic low back pain. Eur Spine J 1:38, 1992.

96. Cooper RG, Stokes MJ, Jayson MIV: Electro- and acoustic myographic changes during fatigue of the human paraspinal muscles in back pain patients. J Physiol (Lond) 438:338, 1991.

97. Fitzmaurice R, Cooper RG, Freemont AJ: A histo-morphometric comparison of muscle biopsies from normal subjects and patients with ankylosing spondylitis and severe mechanical low back pain. J Pathol 163:182, 1992.

98. Bullock-Saxton JE, Janda V, Bullock MI: Reflex activation of gluteal muscles in walking. Spine 18:704, 1993.

99. Janda V: Muscles, central nervous motor regulation, and back problems. In Korr IM (ed): Neurobiologic Mechanisms in Manipulative Therapy. New York, Plenum, 1978.

100. Schaible HG, Grubb BD: Afferent and spinal mechanisms of joint pain. Pain 55:5, 1993.

101. Proske U, Schaible HG, Schmidt RF: Joint receptors and kinaesthesia. Exp Brain Res 72:219, 1988.

102. April C, Bogduk N: The prevalence of cervical zygapophyseal joint pain. Spine 17:744, 1992.

103. Bogduk N, Aprill C: On the nature of neck pain, discography and cervical zygapophyseal joint blocks. Pain 54:213, 1993.

104. Patterson M: Model mechanism for spinal segmental facilitation. Carmel, Academy of Applied Osteopathy Yearbook, 1976.

105. Sturge WA: The phenomena of angina pectoris and their bearing upon the theory of counter irritation. Brain 5:492, 1883.

106. MacKenzie J: Some points bearing on the association of sensory disorders and visceral diseases. Brain 16:321, 1893.

107. Perl ER, Dumuzawa T, Lynn B, et al: Sensitization of high threshold receptors with unmyelinated (C) afferent fibres. In A Iggo and I Liynsky (eds): Somatosensory and Visceral Receptor Mechanisms. Prog Brain Res 43:263, 1974.

108. Kenshalo Jr DR, Leonard RB, Chung JM, et al: Facilitation of the responses of primate spinothalamic cells to cold and mechanical stimuli by noxious heating of the skin. Pain 12:141, 1982.

109. Merskey H: Limitations of pain behavior. APS Journal 2:101, 1992.

110. Merskey H: Regional pain is rarely hysterical. Arch Neurol 45:915, 1988.

111. Nachemson AL: Newest knowledge of low back pain. Clin Orthop 279:8, 1992.

112. Travell J, Rinzler SH: The myofascial genesis of pain. Postgrad Med 11:425, 1952.

113. Cohen ML, Champion GD, Sheaterh-Reid R: Comments on Gracely et al., "Painful neuropathy: altered central processing maintained dynamically by peripheral input" (Pain, 51 (1992) 175–194). Pain 54:365, 1993.

114. Gebhardt GF, Ness TJ: Central mechanisms of visceral pain. Can J Physiol Pharmacol 69:627, 1991.

115. Cervero, F: Somatic and visceral inputs to the thoracic spinal cord of the cat: Effects of noxious stimulation of the biliary system, J Physiol (Lond) 337:52, 1983.

116. Foreman RD, Balir RW, Weber RN: Viscerosomatic convergence onto T2-T4 spinoreticular, spinoreticular-spinothalamic, and spinothalamic tract neurons in the cat. Exp Neurol 85:597, 1984.

117. Yu X-M, Mense S: Response properties and descending control of rat dorsal horn neurons with deep receptive fields. Neuroscience 39:823, 1990.

118. Mense S: Sensitization of group IV muscle receptors to bradykinin by 5-hydroxytryptamine and prostaglandin E2. Brain Res 225:95, 1981.

119. Hoheisel U, Mense S: Long-term changes in discharge behavior of cat dorsal horn neurons following noxious stimulation of deep tissues. Pain 36:239, 1989.

120. Hu JW, Sessle BJ, Raboisson P, et al: Stimulation of craniofacial muscle afferents induces prolonged facilatory effects in trigeminal nociceptive brainstem neurons. Pain 48:53, 1992.

121. Vecciet L, Giamberardino MA, Dragani L, et al: Referred muscular hyperalgesia from viscera: Clinical approach. In Lipton S, et al (eds): Advances in Pain Research and Therapy. Vol. 13. New York, Raven Press, 1990, pp 175–182.

122. Coderre TJ, Katz J, Vaccarino AL, et al: Contribution of central neuroplasticity to pathological pain: Review of clinical and experimental evidence. Pain 52:259, 1993.

123. Henry JA, Montushi E: Cardiac pain referred to site of previously experienced somatic pain. Br Med J 9:1605, 1978.

124. Reynolds OE, Hutchins HC: Reduction of central hyper-irritability following block anesthesia of peripheral nerve. Am J Physiol 152:658, 1948.

125. Brylin M, Hindfelt B: Ear pain due to myocardial ischemia. Am Heart J 107:186, 1984.

126. Willis WD: Mechanical allodynia—A role for sensitized nociceptive tract cells with convergent input from mechanoreceptors and nociceptors? APS Journal 1:23, 1993.

127. LaMotte RH: Subpopulations of "nocisensor neurons" contributing to pain and allodynia, itch and allokinesis. APS Journal 2:115, 1992.

128. Mayer RA, Treed RD, Srinivas NR, et al: Peripheral versus central mechanisms for secondary hyperalgesia. APS Journal 2:127, 1992.

129. Perl ER: Multireceptive neurons and mechanical allodynia. APS Journal 1:37, 1992.

130. Dubner R: Neuropathic pain. APS Journal 1:8, 1993.

131. Willis WD: Mechanical allodynia: A role for nocireceptive tract cells with convergent input from mechanoreceptors and nociceptors? APS Journal 2:23, 1993.

132. Dubner R, Sharav Y, Gracely RH, et al: Idiopathic trigeminal neuralgia: Sensory features and pain mechanisms. Pain 31:23, 1987.

133. Sugimoto T, Bennett GJ, Kajander KC: Transsynaptic degeneration in the superficial dorsal horn after sciatic nerve injury: Effects of a chronic constriction injury, transection, and strychnine. Pain 42:205, 1990.

134. Mogliner A, Grossman JA, Ribary U, et al: Somatosensory cortical plasticity in adult humans revealed by magnetoencephalography. Proc Natl Acad Sci USA 90:3593, 1993.

135. Jull G, Janda V: Muscles and motor control in low back pain. In Twomey LT, Taylor JR (eds): Physical Therapy for the Low Back; Clinics in Physical Therapy. New York, Churchill Livingstone, 1987.

136. Janda V: Some aspects of extracranial causes of facial pain. J Prosthet Dent 56:484, 1986.

137. Sahrmann SA: Posture and muscle imbalance: Faulty lumbar pelvic alignments. Phys Ther 67:1840, 1987.

138. Burke RE: Motor unit types: Functional specialization in motor control. In Evarts EV, Wise SP, Bousfield D (eds): The Motor System in Neurobiology. Amsterdam, Elsevier, 1985.

139. Salmons S: Functional adaptation in skeletal muscle. In Evarts EV, Wise SP, Bousfield D (eds): The Motor System in Neurobiology. Amsterdam, Elsevier, 1985.

140. Janda V: Muscle spasm-a proposed procedure for differential diagnosis. J Manual Med 6:136, 1991.

141. Sarno J: Psychosomatic backache. J Fam Pract 5:353, 1977.

142. Gibson S, Granges G, Littlejohn GO, et al: Increased thermal pain sensitivity in patients with fibromyalgia syndrome. In Bromm B, Desmedt J (eds): Pain and the Brain: Nociception to Cognition. New York, Raven Press, 1994.

143. Janda V: Muscle strength in relation to muscle length, pain and muscle imbalance. In Harms-Rindahl K (ed): Muscle Strength. New York, Churchill Livingstone, 1993.

144. Lewit K: Manipulative therapy in rehabilitation of the motor system. 2nd Ed. London, Butterworths, 1991.

145. Lewit K: Chain reactions in disturbed function of the motor system. Manuelle Med 3:27, 1987.

146. Korr I: The spinal cord as organizer of disease processes: Some preliminary perspectives. J Am Osteopath Assoc 76:35, 1976.

147. Feuerstein M: A multidisciplinary approach to the prevention, evaluation, and management of work disability. J Occup Rehab 1:11, 1991.

148. Bigos S, Bowyer O, Braen G, et al: Acute low back problems in adults. Clinical practice guideline. Rockville, MD: U.S. Department of Health and Human Services, Public Health Service, Agency for Health Care Policy and Research, 1994.

149. Frymoyer L: Back pain and sciatica. N Engl J Med 318:291, 1988.

150. Quebec Task Force on Spinal Disorders: Scientific approach to the assessment and management of activity-related spinal disorders: A monograph for clinicians. Spine 12(Suppl 7):S1, 1987.

151. Delitto A, Cibulka MT, Erhard RE, et al: Evidence for use of an extension-mobilization category in acute low back syndrome: A prescriptive validation pilot study. Phys Ther 73:216, 1993.

152. Schwarzer AC, April CN, Bogduk N: The sacroiliac joint in chronic low back pain. Spine 20:31, 1995.

153. Barnsley L, Lord SM, Wallis BJ, et al: The prevalence of chronic cervical zygapophyseal joint pain after whiplash. Spine 20:20, 1995.

154. Nordin M: Early findings of NIOSH/CDC model back clinic reveal surprising observations on work-related low back pain predictors. Spine Letter 1:5,6, 1994.

155. Kellett J: Acute soft tissue injuries—a review of the literature. Med Sci Sports Exerc 18:489, 1986.

156. Oakes B: Acute soft tissue injuries: Nature and management. Austr Fam Physician Suppl 10:3, 1982.

157. Van DerMeulin JHC: Present state of knowledge on processes of healing in collagen structures. Int J Sports Med 3(Suppl 1):9, 1982.

158. Waddell G: A new clinical model for the treatment of low-back pain. Spine 12:634, 1987.

159. Tarola GA: Whiplash: Contemporary considerations in assessment, management, treatment and prognosis. JNMS 4:156, 1993.

160. Mayer T, Gatchel R, Mayer H, et al: A prospective randomized two year study of functional restoration in industrial low back injury utilizing objective assessment. JAMA 258:1763, 1987.

161. Reis S, Borkan J, Hermoni D: Low back pain: More than anatomy. J Fam Pract 35:509, 1992.

162. Kirkaldy-Willis W: Managing Low Back Pain. New York: Churchill Livingstone, 1983, pp 75–128.

163. Bush K, Cowan NK, Katz DE, et al: The natural history of sciatica associated with disc pathology: A prospective study with clinical and independent radiologic follow-up. Spine 17:1205, 1992.

164. Frymoyer JW: Predicting disability from low back pain. Clin Orthop 221:121, 1987.

165. Cats-Baril WI, Frymoyer JW: Identifying patients at risk of becoming disabled because of low back pain. Spine 16:605, 1991.

166. Waddell G, Newton M, Henderson I, et al. A fear-avoidance beliefs questionnaire and the role of fear-avoidance beliefs in chronic low back pain and disability. Pain 52:157, 1993.

167. Iezzi A, Adams HE, Stokes GS, et al: An identification of low back pain groups using biobehavorial variables. J Occup Rehabil 2:19, 1992.

168. Feuerstein M, Thebarge RW: Perceptions of disability and occupational stress as discriminators of work disability in patients with chronic pain. J Occup Rehabil 1:185, 1991.

169. Bigos SJ, Battie MC, Spengler DM, et al: A prospective study of work perceptions and psychosocial factors affecting the report of back injury. Spine 16:161, 1991.

170. Waddell G, Bircher M, Finlayson D, et al: Symptoms and signs: Physical disease or illness behavior? Br Med J 289:739, 1984.

171. Shekelle PG, Adams AH, Chassin MR, et al: Spinal manipulation for low-back pain. Ann Intern Med 117:590, 1992.

172. Linton SJ, Hellsing AL, Andersson D: A controlled study of the effects of an early intervention on acute musculoskeletal pain problems. Pain 54:353, 1993.

173. Lindstrom A, Ohlund C, Eek C, et al: Activation of subacute low back patients. Phys Ther 72:293, 1992.

174. Hazard RG, Fenwick HW, Kalisch SM, et al: Functional restoration with behavioral support. Spine 14:157, 1989.

175. Sachs BL, David JF, Okimpio D, et al: Spinal rehabilitation by work tolerance based on objective physical capacity assessment of dysfunction. Spine 15:1325, 1990.

176. Alaranta H, Hytokoski U, Rissanen A, et al: Intensive physical and psychosocial training program for patients with chronic low back pain. Spine 19:1339, 1994.

177. Mitchell RI, Carmen GM: Results of a multicenter trial using an intensive active exercise program for the treatment of acute soft tissue and back injuries. Spine 15:514, 1990.

178. Saal JA, Saal JS: Nonoperative treatment of herniated lumbar intervertebral disc with radiculopathy. Spine 14:431, 1989.

179. Cherkin DC: Family physicians and chiropractors: What's best for the patient?. J Fam Pract 35:505, 1992.

180. Cherkin DC, MacCornack FA: Patient evaluations of low back pain care from family physicians and chiropractors. West J Med 150:351, 1989.

181. Bogduk N, Simons DG: Neck pain: Joint pain or trigger points?. In Voeroy H, Merskey H (eds): Progress in Fibromyalgia and Myofascial Pain. Amsterdam, Elsevier Science, 1993, pp 267–273.

182. Haldeman S, Chapman-Smith D, Petersen DM: Frequency and duration of care. In Guidelines for Chiropractic Quality Assurance and Practice Parameters. Gaithersburg, Aspen, 1993, pp 115,130.

183. Turk DC, Rudy TE: Neglected topics in the treatment of chronic pain patients-relapse, noncompliance, and adherence enhancement. Pain 44:5, 1991.

184. Linton SJ: The relationship between activity and chronic back pain. Pain 21:289, 1985.

3 Training and Exercises Science

JEAN P. BOUCHER

Human behaviors are dictated by many laws, constraints, and degrees of freedom. In other words, the human system has limitations. Many limitations in regard to motor behaviors, or movements, are well documented in the field of exercise science or kinesiology, defined as the science of movement in biologic systems. Such limitations as the muscle dynamics and the fundamental factors of performance are discussed in this chapter.

THE LOCOMOTOR SYSTEM

The locomotor system, which is responsible for all motor behaviors involved in locomotion, is composed of fundamental units that must be controlled to achieve complex movements, such as walking or running. Understanding the locomotor system requires then a knowledge of the fundamental units composing it (e.g., bones, joints, and muscles); of the qualities characterizing these units; and of the operations involving them. Concentrating on function, these fundamental units can be labeled as anatomic, mechanical, and functional. It is important initially to consider these units and their motor control that underlies smooth execution of movements before discussing training and exercise topics.

Fundamental Units

Work by Desmarais and Boucher[1] and Boucher and Hodgdon[2] focuses on the need for systematic investigation of the fundamental units activated during any movement. Functionally, these units have been defined in three sets: the anatomic, mechanical, and functional components. The subsequent definition and description of these components of the locomotor system reflect that most of the work concentrating on the fundamental units has centered on the lower limbs and their asymmetries.

ANATOMIC (STRUCTURAL) COMPONENTS

The anatomic components represent the structural units of the system. They dictate the status of the internal environment that must be controlled. These units, the bones or rigid segments, represent the baseline information required by the control system to produce fluid, well-coordinated movements.

For the lower limb asymmetry model, the anatomic factor is defined by the lengths of the segments in the lower limbs,

including the feet, legs, and thighs.[1] Any measurable discrepancies in the measurements from one side to the other are taken as an asymmetry. Traditionally, anatomic asymmetries are derived from differences in the lengths of the bones determined radiographically or on the basis of external tape measurements. The latter technique presents, however, serious limitations.

MECHANICAL (STATIC COMPONENT OF POSTURE) COMPONENTS

The mechanical factor represents the static mechanics or positioning of the joints. The mechanical components are described as the static postural units of the system. These units, the joints and soft tissue holding the bones together, dictate the passive mechanical alignment of the multisegmental links, such as the lower limbs, the trunk, and the upper limbs. These units are then responsible for the passive baseline mechanics that the system must take as a starting point when executing and controlling movements.

The mechanical factor is measured through the bone-bone relationship, or joint angles. A mechanical asymmetry can then be operationally defined as a difference from one side to the other in the lower limb joint angles, or as an above-normal amplitude in a specific joint angle. It is important to measure these angles in a normal weight-bearing situation to appreciate fully the implications of the mechanical factor. With this in mind, the lower limb lengths and pelvic tilt measured in a weight-bearing position are also considered mechanical variables.

FUNCTIONAL COMPONENTS

The functional components, muscles and motor units, are responsible for moving the bones around the joints. In other words, the functional units make it possible for movement of the structural units to occur, starting from the posture dictated by the mechanical or postural units.

The functional factor characterizes the execution of any function. This factor is by far the more complex to assess. The asymmetries in functional patterns can be brought to light only through kinematic,[3] kinetic,[2,4] or electrophysiologic[5,6] analyses conducted during a given normalized function. Hence, functional asymmetries can be operationally defined as any discrepancies revealed between the patterns of the output parameters (e.g., forces, muscle activity) from one side to the other. Such discrepancies are quantified by determining the difference between the patterns, or by establishing side-to-side ratios on specific discrete variables.

According to these definitions, all three factors pertain to mutually exclusive sets of structures. Anatomic factors reveal the status of the bones, the mechanical factors reveal the status of the ligaments holding the bones together, and the functional factors reveal the status of the muscles producing the function or movement of the bones and joints. Using this three-component approach, Desmarais and Boucher[3] and Zarow et al[6] demonstrated that functional components and not anatomic or mechanical components are the major contributor to sacroiliac joint dysfunction and chronic low back pain. Systematic evaluation of the human system according to its fundamental components will allow a better understanding of specific factors underlying any dysfunctions, and a greater chance of efficient treatment.

Motor Control

Following the study of the units composing the human system, a greater challenge is to understand how this system can produce and control voluntary movements. In general, movement control can be divided into two mechanisms: (1) feedforward control and (2) feedback control. These modes of control are also traditionally referred to as open loop and closed loop control. The challenge is to understand not only the different mechanisms, but also how these mechanisms interact to achieve locomotion or any other coordinated movements.

CENTRAL CONTROL (FEEDFORWARD)

The feedforward control mechanism, also referred to as central or suprasegmental control, is described as the direct control of effectors by the central nervous system without interaction with the information from the environment, i.e., the moving limb or segment. Under this type of control, movements are carried out by the execution of motor commands or programs while the system is not concerned by the feedback coming from the afferences activated during the movements. The motor commands are sent down different structures and through pathways or tracts represented schematically in Figure 3.1. Such a mechanism is useful for understanding the execution and control of fast, ballistic movements that are so rapid that feedback contractions cannot modify the movement. Learning or modification of this type of movement can occur only by modifying the motor commands after the fact, by using the knowledge of response information. Information about the error committed can be incorporated through exteroceptors or proprioceptors and the central command can be modified as to reduce the amount of error detected. This type of learning or plasticity is then carried out in an open loop

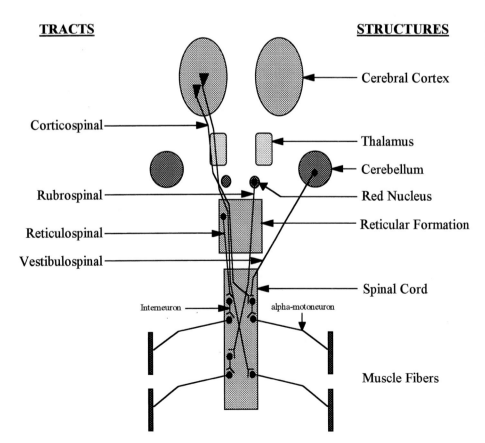

TRACTS

Corticospinal

Rubrospinal

Reticulospinal

Vestibulospinal

Interneuron

alpha-motoneuron

STRUCTURES

Cerebral Cortex

Thalamus

Cerebellum

Red Nucleus

Reticular Formation

Spinal Cord

Muscle Fibers

Fig. 3.1. Neuromuscular structures and pathways or tracts implicated in motor control.

system in which anticipation and knowledge of response are needed to modify future movements. The execution-detection-integration-reexecution loop is said to be open because the detection and integration are not realized on-line while the movement is ongoing, but rather after the movement is terminated.

Furthermore, it is important to note that the motor command responsible for the execution of a movement under feedfoward control is responsible not only for the actual movement, but also for the postural adjustments needed to maintain the equilibrium. Hence, the postural adjustment is not only a reflex reaction to a perturbation caused by the movement; it is programmed within the movement commands and precedes the actual movement. Practically, this fact is important because postural muscles, often involved in dysfunctions, are highly influenced by the execution of movements under voluntary control. Understanding the underlying causes of a dysfunction involving postural muscles must then include the evaluation of movements involving more than the control of posture.

Finally, even though useful to explain some level of control, many movements are certainly controlled and learned differently; i.e., slower movements are corrected as they are performed. The next section is a discussion of the feedback mechanisms involved in this other type of control.

PERIPHERAL CONTROL (FEEDBACK)

Many movements are corrected as they are produced. If the object we are picking up is displaced immediately before we want to grab it, most of the time we will be able to change the trajectory of our hand in order to match the new position of the object and then pick it up. The efficient correction of ongoing movements is made possible through feedback control. The information from the external and internal environments is constantly monitored and compared with the internal goal (e.g., picking up the object) in such a way that the intended movement is executed. The execution-detection-integration-reexecution (or -correction) loop is then closed. The system is able to keep track of the flow of information and fluid movements are organized, executed, and corrected if necessary. The sensory information needed for this control is transmitted through sensory pathways and sent toward the different structures shown in Figure 3.1. Three levels of correction are recognized. First, the short loop or myotactic reflex occurs within the first 25 milliseconds (msec) and is mediated through the spinal cord. Second, the long loop reflex, which occurs in 85 to 125 msec, is controlled by subcortical structures such as the cerebellum. Third, when the reflex contractions are not sufficient to correct the movement, the voluntary command must be triggered from cortical structures.

The role of receptors is fundamental to this type of control. For examples, the eyes provide information on the accuracy, while proprioceptors (e.g., muscle spindles, joint receptors, etc.) provide information relative to the status of the internal environment: joint position, speed of displacement,

relative positions, etc. Receptors play an important role in the control of movement as well as in the learning or modification of motor behavior. The status of the locomotor system, and of the muscles, at any given time is influenced greatly by the discharge of receptors. Their role must then be well understood, especially for functional rehabilitation, which is often based on behavioral approaches.

Behavioral Systems and Approach. A joint adjustment or mobilizations basically a functional stimulus applied to the body. The body, in turn, can be seen as a behavioral system in that it behaves in a stimulus-response mode. In other words, all behaviors of the human system are the result of a stimulus that is perceived and integrated, and then a response is organized and carried out through the effectors (e.g., muscles). Therefore, for a practitioner to be successful, he or she must understand well the stimulus-response relationship associated with any given functional or behavioral technique. A successful practitioner will be able to prescribe and administer the proper treatment because he or she is able to predict, with acceptable accuracy, the outcome of the treatment in the specific case. Naturally, the receptors represent the first line of contact between the environment and the human system. In fact, a stimulus-response reaction will be obtained only if the receptors are simulated and a response is triggered. Therefore, the efficiency of any behavioral approach depends immensely on the ability of stimulating specific receptors. The mechanism triggered that will ultimately produce the desired response is no longer under the control of the stimulus, it is occurring naturally. This explains why several researchers are now interested in the role of different receptors in the modulation of neuromuscular information.

From our study of joint receptors especially, some data suggest that sacroiliac joint adjustments and direct sacroiliac pressure are responsible for a significant modulation of reflex responses.[7,8] Such results confirmed that spinal information or commands can be modulated as a result of a joint adjustment, and that the pressure component especially could be the triggering mechanism. Such a reaction could be mediated through joint receptors. Further, joint receptors, more so than muscle or tendon receptors, are interesting because some are slowly adaptive and nonadaptive receptors. Thus, their effects are longlasting and can then be responsible for long-term dysfunctions or treatment effects.

TRAINING OR EXERCISE SCIENCE

To understand the behaviors and modification in those behaviors of the locomotor system, one must study not only the fundamental units, but also the operations of the system and the qualities of these operations and units.

Fundamental Physiologic Qualities of Performance

The physiologic qualities of the human or locomotor system are divided into three categories: organic, muscular, and perceptivomotor.

ORGANIC QUALITIES

The organic qualities can be presented on a continuum based on the type of metabolic processes underlying the production of energy needed.[9] These qualities are: *endurance, resistance,* and *power.* The *aerobic* processes, underlying the endurance quality, are those realized in the presence of oxygen. On the other hand, resistance and power are based on the *anaerobic* processes available when the oxygen is not present.

MUSCULAR QUALITIES

The muscular qualities of *force, endurance, resistance,* and *power* are best understood using the concept of the strength continuum. This continuum ranks the strength production capabilities from the production of a movement requiring very little force (e.g., moving a limb without an external loading), to the production of the maximal force output. On a relative scale, this continuum ranges from a contraction demanding almost 0% of the maximal force output to a contraction producing 100% of that possible output. A contraction requiring pure force is one that demands 100% of the maximal force output. At the other end of the continuum, contractions demanding below 50% of the maximum can be sustained almost indefinitely and are said to require endurance. If a contraction reaches a level between 70 and 90% of maximum, the blood flow to the muscle will be altered and the amount of oxygen available to fuel the contraction will be drastically reduced or stopped. These conditions represent the resistance quality under which contractions can be maintained for a limited amount of time. Power is a combination of force and speed. A powerful contraction is one that is as strong and as fast as possible. Finally, *flexibility* is also considered a muscular quality. It is in fact a quality that is dictated by the ability of the muscle to relax and let itself stretch passively and by the elasticity of the soft tissue surrounding the joint. Accordingly, flexibility is more accurately called *articulomuscular amplitude,* because it is a function of articular as well as muscular structures.

The qualities are important to consider for exercise or training prescription. In fact, training is highly quality specific. Force training produces a stronger muscle without improving the endurance, i.e., the ability to produce a little contraction for a long time. The reverse is also true. Endurance training increases the efficiency of the muscle at producing small contractions for a long period of time but will not increase pure force. Therefore, knowing that different muscle groups are used differently, one should then realize that they should be trained differently.

For example, postural muscles (e.g., abdominal and dorsal muscles) are used for long periods of time at a low level of force (50% and below). Accordingly, exercise aimed at developing those muscles should involve endurance training (i.e., low intensity and high volume). On the other hand, for muscle groups involved in high intensity contractions (e.g., typically upper and lower limb muscles), or occupations requiring high force levels, exercises should target the force, resistance, and/or power qualities (i.e., high intensity and low

volume). Therefore, when prescribing rehabilitation exercises, one should keep in mind the target quality, the nature of the muscle contraction required in a real-life situation, and the specific nature of muscle training. The prescription of exercise is discussed further in a subsequent section.

Training Considerations. The most important consideration for the prescription of training exercises and programs is the training load or overload. The load is determined with respect to the quality to train and the specific effect desired. Endurance training, for example, requires a low load (e.g., 50 to 60% of the maximum force). At the other end of the continuum, force training requires loads neighboring 100% of maximum force output.

When considering the control of the training load, it is automatic and simple to think about increasing or decreasing the amount of weight used as a training stimulus, as just presented. Two concepts must be addressed, however; (1) the training threshold, and (2) the definition of force (i.e., F = m × a). The concept of training threshold is relatively simple. The training stimulus, i.e., the load, must reach a certain value relative to the subject's capacity in order to have a training effect. The magnitude of this threshold must consider two key parameters: *intensity* (i.e., the load expressed as a percent of maximum force output) and *volume* (i.e., the number of series and repetitions). The specific training stimuli have been described. The second concept concerning the definition of force is important for controlling the training conditions and respecting the training specificity requirements. More specifically, the definition of F = m × a makes us realize that the load (i.e., F for force) can be manipulated by changing the mass (i.e., m) and/or by manipulating the acceleration (i.e., a). The mass can be modified in the usual fashion, by increasing or decreasing the amount of weights. Most people, however, forget that the effective training load can also be manipulated by changing the lever arm used for lifting the load. Placing the load closer or farther away from the joint will decrease or increase the training stimulus, respectively. The technique can be useful when prescribing rehabilitation exercises with surgical tubing or Therabands (Hygenic Corporation, Akron, OH). The last way to control the training load is to manipulate the gravity, which is the acceleration applied on the mass. Because gravity is a vector always oriented in the same direction (i.e., pointing to the center of the earth), modifying the position of the body makes gravity act more or less on the mass, modifying the effective training stimulus. Trunk flexions, or situps, are more demanding when performed on an inclined surface because raising the pelvis relative to the head allows gravity to act more efficiently against the trunk along a greater range of movement, thus producing a more important training stimulus.

PERCEPTUAL OR PERCEPTIVOMOTOR QUALITIES

As the name suggests, the perceptivomotor qualities represent the interaction between perception skills and motor output, qualities specific to the neuromuscular system. The different perceptivomotor qualities are *reaction time, speed of movement, motor accuracy,* and *body image.* While maintaining and focusing on the physiology of motor behavior, it is as important to be preoccupied by the different ways in which the fundamental units can be activated and controlled. The perceptivomotor qualities address how the motor actions are coordinated and how perception is important in the control and execution of any motor task.

Muscle Dynamics

Muscle dynamics focus on the mechanisms underlying muscle function. First, the smallest functional unit of the neuromuscular system must be addressed: the motor unit. Then, the basic mechanisms are discussed in light of the strength continuum, which facilitates the presentation of the contraction types.

MOTOR UNITS

The motor unit is defined as the alpha motor neuron, its axon, and the muscle fibers it innervates.[10] The motor unit and muscle fiber types can be categorized in many different ways. The most objective ways are according to electrophysiology, fatigue resistance, size, and histologic classifications. In all of these quantitative motor unit classifications are three types of units: fast fatigable, fast fatigue resistant (intermediate motor unit), and slow motor units. Edington and Edgerton[11] presented one of the more comprehensive descriptions of the motor unit types (Fig. 3.2).

To fully appreciate the mechanisms underlying the muscle dynamics, the energy sources that fuel the contraction must be discussed (Fig. 3.3). The first source of energy available to the

muscle is the *immediate source* stored in the muscle at the contraction site. This source of energy is short lived and is available for only a few seconds (30 seconds maximum). The *oxidative metabolism* is the result of reactions taking place in the presence of oxygen. This energy production system is responsible for endurance exercises during which smaller contractions are produced. Stronger contractions obstruct the blood flow to the muscle, thus stopping the flow of oxygen and preventing the oxidative processes. Endurance contractions in which blood flow is not obstructed can be carried out almost indefinitely. Finally, the *nonoxidative metabolism* underlies forceful and powerful contractions. During this type of contraction, blood vessels in the muscles are crushed and blood flow is stopped for the duration of the contraction. The oxygen is no longer available and the reactions that can occur to produce energy use glycogen for fuel. These reactions produce byproducts, such as lactic acid, however, that reduce the contractile possibilities of the muscle, especially when they accumulate. Therefore, this type of energy source is available for a few minutes only.

The objective of training is then specific to the type of exercises executed. Endurance exercises increase the efficiency of the muscle in using the oxidative processes. On the other hand, resistance training forces the muscle to work without oxygen and it must increase its capacity to contract with a greater oxygen deficit. Finally, force training is almost independent of the metabolic processes because pure force and power use immediate energy sources almost exclusively. It should then be obvious that parameters such as speed of movement, resistance to movement, and duration influence greatly the depletion of the energy sources and

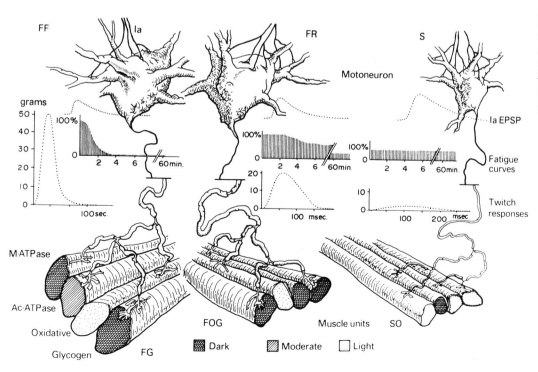

Fig. 3.2. Summary of the motor unit types and characteristics. (From Edington DW, Edgerton VR: The Biology of Physical Activity. Boston, Houghton-Mifflin, 1976.)

Fig. 3.3. Energy sources available for muscle contractions.

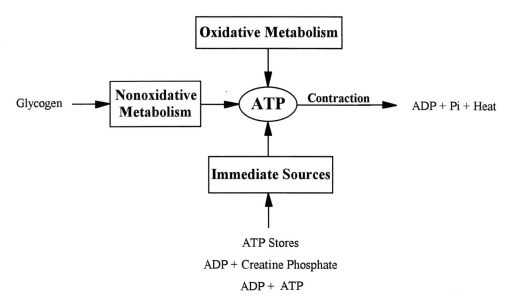

should be considered carefully when exercises or training are prescribed.

Finally, any discussion of the motor units and their control would not be complete without a presentation of the concepts of series elastic and of reflex or spinal control. Studied together, these concepts reveal that the muscle can be perceived as an intelligent elastic that is attached to a simple level. This simple but important definition helps to appreciate the importance of the contraction types and their control.

CONTRACTION TYPES

Simply stated, muscle contractions can occur under only three functional conditions: (1) the external force (F_e) is equal to the contraction or muscular force (F_m) or $F_e = F_m$; (2) the external force is smaller than the muscular force or $F_e < F_m$; and (3) the external force is greater than the muscular force or $F_e > F_m$. The first condition, yielding contractions while no movement occurs, produces *isometric* contractions. The second condition, usually the desired condition, makes it possible for the expected movement to occur because of shortening of the muscle producing a displacement in the expected direction at a given speed. This type is known as *concentric* contraction. The third condition is the exact opposite of the second. *Eccentric* contractions are produced while the muscle is actually being stretched and movement is going in the direction opposite to the one the muscle would normally produce. For that reason, eccentric contractions are often said to be involved in so-called "negative work." These definitions are at the core of the understanding of muscle dynamics. They are fundamental to an important aspect of muscle contraction known as the *force-velocity* relationship or curve.

FORCE-VELOCITY RELATIONSHIP

A schematic representation of a typical force-velocity curve is shown in Figure 3.4. This curve shows clearly that the greatest amount of force is produced in the eccentric condition. This fact could be explained by two distinct mechanisms active simultaneously during muscle lengthening eccentric contractions. One mechanism is the stretching of the elastic components in the muscle. In fact, the muscle acts partly as an elastic; it is able to store energy while being stretched. This storage of energy automatically increases the force output monitored. The second mechanism is based on the neuromuscular control available to the muscle. Receptors, the muscle spindle specifically, are sensitive to stretch. When the muscle is being stretched, the spindle is excited, the Ia afferent fibers that connect directly on the alpha motoneuron responsible for the ongoing contraction are solicited, and the nerve output to the muscle is increased, producing greater force. These two mechanisms are speed dependent. Accordingly, the force-velocity curve levels off at greater levels of negative velocity.

As soon as movement starts in the desired direction (i.e., concentric contraction), the capacity of the muscle to produce force is drastically reduced. At great speeds, force production goes down to 30 to 40% of the isometric force level. This realization is disconcerting, because usually the object of muscle contraction is to produce a given movement and in that very condition the muscle is less efficient

One can ask: so what? What is the relevance of the force-velocity curve? Outside of acknowledging our limitations in producing force during voluntary movements, it is important to consider the force-velocity curve for two reasons: (1) training specificity and (2) recognizing naturally occurring eccentric contractions during which the risk of injury is greater. These aspects of muscle dynamics are discussed subsequently.

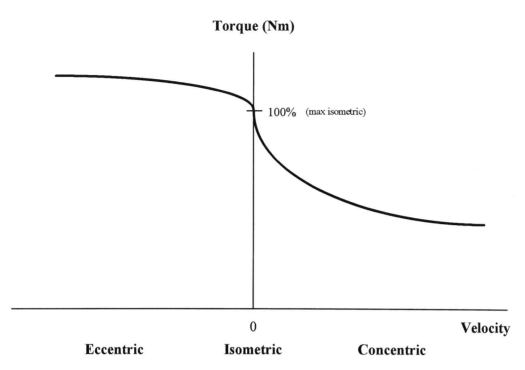

Torque (Nm)

100% (max isometric)

0

Eccentric Isometric Concentric

Velocity

Fig. 3.4. The force-velocity relationship.

FORCE-ANGLE RELATIONSHIP

Figure 3.5 presents an idealized force-angle curve. The importance of this relationship is the demonstration that any muscle, or muscle group and joint system, has an optimal working position. Joint position or angle, related to the length of the muscle, influences the force production capacity of the muscle. For the knee extensor muscle group, for example, the maximum force output is measured at between 80 and 90° of knee flexion. Again, this relationship is important to consider because of its implication in training effects specificity.

TRAINING SPECIFICITY

As suggested previously, training effects are known to be velocity[12,13] and position (i.e., joint angle) specific.[14,15] Training with negative work, for example, increases force output of eccentric contractions without affecting the muscle capacity during concentric contractions. Further, training at a specific joint angle (full joint flexion, for example) will not or may not influence the force output of the muscle group when the joint is near full extension. This fact suggests that a rehabilitation program should be specifically adapted to the muscle, the joint, and the task targeted. Accordingly, a person expected to do static work requiring isometric contractions in a specific joint angle should not be trained or rehabilitated in the same way as a person working in a dynamic situation.

A training overflow, or so-called window of nonspecificity associated with isometric exercises, was measured.[16] We demonstrated that training the knee isometrically at 90° influenced significantly the concentric and eccentric force over a range of up to 46° (i.e., from 54 to 100° of knee flexion). Such findings suggest that a joint can be trained statically at a specific painfree angle to achieve a functional treatment effect within the painful or dysfunctional range of movement.

Further, it has been recognized that the risk of injury associated with eccentric or negative work is greater because of the higher levels of force output achieved in this condition. Do we produce eccentric contractions in real-life situations? In fact, any contraction needed to decelerate a movement requires eccentric work, and the muscle accumulates energy while it is stretched. The best example of that situation is in locomotion, walking or running, when eccentric contractions are executed many times every day. Two muscles especially, the tibialis anterior controlling the fore foot contact during gait, and the hamstrings decelerating knee extension also during gait, are constantly used eccentrically. After an injury or immobilization, those muscles should be retrained using eccentric exercises to ensure that they regain the needed level of strength for their specific daily activity.

Some muscles are used eccentrically because of their bi-articular nature. The gastrocnemius and hamstrings are good examples. Such muscles often are stretched at one joint while they are required to contract to move the other joint. When lifting a load, for instance, the hamstrings are required to extend the hip (shortening contraction) while the knee is being extended (hamstrings being stretched). On the one hand, this synchrony is useful because the energy can be transferred from the knee to the hip by only keeping the hamstrings at the same length. When the knee extends, the hamstrings automatically pull on the ischial tuberosity to produce hip extension if they are able to keep the same length. Bi-articular muscles are indeed good for transferring energy from one joint to the other. On the other hand, this type of sustained and repeated activity can explain why these muscles are often tight

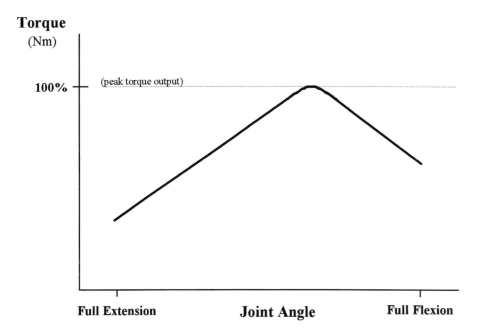

Fig. 3.5. The force-angle relationship.

and prone to contracture. Hence, bi-articular muscles, such as the hamstrings and calf muscles, should be trained to promote elasticity, through endurance and stretching exercises, and not force only.

Finally, the neural adaptation underlying exercise or training effects is often taken lightly. In fact, strength increase can be obtained through modifications at the neural level alone.[17] When morphologic changes do occur, they come into play after the neurophysiologic modifications[18,19] measured, for example, through motor unit recruitment frequency or synchronization of motor units. Further, the highest level of training specificity may be in the neural adaptation underlying the motor programming or learning associated with exercise. The motor control levels achieved with a specific exercise can be totally inappropriate for a given functional task, even if the same muscle groups are used. A strong recommendation is to select training or rehabilitation exercises according to specific motor tasks taken from the patient's daily activities.

EXERCISE AND/OR TRAINING PRESCRIPTION

Professionals dealing to a great extent with functional problems (e.g., pathologic or traumatic) or dysfunctions are often called on to evaluate, treat, and rehabilitate muscular functions. Exercise and/or training prescription is then a common demand. The basic training in exercise science or kinesiology is often limited, however. In that respect, the information relative to the force-velocity and force-angle relationships and training specificity are fundamental to the practice of exercise prescription.

More specifically, when confronted with exercise or training prescription, I always consider the following: (1) the objectives or goals pursued by the exercise program and the concerned individual (e.g., rehabilitation, well-being, competition); (2) training specificity (e.g., velocity and position); (3)

population segment to which the concerned individual belongs (e.g., age, sex); and (4) the targeted quality (i.e., where on the continuum will the person exercise in function of the specific task to be executed?).

USE, OVERUSE, MISUSE, AND IMMOBILIZATION

Dysfunctions are often associated with use, overuse, misuse, or immobilization. It appears that too much or too little movement brings about a functional problem.

Movement in men and women is neither accidental nor incidental. Movement is certainly essential to healthy life, if not its essence. Realizing that both use and immobilization, two opposites, can or will cause functional problems leading to discomfort, dysfunction, or dys-ease, highlights the need to define what can be called a *window of optimal activity*. On a *performance continuum* (Fig. 3.6), this window should be placed in a functional zone between reactivation and activation. This concept of performance continuum, including the levels of intervention (i.e., rehabilitation, reactivation, and activation), the types of intervention increasing performance, and the events leading to decreasing performance (see Fig. 3.6), should help to organize the research needed to understand the complexity of functional health or pathologic change to organize the intervention needed to maintain an individual in an optimal position along that continuum, and to reveal the importance of overuse and immobilization.

Such a conceptual framework is the basis for the research, in chiropractic, kinesiology, and sports medicine, produced in our laboratory. Our focus is on imbalances, knee dysfunctions, and the relationship existing between the mechanical and neuromuscular components of function. This research program should help to understand this window of optimal activity and the consequences of being outside of it.

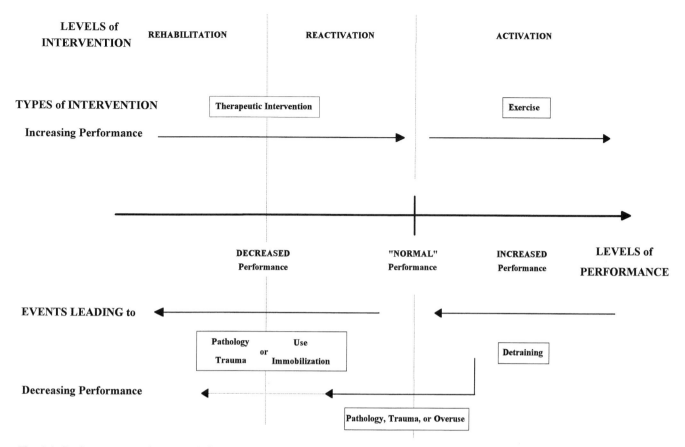

Fig. 3.6. Performance continuum including the relative position of the levels of intervention (rehabilitation, reactivation, and activation) and the different phenomena responsible for increasing and decreasing performance.

CONCLUSION

All exercise science approach outlined in this chapter should be useful in guiding functional evaluations. All three fundamental components of the system—anatomic, mechanical, and functional—should be investigated systematically to determine objectively the course of events after the evaluation. This course of events, leading to the restoration of the dysfunction, most probably includes reactivation and activation of the functional units. The exercises or techniques used to achieve the reactivation goals should be guided by:

- The type of muscle involved (i.e., fiber type composition)
- The type of demand or work normally imposed on the muscle (i.e., concentric, isometric, or eccentric contractions for postural or volitional work)
- The normal work range of motion (i.e., angle specificity)
- The load required for the specific development targeted (i.e., specific muscular quality, endurance, resistance, force, power, or articulomuscular amplitude)

Only when all these aspects are considered carefully are the reactivation and activation goals reached systematically. Therapists lacking background in the exercise sciences which is needed to appreciate all the important details underlying the reactivation and activation techniques, should seek a multi-disciplinary approach to enlist and benefit from the assistance of an exercise scientist or kinesiologist.

REFERENCES

1. Desmarais F, Boucher JP: A lower limb asymmetry model: Anatomical, mechanical, and functional factors. In Proceedings of the 1991 International Conference on Spinal Manipulation. FCER, Arlington, VA, 1991, pp 129–133.
2. Boucher JP, Hodgdon JA: Anatomical, mechanical, and functional factors in patello-femoral pain syndromes. Chiropract Sports Med 7:1, 1992.
3. Desmarais F, Boucher JP: Anatomical, mechanical and functional characterization of sacroiliac joint fixation. In Proceedings of the 1993 International Conference on Spinal Manipulation. FCER, Arlington, VA, 1993, pp 52–53.
4. Herzog W, Nigg BM, Read JL: Quantifying the effects of spinal manipulations on gait, using patients with low back pain. J Manipulative Physiol Ther 11:151, 1988.
5. Roy SH, De Luca CJ, Casavant DA: Lumbar muscle fatigue and chronic low back pain. Spine 14:992, 1989.
6. Zarow FM, Boucher JP, Hsieh J: Anatomical, mechanical and functional characterization of chronic low back pain. In Proceedings of the 1993 International Conference on Spinal Manipulation. FCER, Arlington, VA, 1993, pp 54–55.
7. Charbonneau M, Boucher JP: Segmental modulation of T and H reflexes and M wave following a chiropractic adjustment: A pilot study.

In Proceedings of the 1990 International Conference on Spinal Manipulation. FCER, Arlington, VA, 1990, pp 393–398.

8. Lefebvre S, Charbonneau M, Boucher JP: Modulation of segmental spinal excitability by mechanical stress upon the sacro-iliac joint: Preliminary report. In Proceedings of the 1993 International Conference on Spinal Manipulation. FCER, Arlington, VA, 1993, pp 56–57.

9. Astrand PO, Rodahl K: Textbook of Work Physiology. New York, McGraw Hill, 1977.

10. Basmajian JV, DeLuca CJ: Muscle Alive. 5th ed. Baltimore, Williams & Wilkins, 1985.

11. Edington DW, Edgerton VR: The Biology of Physical Activity. Boston, Houghton Mifflin, 1976.

12. Moffried MT, Whipple RH: Specificity of speed exercise. Phys Ther 50:1693, 1970.

13. Caizzo VJ, Perine, JJ, Edgerton VR: Training-induced alterations of the in vivo force-velocity relationship of human muscle. J Appl Physiol 51:750, 1981.

14. Bender JA, Kaplan HM: The multiple angle testing method for the evaluation of muscle strength. J Bone Joint Surg [Am] 45A:135, 1963.

15. Meyers C: Effects of 2 isometric routines on strength, size and endurance of exercised and non-exercised arms. Res Q 38:430, 1967.

16. Boucher JP, Cyr A, King MA, et al. Isometric training overflow: Determination of a non-specificity window. Med Sci Sports Exerc, 25: S134, 1993.

17. Enoka RM: Neuromechanical Basis of Kinesiology. Champaign, IL, Human Kinetics Books, 1988.

18. Sale D, MacDougall D: Specificity in strength training: A review for the coach and athlete. Can J Sport Sci 6:87, 1981.

19. Rutherford OM: Muscular coordination and strength training, implications for injury rehabilitation. Sports Med 5:196, 1988.

II

ASSESSMENT OF
MUSCULOSKELETAL FUNCTION

4 Pain and Disability Questionnaires in Chiropractic Rehabilitation

HOWARD VERNON

"An old joke: Which is better to have, a watch that's stopped, or a watch that's always five minutes fast? Answer: The watch that's stopped—because at least it's right twice a day!"

Evaluation is the cornerstone of clinical medicine. No diagnosis can be reached and no effective treatment can be rendered without conducting a clinical evaluation, which allows for the identification of salient signs and symptoms of the presenting disorder. This form of clinical assessment is conducted by using a time-honored system comprising a patient interview or history, observation, and clinical examination procedures. These procedures often include established and traditional "tests" to, for example, provoke pain, feel for tissue changes, visualize the structures, and otherwise diagnose the condition. In the biomedical disease model,[1] some physical disorder must account for the disease, and the process of clinical evaluation permits the most precise and trustworthy determination of the nature and underlying cause of the disorder.

New clinical models challenge the limits of the traditional "disease model"[2,3] and of its classical forms of clinical evaluation. One important new way of viewing disorders of health is called the "functional model."[4–8] In this model, it is recognized that although two patients may have the same diagnosed condition, each may have different alterations of function, especially in relevant areas of daily living and work. These alterations are typically defined as levels of disability, and they are not always fully measured in the classical clinical evaluation.

Also of importance is the "illness behavior model,"[9–11] in which the distinction is made between "disease," defined in a mechanistic sense as disordered physiology, and "illness," defined as the manner in which the person with the disordered physiology adapts to his or her own environment. These two models are particularly appropriate when applied to rehabilitation of painful disorders of the musculoskeletal system.

CONCEPTUAL BACKGROUND

It is useful for this discussion to start with a definition of pain, as originally adopted by the International Association for the Study of Pain: "Pain is that association of stimuli with responses which result in an unpleasant experience which hurts a person and from which they want to be freed."[12] Although definitions are helpful, a conceptual model aids greatly in clarifying the complexities involved. Loeser's model depicts pain as a multidimensional hierarchy, beginning at its lowest level with nociception, which leads to pain, which leads to pain behavior and ultimately to suffering.[13] Each of these dimensions lends itself to particular kinds of assessments. On the other hand, the further we ascend in the multidimensional hierarchy, the more it is that any particular phenomenon is a product of each of the dimensions subserving it. For example, tenderness levels measured in the somatic tissues may reveal something about nociceptive activity and its interpretation as pain, especially in terms of the threshold to perception by the patient. This particular measurement, however, may have little to do with other pain outcomes, such as return to work. Return to work is a function of the social dimension of pain and is therefore influenced by a host of factors beyond that of the current quantum of nociception experience by the patient.

Also warranting considering is the currently accepted model of parallel and interactive processing of sensory as compared to affective motivational dimensions of pain.[14] It is generally accepted that tests and measures that evaluate one of these crucial dimensions may not be applicable to the other.

When considering pain and loss of function, especially in regard to low back pain, a crucial distinction must be drawn between disease and illness.[3,11] The illness behavior model provides a framework within which the subjective experience of disease becomes legitimized conceptually as illness, which is then viewed operationally as disability. The physical components of disease require treatment, whereas the illness component of disability requires care. Treatment and care become two distinct operational domains with different objectives, different measurements of assessment and diagnosis, different strategies of management and, most important for this discussion, different outcomes. Gaining separate but integrated perspectives on the outcomes of treatment as opposed to those of care will substantially improve the delivery of rehabilitation services.

Properties of Measurements

As a preface to a discussion of tests for pain and disability, the reader should appreciate several axes around which tests such as these are configured (subjective vs. objective, qualitative vs. quantitative). Measurements are ideally designed to mini-

Table 4.1. Attributes of Tests in Clinical Rehabilitation

• Reliability	• Specificity
• Validity	• Responsivity
• Sensitivity	

mize error and to reduce variability. In the clinical setting, the involvement of the patient in the process of measurement of pain creates a great deal more variability than many scientists are willing to tolerate.[15-17] Nonetheless, by its very definition as an experience and not an objectifiable state, pain eludes such rigorous analysis. Often, the best we can do is to manage systematically the high degree of variability in patient groups. When discussing the issue of outcomes measures in chiropractic rehabilitation, numerous attributes of such measures must be understood.[18,19] Table 4.1 lists some of these attributes.

Measurement Scales

All instruments use a scale to measure a specific parameter.[20,21] Typically, the scale is only representative of the phenomenon itself. For example, the increase of temperature is really measured in linear units of increase in a column of mercury—a thermometer. Similarly, the visual analog scale (VAS) uses a 100-mm line to represent pain intensity. In this instance, the anchors or end points of the scale are both absolute and arbitrary. They are absolute because they are intended to measure the phenomenon from its lowest to its highest level. On the other hand, they are arbitrary because the numbers assigned to these and any intermediate states are purely a matter of the choice of the designer of the scale. In fact, many pain scales use the numbers 0-5, 0-10, or even 0-101, when, all the while, there is no more pain with one scale than with the next!

The manner in which numbers or units are used in a scale is organized according to the degree to which the scale actually represents the quality or quantity being measured. The first scale uses a numeric code to represent the response category. If only two answers—yes or no—are possible on a certain scale, and numbers such as 1 or 2 are assigned to represent these answers, then these data are said to be *nominal data.* In this respect, the numbers actually represent a code for other data. Nominal data are said to be the lowest order of data in that little of the actual parameter measured is revealed by the data. All the qualities of the parameter that are measurable are reduced to one of two states—present or absent, yes or no, male or female, etc. As such, this type of data is also referred to as "dichotomous data" (Table 4.2).

On the *ordinal scale,* numbers are still used as codes for other characteristics, but the numbers are used to rank the level of the characteristic and, therefore, bear some (if only indirect) relationship to the measured value. On an ordinal scale, the number 2 represents a greater value than 1; however, the true intervals of such a scale are really unknown. In other words, whether 2 really represents twice as much of the value as one, or, on a scale from 1 to 5, whether each interval really represents 25% of the total value is, at best, uncertain. Nonetheless, this relationship of an ordinal scale to the value measured is often assumed by users, prompting some inappropriate conclusions.

In the *interval scale,* numbers do not merely represent units of value, they constitute the units of value. This scale is synonymous with a type of data known as "continuous data." On the interval scale, data points are true numeric representations of the value of the parameter in question. These data points can be subdivided (at least theoretically) into infinitely smaller units, each of which would still represent a true unit of measurement of the parameter. For example, temperature is measured on a continuous scale, whereby a measurement of 10° is hotter than 9°, and colder than 11°, and the difference between 10° and 10.5° is real. On an interval scale, however, there may not be a true zero point; there are three different temperature scales, each with their own zero point. As such, at least on the Fahrenheit and Celsius scales, there may not be an absolute representation of the measured value by the scale, in that 20° may not be twice as hot as 10°.

The latter aspect is the feature of scales known as *ratio scales.* When measuring the angle of the straight leg raising test, the angular scale from 0° to (typically) 90 to 100° is used. Data are continuous and ratios can be formed such that 20° of angle is, indeed, twice as much as 10°. This scale allows the observer to make true comparisons between measured results of a test under a variety of conditions.

As an example of appropriately ratio scale comparisons, consider a patient with low back pain who scores 30 out of 50 on an ordinally scaled disability questionnaire, and whose straight leg raising signs, bilaterally, are limited to 45°. If, after a course of treatment and rehabilitation, the disability score drops to 15 out of 50 and the straight leg raising signs increase to 90°, it is reasonable to say that an increase of 100% has occurred. Because the disability scale uses ordinal data, however, we are advised to conclude that a substantial decrease in score has occurred, but not one that really represents 50% less disability.

Table 4.2. Scaling in Pain and Disability

Questionnaires
  Nominal Scale:
    "Do you have pain?"   Yes/No
                                                   1   2

  Ordinal Scale:
    "How severe is your pain?"
          0 2 4 6 8 10
      none   awful
Testing
  Interval Scale:
    Determine the thermal pain threshold in a pain patient (Range: 40 to 55°)
  Ratio Scale:
    Determine the pressure pain threshold in a pain patient (Range: 0 to 10 kg/cm²)

Sources of Bias

One fundamental premise underlying clinical measurement is the notion that error and bias may exist at all levels and from all sources throughout the measurement process.[21,22] These sources include the subject, the instrument, and the examiner.

THE SUBJECT

Emotional, psychologic, and personality factors inevitably play a part in the subject's response to measurement,[23] be it self-rating questionnaires or physical performance tests. Such factors as pain tolerance, self-image, beliefs and attitudes about health and health practitioners, mood, and underlying motivation may all influence the participation of an individual in functional measurement.

Physiologic factors certainly play a role in physical performance testing. For example, fatigue, neurologic status, and pain levels may all influence testing.

Cognitive factors play a crucial role, especially in the area of instructions for test activities. Language and cultural and educational factors all impact the subject's comprehension of the overall purpose of any test, as well as the manner in which it is to be conducted.

Finally, traditional sources of *psychometric bias* exist,[24] such as in the tendency of subjects to choose responses in the mid-range or at the extremes of a scale; the effects of the order of different responses, items, and, indeed, of different tests when using a battery of tests; and the tendency of subjects to over- or underestimate depending on their perception of the responses expected in the test.

THE INSTRUMENT

The *content domain* of self-reporting instruments may be insufficient to capture all necessary characteristics of the parameter to be measured. The *format of questions* can introduce errors or response biases by providing too much or too little prompting information. If questions are always ranked in a similar order, then order bias may creep into a patient's responses. Finally, the *instructions,* either on the form or by the examiner, may be insufficient, misleading, or poorly understood by the patient.

THE EXAMINER

The *context of the clinical setting* is an important aspect of the measurement. Questionnaires may be filled out differently before relative to after seeing a health practitioner. The quality of the overall health care experience of the patient may influence their responses.

The *presence or absence of an examiner* while the patient is completing various tests may influence their responses. Response expectations may be operative, such as the Hawthorne effect,[21,25] in which the patient's responses may be influenced by the knowledge that they are being tested, or the Pygmalion effect,[21,25] in which the patient may erroneously assume that the practitioner or examiner has a certain response expectation that the patient merely fulfills. The demeanor of the examiner and the cues and instructions they give are all important in minimizing this sort of error.

Reliability

Reliability may be defined most technically as the degree to which random error in a test is reduced. More colloquially, reliability is characterized by the degree of consistency in the results obtained with repeated testing. The data obtained from only one application of a test can reflect results from anywhere in the typical range of the test. With repeated applications of the test, the results tend to narrow in their variation. In fact, in classic measurement theory, the reliability of a statistic increases in proportion to the square root of the number of additional data (or test applications). The mean of 16 data points is four times more reliable than that of a single data point.

In regard to pain and disability questionnaires, the most important form of reliability is *test-retest reliability,* which measures stability over time in repeated applications of the test. Some assumptions must be made when considering this form of reliability. In determining if the test itself is a source of error, all other factors that can contribute to variability in the test result must remain constant. In clinical settings, the natural history of the condition under investigation is a variable. Changes in the course of the condition will naturally introduce variability with repeated applications of the test, making it difficult to determine the reliability of the test itself.

Typically, two applications of the test are made in an interval of time that is suitable for the natural history of the condition itself (typically within hours to 1 or 2 days). The results of these tests are compared using some form of reliability statistic, such as Pearson's R or the Intraclass Coefficient. Acceptable levels of reliability range from 0.70 to 0.90 and up.

Other means of determining the reliability of questionnaires for pain and disability include the "split-half" method, in which the responses of one half of the test are compared to those of the other half, and other tests for what is known as "internal consistency," or the degree to which answers to individual items reflect the total score of the questionnaire.[26]

Another important type of reliability is the consistency of findings between different raters (inter-examiner reliability) or in measurements made by the same rater (intra-observer reliability). Depending on the type of data used in the instrument, reliability statistics, such as Pearson's R, Intraclass Coefficient, or the Kappa Concordance statistic, can be used.[27]

Validity

The concept of validity pertains to the accuracy of any test, or the degree to which it truly measures the attribute under investigation. McDowell and Newell propose a somewhat broader definition of validity to include the context in which the measurement occurs, "the range of interpretations that may be placed upon the test; what do the results mean!"[21] This definition also has the advantage of connecting results (data) of the test to the theoretic constructs underlying the use of the test. In this way, data plus meaning becomes something useful; i.e., information.

FACE VALIDITY

Face validity, or content validity, refers to the degree to which the questions or procedures incorporated within a test make sense to its users. Typically, a group of experts is asked to review a test and come to a consensus on the overall sensibility of its components.

CONSTRUCT VALIDITY

This term refers to the degree to which a test and its result fit with accepted theory. As an example, lift strength testing has a high degree of construct validity when used in assessing an injured worker with low back pain whose job involves significant manual handling and carrying. Assessing small differences in the length of the legs in such a worker has poor construct validity given that no evidence suggests that a small leg length difference equates with work impairment.

CONCURRENT VALIDITY

One way of determining the validity of one test is to correlate it with another test done at the same time. In some cases, different tests have been designed to measure similar attributes. For example, a VAS for pain intensity can be validated by comparison to a verbal rating scale for pain severity. In this context, relatively higher correlations are expected between tests of similar attributes. On the other hand, a test of one attribute can be correlated with tests of another attribute that is related, at least theoretically if not empirically; for example, reduction in levels of activities of daily living with levels of pain severity. In such a circumstance, the levels of expected correlation are usually lower.

CRITERION VALIDITY

One form of concurrent validity that is particularly robust is to compare the results of one test with the best test available at the time—known as the gold standard. If the new test performs in a relatively similar fashion, then it can be said to have good criterion validity.

DISCRIMINANT VALIDITY

This attribute of a test refers to its ability to discriminate between major categories of test findings, often referring to categories such as "normal or abnormal," positive or negative, symptomatic or asymptomatic. *Sensitivity* is the attribute of a test whereby a positive test result is highly correlated with the true diseased or abnormal state; i.e., high true-positive rate/low false-negative rate. *Specificity* is the

opposite, wherein test negatives equate highly with true negatives (with low false positives).

Responsivity. One form of discriminant validity involves the performance of a test over time. It is reasonable to determine if the test accurately measures the amount of change in a condition or attribute when such change truly occurs. In the development of the Neck Disability Index (NDI),[28] we studied 10 subjects with neck pain who had undergone chiropractic treatment for 3 to 4 weeks. All 10 individuals reported improvement. They were asked to complete two instruments—the NDI and a visual analog pain scale (VAS)—at the beginning of treatment and again at the end of the treatment period. We correlated the change in VAS scores (as a percentage) with the change in the NDI scores. The average change in VAS scores was approximately 75%, whereas the change in NDI scores averaged only about 50%. These data correlated at 0.62, which is a relatively good level of correlation. Which test result reflected the true level of improvement? Which was the more responsive? Only further research using statistical techniques designed specifically to study responsivity[29–31] will provide answers to these questions.

MEASUREMENTS FOR PAIN AND DISABILITY

Each instrument discussed subsequently is representative of a greater number in each category. This section provides a summary of the content and description of each instrument and then a discussion of its reliability and validity.

Location

Pain may be localized by using the *pain diagram*[32–37] (Fig. 4.1), a standardized self-report measurement of the location, extent, and, to some degree, the quality of pain. As well as these descriptive features, the manner in which a patient depicts his or her pain has been shown to reveal a great deal about interpretations of the pain experience, mood, and psychologic state and behavior while in pain. In this respect, filling out the pain diagram becomes a pain behavior, and it can demonstrate an appropriate as opposed to an inappropriate manner on the part of the patient.[35]

Outcomes are derived from the pain diagram in a number of ways. First, subjective ratings by trained observers can be made from the appearance of the diagrams. These ratings, in fact, can be systematized, using rankings from more organic/more realistic to less organic/less realistic and, perhaps, psychogenic or inorganic.[35] Second, scores from a checklist of penalty points, which rate the anatomic fidelity, the presence of extraneous markings within and outside the body, etc., are compiled. The higher the score, the more likely it is to reflect inappropriate pain behavior.[35,36] Third, body area charts can be used to quantify the size of the painful area so a single measure can be derived from the pain diagram.[37]

High reliability of the pain diagram has been reported. Margolis et al[33] reported test/retest correlations for body area to range between 0.83 and 0.93; for pain location, they found

PAIN DIAGRAM
INSTRUCTIONS

On the following diagrams, indicates all areas of :

pain	- XXXX
stiffness	- / / / /
numbness	- OOOO
other	- _____
(specify)	

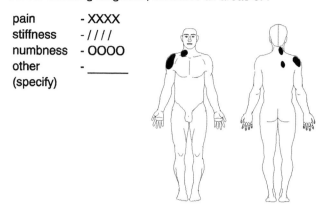

A

PAIN DIAGRAM
INSTRUCTIONS

On the following diagrams, indicates all areas of :

pain	- XXXX
stiffness	- / / / /
numbness	- OOOO
other	- _____
(specify)	

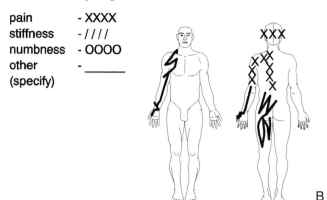

B

Fig. 4.1. Pain diagram. **A,** Example of a well–delineated, anatomically correct depiction. **B,** Example of a poorly delineated, anatomically incorrect, exaggerated depiction.

test/retest agreement to be 76%. These authors found no age or gender differences in the degree of reliability.

With regard to validity, high pain drawing scores have been correlated with elevated hysteria and hypochondriasis scores on the Minnesota Multiphasic Personality Index (MMPI); greater chronicity of low back pain and higher hospitalization rates; and high McGill Pain Questionnaire (MPQ) scores.[35]

Finally, with regard to its usefulness, the strengths of the pain diagram are ease of administration, relative ease of interpretation, and implicit face validity as a tool with which patients can effectively communicate their complaint to health care practitioners.

Intensity

Several simple scales exist that are designed for the self-rating of pain intensity. The visual analog scale (VAS), devised by Huskisson in 1974,[38] (Fig. 4.2), is a numerically continuous scale that requires that pain level be identified by making a mark on a 100-mm line. The uniformity and density of this type of pain scale creates a high level of sensitivity to variations in pain ratings.

Verbal descriptive scales (VDS) also exist[39–41] (Fig. 4.3); some are ordinally scaled, like the Present Pain Index of the MPQ,[14] and others are ratio scaled, like the Borg pain scale.[42] The numeric rating scale and the Borg pain scale are 10-point scales. In the newer Numerical Rating Scale (NRS) 101, which is a version of the VAS, a patient chooses a number between 1 and 100 to rate the severity of their pain.[43]

With regard to reliability, these pain scales are the mainstay of most pain studies and clinical trials. The original reports of reliability included correlations between the vertical and the horizontal forms of the VAS, which are reported as high as 0.99, with similarly high test/retest reliability.[38,44–46]

Concurrent validity among these scales and with other measures of pain and loss of function is reportedly high. Scott and Huskisson[47] reported comparisons of the VAS and the VDS-type scales that correlated at 0.75, whereas a coefficient of 0.63 was reported between the VAS scores and MPQ scores.[47] The VAS has been shown time and again to be sensitive to treatment effects,[48] although Scott and Huskisson cautioned that providing the original score or using a VAS for relief or improvement may be more appropriate.[49] Other authors disagree with this strategy, however, and require an absolute measurement.[50,51]

The scales just described are easy to administer and to score, although the ordinal scales of the VDS-type scales should be approached with caution, especially in regard to intergroup comparisons. There is a high degree of sensitivity to change, especially on the linear scales.

Quality

In 1975, Melzack introduced the McGill Pain Questionnaire (MPQ),[52] and it has since been used in numerous studies of musculoskeletal and other pain syndromes. It has undergone a great deal of replication and is acknowledged as one of the gold standards in the field of pain assessment. The MPQ consists of 20 category scales of verbal descriptors of pain,[53,54] ranked in order of severity and clustered into four subscales: sensory, affective, evaluative, and miscellaneous scales, as well as a five-point "present pain rating index." Scores can be obtained on the rank scores added for the total instrument or for each of the subscales. Of greatest interest to researchers has been the ability to distinguish the sensory and the affective domains of the pain experience.

Test/retest reliability had been confirmed as high from the outset, with Melzack's first report indicating a 70% consistency of responses of three trials over a 3-day period.[52] Allen

Fig. 4.2. Visual analog scales for rating pain (**A**) and visual analog scale for rating improvement (**B**).

Make a mark (/) along the line which you think represents your current level of pain in your major area of injury, somewhere between "No Pain At All" and "Pain As Bad As It Could Be".

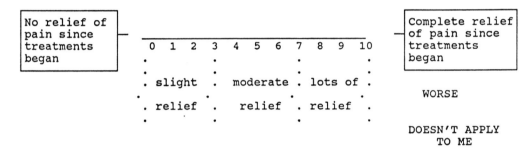

No Pain
A At All

Pain As Bad
As It Could Be

ARE YOU BETTER SINCE YOUR FIRST TREATMENT?

Name _____   Date _____

Please try to remember back to the first day when you started these treatments and tell us how much you have improved since that first day. Please do this page before today's treatment begins.

1. PAIN RELIEF

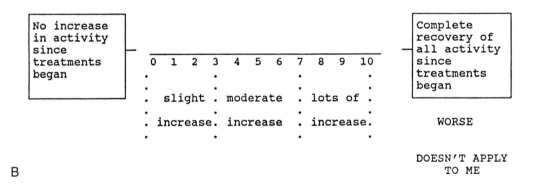

2. ACTIVITY INCREASE (walking, standing, working, exercising, etc)

B

and Weinmann[55] reported similar results over four trials within 1 week. Phillips and Hunter[56] studied test/retest reliability of the MPQ in patients with headache and reported correlation coefficients as follows: for the Present Pain Index, which is the total score, an R of 0.94; for the sensory scale, 0.83; and for the affective scale, 0.95. These findings indicate that people can, within a relatively short period of time, remember their pain state from one measurement interval to another.

The greatest interest with the MPQ has been in the area of validity. Numerous factorial analyses have confirmed the fac-

torial structure, especially of the sensory and the affective scales.[57–60] The concurrent validity has been confirmed between the MPQ and the MMPI and many other instruments that measure pain intensity, mood state in pain, and psychosocial disturbance. Phillips and Hunter reported an interesting and significant correlation between MPQ scores and the pain diary in headache subjects.[56]

With regard to discriminant validity, Dubuisson and Melzack[54] found that 77% of 95 pain patients could be correctly classified into diagnostic groups on the basis of their MPQ score alone. Reading[57] studied patients with acute and

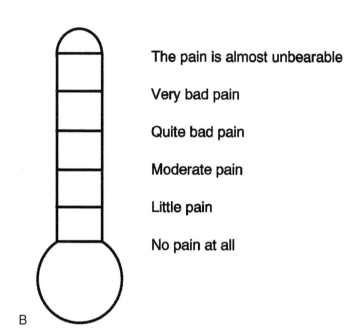

Patient Directions:

On a scale of 1 - 10 place an X in your current pain level

NORMAL	LOW PAIN	MODERATE PAIN	INTENSE PAIN	EMERGENCY
( ) 0	( ) 1	( ) 4	( ) 7	( ) 10
	( ) 2	( ) 5	( ) 8	
	( ) 3	( ) 6	( ) 9	

A

The pain is almost unbearable

Very bad pain

Quite bad pain

Moderate pain

Little pain

No pain at all

B

Fig. 4.3. Borg verbal rating pain scale (**A**) and verbal pain rating scale (**B**) (from the Roland-Morris scale).

chronic disorders and found that the former used more sensory words whereas the latter, as predicted by the theory, used more affective and evaluative words.

Finally, the MPQ has been used in a many treatment trials and has been found to be sensitive to treatment effects.[61] Its usefulness lies in its relative ease of administration. Also, it is easy to score and rich in data, particularly with regard to the subscales and how their scores may apply to the theoretic concerns mentioned previously. Because of its strengths, it has taken on the status of a gold standard in pain assessment.

Course

The course of the complaint can be monitored by using the pain diary (Fig. 4.4). The diary is an often-used tool for ongoing patient self-report. It allows for continuous recording of a wide range of pain-related outcomes, such as the frequency of painful episodes; the time course of constant pain complaints, which can be recorded over daily and hourly inter-

vals; the severity and actual duration of these episodes; medication usage; and effect on activities of daily living. All of these parameters can be combined into a compact instrument. These various categories are typically combined into ordinal or continuous scales with frequency counts and continuous data on the time, course, and duration.

Blanchard reviewed the stability of pain diary data, especially for headache (an episodic complaint), and determined that an average of 2 weeks is sufficient to obtain stable baseline values from the diary.[62] For constant pain syndromes, such as those involving the low back or neck, stable values ought to be obtained within days of administration. The drawbacks of the pain diary are the bias and Hawthorne effects that are likely to creep into the data recording process, as well as the rare instance of completely false and misleading recordings, which are more likely from a complete malingerer. As such, pain diary data should, if at all possible, be cross-checked with some comparable observer-based data as to the pain behavior or clinical status of the patient.

PAIN DIARY   **PAIN MAP**

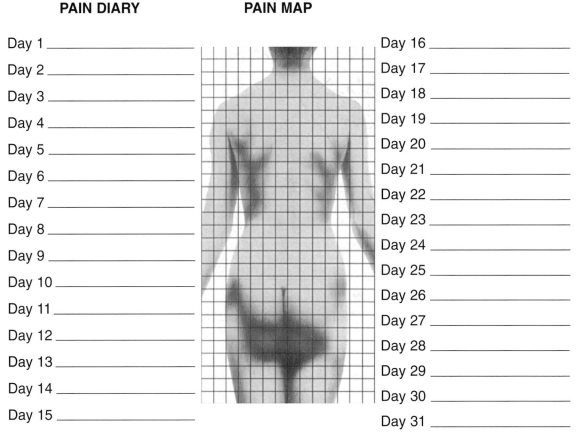

Day 1 _____	Day 16 _____
Day 2 _____	Day 17 _____
Day 3 _____	Day 18 _____
Day 4 _____	Day 19 _____
Day 5 _____	Day 20 _____
Day 6 _____	Day 21 _____
Day 7 _____	Day 22 _____
Day 8 _____	Day 23 _____
Day 9 _____	Day 24 _____
Day 10 _____	Day 25 _____
Day 11 _____	Day 26 _____
Day 12 _____	Day 27 _____
Day 13 _____	Day 28 _____
Day 14 _____	Day 29 _____
Day 15 _____	Day 30 _____
	Day 31 _____

Fig. 4.4. Pain diary.

PAIN BEHAVIOR

This section addresses five instruments, the purposes of which are less to describe the pain complaint itself than to assess the behavior of the individual in pain and come to an understanding of the motivational components of that pain state, i.e., to assess the illness/disability component of the disorder. The focus of this discussion is on systematic behavioral observation, and then four scales that measure activities of daily living: Oswestry,[63] Roland-Morris,[64] Neck Disability,[28] and Pain Disability.[65]

Systemic Behavioral Observation

Keefe et al[66] devised a method of observing a patient's pain behavior in order to provide quantifiable data regarding the patient's disability that would be directly relevant to functioning. They identified a group of overt behaviors that appeared to be unique for the pain experience: grimacing, bracing, guarded movements, rubbing, and sighing.

The protocol of Keefe et al consists of a 10-minute video of the patient undergoing a standardized series of movements. They walk, sit, recline, and stand up again, and the frequency of various pain behaviors is recorded by trained observers. With regard to reliability, Keefe et al reported interexaminer agreement levels as high as 88%.[66] Findings from a study of patients with chronic low back pain by Jensen et al[67] con-

firmed the high degree of reliability of the protocol. They reported inter-rater agreement Kappa coefficients between 0.80 and 0.93. Test/retest correlations over 12 days were at 0.78.

With regard to validity, Keefe et al[66] reported sensitivity to treatment changes as well as high correlations with pain intensity ratings, physical findings, and functional disability scores. They also demonstrated high correlation between scores of trained versus naive observers, so these pain behaviors are consistent across evaluators.

The pain behavior scores discriminate between pain patients and control subjects. Authors of a recent study found that the observational method can actually discriminate four subgroups of back pain with different patterns of pain behavior; in other words, people who have a homogeneous problem, like back pain, appear to behave differently, and, in fact, consistently in those differences. In this study, guarding and rubbing were the behaviors observed most often.[67]

In a report by Jensen et al,[67] the total pain behavior scores correlated significantly with the VAS and the Borg pain scales, as well as with measures of reduced spinal mobility (i.e., where flexion and extension were reduced) and increased medication usage. In their study, correlation with depression and two scales of the Sickness Impact Profile (SIP) were also investigated. The only pain behavior to correlate consistently with these psychosocial parameters was "sighing," which was actually the least observed behavior.

Nonetheless, the link between pain behaviors and pain severity is not firmly established, even at the theoretical level. Observers have noted a great deal of pain behavior in the absence of high levels of pain severity itself, as well as diminished pain behavior and even recovery of relatively normal function in the presence of severe pain. So, theoretically and empirically, behavior and severity may not be absolutely linked.

Oswestry Low Back Pain Index (Fig. 4.5)

This index was reported by Fairbank et al in 1980.[63] It is a 10-item scale in which each item has six ranked detractors, scored from 0 to 5, so a total score of 50 can be compiled. The first section is a pain-rating scale. The other sections deal with various daily activities deemed relevant to low back disability by the consensus team.

In their original report, Fairbank et al included a test/retest reliability coefficient of 0.99 and a split-half coefficient reported as "good." Regarding validity, Fairbank et al reported only that Oswestry scores lowered after a 3-week rest period, which is presumed to indicate sensitivity to treatment effects.

Triano et al[68] provided a much needed study of concurrent validity. They compared Oswestry scores to measures of muscle dysfunction and reported a good correlation between higher Oswestry scores and the presence of signs of abnormal muscle function, with the converse correlation existing as well. This finding speaks, if only implicitly, to the sensitivity and specificity of this instrument.

Roland Morris Scale[64] (Fig. 4.6)

This scale consists of a set of 24 questions pertaining to work, time at home, walking, personal care, sitting, etc.—a wide range of activities relevant to patients with low back pain. The test/retest coefficient (half-day interval) was originally reported as 0.91. The internal consistency of the items, measured using an "agreement percent coefficient," was calculated as 0.83.

To test the validity of the instrument, the original authors compared test results to a verbal pain rating instrument and reported these to be in "good agreement." Some test questions were compared to doctors' physical findings, with generally good-to-equivocal agreement. Scores were not related to age, gender, or social class, indicating that wide use in general practice was probably well supported.

One criticism of this instrument is that it uses the nominal scale, and therefore may miss important information about clinical status. Patients are forced to agree or disagree completely with each of the test items, when, in fact, the status of most patients is usually a matter of degree of some limitation, not whether it is present or absent. Nonetheless, this attribute of the instrument may lend itself to an improved level of responsivity. Hsieh et al found the Roland-Morris scale superior in its responsivity compared to the Oswestry Index (which uses an ordinal scale) in determining levels of improvement in patients with low back pain.[69]

Neck Disability Index (NDI)[28] (Fig. 4.7)

This index, a revision of the Oswestry Index, was developed at the Canadian Memorial Chiropractic College by Vernon and Mior to address the need for an instrument specifically designed to measure reduced activities of daily living in patients with neck pain. The test/retest reliability was found, in a suitable sample of subjects, to be 0.89. The total Cronbach's alpha, which is a measure of internal reproducibility, was 0.80, and all of the items achieved alpha levels above 0.75.

Regarding the construct validity, scores were normally distributed and clustered at the moderate severity level, which was appropriate for an ambulatory clinical population. With regard to concurrent validity, we compared NDI to MPQ scores at an R value of 0.73, and sensitivity to change was measured by comparing changes on the NDI to visual analog scale rating changes. This correlation was 0.60.

Pain Disability Index (PDI)

The PDI was first reported by Pollard in 1984.[65] It is a seven-item scale using VAS to rate intensity of disturbances to a variety of psychosocial variables and activities of daily life. Tait et al[70] reported a Cronbach's alpha value of 0.87. As for validity, PDI scores for inpatient groups were higher than those for outpatient groups, and more recently, Tait et al[71] found that high PDI scores correlated well with higher psychologic distress states, higher disability levels, high pain description scores (from the MPQ), and higher pain behavior scores from the protocol of Keefe and colleagues.[66] The advantage of the PDI as opposed to the other indices is that it is not specific for one type of pain and the seven categories can be applied to virtually any pain syndrome.

ILLNESS BEHAVIOR

The psychosocial indices of illness behavior warrant discussion.

Back Pain Classification Scale

Leavitt and Garron first published this scale in 1979.[72] It is a subscale of a larger check list of symptoms applicable to back pain. Of the large list, 13 words were found to discriminate pain of organic origin reliably and accurately. These words include the negatively scored items: nagging, dull, throbbing, intermittent, shooting, and punishing. These terms as a group pose some interesting paradoxes. Conversely, the words squeezing, exhausting, sickening, troublesome, tender, numb, and tiring indicate a high likelihood of a psychogenic origin for the pain complaints.

Test/retest reliability after 1 day achieved a correlation coefficient of 0.86, whereas the split-half reliability score was reported at 0.89. Cross-validation with the MMPI scales is high. Improvement ratings correlate highly with the Back Pain Classification Scale; that is, "organics" respond better than "psychogenics."[72,73]

Please rate the severity of your low back pain by circling a number below:

0	1	2	3	4	5	6	7	8	9	10

No pain   *Unbearable pain*

Name _____   Date ____/____/____   File # _____

Instructions: Please mark the ONE BOX in each section which most closely describes your problem.

Section 1 - Pain Intensity

☐ 1. The pain comes and goes and is very mild.

☐ 2. Th pain is mild and does not vary much.

☐ 3. The pain comes and goes and is moderate.

☐ 4. The pain is moderate and does not vary much.

☐ 5. The pain comes and goes and is severe.

☐ 6. The pain is severe and does not vary much.

Section 2 - Personal Care (Washing, Dressing, etc.)

☐ 1. I would not have to change my way of washing or dressing in order to avoid pain.

☐ 2. I do not normally change my way of washing or dressing even though it causes some pain.

☐ 3. Washing and dressing increase the pain but I manage not to change my way of doing it.

☐ 4. Washing and dressing increase the pain and I find it necessary to change my way of doing it.

☐ 5. Because of the pain I am unable to do some washing and dressing without help.

☐ 6. Because of the pain I am unable to do any washing or dressing without help.

Section 3 - Lifting

☐ 1. I can lift heavy weights without extra pain.

☐ 2. I can lift heavy weights but it gives extra pain.

☐ 3. Pain prevents me lifting heavy weights off the floor.

☐ 4. Pain prevents me lifting heavy weights off the floor, but I can manage if they are conveniently positioned, e.g., on a table.

☐ 5. Pain prevents me from lifting heavy weights but I can manage light to medium weights if they are conveniently positioned.

☐ 6. I can only lift very lights weights at the most.

Section 4 - Walking

☐ 1. I have no pain on walking.

☐ 2. I have some pain on walking but it does not increase with distance.

☐ 3. I cannot walk more than one mile without increasing pain.

☐ 4. I cannot walk more than 1/2 mile with increasing pain.

☐ 5. I cannot walk more than 1/4 mile without increasing pain.

☐ 6. I cannot walk at all without increasing pain.

Section 5 - Sitting

☐ 1. I can sit in any chair as long as I like.

☐ 2. I can sit only in my favorite chair as long as I like.

☐ 3. Pain prevents me sitting more than 1 hour.

☐ 4. Pain prevents me from sitting more than 1/2 hour.

☐ 5. Pain prevents me from sitting for more than 10 minutes

☐ 6. I avoid sitting because it increases pain immediately.

Section 6 - Standing

☐ 1. I can stand as long as I want without pain.

☐ 2. I have some pain on standing but it does not increase with time.

☐ 3. I cannot stand for longer than one hour without increasing pain.

☐ 4. I cannot stand for longer than 1/2 hour without increasing pain.

☐ 5. I cannot stand for longer than 10 minutes without increasing pain.

☐ 6. I avoid standing because it increases the pain immediately.

Section 7 - Sleeping

☐ 1. I get no pain in bed.

☐ 2. I get pain in bed but it does not prevent me from sleeping well.

☐ 3. Because of pain my normal nights sleep is reduced by less than 1/4

☐ 4. Because of pain my normal nights sleep is reduced by less than 1/2

☐ 5. Because of pain my normal nights sleep is reduced by less than 3/4

☐ 6. Pain prevents me from sleeping at all.

Section 8 - Social Life

☐ 1. My social life is normal and gives me no pain.

☐ 2. My social life is normal but increases the degree of pain.

☐ 3. Pain has no significant effect on my social life apart from limiting my more energetic interests, e.g., dancing, etc.

☐ 4. Pain has restricted my social life and I do not go out very often.

☐ 5. Pain has restricted my social life to my home.

☐ 6. I have hardly any social life because of the pain.

Section 9 - Traveling

☐ 1. I get no pain when traveling.

☐ 2. I get some pain when traveling but none of my usual forms of travel make it any worse.

☐ 3. I get extra pain while traveling but it does not compel me to seek alternative forms of travel.

☐ 4. I get extra pain while traveling which compels me to seek alternative forms of travel.

☐ 5. Pain restricts me to short necessary journeys under 30 minutes.

☐ 6. Pain restricts all forms of travel.

☐ 7. Pain prevents all forms of travel except that done lying down.

Section 10 - Changing Degree of Pain

☐ 1. My pain is rapidly getting better.

☐ 2. My pain fluctuates but overall is definitely getting better.

☐ 2. My pain seems to be getting better but improvement is slow.

☐ 3. My pain is neither getting better nor worse.

☐ 4. My pain is gradually worsening.

☐ 5. My pain is rapidly worsening.

Fig. 4.5. Oswestry Low Back Pain Scale.

❏ 1. I stay home most of the time because of my back.

❏ 2. I change position frequently to try and get my back comfortable.

❏ 3. I walk more slowly than usual because of my back.

❏ 4. Because of my back, I am not doing any of the jobs that I usually do around the house.

❏ 5. Because of my back, I use a handrail to get upstairs.

❏ 6. Because of my back, I lie down to rest more.

❏ 7. Because of my back, I have to hold on to something to get out of an easy chair.

❏ 8. Because of my back, I try to get other people to do things for me.

❏ 9. I get dressed more slowly because of my back.

❏ 10. I only stand up for short periods of time because of my back.

❏ 11. Because of my back, I try not to bend or kneel.

❏ 12. I find it difficult to get out of a chair because of my back.

❏ 13. My back is painful almost all of the time.

❏ 14. I find it difficult to turn over in bed because of my back.

❏ 15. My appetite is not very good because of my back.

❏ 16. I have trouble putting on my socks {stockings} because of my back.

❏ 17. I only walk short distances because of my back pain.

❏ 18. I sleep less well because of my back pain.

❏ 19. Because of my back pain, I get dressed with help from someone else.

❏ 20. I sit down for most of the day because of my back.

❏ 21. I avoid heavy jobs around the house because of my back.

❏ 22. Because of my back pain, I am more irritable and bad tempered with people than usual.

❏ 23. Because of my back, I go upstairs more slowly than usual.

❏ 24. I stay in bed most of the time because of my back.

Fig. 4.6. Roland-Morris Back Pain Scale.

NECK DISABILITY INDEX

This questionnaire has been designed to give the doctor information as to how your neck pain has affected your ability to manage in everyday life. Please answer every section and mark in each section only the ONE box which applies to you. We realize you may consider that two of the statements in any one section relate to you, but please just mark the box which most closely describes your problem.

Section 1 - Pain Intensity
- ☐ I have no pain at the moment.
- ☐ The pain is very mild at the moment.
- ☐ The pain is moderate at the moment.
- ☐ The pain is fairly severe at the moment.
- ☐ The pain is very severe at the moment.
- ☐ The pain is the worst imaginable at the moment.

Section 2 - Personal Care (Washing, Dressing etc.)
- ☐ I can look after myself normally without causing extra pain.
- ☐ I can look after myself normally but it causes extra pain.
- ☐ It is painful to look after myself and I am slow and careful.
- ☐ I need some help but manage most of my personal care.
- ☐ I need help every day in most aspects of self care.
- ☐ I do not get dressed, I wash with difficulty and stay in bed.

Section 3 - Lifting
- ☐ I can lift heavy weights without extra pain.
- ☐ I can lift heavy weights but it gives extra pain.
- ☐ Pain prevents me from lifting heavy weights off the floor, but I can manage if they are conveniently positioned, for example on a table.
- ☐ Pain prevents me from lifting heavy weights, but I can manage light to medium weights if they are conveniently positioned.
- ☐ I can lift very light weights.
- ☐ I cannot lift or carry anything at all.

Section 4 - Reading
- ☐ I can read as much as I want to with no pain in my neck.
- ☐ I can read as much as I want to with slight pain in my neck.
- ☐ I can read as much as I want with moderate pain in my neck.
- ☐ I can't read as much as I want because of moderate pain in my neck.
- ☐ I can hardly read at all because of severe pain in my neck.
- ☐ I cannot read at all.

Section 5 - Headaches
- ☐ I have no headaches at all.
- ☐ I have slight headaches which come in-frequently.
- ☐ I have moderate headaches which come in-frequently.
- ☐ I have moderate headaches which come frequently.
- ☐ I have severe headaches which come frequently.
- ☐ I have headaches almost all the time.

Section 6 - Concentration
- ☐ I can concentrate fully when I want to with no difficulty.
- ☐ I can concentrate fully when I want to with slight difficulty.
- ☐ I have a fair degree of difficulty in concentrating when I want to.
- ☐ I have a lot of difficulty in concentrating when I want to.
- ☐ I have a great deal of difficulty in concentrating when I want to.
- ☐ I cannot concentrate at all.

Section 7 - Work
- ☐ I can do as much work as I want to.
- ☐ I can only do my usual work, but no more.
- ☐ I can do most of my usual work, but no more.
- ☐ I cannot do my usual work.
- ☐ I can hardly do any work at all.
- ☐ I can't do any work at all.

Section 8 - Driving
- ☐ I can drive my car without any neck pain.
- ☐ I can drive my car as long as I want with slight pain in my neck.
- ☐ I can drive my car as long as I want with moderate pain in my neck.
- ☐ I can't drive my car as long as I want because of moderate pain in my neck.
- ☐ I can hardly drive at all because of severe pain in my neck.
- ☐ I can't drive my car at all.

Section 9 - Sleeping
- ☐ I have no trouble sleeping.
- ☐ My sleep is slightly disturbed (less than 1 hr. sleepless).
- ☐ My sleep is mildly disturbed (1-2 hrs. sleepless).
- ☐ My sleep is moderately disturbed (2-3 hrs. sleepless).
- ☐ My sleep is greatly disturbed (3-5 hrs. sleepless).
- ☐ My sleep is completely disturbed (5-7 hrs. sleepless).

Section 10 - Recreation
- ☐ I am able to engage in all my recreation activities with no neck pain at all.
- ☐ I am able to engage in all my recreation activities, with some pain in my neck.
- ☐ I am able to engage in most, but not all of my usual recreation activities because of pain in my neck.
- ☐ I am able to engage in a few of my usual recreation activities because of pain in my neck.
- ☐ I can hardly do any recreation activities because of pain in my neck.
- ☐ I can't do any recreation activities at all.

© 1987 Vernon/Hagino, modified from Fairbanks et al; Physiotherapy, 1980

Fig. 4.7. Neck Disability Index.

ILLNESS BEHAVIOR QUESTIONNAIRE (IBQ)

First reported by Pilowsky and Spence in 1976,[74,75] the IBQ was designed to assess fundamental attitudes toward sickness, the role of doctors, and a variety of other psychosocial variables considered important in explaining abnormal illness behavior. It consists of 62 items answered in a yes/no fashion and comprises seven factor scales. The reliability of these scales on test/retest correlations has been between 0.67 and 0.87.

The following facts have been reported about the IBQ. It has good correlation between patient and spousal evaluations, so it seems to be consistent. Factor analyses have confirmed the seven scale structure and, in fact, other scales have been found by Main and Waddell.[76] Comparative and control studies demonstrated differences between symptomatic and control subjects, between various clinical groups, and between responders and nonresponders. Concurrent validity has been established between the IBQ and the Zung depression scale[77] as well as other measures of anxiety. Waddell, Pilowsky, and Bond[78] correlated the IBQ to previously determined abnormal illness behavior, which included the nonorganic signs of Waddell.[79] One of the strongest findings in that study is the importance of the disease conviction scale of the IBQ in distinguishing patients with low back pain who demonstrate abnormal illness behavior. In other words, they believe strongly that they have a serious problem, even though they may not.

Sickness Impact Profile (SIP)

The SIP[80–82] consists of 136 statements clustered into 12 categories that involve issues ranging from those from the simpler ADL scales as well as those from the abnormal illness behavior realm. To address the reliability of the SIP, Pollard et al[83] reported test/retest coefficients between 0.88 and 0.92, with an interviewer-administered approach achieving a higher reliability than the self-administered approach. The shorter version of the SIP has been reported as equally reliable.[84]

Nonorganic Signs

The *nonorganic signs* of Waddell and colleagues[79] are useful in distinguishing those patients who manifest abnormal illness behavior. These signs are the patient responses to seven different tests performed by the practitioner and include (1) tenderness that is superficial or nonanatomic in location; (2) pain with axial loading or (3) full trunk rotation in the standing position; (4) lack of pain on sitting straight leg raising (when supine, test was positive); (5) unexplained weakness and/or (6) sensory disturbance; and finally, (7) a pattern of exaggeration to all provocative testing.

The higher the number of positive signs, the higher the likelihood of response bias to the pain phenomenon and an exaggerated response representing critical factors in the patient's condition.

USES OF PAIN AND DISABILITY QUESTIONNAIRES IN CASE MANAGEMENT (Table 4.3)

Timing

Baseline. Total scores for each test help to clarify and quantify the extent of pain and disability. These scores can be compared to expected values in the literature or within one's own clinical population.

Individual items can provide meaningful information on worst-case issues. For example, on the Oswestry or NDI scales, any item scoring 4 or 5 represents a key issue in the patient's life. Identifying that item (i.e., driving or lifting, etc.) as important and more highly impaired allows for individualized goal setting in the rehabilitation plan of management.

Sequential testing. Serial testing at appropriate intervals (i.e., weekly for acute conditions, biweekly for chronic cases) allows for ongoing evaluation of progress. Providing feedback to the patient can be an important source of motivation to sustain their compliance with the program requirements.

After treatment/discharge. The final evaluation can be compared to baseline levels for a determination of total in-program benefit.

Mode of Application

Doctor-only. Patients may fill out a variety of forms, the results of which may never be disclosed to them. This practice is suitable for cohort research, in which some level of patient blinding is useful to reduce bias in self-reporting.

Doctor plus patient feedback. Ongoing results, especially in the form of simple serial comparisons (i.e., "Your pain level is 50% reduced"), are provided to the patient for motivation and encouragement and as part of the learning process that underlies the application of a rehabilitation program (i.e., learning to comply with instructions, learning the meaning of various disability issues relevant to their own condition). This discussion is especially useful for the key items identified at baseline (i.e., "I see your level of comfort while driving is increasing. That's good.").

Doctor plus patient plus staff. In programmatic care, all levels of the clinical rehabilitation team share in the serial data collection and feedback process. This approach maximizes opportunities for positive reinforcement for identifying areas of poorer response, and for risk-managing "redflag" areas. Program staff should use the ongoing data for modifying the plan of management as necessary and for keeping the program on target for the patient's individualized goals.

Table 4.3. Uses of Pain and Disability Questionnaires in Patient Care

Timing	Application
• Measures of post-treatment outcome	• Doctor-only
	• Doctor plus patient feedback
• Measures of ongoing improvement	• Doctor plus patient plus staff

CONCLUSION

As rehabilitation programs develop and expand within chiropractic, a corresponding need arises to document both the progress of the patient and the outcome of the care provided,[85,86] regardless of its specific components. The instruments discussed in this chapter will help the modern chiropractor meet the challenges of outcome assessment.

REFERENCES

1. Vallis TM, McHugh S: Illness behavior: Challenging the medical model. Humane Med 3:2, 1987.
2. Engel GL: The need for a new medical model: A challenge for biomedicine. Science 196:129, 1977.
3. Waddell G: A new clinical model for the treatment of low back pain. Spine 12:632, 1987.
4. Frey WD: Functional assessment in the '80s: A conceptual enigma, a technical challenge. In Halpern HS, Fuhrer MJ (eds): Functional Assessment in Rehabilitation. Baltimore, Paul Brooks, 1984.
5. Forer SK: Functional assessment instruments in medical rehabilitation. J Organizational Rehabil Evaluators 2:29, 1982.
6. Williams RGA, Johnston M, Willis LA, et al: Disability: A model and measurement technique. Br J Prev Soc Med 30:71, 1976.
7. Gallin RS, Given CW: The concept and classification of disability in health interview surveys. Inquiry 13:395, 1976.
8. Harper AC, Harper DA, Lambert LJ, et al: Symptoms of impairment, disability and handicap in low back pain: A taxonomy. Pain 50:189, 1992.
9. Mechanic D, Volkhart EH: Illness behavior and medical diagnosis. J Health Hum Behav 1:86, 1960.
10. Pilowsky I: Abnormal illness behavior. Br J Med Psychol 42:347, 1969.
11. Vernon H: Chiropractic: A model of incorporating the illness behavior model in the management of low back pain patients. J Manipulative Physiol Ther 14:379, 1991.
12. Vernon HT: Applying research-based assessments of pain and loss of function to the issue of developing standards of care in chiropractic. J Chiro Tech 2:121, 1990.
13. Loeser JD: Concepts of pain. In Stanton HM, Boas RA (eds): Chronic Low Back Pain. New York, Raven Press, 1982.
14. Melzack R: The Puzzle of Pain. New York, Basic Books, 1973.
15. Koran LM: Reliability of clinical methods, data, and judgments. N Engl J Med 293:642, 1975.
16. Waddell G, Main CJ, Morris EW, et al: Normality and reliability in clinical assessment of backache. Br Med J 284:1519, 1982.
17. Nelson MA, Allen P, Clamp SE, et al: Reliability and reproducibility of clinical findings in low back pain. Spine 4:97, 1979.
18. Hanson DT, Ayres JR: Chiropractic outcome measures. J Chiro Tech 3:53, 1991.
19. Deyo RA: Measuring the functional status of patients with low back pain. Arch Phys Med Rehabil 69:1044, 1988.
20. Torgerson WS: Theory and Methods of Scaling. New York, McGraw–Hill, 1958.
21. McDowell I, Newell C: Measuring Health: a Guide to Rating Scales and Questionnaires. New York: Oxford Press, 1987.
22. Bennett AE, Ritchie K: Questionnaires in Medicine: A Guide to Their Design and Use. London, Oxford University Press, 1975.
23. Fordyce WE: Behavioral Methods in Chronic Pain and Illness. St. Louis, CV Mosby, 1976.
24. Bradburn NM, Sudman S, Blair E, et al: Question threat and response bias. Public Opinion Q 42:221, 1978.
25. Philips RB: The challenge of proving the efficacy of chiropractic: Placebo, Hawthorne and Pygmalion effects in research. ACA J Chiro 20:30, 1983.
26. Cronbach LJ: Essentials of Psychological Testing. 3rd Ed. New York, Harper, 1970.
27. Keating J, Bergmann T, Jacobs G: Inter–examiner reliability of eight evaluative dimensions of lumbar segmental abnormality. J Manipulative Physiol Ther 13:463, 1990.
28. Vernon HT, Mior S: The neck disability index: A study of reliability and validity. J Manipulative Physiol Ther 14:409, 1991.
29. Guyatt G, Walter S, Norman G: Measuring change over time: Assessing usefulness of evaluation instruments. J Chronic Dis 40:171, 1987.
30. Bombardier C, Tugwell P: Methodological considerations in functional assessment. J Rheumatol 14(Suppl 15):6, 1987.
31. Kirschner B, Guyatt G: A methodological framework for assessing health indices. J Chronic Dis 38:27, 1985.
32. Keele KD: The pain chart. Lancet 2:6, 1948.
33. Margolis RB, Chibnall JT, Tait RC: Test-retest reliability of the pain drawing instrument. Pain 33:49, 1988.
34. Margolis RB, Tait RC, Krause SJ: Rating system for use with patient pain drawings. Pain 24:57, 1986.
35. Tait RC, Chibnall JT, Margolis RB: Pain extent: Relations with psychological state, pain severity, pain history and disability. Pain 41:295, 1990.
36. Ransford HV, Cairns D, Mooney V: The pain drawing as an aid to psychological evaluation of patients with low back pain. Spine 1:127, 1976.
37. Uden A, Hstrom M, Bergenudd H: Pain drawings in chronic back pain. Spine 13:389, 1988.
38. Huskisson EC: Measurement of pain. Lancet 2:127, 1974.
39. Reading AE: Comparison of pain rating scales. J Psychosom Res 24:119, 1980.
40. Ohnhaus EE, Adler R: Methodological problems in the measurement of pain: A comparison between the verbal rating scale and the visual analogue scale. Pain 1:379, 1975.
41. Duncan GH, Bushnell MC, Lavigne GJ: Comparison of verbal and visual analogue scales for measuring the intensity and unpleasantness of experimental pain. Pain 37:295, 1989.
42. Jensen MP, Karoly P, Braver S: The measurement of clinical pain intensity: A comparison of six methods. Pain 27:117, 1986.
43. Downie WW, Leatham PA, Rhind VM, et al: Studies with pain rating scales. Ann Rheum Dis 37:378, 1978.
44. Huskisson EC: Measurement of pain. J Rheumatol 9:768, 1982.
45. Huskisson EC: Visual analogue scales. In Melzack R (ed): Pain Measurement and Assessment. New York, Raven Press, 1983.
46. Dixon JS, Bird HA: Reproducibility along a 10-cm vertical visual analogue scale. Ann Rheum Dis 40:87, 1981.
47. Scott J, Huskisson EC: Vertical or horizontal visual analogue scales. Ann Rheum Dis 38:560, 1979.
48. Maxwell C: Sensitivity and accuracy of the visual analogue scale. Br J Clin Pharmacol 6:15, 1978.
49. Scott J, Huskisson EC: Accuracy of subjective measurements made with or without previous scores: An important source of error in serial measurement of subjective states. Ann Rheum Dis 38:558, 1979.
50. Cheng RSS, Pomeranz B: Electrotherapy of chronic musculoskeletal pain: Comparison of electroacupuncture and acupuncture-like transcutaneous electrical nerve stimulation. Clin J Pain 2:143, 1987.
51. Marchin D, Lewith GT, Wylson S: Pain measurement in randomized clinical trials: A comparison of two pain scales. Clin J Pain 4:161, 1988.
52. Melzack R: The McGill Pain Questionnaire: Major properties and scoring methods. Pain 1:277, 1975.
53. Melzack R, Torgerson WS: On the language of pain. Anaesthesiology 34:50, 1971.
54. Dubuisson D, Melzack R: Classification of clinical pain descriptions by multiple group discriminant analysis. Exp Neurol 51:480, 1976.
55. Allen RA, Weinmann RL: The MPQ in the diagnosis of headache. Headache 22:20, 1982.
56. Phillips HC, Hunter MS: Pain behavior in headache patients. Behav Anal Mod 19:251, 1981.
57. Reading AE: The internal structure of the McGill Pain Questionnaire in dysmenorrhoea patients. Pain 7:353, 1979.
58. Prieto EJ, Geisinger KF: Factor-analytic studies of the McGill Pain Questionnaire. In Melzack R (ed): Pain Measurement and Assessment. New York, Raven Press, 1983, pp 63–70.
59. Byrne M, Troy A, Bradley LA, et al: Cross-validation of the factor structure of the MPQ. Pain 13:193, 1982.
60. Pearce J, Morley S: An experimental investigation of the construct validity of the McGill Pain Questionnaire. Pain 39:115, 1989.

61. Burkhardt CS: The use of the McGill Pain Questionnaire in assessing arthritis pain. Pain 19:305, 1984.
62. Andrassik F, Blanchard EB, Ahles T, et al: Assessing the reactive as well as the sensory component of headache pain. Headache 21:218, 1981.
63. Fairbank JCT, Couper J, Davies JB, et al: The Oswestry Low Back Pain Index. Physiotherapy 66:271, 1980.
64. Roland M, Morris R: A study of the natural history of low back pain. Part I. Development of a reliable and sensitive measure of disability in low back pain. Spine 8:141, 1983.
65. Pollard CA: Preliminary validity study of the Pain Disability Index. Percept Mot Skills 59:974, 1984.
66. Keefe FJ, Wilkins RH, Cook WA: Direct observation of pain behavior in low back pain patients during physical examination. Pain 20:59, 1984.
67. Jensen IB, Bradley LA, Linton SJ: Validation of an observation method of pain assessment in non-chronic back pain. Pain 39:267, 1989.
68. Triano JJ, Schultz AB: Correlation of objective measures of trunk motion and muscle function with low back disability ratings. Spine 12:561, 1987.
69. Hsieh CJ, Phillips RB, Adams AH, et al: Functional outcomes of low back pain: Comparison of four treatment groups in a randomized controlled trial. J Manipulative Physiol Ther 15:4, 1992.
70. Tait RC, Pollard CA, Margolis RB, et al: The Pain Disability Index: Psychometric and validity data. Arch Phys Med Rehabil 68:438, 1987.
71. Tait RC, Chibnall JT, Krause S: The Pain Disability Index: Psychometric properties. Pain 40:171, 1990.
72. Leavitt F, Garron DC: Validity of a Back Pain Classification Scale among patients with low back pain not associated with demonstrable organic disease. J Psychosom Res 23:301, 1979.
73. Leavitt F, Garron DC. Validity of a Back Pain Classification Scale for detecting psychological disturbance as measured by the MMPI. J Clin Psychol 36:186, 1980.

74. Pilowsky I, Spence ND: Pain and illness behavior: A comparative study. J Psychosom Res 20:131, 1976.
75. Pilowsky I, Spence ND: Manual for the Illness Behavior Questionnaire (IBQ). 2nd Ed. Adelaide, Australia: University of Adelaide, 1983.
76. Main CJ, Waddell G: A comparison of cognitive measures in low back pain: Statistical structure and clinical validity at initial assessment. Pain 46:287, 1991.
77. Pilowsky I, Chapman CR, Bonica JJ: Pain, depression and illness behavior in a pain clinic population. Pain 4:183, 1977.
78. Waddell G, Pilowsky I, Bond MR: Clinical assessment and interpretation of abnormal illness behavior in low back pain. Pain 39:41, 1989.
79. Waddell G, McCulloch JA, Kummel E, et al: Nonorganic physical signs in low back pain. Spine 5:117, 1980.
80. Bergner M, Bobbitt RA, Pollard WE, et al: The Sickness Impact Profile validation of a health status measure. Med Care 14:57, 1976.
81. Bergner M, Bobbitt RA, Kressels, et al: The Sickness Impact Profile: A conceptual formulation and methodology for the development of a health status questionnaire. Int J Health Serv 6:393, 1976.
82. Bergner M, Bobbitt RA, Carter WB, et al: the Sickness Impact Profile: Development and final revision of a health status measure. Health Care 19:787, 1981.
83. Pollard WE, Bobbitt RA, Bergner M, et al: The Sickness Impact Profile: Reliability of a health status measure. Med Care 14:146, 1976.
84. Deyo RA: Comparative validity of the Sickness Impact Profile and shorter scales for functional assessment in low back pain. Spine 11:951, 1986.
85. Millard RW: A critical review of questionnaires for assessing pain—related disability. J Occup Rehab 1:289, 1991.
86. Bombardier C, Tugwell P: Methodological considerations in functional assessment. J Rheumatol 14(Suppl 15):6, 1987.

5 Outcomes Assessment in the Small Private Practice

CRAIG LIEBENSON and JEFF OSLANCE

Determining the most cost-effective treatment depends on appropriate measurement of treatment results. Such measurement is called *outcomes assessment*. The development of outcome assessment tools for objective measurement of a patient's response to care has become a major research endeavor. For musculoskeletal problems, it is essential to assess objectively deficits in biomechanical function, including range of motion, muscle strength/endurance, and cardiovascular fitness. Questionnaires, algometry, and other tools also make it possible to quantify disability and the subjective experience of pain. Using functional outcome assessment tools to evaluate the progress of an injured worker or patient allows a shift in emphasis away from subjective factors of pain toward more realistic functional measures.

In the majority of soft tissue injuries, functional changes are the only objective findings on which to base treatment and to judge progress. Unfortunately, most orthopedic examinations rely on tests that search for structural lesions (i.e., nerve root compression or tension). Although structural lesions are present in only about 20% of cases, overuse of expensive diagnostic tests (i.e., magnetic resonance imaging) is typical in the search to diagnose such structural pathology.[1] The remaining 80% of patients have no identifiable structural pathologic abnormality and require treatment based on the evaluation of functional deficits. Outcomes assessment that includes objective functional testing gives third party payers, the patient, and the doctor a way to measure progress over time and thus adjudicate the prescribed treatment approach.

Treatment of functional deficits is addressed with functional reactivation/restoration programs. Studies have demonstrated that more than 80% of chronically disabled individuals can return to work if rehabilitation based on objective quantification of function is used as the standard of care.[2–4] Although quantification of functional deficits is the goal, this attempt is only in its infancy. Many physiologic parameters of the musculoskeletal system cannot be realistically measured quantifiably. Intersegmental accessory motion between articulations is palpated regularly, but interexaminer reliability is poor and no quantification is possible. Palpation of areas of tenderness by an algometer does not resemble manual palpation, although it is quantifiable. Visual inspection of the posture, gait, and movement skills of a patient is part of a qualitative examination that is clinically invaluable. While we strive toward objective quantification and measurement, we should not limit ourselves to quantification alone.

Objective outcome measurements are increasingly required to ensure reimbursement for care provided. They help to document the patient's status in terms of their subjective complaint, functional loss, changes in activities of daily living, psychosocial problems, and time off work. They also provide objective baselines that can be used to show the patient their progress over time. This feedback is a motivational aid the provider can use to encourage the patient.

MEASUREMENT OF PAIN, DISABILITY, AND PSYCHOSOCIAL STATUS

Rehabilitation begins with a thorough history from the patient. The history should identify various features about the pain, occupation, lifestyle, and psychosocial status of the individual. Certain objective tools that complement the traditional history-taking process are shown in Table 5.1.

Waddell's signs of abnormal illness behavior are important in patient evaluation. The presence of three of five of these signs is significantly correlated with disability.[14]

Superficial or nonanatomic tenderness: Widespread sensitivity to light touch in the lumbar region and pain referred to other areas, such as thorax, sacrum, or pelvis.
Simulation: Axial loading (light pressure to the skull) should not significantly increase low back pain. Passive rotation of the shoulders and pelvis together in a standing patient should not reproduce low back pain.
Distractions: Difference of 40 to 45° between the supine and seated straight leg raising tests.
Regional disturbances: Sensory or motor disturbance ("giving way") that is not neurologically correlated.
Overreaction: Inappropriate overreaction, such as guarding, limping, rubbing the affected area, bracing oneself, grimacing, or sighing, are all signs of illness behavior.

Wernecke et al found that these behavioral signs could be improved in individuals in a physical rehabilitation program.[14]

Measuring pain intensity and functional loss as a result of pain at 2- or 4-week intervals helps to document a patient's progress under care. The Visual Analog Scale (VAS) can even be used with each visit along with a pain drawing (see also Chapter 4). The VAS can be used to assess characteristic pain intensity "right now," "average pain," and "worst pain."[25–27]

Table 5.1. Objectification of Subjective Factors

Pain
　　Visual Analog Scale (intensity)[5]*
　　Pain drawing (location)[6]*
　　McGill (quality)[7]
Psychosocial
　　Beck[8]*
　　Zung[9,10]
　　Back Pain Classification Scale[11]
　　SCL-90-R[12]
　　FABQ[13]
　　Waddell's behavioral signs[14]*
Lifestyle/Disability
　　Oswestry[15]*
　　Neck Disability Index[16]*
　　Million[17]
　　Vermont[18]
　　Roland-Morris[19]*
　　Dallas Pain Questionnaire[20]*
　　Sickness Impact Profile[21,22]
　　Pain Disability Index[23]
Job Dissatisfaction
　　Apgar[24]

*Especially simple and practical tool for office use.

Average and worst pain should refer to the previous 6 months in the case of a chronic patient. If measurements are made at intervals during the provision of care, it should refer to the period since the last assessment.

The mean of the three pain intensity measurements should be multiplied by 10 to yield a 0 to 100 score. Characteristic pain intensity less than 50 is classified as low intensity; anything above 50 is classified as high intensity.[27]

Questionnaires such as the Oswestry or Neck Disability Index, pain diagrams, and the VAS should be used from the outset of care. A good rule of thumb is to obtain baselines at the patient's initial office visit and repeat the outcome measurements at weeks 2, 4, and 6. After 6 weeks, most patients are well. When treating a complicated patient (one prone to chronicity), however, it is reasonable to continue tracking their outcomes every 4 weeks. These measurements can help immeasurably with stubborn insurance adjusters or utilization reviewers because they document the patient's progress under your care.

Quantification of soft tissue tenderness is also possible with a pressure algometer.[28] This device measures soft tissue compliance. Pre- and post-treatment checks of tenderness can thus be quantified. Qualifiable assessment of soft tissue tenderness is also possible[29,30] by applying 4 kg of digital pressure (enough pressure to blanch the tip of the thumbnail when pressing the palmar surface of the thumb against a rigid surface). The grading scheme shown in Table 5.2 is adapted from Wolfe et al[29] and Hubbard et al.[30]

It is also of value to note the presence or absence of referred pain (expanded receptor field) associated with soft tissue palpation of an area of tenderness. Documenting areas of soft tissue tenderness, along with their potential patterns of referred pain, serves a number of purposes. First, it helps to establish a baseline level of soft tissue tenderness or sensitivity. Second, it helps identify trigger points (+ Jump sign and re-

ferred pain). Finally, it helps to identify signs of neuropathic pain (hyperalgesia to non-noxious stimuli).

FUNCTIONAL CAPACITY EVALUATION

A key to successful rehabilitation of the musculoskeletal system is functional assessment. In contrast to the clinical examination, this evaluation is not important until the patient is "out" of the acute episode. As soon as a patient emerges from the acute stages of an injury, objective measurement of functional outcomes is necessary. This information gives the doctor, patient, and third party payor means by which to communicate the status of the patient and to identify the goals of care.

The chief purpose of the functional capacity evaluation (FCE) is to demonstrate objectively an individual's level of impairment as it relates to both pain and disability.[31,32] This evaluation gives objective information to the health care provider who can then rationally prescribe treatment and then monitor its results. In addition, it provides the patient with objective feedback on how their injury and/or pain affects their ability to perform normal activities, as well as an objective way to see their progress. Finally, the FCE provides the third party payor with objective, quantifiable evidence of impairment from injury or subjective complaint.

According to Mooney, an FCE is recommended 2 weeks after injury to identify the "weak functional link" (see Chapter 21). Triano suggests 4 weeks as an appropriate time to begin testing (personal communication, 1994). Hart, Isernhagen, and Matheson wrote that the indications for functional testing include plateau of treatment progress, discrepancy between subjective and objective findings, difficulty returning to gainful employment, and vocational planning or medicolegal case settlement.[33] *Functional testing in the subacute stage can provide ideal outcomes as well as help to identify key functional pathologies that should be addressed with manipulation, advice, and exercise.*

The FCE allows objective confirmation of patient status to complement the patient's subjective self-report of their symptoms. It also documents patient progress over time, which helps to motivate the patient to pursue reactivation after injury. Prolonged passive care (e.g., hot packs, massage, ultrasound) directed at providing symptomatic relief may only achieve short-term results.[34,35] When symptomatic, not functional, outcomes are the patient's only goal, incomplete healing, chronic pain, and overtreatment often result.[34,35] This

Table 5.2. Soft Tissue Tenderness Grading Scheme[29,30]*

Grade 0–no tenderness
Grade I–tenderness with no physical response
Grade II–tenderness with grimace and/or flinch
Grade III–tenderness with withdrawal (+Jump sign)
Grade IV–withdrawal to non-noxious stimuli (i.e., superficial palpation, pin prick, gentle percussion)†

*Adapted from Wolfe et al[29] and Hubbard et al.[30]
†In noninjured tissue, a sign of neuropathic pain.

common situation is the albatross of employers and insurance companies alike.

The "sports medicine" approach, which measures functional impairment and uses active exercise to rehabilitate injured tissues, is recognized as the "standard of care" for soft tissue injuries.[2,32,36] This active approach is better suited to alleviating pain, completing soft tissue healing, and preventing reoccurrences.

The FCE should be mandatory for any patient still experiencing pain after 6 to 7 weeks (see Chapter 21).[1] The FCE is composed of measurable functional tests and complements previously described questionnaires (see Chapter 4). The functional tests measure flexibility, strength, coordination, endurance, aerobic capacity, posture, and balance.

The FCE identifies intrinsic impairments in the individual. Often, the extrinsic demands of the work environment are the overloading or injurious factor. A work capacity evaluation (WCE) or job analysis may be required to identify such potential sources of repetitive overload or injury. The combination of an FCE, a job analysis, and a WCE will help to identify return-to-work outcomes and specific ergonomic and exercise instructions for safe sitting, lifting, or other repetitive tasks in the workplace.[37,38]

The focus of the FCE should be on relevant functions that can be safely and reliably measured. Normative data bases, where they exist, are most helpful. Whenever possible, quantification is ideal. The most valid tests are those that most closely resemble the actual way the body is used. Unfortunately, validity is often ignored as evaluators become infatuated with highly technical tests possessing high reproducibility and reliability. Matheson says, "The interpretation of the test score should be able to predict or reflect the evaluee's performance in a target task."[39] If an effort factor can be measured, this information will help to unmask a malingerer. Matheson indicates that the best test is one that is valid, reliable, and safe,[39] Tables 5.3 and 5.4 provide the important aspects of functional tests and the key functions of the musculoskeletal system that are necessary to evaluate.

An FCE does not require great expense of time or money in that it can be accomplished with low technology instruments such as a tape measure or inclinometer. A "low-tech" approach can be accomplished in about 20 minutes of office time. Highly technologic dynametric assessment of low back function has become the gold standard of lumbar spine functional assessment. Because it is reliable and reproducible, it serves as an excellent outcome assessment tool. The validity of a number of technologically advanced tests, however, is questionable. Grabiner et al demonstrated that normal strength measurements alone do not necessarily correlate with

Table 5.4. Key Aspects of Musculoskeletal Function

Static (Maintenance of Posture)
  Posture
  Balance
Dynamic (Production and Control of Movement)
  Mobility/flexibility
  Strength
  Coordination
  Endurance
  Cardiovascular fitness

normal function.[40] Using electromyographic (EMG) evaluation during isometric trunk extension, they demonstrated decoupling or asymmetric lumbar paraspinal muscular activity in patients with low back pain who were considered normal on dynamometric tests. This decoupling was also useful in differentiating pain and nonpain subjects.

The study by Grabiner and colleagues points out that musculoskeletal function involves coordination as well as strength during performance of a specific task. Simply because a patient passes a battery of technologically advanced tests does not necessarily mean their spinal function is normal. The EMG test not only points out the limitations of high-technology dynamometric testing of muscle strength and endurance, but suggests that overly harsh criticism of lower technology evaluations of coordination may be unjustified.

As Lewit puts it " . . . in many fields of medicine the importance of changes in function is now well recognized, whereas in the motor system, where function is paramount, this fundamental aspect is rarely considered. However, the functioning of the locomotor system is extremely complex, . . . and diagnosis of disturbed function is a highly sophisticated proceeding carried out, as it were, in a clinical no man's land."[41]

In the Presidential Address to the Cervical Spine Research Society Annual Meeting in December of 1991, LaRocca criticized his colleagues for jumping to a psychologic diagnosis when they cannot find a structural cause for a patient's persistent pain: " . . . The error here is the automatic leap to psychology. It assumes that all organic factors have been considered, when in reality the clinician's appreciation of the complexity of such factors in often severely limited."[42] Newton and Waddell said, "There is no convincing evidence that isokinetic or any other iso-measure has greater clinical utility in the patient with low back pain than either clinical evaluation of physical impairment, isometric strength, simple isoinertial lifting or psychophysical testing."[43]

At present, the quality of high technology tests is not demonstrated sufficiently to lead to the abandonment of lower technology tests of spinal function. Many low technology ways to identify functional pathology are reliable (see Chapter 8).[44–71] Often, if the musculoskeletal function of a patient cannot be quantified, qualifiable tests may be performed that give insight into valid muscle imbalances, joint stiffness, postural dysfunctions, and movement incoordination.

Table 5.3. Critical Factors for Functional Tests

Valid/relevant	Normative database
Reliable/reproducible	Cost/ practicality
Safe	

In 1987, the NIOSH Low Back Atlas identified 19 tests with significant reliability <.74 Cohen's Kappa and >.79 co-efficients for interclass correlation coefficient [ICC]).[60,66] Moffroid and colleagues found that 23 of 53 NIOSH tests could discriminate between subjects with and without low back pain.[67] They also found that the seven strongest tests together had a sensitivity of 87% and a specificity of 93%. The most important measurements were of symmetry, strength, passive mobility, and dynamic mobility. Rissanen and co-workers found that nondynamometric tests correlated better with pain and disability than did isokinetic tests,[68] They con-

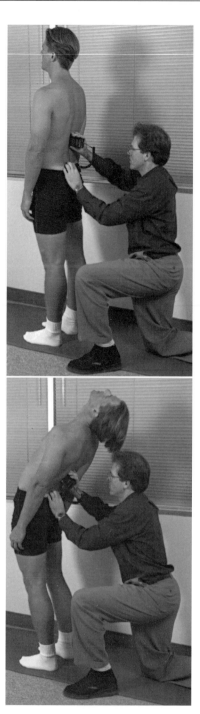

Fig. 5.2. Dorsolumbar extension.

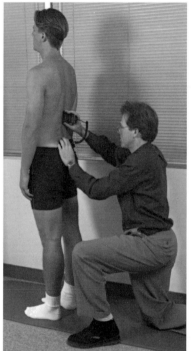

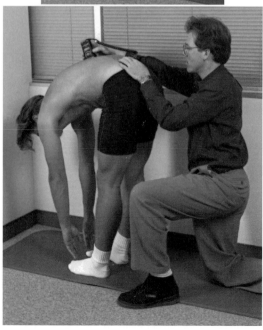

Fig. 5.1 Dorso-lumbar flexion. *Inclinometer used is the Dualer from JTech (324 West 1120, North American Fork, UT 84003).

cluded, "The non-dynamometric tests are still useful in clinical practice in spite of the development of more accurate muscle strength evaluation methods."[68] In another study, Harding and colleagues found a battery of low technology tests safe, reliable, and valid for assessing physical functioning in patients with chronic pain.[69] Alaranta and co-workers showed reliability and established a normative database for low technology tests on more than 500 individuals.[71]

Assessing impairment is crucial to rating the level or percent of impairment a patient has suffered. It is also the only objective way to show progress and to document the need for further treatment. It is absolutely essential in cases involving medicolegal challenge, but it is also useful to document all insurance claims, which are coming under greater and greater scrutiny. As standards are elucidated, these industries will rely on universal outcomes assessment tools, and quantifiable measurement is absolutely key to this process.

Functional Tests

During functional testing, the effects of movement and position on the behavior of pain, the painful or painfree range, and the effects of repeated testing should be determined. Sensitivity to various movements and positions, along with any weight-bearing intolerance, should also be determined. This information helps to establish the functional or training range of the patient (see Chapter 14). Evaluation of posture, gait, and muscle length are not discussed in this chapter, but this assessment is considered important clinically (see Chapters 6 and 18).

Objective, Quantifiable Tests[1]

STANDING

Lumbar Spine Range of Motion
Flexion (erector spinae flexibility) (Fig. 5.1)

- Patient stands with knees straight and feet slightly apart
- Sensors are placed on the sacral apex and T12 spinous process (use skin marking pencil)

---

[1]A videotape and updated examination forms on the functional capacity evaluation by S. Yoemans are available from 800–393–7255.

- Sensors are zeroed and patient is requested to flex maximally, the new angle is recorded
- If hamstrings are tight, patient may bend knees[54]
- Note: if lesser of straight leg raise angle exceeds trunk flexion, then test is invalid.[54]

Extension (Fig. 5.2)

- Starting position is the same as for flexion
- Patient is requested to extend maximally, and the angle is recorded

Lateral flexion (Fig. 5.3)

- Starting position is the same as for flexion
- Patient is requested to side bend maximally to the right/left
- To minimize rotation, patient is instructed to slide fingers along the side of their leg
- Angle is recorded

Quantification

- Final angles are recorded
- Normal values[54]
    Trunk flexion, 60°
    Trunk extension, 25°
    Trunk lateral flexion, 25°

Purpose

- Screening tests for erector spinae (flexion) or quadratus lumborum (lateral flexion) tightness
- Screening test for lumbar joint stiffness

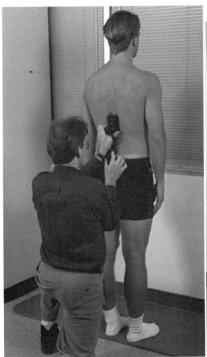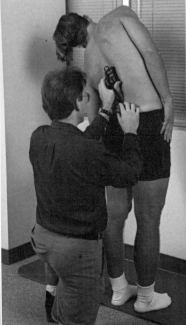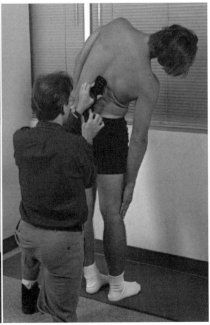

Fig. 5.3. Dorsolumbar lateral flexion.

Thoracic Spine Range of Motion (Flexion/Extension) (Fig. 5.4)

- Patient stands with knees straight and feet slightly apart
- Sensors are placed on T1 and T12 spinous processes (use skin marking pencil)
- Sensors are zeroed and patient is requested to flex maximally, the new angle is recorded
- Sensors are zeroed again after patient returns to upright posture and patient is asked to extend maximally and final angle is recorded

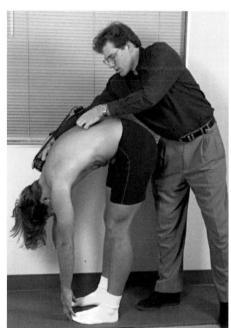

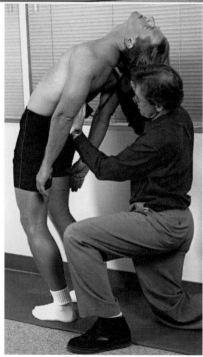

Fig. 5.4. Thoracic flexion/extension.

Quantification

- The two angles are combined for total measurement
- Normal value, 60°[54]

Purpose

- Screen for decreased thoracic spine mobility

SEATED

Trunk Rotation Range of Motion (Fig. 5.5)

- Patient is seated straddling the table
- Patient turns shoulders and torso as far as possible while avoiding trunk flexion or extension (may use stick behind back to help visualize asymmetry)

Note

- If asymmetry of trunk rotation is present
- If less than 90° of trunk rotation is possible

Quantification

- Possible in standing position with trunk flexed as described in A.M.A. Guidelines[52]

Qualification

- Pass/fail
- Fail if less than 90° of trunk rotation is possible
- If asymmetry is present

Purpose

- To identify if asymmetric trunk rotation mobility is present, indicating probable thoracolumbar joint dysfunction

Cervical Spine Range of Motion[54,62,63]

Flexion/Extension (Fig. 5.6)

- Place one sensor at T1 and the other on the occiput (or strap to head with a Velcro strap)
- Patient sits erect
- Patient is requested to flex neck maximally and angle is recorded
- Patient is requested to extend neck maximally and angle is recorded

Lateral Flexion (Fig. 5.7)

- Patient and sensor position same as flexion/extension
- Patient is instructed to side-bend maximally to the left and right; angles are recorded

Rotation (Fig. 5.8)

- In A.M.A. tests, patient is supine; gravity inclinometer is used[54]
- Patient rotates head fully and angle is recorded

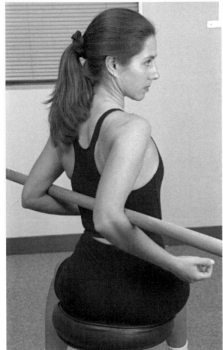

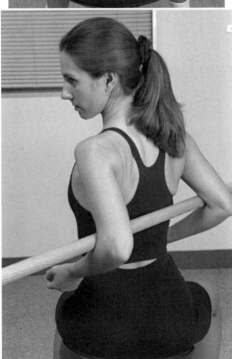

Fig. 5.5. Trunk rotation.

Quantification

- Final angles are recorded
- Normal values[62]
    Flexion 50°
    Extension 70°

Lateral flexion 45°
Rotation 85°

Purpose

- Measure cervical spine mobility

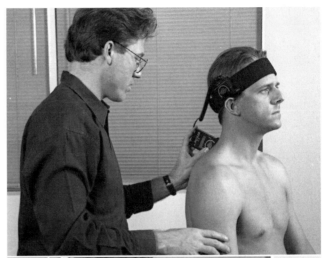

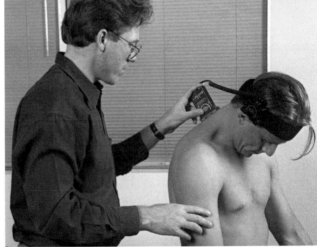

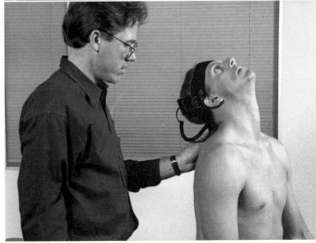

Fig. 5.6. Cervical flexion/extension.

- Sensor is zeroed on table and then placed on proximal or distal end of the femur
- While holding flexed knee toward chest, doctor applies passive overpressure to the tested thigh, and the angle is recorded
- With thigh passively extended, re-zero inclinometer on thigh and then record knee angle by placing sensor on distal end of tibia

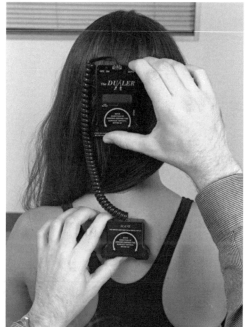

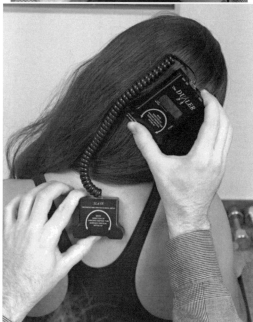

Fig. 5.7. Cervical lateral flexion.

SUPINE

***Hip Flexor (Psoas* [Fig. 5.9],** *Rectus Femoris* **[Fig. 5.10])** *Flexibility Test* [41,44,45,51,57,60,64,66]

Modified Thomas Test

- A firm table is required for accurate measurement
- Patient sits at edge of table and brings knee to chest firmly to flatten low back
- Doctor helps patient assume supine position
- Allow tested leg to extend off table

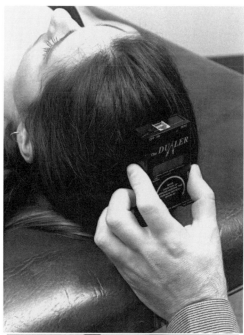

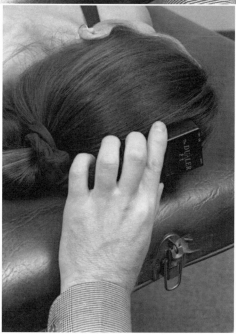

Fig. 5.8. Cervical rotation.

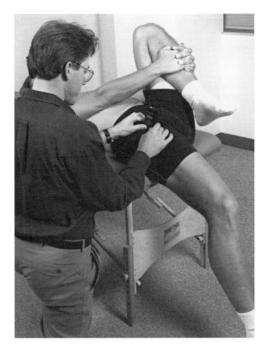

Fig. 5.9. Hip extension and psoas.

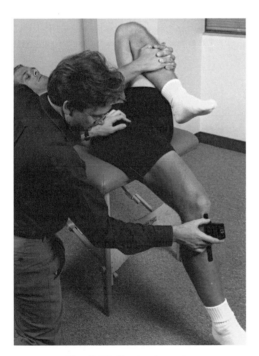

Fig. 5.10. Rectus femoris.

Quantification

- Hip angle is recorded after passive overpressure into hip extension
- Knee angle is recorded with addition of passive overpressure into knee flexion

    Add hip angle to knee angle to obtain rectus femoris measurement

- Normal[41,44,57]

    Hip extension −10°

    Knee flexion 90°

Purpose

- Identify psoas shortening
- Identify rectus femoris shortening (normal is 90° knee flexion)
- If hip flexes without knee extension or thigh abduction (psoas)
- If hip flexes with knee extension (rectus femoris)
- If hip flexes with thigh abduction (TFL)

Note

Wang et al[44] test the psoas by extending the hip while keeping the knee extended. They measure the rectus femoris by extending the hip with the knee bent at a 90° angle. For both tests, they place the inclinometer just superior to the patellae.

Straight Leg Raise (Hamstring Flexibility) Test (Fig. 5.11)[44,45,51,54,58,60,64,66]

- Patient lies supine on a firm table; sensor is placed mid tibia and zeroed (or strapped to lower leg with Velcro)
- Patient's calf is placed in crook of doctor's elbow
- Doctor holds inclinometer in place with one hand while opposite hand stabilizes opposite pelvis (if Thomas' test is positive, place a pillow under opposite knee)
- Patient's leg is flexed without permitting any knee flexion to occur
- Angle is recorded when pelvic rocking is apparent

Quantification

- Record angle of hip flexion
- Normal is 70 to 90°[44,45,58]

Purpose

- Establish hamstring flexibility

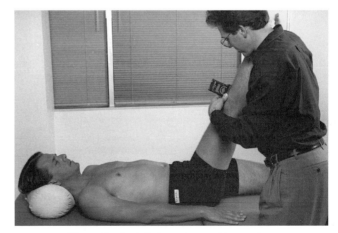

Fig. 5.11. Straight leg raise and hamstring.

PRONE

***Knee Flexion (Quadriceps) Flexibility (Nachlas Test)
(Fig. 5.12)***[45,58]
- Patient is prone on table
- Doctor places sensor at back of midcalf and zeroes it
  (alternate position is on anterior shin after being zeroed
  to bottom of table or desk)
- Patient's knee is passively flexed
- Angle is measured at point just before lumbar spine be-
  gins to extend or hip raises up

Quantification

- Angle of knee flexion is recorded
- Normal is 140 to 150°[58]

Purpose

- Measure flexibility of quadriceps muscles

Hip Rotation Range of Motion[56,60,66] **(Figs. 5.13 and
5.14)**
- Patient lies prone with nontested leg in 30° abduction
  and tested leg at 0° abduction
- Doctor firmly stabilizes pelvis
- Patient's knee is placed in 90° flexion so that sole faces
  the ceiling
- Sensor is placed midtibia (laterally for measuring exter-
  nal rotation and medially for internal rotation) and zeroed
- Doctor passively internally/externally rotates leg until
  opposite pelvis starts to move
- Angle is recorded

Quantification

- Angle of hip internal/external rotation is measured
- Normal[56,60]
  - 38 to 45° internal rotation
  - 35 to 45° external rotation

Purpose

- To quantify hip internal/external rotation mobility

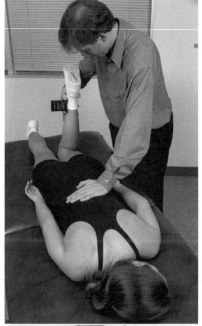

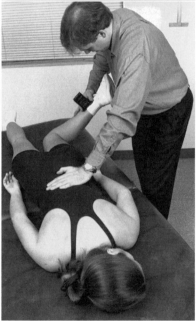

Fig. 5.13. Hip internal rotation.

Note

- A.M.A. guidelines test hip rotation while patient is
  supine, with knee extension and no pelvic stabilization[54]
- May also be tested with patient seated[56,57]
- Supine test with hip and knee at 90° may be used to estimate mobility. Also allows for testing of hip capsule
  integrity (capsular dysfunction manifests with pain in
  internal rotation in this position)

Gastrocnemius Flexibility Test[44,45] **(Fig. 5.15)**
- Patient is supine with feet off edge of table
- Sensor is zeroed to vertical plane and then placed on
  sole of foot

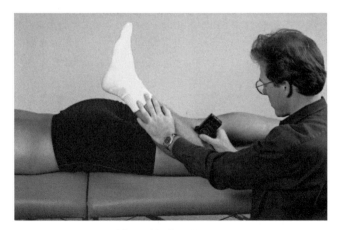

Fig. 5.12. Quadriceps.

- Foot is maximally dorsiflexed, making sure to pull on heel fully (knee is kept in extension)
- Angle is measured

Quantification

- Angle of dorsiflexion is recorded
- Normal is 10 to 15°[44]

Purpose

- Quantify gastrocnemius flexibility

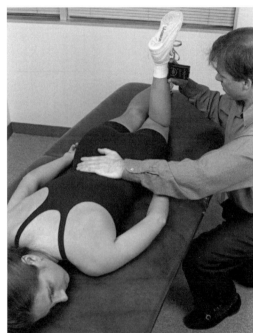

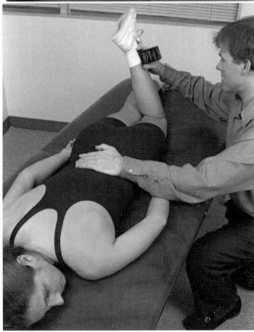

Fig. 5.14. Hip external rotation.

Note

- May also be tested with patient standing or prone

Soleus Flexibility Test[44,45] **(Fig. 5.16)**

- Patient is prone with knee bent to 90°
- Sensor is zeroed to horizontal plane and then placed on sole of foot
- Foot is maximally dorsiflexed, making sure to pull on heel fully (knee is kept at 90°)
- Angle is measured

Quantification

- Angle of dorsiflexion is recorded
- Normal is 25 to 30°[44]

Purpose

- Quantify soleus flexibility

Note

- May also be tested with patient standing

Qualifiable Functional Tests

STANDING

One Leg Standing Test[59,61,69] **(Fig. 5.17)**

- Patient stands on one foot with eyes open
- Foot on raised leg is at knee level
- Arms are relaxed at the side
- Patient fixes gaze on a point on wall
- Patient then closes eyes and attempts to maintain balance for 10 seconds

Quantification

- Record seconds until patient loses balance
  - Reaches out for stability
  - Touches foot to floor
  - Slides supporting foot
- With force platform[59]

Purpose

- Identify need for propriosensory re-education
- Screening test for gluteus medius weakness

Stand to Kneel (Lunge Coordination) Test **(Fig. 5.18)**

- Patient stands with feet about shoulder width apart
- Patient is instructed to perform a lunge to kneeling position
- One foot steps forward with knee flexing to 90° and back knee just touches floor
- Back should remain straight with arms at the side

Quantification

- None, except with Chattanooga lumbar motion monitor

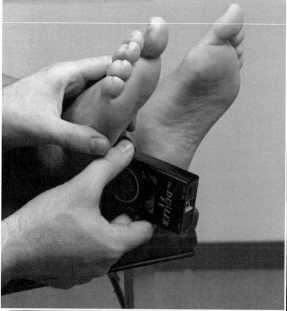
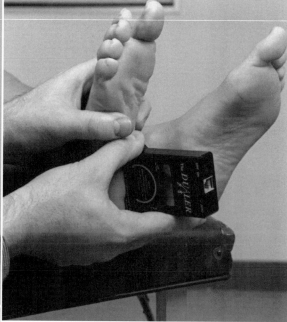
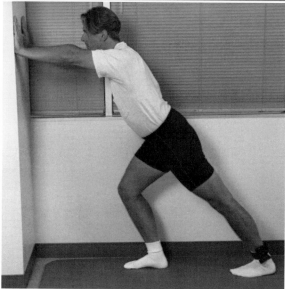

Fig. 5.15. Gastrocnemius.

Qualification

- Pass/fail
- Positive test if patient flexes trunk while performing test
- Also note:
  Balance of forward foot
  Strength of quadriceps
  Mobility of hip joint and flexibility of hip flexors of
  back leg

Purpose

- Qualifiable test for balance, coordination, hip extension
  mobility, and quadriceps strength

Squat Strength/Coordination Test [68,71] **(Fig. 5.19)**

- Patient stands with feet about shoulder width apart and
  is instructed to perform a squat

- Patient should do a deep knee bend with their back
  straight to about 90° of knee flexion

Quantification [71]

- Record number of repetitions patient can perform
- Alaranta et al has published normative database for different ages and genders. [71]

Qualification

- Pass/fail
- Positive test if patient flexed their trunk or cannot reach
  90° knee flexion

Note

- If heels raise off floor (soleus tightness)

Purpose

- Qualifiable test for balance, coordination, quadriceps strength, soleus flexibility

SEATED

Shoulder Abduction Coordination Test [41,69] (Fig. 5.20)
- Patient is seated with elbow flexed to 90° to limit unwanted rotation
- Patient is instructed to slowly abduct arm

Quantification

- Only possible with dynamic electromyography

Qualification

- Pass/fail
- Positive test if scapular elevation or rotation (laterally) occurs in first 30 to 60°

Purpose

- Identify loss of normal glenohumeral rhythm attributable to overactivity of upper trapezius and/or levator scapulae muscles

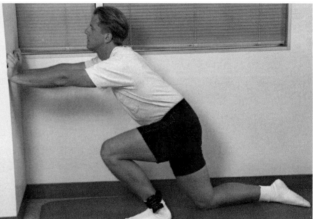

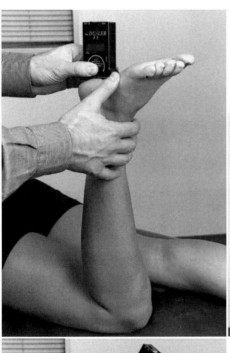

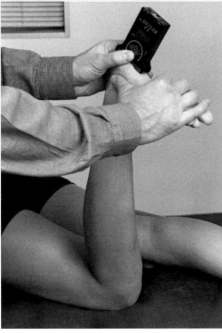

Fig. 5.16. Soleus.

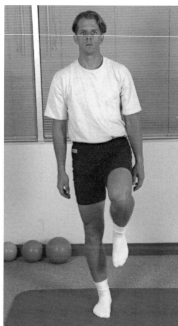

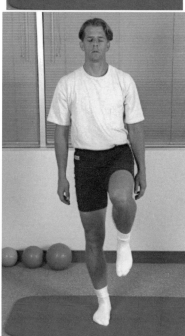

Fig. 5.17. One leg balance test.

Quantification

- None

Qualification

- Grade I able to perform A, B, and C
- Grade II able to perform A and B
- Grade III able to perform only A
- Grade IV unable to perform A, B, or C

Purpose

- Evaluate lumbopelvic coordination and control
- Lower abdominal strength test

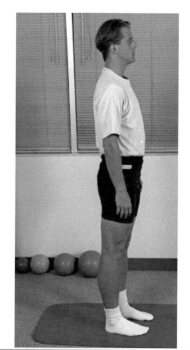

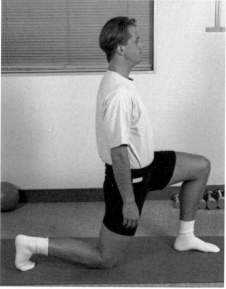

Fig. 5.18. Lunge test.

SUPINE

Pelvic Tilt (Supine Hook Lying) **(Figs. 5.21 and 5.22)**
- Patient is supine with knees bent
- Doctor places hand under lumbar spine and instructs patient to first arch, then flatten low back without raising buttocks off the table (A)
- Doctor may cue movement or offer counter resistance to facilitate coordination
- Patient then asked to hold back flat (posterior pelvic tilt) while sliding legs to extended position (B)[57]
- Patient then asked to raise both legs while holding back flat (legs should be held for 2 to 3 seconds) (C)

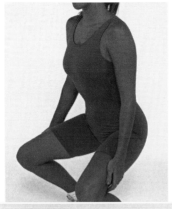

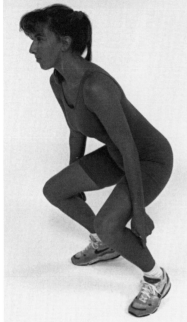

Fig. 5.19. Squat test.

Trunk Flexion Coordination and Strength[41,60,68,69,71] **(Fig. 5.23)**

- Patient is supine with knees bent, arms forward, across chest or behind neck (without pulling)
- Doctor may contact patient's heels or place hand under the patient's lumbar spine
- Patient is instructed to perform posterior pelvic tilt and to raise trunk up until scapulae are off table and then hold for 2 seconds
- Patient should hold pelvic tilt while lowering back to table
- Patient is asked to perform 10 repetitions
- Last repetition is held for 30 seconds

Note

- If heels rise off table (positive test)
- If cannot maintain pelvic tilt (positive test)
- If excessive shaking occurs
- If head is forward of trunk

Quantification

- Alaranta determined a normative database for both genders and most age groups.[71] Test is performed holding down both feet and recording number of repetitions until failure.

Qualification

- Pass/fail
- Fail if unable to perform 10 repetitions without heels or lumbar spine rising off table

Purpose

- Quantify rectus abdominus strength/endurance and coordination

Head/Neck Flexion Strength/Coordination Test[41,70,72] **(Fig. 5.24)**

- Patient is supine and is instructed to bring chin to chest Back of head should be only 1 to 2 cm off of table
- Overpressure may be added at end point

Note

- If chin juts forward during movement
- If shaking occurs during movement
- If chin jutting or shaking occurs with overpressure added

Quantification[70,72]

- Strain gauge may be used[72]
- Record time patient can hold a position with head 1 cm off the table and maintaining constant force of the head into a pressure cuff[70]

Qualification

- Pass/fail
- Fail if chin juts forward during movement
- Fail if cannot hold head just 1 to 2 cm off of table but raises up further

Purpose

- To identify if neck flexor weakness or incoordination is present
- In particular, to identify if deep neck flexors are weak and sternocleidomastoid (SCM) muscle is overactive

Sternocleidomastoid Strength Test **(Fig. 5.25)**

- Patient is supine and is asked to rotate head to one side
- Then to raise head up while maintaining rotation and hold for 2 to 3 seconds

Note

- If can reach full rotation
- If cannot maintain rotation while lifting head
- If cannot lift head

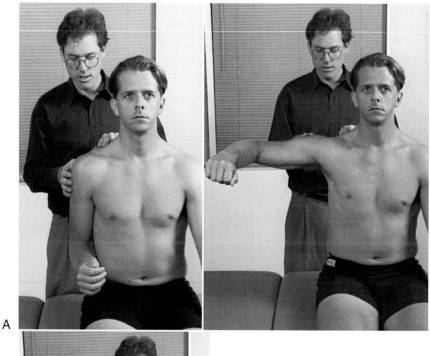

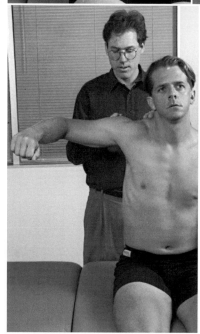

Fig. 5.20. Shoulder abduction test. Correct (A and B) and incorrect (C).

Quantification

- None

Qualification

- Pass/fail
- Fail if cannot lift head or maintain head rotation
- Grading
  I-Normal
  II-Head is lifted, but without full rotation or it cannot be maintained for 3 seconds
  III-Head cannot be lifted

Purpose

- To identify weakness of SCM muscles
  Respiration Coordination Test[41] **(Fig. 5.26)**
- Supine patient is asked to take in a deep breath

Note

- Doctor observes for excessive chest breathing
- Also notes lateral chest excursion
- Note if scalene muscles are visibly active during respiration

Quantification

- None

Qualification

- Pass/fail
- Fail if chest raises more than abdomen

Purpose

- To identify presence of paradoxic breathing (chest breathing predominates over diaphragm)

SIDE LYING

Hip Abduction (Gluteus Medius, TFL, QL) Coordination Test [41,66] (Fig. 5.27)
- Patient side lying with lower knee flexed and upper leg extended
- Pelvis placed in slightly untucked position

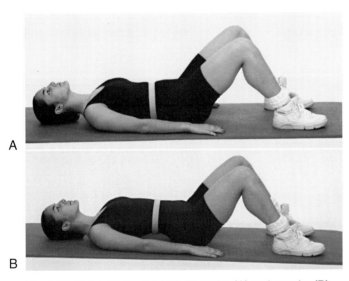

Fig. 5.21. Pelvic tilt (hook lying). Posterior **(A)** and anterior **(B).**

Concentric Test

- Upper leg is raised into abduction and held for 2 seconds
  Note
  - If patient can raise leg
  - Shaking or twisting
  - Any hip flexion or hip external rotation
  - Excessive hip hiking
  - Posterior rotation of upper ilium
  Quantification
  - Only with dynamic electromyography
  Qualification
  - Pass/fail
  - Fail if cannot abduct leg without hip flexion, if foot raises less than 6 inches, if hip externally rotates, pelvis rotates, or hip hiking occurs

Isometric Test

- Pre-position leg in abduction without flexion and ask patient to hold leg for 5 seconds
  Note
  - If shaking occurs
  - Hip flexion, external rotation, pelvic rotation, or hip hiking (positive test)
  Quantification
  - None
  Qualification
  - Pass/fail
  Purpose
  - To identify coordination of hip abduction
  - To identify tightness/overactivity of quadratus lumborum (hip hiking), tensor fascia latae, and psoas (hip flexion and external rotation), thigh adductors (limited abduction range), and piriformis (external rotation)
  - To identify poor hip joint mobility (decreased extension)
  - To identify weakness of gluteus medius

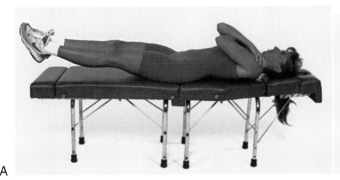
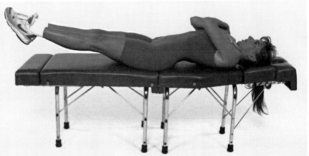

Fig. 5.22. Double leg raise with posterior pelvic tilt. Correct **(A)** and incorrect **(B).**

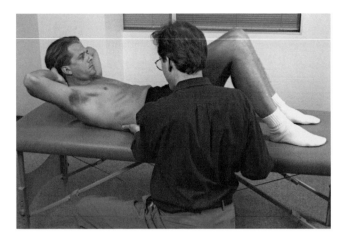

Fig. 5.23. Trunk flexion test.

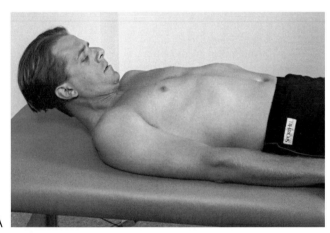

A

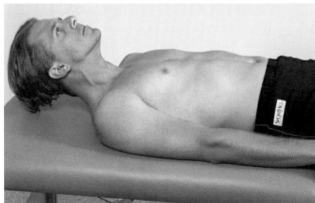

B

Fig. 5.24. Neck flexion test. Correct **(A)** and incorrect **(B).**

Note
- If patient can raise trunk
- If patient twists backward (recruiting oblique abdominals)
- Shaking

Quantification
- None

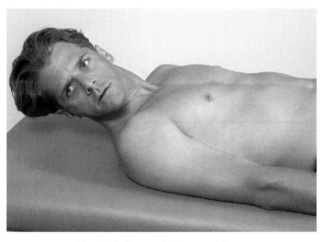

Fig. 5.25. Sternocleidomastoid test.

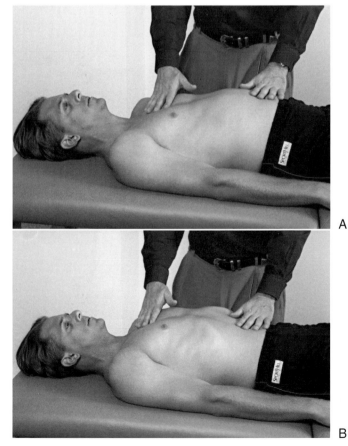

A

B

Fig. 5.26. Respiration test. Correct **(A)** and incorrect **(B).**

Trunk Side Raising Strength Test [65] **(Fig. 5.28)**
- Patient is side lying with knees bent and upper arm fully adducted while hand of lower arm rests on upper shoulder
- Doctor anchors both feet
- Patient attempts to raise trunk off table without using arms for assistance
- Patient is asked to hold for 10 seconds

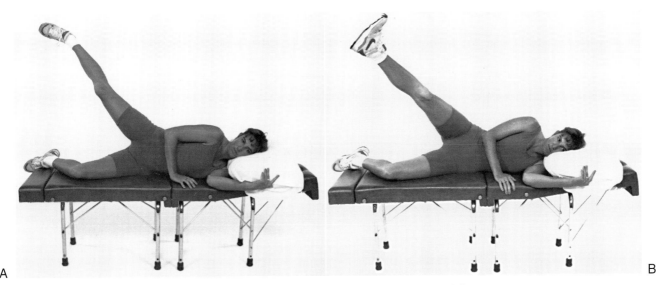

Fig. 5.27. Hip abduction test. Correct **(A)** and incorrect **(B)**.

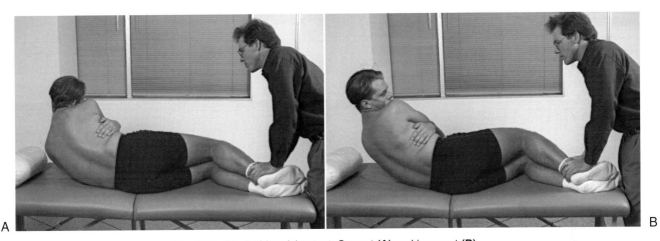

Fig. 5.28. Trunk side raising test. Correct **(A)** and incorrect **(B)**.

Qualification

- Pass/fail

Purpose

- To identify strength/stability of trunk side bending muscles (quadratus lumborum)

PRONE

Hip Extension Coordination/Strength[41] **(Fig. 5.29)**

- Patient prone
- Patient attempts to raise leg into extension with knee held in extended position
- Positive test if erector spinae musculature contracts before gluteus maximus
- Doctor should observe activation sequence of (1) hamstrings and gluteus maximus, (2) contralateral lumbar erector spinae, and (3) ipsilateral erector spinae
- Palpation used only to confirm results

Quantification

- With dynamic electromyography

Qualification

- Pass/fail
- Fail if erector spinae contracts before gluteal maximus
- Record activation sequence or firing order of gluteal maximus, hamstrings, lumbar erector spinae, thoracolumbar erector spinae (ipsilateral and contralateral)
- Note if contralateral shoulder/neck musculature contracts

Purpose

- To identify incoordination of hip extension
- To determine if gluteal maximus is weak or inhibited
- To determine if erector spinae is overactive
- To determine if hamstring is overactive
- To determine if hip joint has reduced extension mobility or if psoas is shortened

Trunk Extension Strength Test [47,68,71] **(Fig. 5.30)**

- Patient is prone with hands behind head and elbows held horizontally
- Patient is instructed to lift chest off table (about 2 inches) 15 times (with 1- to 2-second pause) and hold 15th repetition for 30 seconds

Note

- If patient can raise trunk into extension
- Shaking or twisting
- If feet raise up off table

Quantification

- Strain gauge testing [73,74]
- Alaranta et al described repetitive and isometric endurance tests.[71] In the former, patient assumes slightly flexed position and raises trunk to neutral position until no more repetitions are possible.[71] A normative database has been established. The isometric test is a predictor of recurrences.[47] Alaranta et al reported both reliability and a normative database for this timed endurance test.

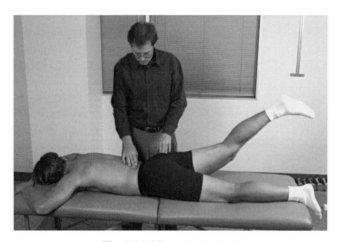

Fig. 5.29. Hip extension test

Qualification

- Pass/fail
- Pass if patient can perform 15 repetitions and then hold position for 30 seconds

Purpose

- To establish baseline measurement of trunk extension strength/endurance

OTHER TESTS

Simple tests that identify whether a certain movement provokes symptoms have been found useful clinically. More advanced approaches have proven valuable for establishing trunk flexor/extensor ratios, lifting capacity, neck flexor strength and endurance, and cardiovascular fitness.

Provocative Testing

Movements that provoke, relieve, or are status quo with respect to presenting symptoms represent a reliable way to test patients.[75] These tests have been used clinically to classify patients into different treatment groups.[76] This evidence validates the McKenzie system of prescribing exercises based on the response of pain to various loading strategies (see Chapter 12). The specific tests adjudicated are discussed in Chapter 18. Being able to provoke pain with active trunk movements in more than one direction has been found to be a predictor of chronicity.[77]

Strain Gauge Testing of Trunk Flexion/Extension Strength

A simple, low-cost protocol exists for quantifiably measuring isometric trunk flexion and extension strength. A ratio of 1.3 : 1.0 extension : flexion is normal for this test,[73,74,78] although reliability is questionable.

Lifting

STRAIN GAUGE TESTING OF ISOMETRIC LIFTING STRENGTH

A simple, low-cost protocol following the NIOSH guidelines exists for quantifiably measuring lifting strength.[52]

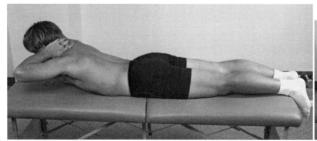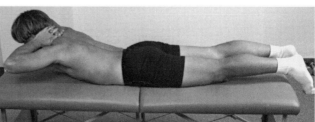

A   B

Fig. 5.30. Trunk extension test. Correct **(A)** and incorrect **(B)**.

ISOTONIC TESTING OF LIFTING STRENGTH

Mayer and co-workers developed the P.I.L.E. test,[53] and Matheson developed the E.P.I.C. test (see Chapter 8), both of which are low-cost, quantifiable methods. They offer standardized protocols with normative databases established.

Neck Flexor Strength/Endurance

Watson and Trott found that decreased isometric strength and endurance of neck flexors along with a forward head posture could differentiate headache from nonheadache sufferers.[72] Treleaven and colleagues described the same distinguishing features of postconcussional headache patients.[79] Treleaven and co-workers showed that observation of supine, neck flexion, as just discussed, was as reliable as the strain gauge for identifying neck flexor weakness.

Cardiovascular Fitness

Simple protocols exist for measuring aerobic capacity using treadmills, bicycles, and other ergometric instruments.[80,81]

High Technology Tests

High technologic quantification of functional deficits can cost from $10,000 to $100,000. Use of equipment from Dynatronics, Lido, Cybex, MedX, etc. can isolate specific movements and results are highly repeatable and reliable. Costs make these units prohibitive for most small private practitioners. Electromyographic units are also cost prohibitive for the average field practitioner, although in medicolegal practices or research settings, such equipment can be beneficial.

Work Capacity Evaluation

It is the duty of the occupational physician to rate impairment, determine functional limitations, and establish the patient's work capacity.[82,83] Translating functional capacity into work capacity has been a great challenge. Fishbain et al outlined the reasons for this difficulty: (1) normal values for functional capacity are needed for the individual (for age and sex and type of worker); (2) many functional capacities are difficult to translate into job skills or traits (i.e., isokinetic abdominal strength); and (3) it is hard to translate functional capacity into a "demand minimum functional capacity" for a specific job or job category.[83,84]

To correlate functional capacity with work capacity, the Dictionary of Occupational Title (DOT) may be used as the standard of physical demands of a specific job or job factor.[83,85,86] Twenty job factors detailed: standing, balancing walking, sitting, carrying, climbing, squatting, lifting, kneeling, stooping, crouching, crawling, reaching, handling, fingering, feeling, pushing, pulling, talking, seeing, and hearing. A standard WCE delineates a worker's readiness to return to work based on their ability to perform job factors.[87]

The DOT lists the job factors that are important for most jobs in the United States.[85,86] According to Fishbain et al, "the

DOT thus, has defined the demand minimum functional capacity of most jobs in the U.S."[83] Jobs are further categorized as sedentary, light, medium, heavy, or very heavy according to the maximum weight lifted during lifting or carrying.[85,86] Unfortunately, strength factors have not been defined for any other job factors. An additional problem with WCE is that a one-time test does not reflect an individual's ability to perform a task over the course of an 8-hour day.[83]

These problems aside, as many job factors as possible should be included in the FCE. Sitting tolerance can be tracked as an outcome. Walking can be evaluated for pain provocation (sensitivity) and examined qualitatively. Lifting can be evaluated as described by Matheson (see Chapter 8). Squatting can be assessed using Alaranta's test or as shown in this chapter.[71] Standing can be evaluated for pain provocation and qualitatively with postural analysis (see Chapter 6). Stooping can be assessed with trunk flexion range of motion tests and by pain provocation (see Chapter 12). Balancing can be evaluated quantitatively with the one-leg standing test.[69] Kneeling can be assessed with the lunge test, and reaching with the shoulder abduction test. Carrying can be examined with specific protocols.[88,89] Pushing, pulling, and other job factors can be evaluated as well.[88,89]

During functional testing and exercise training, it is important to evaluate an individual's performance potential for activities of daily living (ADL), athletic activities, and demands of employment. Many of the traits just described should be objects of rehabilitation that can guide the functional training of patients. An individual who can sit, stand, balance, walk, squat, climb, carry, reach, grasp, kneel, etc. with minimum discomfort and adequate strength, endurance, flexibility, and coordination is an individual who is not impaired. He or she therefore has little or no limitation in ADL or work capacity. Functional restoration should strive to promote the development of these functional traits as the final goal of a successful rehabilitation program.

CONCLUSION

Functional restoration addresses the deconditioning syndrome. It does not require expensive testing or training equipment. Small practitioners in private practice can begin to train patients with customized exercises programs using simple equipment. Measurable functional outcomes are of growing importance both for patient motivation and reimbursement. Directing the focus of the patient toward functional outcomes rather than pain relief is essential to this process. This approach is appropriate in the subacute phase of care as well as with patients with recurrent or chronic pain.

REFERENCES

1. Spitzer WO, Le Blanc FE, Dupuis M, et al: Scientific approach to the assessment and management of activity-related spinal disorders: A monograph for clinicians. Report of the Quebec Task Force on Spinal Disorders. Spine 12(Suppl 7):,S1, 1987.
2. Mayer TG, Gatchel RJ, Mayer H, et al: A prospective two-year study of functional restoration in industrial low back injury. JAMA 258:1763, 1987.

3. Hazard RG, Fenwick JW, Kalisch SM, et al: Functional restoration with behavioral support. Spine 14:157, 1989.

4. Sachs BL, David JF, Olimpio D, et al: Spinal rehabilitation by work tolerance based on objective physical capacity assessment of dysfunction. Spine 15:1325, 1990.

5. Reading AE: A comparison of pain rating scales. J Psychosom Res 24:119, 1979.

6. Mooney V, Cairns D, Robertson J: A system for evaluating and treating chronic back disability. West J Med 124:370, 1976.

7. Melzack R: The short-form McGill Pain Questionnaire. Pain 30:191, 1987.

8. Beck A: Depression: Clinical, Experimental and Theoretical Aspects. New York, Harper & Row, 1967.

9. Zung WWK: A self-rated depression scale. Arch Gen Psychiatr 32:63, 1965.

10. Main CJ, Wood PLR, Hollis S, et al: The distress and risk assessment method. Spine 17:42, 1992.

11. Leavitt F, Garron DC, Whisler WW, et al: A comparison of patients treated by chymopapain and laminectomy for low back pain using a multidimensional pain scale. Clin Orthop 146:136, 1980.

12. Bernstein IH, Jaremko ME, Hinkley BS: On the utility of the SCL-90-R with low-back pain patients. Spine 19:42, 1994.

13. Waddell G, Newton M, Henderson I, et al: A fear-avoidance beliefs questionnaire (FABQ) and the role of fear-avoidance beliefs in chronic low-back pain and disability. Pain 52:157, 1993.

14. Werneke MW, Harris DE, Lichter RL: Clinical effectiveness of behaviorial signs for screening chronic low-back pain patients in a work-oriented physical rehabilitation program. Spine 18:2412, 1993.

15. Fairbank JC, Davies JD, Couper J, et al: The Oswestry low back pain disability questionnaire. Physiotherapy 66:271, 1980.

16. Vernon H, Mior S.: Neck Disability Index. J Manipulative Physiol Ther 14:409, 1991.

17. Million R, Nilsen K, Jayson MIV, et al: Evaluation of low back pain and assessment of lumbar corsets with and without back supports. Ann Rheum Dis 40:449, 1981.

18. Vermont Rehabilitation Engineering Center: Low Back Pain Questionnaire. University of Vermont, 1988.

19. Roland M, Morris R: A study of the natural history of back pain. Spine 8:141, 1983.

20. Lawlis GF, Cuencas R, Selby D, et al: The development of the Dallas Pain Questionnaire for illness behavior. Spine 14:511, 1989.

21. Deyo RA, Diehl AK: Measuring physical and psychosocial function in patients with low-back pain. Spine 8:635, 1983.

22. Evans JH, Kagan A II: Development of functional rating scale to measure treatment outcomes of chronic spinal patients. Spine 11:277, 1986.

23. Tait RC, Pollard CA, Margolis RB, et al: Pain disability index: Psychometric and validity data. Arch Phys Med Rehabil 12:561, 1987.

24. Bigos S., Battie, Spengelere DM, et al: A prospective study of work perceptions and psychosocial factors affecting the report of back injury. Spine 16:1, 1991.

25. Von Korff M, Deyo RA, Cherkin D, et al: Back pain in primary care: Outcomes at 1 year. Spine 18:855, 1993.

26. Dworkin SF, Von Korff, Whitney WC, et al: Measurement of characteristic pain intensity in field research. Pain Suppl 5:S290, 1990.

27. Von Korff M, Ormel J, Keefe F, et al: Grading the severity of chronic pain. Pain 50:133, 1992.

28. Waldorf T, Devlin L, Nansel DD: The comparative assessment of paraspinal tissue compliance in asymptomatic female and male subjects in both prone and standing positions. J Manipulative Physiol Ther 14:457, 1991.

29. Wolfe F, Smythe HA, Yunnus MB, et al: The American College of Rheumatology 1990 Criteria for Classification of Fibromyalgia. Arthritis Rheum 33:160, 1990.

30. Hubbard DR, Berkoff GM: Myofascial trigger points show spontaneous needle EMG activity. Spine 18:1803, 1993.

31. Waddell G, Main CJ: Assessment of severity in low-back disorders. Spine 9:204, 1984.

32. Waddell G: A new clinical model for the treatment of low-back pain. Spine 12:634, 1987.

33. Hart DL, Isernhagen SJ, Matheson LN: Guidelines for functional capacity evaluation of people with medical conditions. J Orthop Sports Phys Ther 18:682, 1993.

34. Mitchell RI, Carmen GM: Results of a multicenter trial using an intensive active exercise program for the treatment of acute soft tissue and back injuries. Spine 15:514, 1990.

35. Andersson GBJ, Pope MH, Frymoyer JW: Epidemiology. In Pope MH, Frymoyer JW, Andersson G (eds): Occupational Low Back Pain. New York, Praeger, 1984, pp 101–114.

36. Frymoyer JW: Epidemiology. In Frymoyer JW, Gordon SL (eds): Symposium on New Perspectives on Low Back Pain. Park Ridge, American Academy of Orthopaedic Surgeons, 1989, pp 19–33.

37. Gundewall B, Liljeqvist M, Hansson T: Primary prevention of back symptoms and absence from work. Spine 18:587, 1993.

38. Videman T, Rauhala S, Asp K, et al: Patient-handling skill, back injuries, and back pain. Spine 14:148, 1989.

39. Matheson L: Basic requirements for utility in the assessment of physical disability. APS Journal 3:195, 1994.

40. Grabiner MD, Koh TJ, Ghazawi AE: Decoupling of bilateral paraspinal excitation in subjects with low back pain. Spine 17:1219, 1992.

41. Lewit K: Manipulative Therapy in Rehabilitation of the Motor System. 2nd Ed. London, Butterworths, 1991.

42. LaRocca H: A taxonomy of chronic pain syndromes: 1991 Presidential Address, Cervical Spine Research Society Annual Meeting, December 5, 1991. Spine 10S:S344, 1992.

43. Newton M, Waddell G: Trunk strength testing with isomachines. Part 1: Review of a decade of scientific evidence. Spine 18:801, 1993.

44. Wang S, Whitney SL, Burdett RG, et al: Lower extremity muscular flexibility in long distance runners. J Orthop Sports Phys Ther 2:102, 1993.

45. Ekstrand J, Wiktorsson M, Oberg B, et al: Lower extremity goniometric measurements: A study to determine their reliability. Arch Phys Med Rehabil 63:171, 1982.

46. Mayer T, Gatchel R, Kishino N, et al: Objective assessment of spine function following industrial injury: A prospective study with comparison group and one-year follow-up. Spine 10:482, 1985.

47. Biering-Sorensen F: Physical measurements as risk indicators for low-back trouble over a one-year period. Spine 9:106, 1984.

48. Troup JDG, Martin JW, Lloyd DCEF: Back pain in industry: A prospective study. Spine 6:61, 1981.

49. Vernon H, Aker P, Aramenko M, et al: Evaluation of neck muscle strength with a modified sphygmomanometer dynamometer: Reliability and validity. J Manipulative Physiol Ther 15:343, 1992.

50. Cassidy JD, Lopes AA, Yong-Hing K: The immediate effect of manipulation versus mobilization on pain and range of motion in the cervical spine: A randomized controlled trial. J Manipulative Physiol Ther 15:570, 1992.

51. Toppenberg RM, Bullock MI: The interrelation of spinal curves, pelvic tilt and muscle lengths in the adolescent female. Aust J Physiother 32:6, 1986.

52. Konz S: NIOSH lifting guidelines. Am Ind Hyg Assoc J 43:931, 1982.

53. Mayer T, Barnes D, Kishino N, et al: Progressive isoinertial lifting evaluation. I. A standardized protocol and normative database. Spine 13:993, 1988.

54. Guides to the Evaluation of Permanent Impairment. 3rd Ed. Chicago, American Medical Association, 1988.

55. Nansel D, Jansen R, Cremata E, et al: Effects of cervical adjustments on lateral-flexion passive end-range asymmetry and on blood pressure, heart rate and plasma catecholamine levels. J Manipulative Physiol Ther 14:450, 1991.

56. Ellison JB, Rose SJ, Sahrmann SA: Patterns of rotation range of motion: A comparison between healthy subjects and patients with low back pain. Phys Ther 70:537, 1990.

57. Reid DC, Burnham RS, Saboe LA, et al: Lower extremity flexibility patterns in classical ballet dancers and their correlation to lateral hip and knee injuries. Am J Sports Med 15:347, 1987.

58. Ekstrand J, Gillquist J: The frequency of muscle tightness and injuries in soccer players. Am J Sports Med 10:75, 1982.

59. Inamura K: Re-assessment of the method of analysis of electrogravitograph and the one foot test. Aggressologie 24:107, 1983.

60. Nelson RM: NIOSH Low Back Atlas of Standarized Tests/measures. U.S. Department of Health and Human Services, National Institute for Occupational Safety and Health. December 1988.

61. Hirasawa Y: Left foot to support human standing and walking. Sci Am (Japan) 6:33, 1981.

62. Mayer T, Brady S, Bovasso E, et al: Noninvasive measurement of cervical tri-planar motion in normal subjects. Spine 18:2191, 1994.

63. Youdas J, Carey J, Garret T: Reliability of measurements of cervical spine range of motion-comparison of three methods. Phys Ther 71:98, 1991.

64. Gajdosik RL, Rieck MA, Sullivan DK, et al: Comparison of four clinical tests for assessing hamstring muscle length. JOSPT 18:614, 1993.

65. Grice A: Lumbar exercises for kinesiological harmony and stability. JCCA, Dec. 1976.

66. Nelson RM, Nestor DE: Standardized assessment of industrial low-back injuries: Development of the NIOSH low-back atlas. Top Trauma Acute Care Rehabil 2:16, 1988.

67. Moffroid MT, Haugh LD, Henry SM, et al: Distinguishable groups of musculoskeletal low back pain patients and asymptomatic control subjects based on physical measures of the NIOSH low back atlas. Spine 19:1350, 1994.

68. Rissanen A, Alaranta H, Sainio P, et al: Isokinetic and non-dynamometric tests in low back pain patients related to pain and disability index. Spine 19:1963, 1994.

69. Harding VR, de C Williams AC, Richardson PH, et al: The development of a battery of measures for assessing physical functioning of chronic pain patients. Pain 58:367, 1994.

70. Treleaven J, Jull G, Atkinson L: Cervical musculoskeletal dysfunction in post-concussional headache. Cephalgia 14:273, 1994.

71. Alaranta H, Hurri H, Heliovaara M, et al: Non-dynametric trunk performance tests: Reliability and normative data. Scand J Rehab Med 26:211, 1994.

72. Watson DH, Trott PH: Cervical headache: An investigation of natural head posture and upper cervical flexor muscle performance. Cephalgia 13:272, 1993.

73. Triano JJ, Skogsbergh DR, Kowalski MH: The use of instrumentation and laboratory examination procedures by the chiropractor. In Haldeman S (ed): Principles and Practice of Chiropractic. 2nd Ed. Norwalk, CT, Appleton & Lange, 1992.

74. Sinaki M, Grubbs N: Back strengthening exercises: Quantitative evaluation of their efficacy for women aged 40-65 years. Arch Phys Med Rehabil 70:16, 1989.

75. Delitto A, Cibulka MT, Erhard RE, et al: Evidence for use of an extension-mobilization category in acute low back syndrome: a prescriptive validation pilot study. Phys Ther 73:216, 1993.

76. Erhard RE, Delitto A, Cibulka MT: Relative effectiveness of an extension program and a combined program of manipulation and flexion and extension exercises in patients with acute low back syndrome. Phys Ther 74:1093, 1994.

77. Hellsing AL, Linton SJ, Kalvemark M: A prospective study of patients with acute back and neck pain. Phys Ther 74:116, 1994.

78. Beimborn DS, Morrissey MC: A review of the literature related to trunk muscle performance. Spine 13:655, 1988.

79. Treleaven J, Jull G, Atkinson L: Cervical musculoskeletal dysfunction in post-concussional headache. Cephalgia 14:273, 1994.

80. Parker DL: A new submaximal treadmill for predicting VO2 max: Rationale and validation. Ann Sports Med, Submitted for publication.

81. Astrand P-O, Rodahl K: Textbook of Work Physiology. 3rd Ed. New York, McGraw-Hill, 1986.

82. Spektor S: Chronic pain and pain-related disabilities. J Disability 1:98, 1990.

83. Fishbain DA, Khalil TM, Abdel-Moty A, et al: Physician limitation when assessing work capacity: A review. J Back Musculoskelet Rehabil 5:107, 1995.

84. Batista ME: Disability evaluations: Expectations of insurers and payors. J Disability 1:168, 1990.

85. U.S. Department of Labor, Employment and Training Administration: Dictionary of Occupational Titles. 4th Ed., Supplement. Washington, DC, U.S. Government Printing Office, 1986.

86. U.S. Department of Labor, Employment and Training Administration: Selected Characteristics of Occupations defined in the Dictionary of Occupational Titles. Washington, DC, U.S. Goverment Printing Office, 1981.

87. Isernhagen SJ: Physical therapy and occupational rehabilitation. J Occup Rehabil 1:71, 1991.

88. Fishbain DA, Abdel-Moty A, Cutler R, et al: A method for measuring residual functional capacity in chronic low back pain patients based on the dictionary of occupational titles. Spien 19:872, 1994.

89. Mooney V, Mathsson LN: Objective Measurement of Soft Tissue Injury: Feasibility Study Examiner's Manual. Industrial Medical Council, State of California, 1994.

6 Evaluation of Muscular Imbalance

VLADIMIR JANDA

Muscle imbalance describes the situation in which some muscles become inhibited and weak, while others become tight, losing their extensibility. Moderately tight muscles are usually stronger than normal, although in the case of pronounced tightness, some decrease of muscle strength occurs. This is called "tightness weakness."[1] The treatment of tightness is not in strengthening, which would increase tightness and possibly result in more pronounced weakness, but in stretching, oriented toward influencing the noncontractile but retractile connective tissue of the muscle. Stretching of tight muscles also results in improved strength of inhibited antagonistic muscles, probably mediated via the Sherrington's law of reciprocal innervation.

The terms *muscle tightness* (stiffness, tautness, loss of flexibility) and *muscle spasm* should not be confused. A detailed differential diagnosis is necessary because each condition requires a different type of treatment.[2] Unfortunately, a precise and adequate analysis is often neglected.

The tendency for some muscles to develop weakness or tightness does not occur randomly; rather, typical "muscle imbalance patterns" can be described. Further, the development of these patterns can be predicted clinically and, therefore, preventative measures may be taken.

Muscle imbalance does not remain limited to a certain part of the body, but gradually involves the whole striated muscular system. Because the muscle imbalance usually precedes the appearance of pain syndromes, a thorough evaluation can help in introducing preventive measures.

Muscle imbalance develops mainly between *muscles prone to develop tightness* (triceps surae, hamstrings, one-joint thigh adductors, rectus femoris, iliopsoas, tensor fasciae latae, piriformis, quadratus lumborum, erectors of the spine, pectoralis major and minor, upper trapezius and levator scapulae, sternocleidomastoideus, short deep neck extensors, flexors of the upper extremities) and *muscles prone to develop inhibition* (tibialis anterior; vasti, in particular the medialis; the entire gluteal group; abdominal muscles [the obliques, however, are controversial]; lower stabilizers of the scapula; deep neck flexors [they tend to spasm, however, which is often misdiagnosed]; mainly the extensors of the upper extremities).

Although muscle imbalance involves the whole body, the imbalance is more evident or starts to develop gradually and predictably in the pelvic region, where we speak about the pelvic or distal crossed syndrome, and the shoulder girdle/neck region, associated with a proximal or shoulder girdle crossed syndrome.

The proximal crossed syndrome is characterized by development of tightness in the upper trapezius, levator, and pectoralis major and, on the other hand, inhibition in the deep neck flexors and lower stabilizers of the scapula. Topographically, when the inhibited and tight muscles are connected, they form a cross. This pattern of muscle imbalance produces typical changes in posture and motion. In standing, elevation and protraction of the shoulders are evident, as well as counterclockwise rotation and abduction of the shoulder blades and a push-forward head position. This altered posture is likely to stress the cervicocranial and the cervicothoracic junctions. In addition, the stability of the shoulder blades is decreased and, as a consequence, all movement patterns of the upper extremity are altered.

The distal crossed syndrome is characterized by tightness of the hip flexors and spinal erectors and inhibition and weakness of the gluteal and abdominal muscles. Again, connection of tight and inhibited muscles form a cross. This imbalance results in an anterior tilt of the pelvis, increased flexion of the hips, and a compensatory hyperlordosis. This situation is a presumption to overstress of both hip joints as well as of the lower back.

The examination of joints must precede muscle evaluation of muscles.

In clinical practice, it is advisable to start by analyzing erect standing and gait. This analysis requires experience, however, and an observation skill in particular. On the other hand, it gives fast and reliable information that can save time by indicating those tests that need to be performed in detail and those that can be omitted. The observer is afforded an overall view of the patients muscle function and is encouraged to think comprehensively about the patient's entire motor system and not to limit attention to the local level of the lesion.

Evaluation of muscle imbalance in a patient with an acute pain syndrome is unreliable and must be undertaken with precaution. A precise evaluation of tight muscles and movement patterns can be performed only if the patient is or is almost painfree. Its use is typical in the chronic phase or in patients with recurrent pain after the acute episode has subsided.

SURVEY OF EVALUATION OF TIGHT MUSCLES

Upper trapezius (Fig. 6.1) is tested with the patient supine, the head passively flexed and inclined to the contralateral side. From this position, the shoulder girdle is pushed distally. Normally, a soft barrier is at the end of the push; when the movement is restricted, it is hard.

Levator scapulae (Fig. 6.2) is examined in a similar manner, only the had is in addition rotated to the contralateral side.

Pectoralis major (Fig. 6.3) is tested with the patient supine, the arm moved passively into abduction. The trunk must be stabilized before the arm is placed into abduction because a possible twist of the trunk might mimic the normal range of movement. The arm should reach the horizontal level. To estimate the clavicular portion, the arm is allowed to hang down loosely and the examiner pushes the shoulder downward. Normally, only a slight soft barrier is felt.

Deep posterior neck muscles can be tested only by thorough palpation. Evaluation of the *sternocleidomastoid* is not reliable because it crosses too many segments (Fig. 6.4).

Hip flexors (iliopsoas (Fig. 6.5), *rectus femoris* (Fig. 6.6) are tested with the patient in a modified Thomas position. The presented modification also allows examination of the *short thigh adductors* and the *tensor fascia latae*.

The patient is supine with the torso on the plinth and the tested leg loosely hanging. The nontested leg is maximally flexed to stabilize the pelvis and flatten the lumbar spine. The flexion position in the hip joint indicates the tightness of the iliopsoas, the oblique position of the lower leg indicates the tightness of the rectus. The inability to achieve passively the hyperextension in the hip joint and the inability to achieve full flexion of the knee (135°) confirms the tightness of the iliopsoas and the rectus, respectively. Limitation of a passive hip

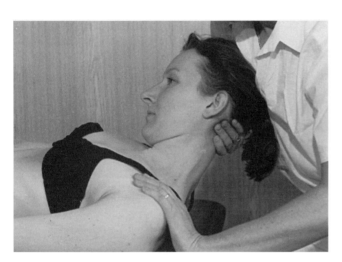

Fig. 6.1. Upper trapezius.

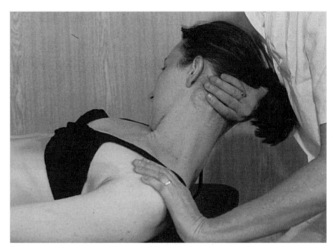

Fig. 6.2. Levator scapulae.

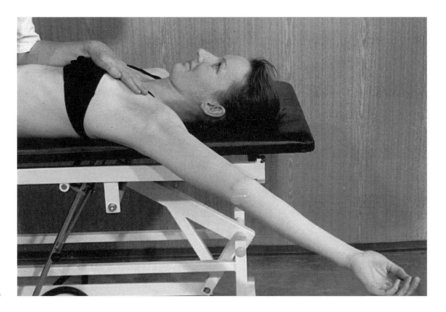

Fig. 6.3. Pectoralis major.

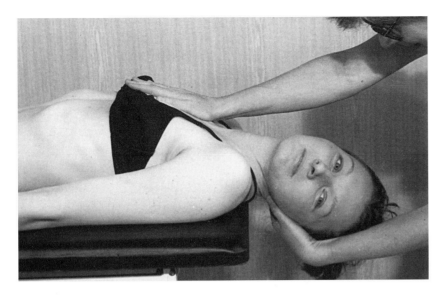

Fig. 6.4. Screening test for sternocleidomastoid tightness.

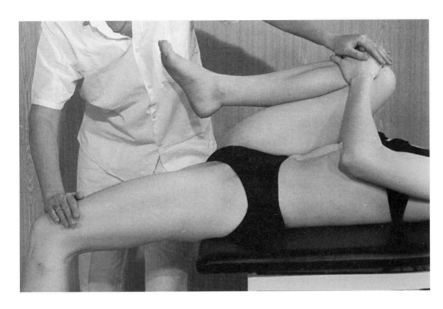

Fig. 6.5. Iliopsoas.

adduction to 15° or less indicates the tightness of the tensor fascia lata (Fig. 6.7); abduction less than 25° indicates shortness of the short one-joint thigh adductors. This test can be influenced by the stretch of the joint capsule, however, and thus the more specific test should be used to confirm the tightness of the adductors (Fig. 6.8).

Confirmation of tightness is clear when excessive soft tissue resistance and decreased range of motion are encountered on application of pressure in the following directions:

Hip flexion—less than 10 to 15°—iliopsoas. A simultaneous extension of the knee joint points out the shortening of the rectus femoris.

Knee flexion—less than 100 to 105°—rectus femoris. Compensatory hip flexion may occur during the test.

Hip adduction—less than 15 to 20°—tensor fascia lata and the iliotibial band. An associated deepening

of the groove on the outside of the thigh is noted.

Hip abduction—less than 15 to 20°—short hip adductors. The tendency toward compensatory hip flexion should be controlled during the test.

Hamstrings (Fig. 6.9) tightness is evaluated by the leg raising test. To avoid the influence of the eventually tight iliopsoas on the position of the pelvis and thus on the range of hip flexion, the nontested leg should be in flexion. Under these circumstances, the normal range of motion is 90°.

Thigh adductors are tested with the patient lying supine at the edge of the plinth (Fig. 6.10). The passive abduction in the hip joint should be at least 45°. Tight hamstrings may contribute to the range limitation. If this situation occurs, bending the knee should increase the range of movement.

M. piriformis is tested with the patient supine. The tested leg is placed with the hip joint in flexion not over 60°, in maximal adduction, and the pelvis is stabilized by pushing the knee in the long axis of the femur (Fig. 6.11). Then, the internal rotation in the hip is performed. Normally, soft, gradually increasing resistance is noted at the end of the range of motion. If the muscle is tight, the end feeling is hard and may be associated with pain deep in the buttocks.

Quadratus lumborum is difficult to examine because too many spine segments enter the play. In principle, passive trunk side bending is tested while the patient assumes a side-lying position (Fig. 6.12). The reference point is the level of the inferior angle of the scapula, which should be raised from the floor for about 2 inches.

Spinal erectors are again difficult to examine. As a screening test, forward bending in a short sit allows observation of the gradual curvature of the spine (Fig. 6.13). More reliable, however, is Schober's test. Any increase of distance under 3 cm should be considered as limitation of the range of motion.

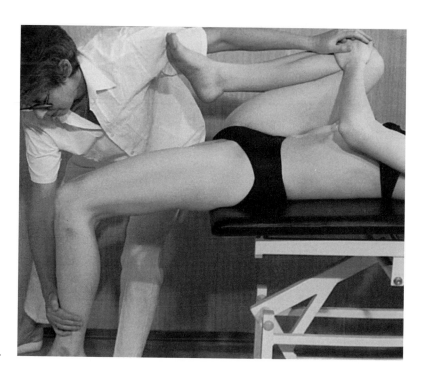

Fig. 6.6.   Rectus femoris.

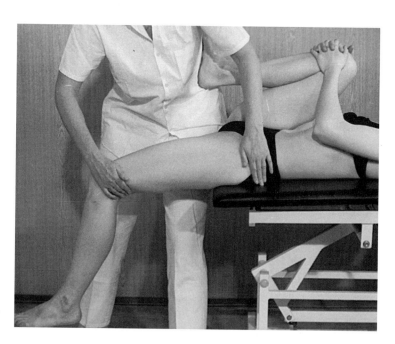

Fig. 6.7.   A screening test for tensor fascia lata tightness.

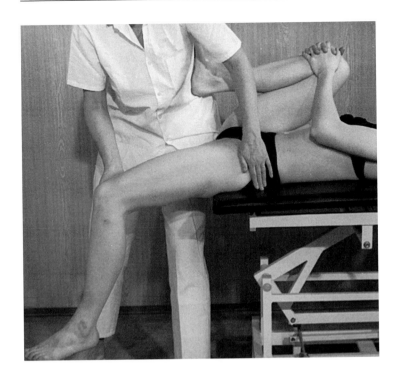

Fig. 6.8. Screening test for the short hip adductors.

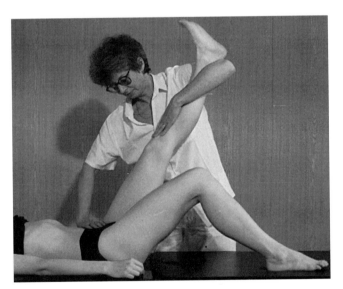

Fig. 6.9. Hamstrings.

Triceps surae are tested by performing passive dorsiflexion of the foot. Normally, the therapist should be able to achieve passive dorsiflexion to 90° (Figs. 6.14 and 6.15).

More detailed description of the tests is available elsewhere.[3]

EVALUATION OF INHIBITED MUSCLES

To examine the inhibited muscles is difficult, because the classical muscle strength testing does not give sufficient and reliable information. The focus of this evaluation is less on the strength of the particular movement and more in sequenc-

ing of activation of the most important muscles that take part in a particular movement and in the degree of activation of the prime movers and their synergists. In this respect, the beginning of the movement is more important than the end of the movement. Poor quality and control of movement can be of major importance in either the production or perpetuation of adverse stresses on the spine. Although the movement patterns are individualized, the typical abnormal patterns can be observed.

In principle, six basic movement patterns give overall information about the movement quality of the particular subject: hip (hyper)extension, hip abduction, curl up, push up, neck flexion, and shoulder abduction.

Hip extension (Fig. 6.16) is examined in order to analyze one of the most important phases (related to low back pain) of the gait cycle—hyperextension of the hip. The patient is prone. During straight leg lifting, the relation between the activation of the gluteus maximus, hamstrings, spinal extensors, and shoulder girdle muscles is observed. The first sign of altered patterning is when the hamstrings and erector spinae are readily activated during the movement and contraction of the gluteus maximus is delayed. The poorest pattern occurs when the erector spinae on the ipsilateral side or even the shoulder girdle muscles initiate the movement and activation of the gluteus maximus is weak and substantially delayed. In this situation, the entire motor performance is changed. Little if any extension in the hip joint is noted and the leg lift is achieved through pelvic forward tilt and hyperlordosis of the lumbar spine, which undoubtedly overstresses this region.

Hip abduction (Fig. 6.17) gives information about the quality of the lateral muscular pelvic brace and thus indirectly

Fig. 6.10. Thigh adductors **(A)**; test if hamstrings are tight **(B)**.

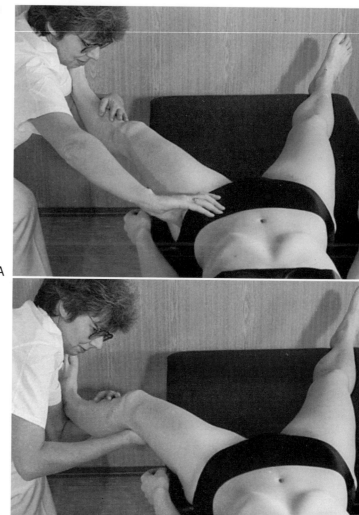

A

B

about the stabilization of the pelvis in walking. It is tested with the patient in the side-lying position. The gluteus medius and minimus together with the tensor fasciae latae act as prime movers while the quadratus lumborum stabilizes the pelvis. The first sign of an altered abduction pattern is a tensor mechanism of hip abduction; instead of pure abduction, the movement is combined as abduction, lateral rotation, and flexion. The poorest pattern of hip abduction occurs when the quadratus lumborum acts not only to stabilize the pelvis, but also to initiate the movement through a lateral pelvic tilt. This pattern again can cause excessive stress to the lumbar and lumbosacral segments during walking.

Trunk curl up (Fig. 6.18) is tested to estimate the interplay between the usually strong iliopsoas and the abdominal muscles. With the patient supine, the test involves active plantar flexion of the feet against resistance. Initially, the examiner observes the patient's spontaneous pattern of sitting up. If the iliopsoas is strong and dominant, curling movement of the trunk is minimal and the movement will be performed with an almost straight back and anterior tilting of the pelvis. The

movement is thus performed mostly in the hip joint rather than by kyphosis of the trunk.

Push up (Fig. 6.19) from the prone position gives information about the quality of stabilization of the shoulder blade. If stabilization is impaired, the scapula glides over the thorax, shifting upward and/or rotates, and/or winging of the scapula occurs.

Head flexion (Fig. 6.20) is tested with the patient supine. The subject is requested to raise the head slowly in the usual way. If the deep neck flexors are weak and the sternocleidomastoideus is strong, the jaw juts forward at the beginning of the movement with hyperextension in the cervicocranial junction. The test provides information about the interplay between the sternocleidomastoideus and the deep neck flexors. This information is essential in estimating the dynamics of the cervical spine.

Shoulder abduction (Fig. 6.21) provides information about the coordination of muscles of the shoulder girdle. It is tested while the patient is sitting, with the elbow flexed to control undesired rotation. Shoulder abduction is a result of three components: abduction in the glenohumeral joint, rota-

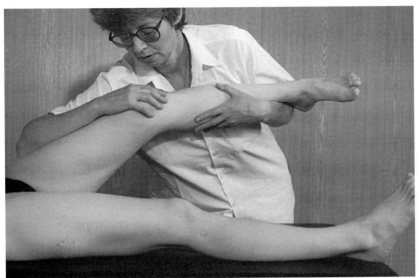

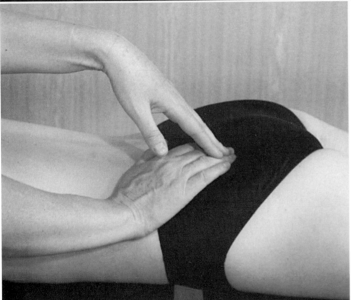

Fig. 6.11. Screening test for piriformis tightness (A); palpation test for piriformis tension or irritability (B).

A

B

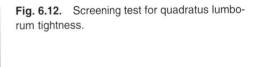

Fig. 6.12. Screening test for quadratus lumborum tightness.

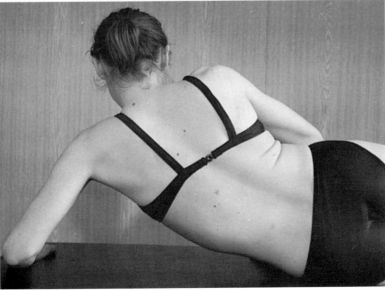

Fig. 6.13. Screening test for erector spinae tightness.

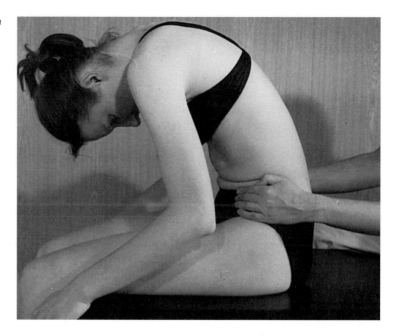

Fig. 6.14. Gastrocnemius.

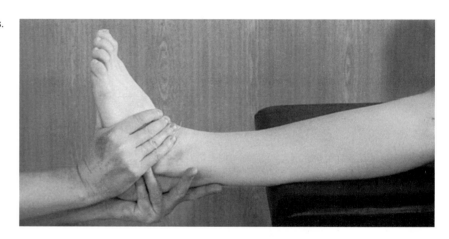

Fig. 6.15. Soleus.

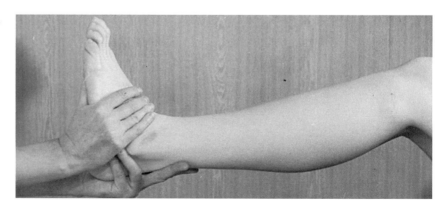

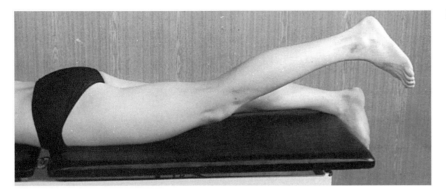

Fig. 6.16. Hip extension.

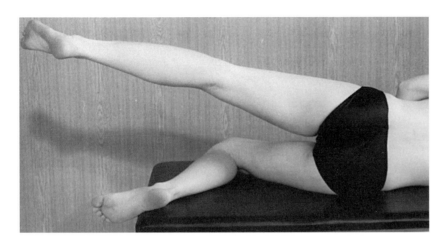

Fig. 6.17. Hip abduction.

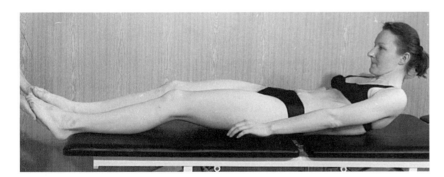

Fig. 6.18. Trunk curl up.

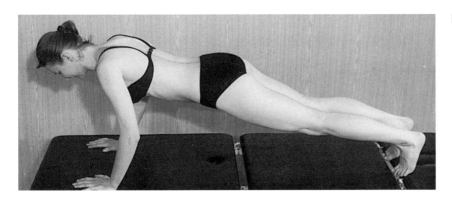

Fig. 6.19. Push up.

tion of the scapula, and elevation of the shoulder girdle. The decisive movement is identifying incoordination is the elevation that normally starts to occur at about 60° of abduction. In an individual with shoulder dysfunction, elevation starts earlier or may even initiate the movement.

ANALYSIS OF MUSCULAR IMBALANCE IN STANDING

In an analysis of standing, an attempt is made to differentiate between possible provocative causes, including structural variations, age, altered joint mechanics, and residual effects of pathologic processes. In this chapter, only muscular changes are described. In muscular analysis, the main concern is with size, shape, and tone of the superficial muscles known to react by hyperactivity and tightness or by weakness and inhibition. The role of deeper muscles

may need to be confirmed or negated in subsequent muscle length tests.

The patient is first observed from behind and an overall impression of posture is determined. Attention is then directed toward the position of the pelvis, because abnormalities of other structures such as the lumbar spine, sacroiliac joints, and lower limbs are, as a rule, reflected in pelvic position. An increase or decrease in sagittal tilt, a lateral shift, an oblique position, rotation, and torsion should be observed. The pelvic crossed syndrome may be responsible for the increased anterior tilt of the pelvis. This condition is usually associated with increased lumbar lordosis. The pelvic twist is usually associated with shortness of the piriformis and/or iliopsoas; an oblique position of the pelvis is associated mostly with leg length asymmetry. Shortness of thigh adductors and tightness of the quadratus lumborum and of the iliopsoas

Fig. 6.20. Head flexion "correct" **(A)** and "incorrect" **(B).**

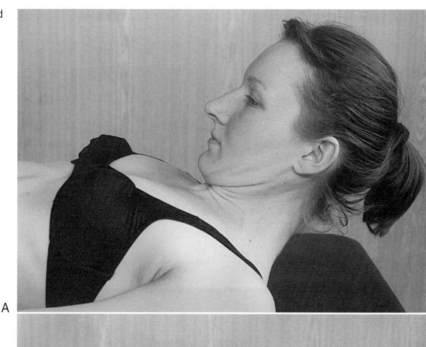

A

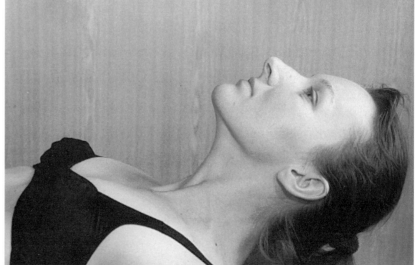

B

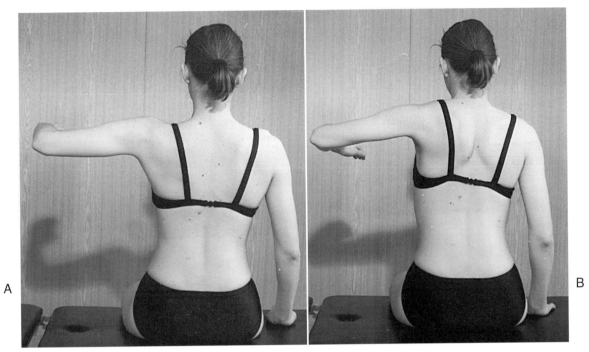

Fig. 6.21. Shoulder abduction "correct" **(A)** and "incorrect" **(B).**

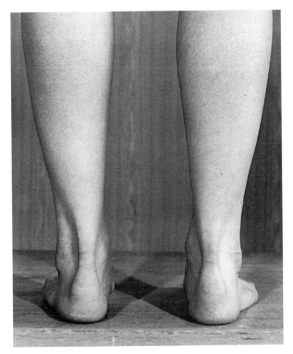

Fig. 6.22. Soleus tightness on the right.

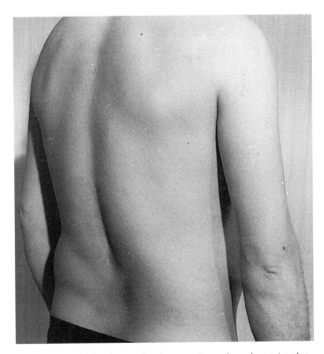

Fig. 6.23. Right thoracolumbar erector spinae hypertrophy.

shorten the leg, whereas tightness of the piriformis makes the leg longer.

Next, the shape, size, and tone of the buttock are observed. Usually, the gluteus is hypotonic and inhibited on the side where the sacroiliac joint is blocked.

The hamstrings are usually well developed, but it is important to look at their bulk relative to that of the glutei, because when the latter is inhibited, the hamstrings often become predominant. This change is readily evident if the impairment is unilateral.

The shape of the line of the medial aspect of the thigh gives important information about the thigh adductors. In individuals with adductor tightness, the one-joint adductors form a distinct bulk in the upper one third of the thigh. The one-joint adductors are, as a rule, short in patients with painful hip joint afflictions.

On the calf, differentiation must be made between the gastrocnemius and the soleus. If the whole triceps is short, the Achilles tendon seems broader, and if the soleus is tight, in addition, the lower leg becomes cylindric (Fig. 6.22).

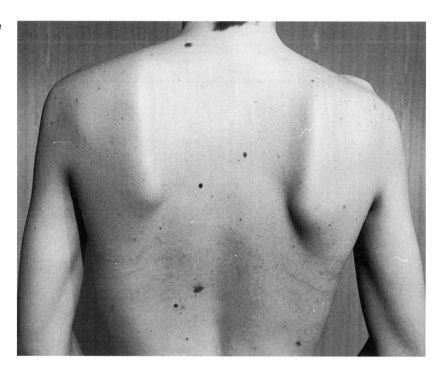

Fig. 6.24. Abduction and winging of the right scapula.

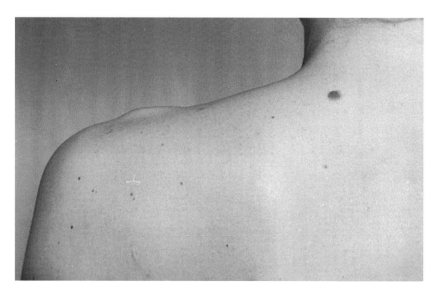

Fig. 6.25. Tightness of the levator scapulae.

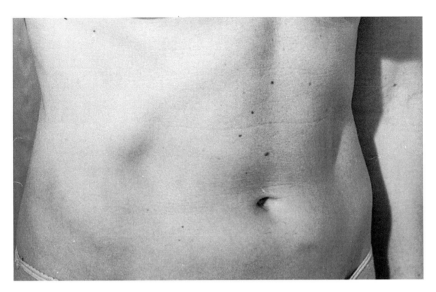

Fig. 6.26. Oblique abdominal dominance.

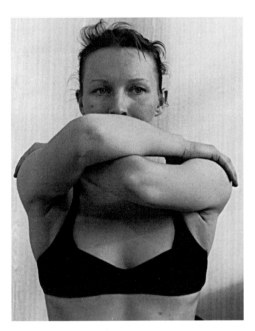

Fig. 6.27. High arm cross.

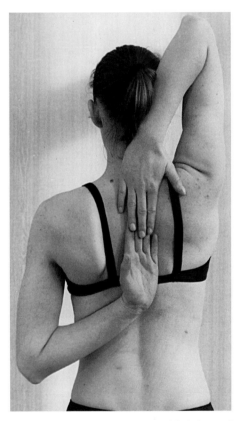

Fig. 6.28. Touching the hands behind the neck.

Careful examination of the back muscles is warranted. The bulk of the erector spinae should be compared from side to side as well as from the lumbar to the thoracolumbar region. There should be no evident difference between sides and regions. Prevalence of the thoracolumbar portions of the rector is a poor sign. It may be indicative of poor muscle stabilization in the lumbosacral region (Fig. 6.23).

The interscapular space and the position of the shoulder blades give information about the quality of the lower stabilizers of the scapula. If these muscles are weak and/or inhibited, slight abduction, elevation, and winging of the shoulder blade are observed (Fig. 6.24).

Tightness of the upper trapezius and levator scapulae (Fig. 6.25) can be seen on the neck shoulder line. In areas of tightness, the contour straightens. If tightness of the levator predominates, the contour of the neck line appears as a double wave in the area of insertion of the muscle on the scapula. This straightening of the neck shoulder line is sometimes described as "Gothic shoulder" in that it is reminiscent of the form of Gothic church tower.

Viewing the patient from the front, the quality of the abdominals is observed first. Ideally, the abdominal wall is flat. A sagging and protruded abdomen may reflect generalized weakness of the abdominals. When the obliques are domi-

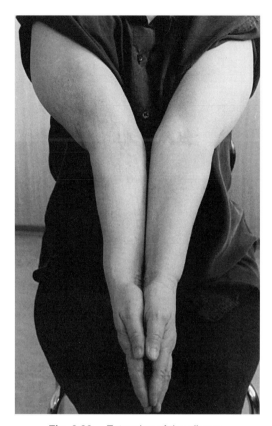

Fig. 6.29. Extension of the elbows.

Fig. 6.30. Hyperextension of the thumb.

nant, a distinct groove is apparent on the lateral side of the recti. This finding indicates a possible decrease in the stabilizing function of the recti in the anteroposterior direction, an important factor for stabilization of the spine (Fig. 6.26).

The two anterior thigh muscles that can influence the lumbopelvic posture are the tensor fasciae latae and the rectus femoris. Normally, the bulk of the tensor is not distinct. Its visibility, coupled with the appearance of a groove on the lateral side of the thigh, usually indicates that this muscle is overused and short. When the rectus femoris is tight, the position of the patella moves slightly upward and also laterally in the case of concurrent tightness of the iliotibial tract.

Tightness of the pectoralis major is characterized by a more prominent muscle belly and thickness of the anterior axillar fold.

Much information can be obtained from observation of the anterior aspect of the neck and throat. Normally, the sternocleidomastoid muscle is just visible. Prominence of the insertion of the muscle, particularly its clavicular portion, is a sign of tightness. A groove along this muscle is an early sign of weakness of the deep neck flexors. Straightening of the throat line is usually a sign of increased tone of the suprahyoid muscles.

Additionally, head posture should be observed. From a muscular point of view, a forward head posture is attributable to weakness of the deep neck flexors and dominance or even tightness of the sternocleidomastoid.

From this brief description, it is evident that neglecting the analysis of the muscular system in standing leads to a loss of a substantial amount of information. Only the main changes or most frequent findings are mentioned in this chapter; however, other less common signs bring additional data.

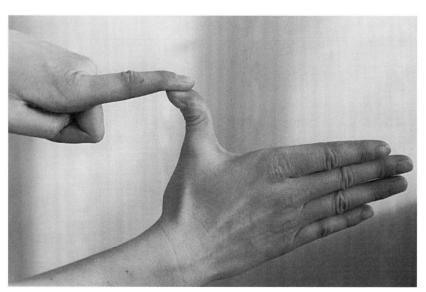

HYPERMOBILITY

Muscles can be involved in many other afflictions. One of the most common situations is constitutional hypermobility. This vague, nonprogressive clinical syndrome, not really a disease, is of unknown origin. It is characterized by a general laxity of tissues, in particular of ligaments. Muscle strength in affected individuals usually is low, and even a vigorous strengthening

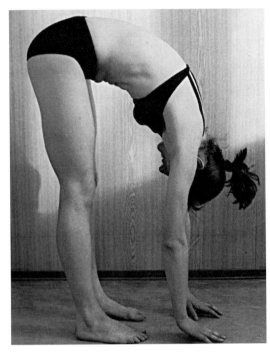

Fig. 6.31. The forward bending test.

exercise does not lead to evident hypertrophy. The muscle tone is decreased when assessed by palpation and the range of movement in joints is comparatively increased. In spite of joint instability, it has not been confirmed that "hypermobile" subjects are more prone to develop musculoskeletal pain syndromes.

Constitutional hypermobility involves the entire body, although all areas may not be affected to the same extent and slight asymmetry can be observed. This syndrome is noted more frequently in women and it typically involves the upper part of the body. With aging, hypermobility decreases.

Patients with constitutional hypermobility may develop muscle tightness as well, although it is never so evident. Mostly, this tightness is considered a compensatory mechanism to stabilize, in particular, the weight-bearing joints. Therefore, stretching, if necessary, should be performed gently and only in key muscles that are supposed to be decisive in a particular syndrome. Because the muscles generally are weak, they may be easily overused and, therefore, trigger points in muscles and ligaments develop easily.

Assessment of hypermobility is in principle based on estimation of muscle tone by palpation and range of motion of the joints. In clinical practice, orientation tests usually are sufficient. In the upper part of the body, the most useful tests are head rotation, high arm cross (Fig. 6.27), touching the hands behind the neck (Fig. 6.28), extension of the elbows (Fig. 6.29), and hyperextension of the thumb (Fig. 6.30). In the lower part of the body, the best choices are the forward bending test (Fig. 6.31), lateral flexion test, leg raising test, and dorsiflexion of the foot (Fig. 6.32).

SUMMARY

Muscle imbalance is an essential component of dysfunction syndromes of the musculoskeletal system. Important ap-

Fig. 6.32. Dorsiflexion of the foot.

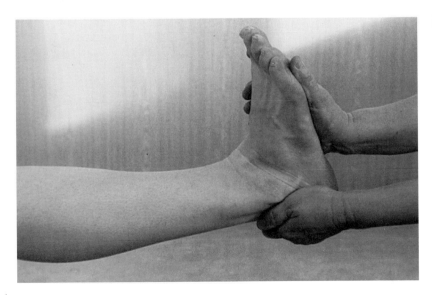

proaches in the overall therapeutic program lie in the recognition of factors that perpetuate the dysfunction and normalization. This fact is true regardless of whether muscle imbalance is considered to cause the joint dysfunction or to occur parallel to it.

REFERENCES

1. Janda V: Muscle strength in relation to muscle length, pain and muscle imbalance. In Harms-Rindahl K (ed): Muscle Strength. New York, Churchill Livingstone, 1993.
2. Janda V: Muscle spasm—a proposed procedure for differential diagnosis. J Manual Med 6:136, 1991.
3. Janda V: Muscle Function Testing. Butterworths, London, 1983.

7 Diagnosis of Muscular Dysfunction by Inspection

LUDMILA F. VASILYEVA and KAREL LEWIT

This chapter is devoted to the art of inspection. On the basis of work by Janda concerning movement patterns and that of Travell and Simons dealing with the musculature, the authors show how much can be gained by inspection. It is no coincidence that findings primarily concern muscles, for they are most important for the shape of the human body. Their hyperactivity and shortening results in visible hypertonus, their weakness in flabbiness. These changes not only are patent but also significantly change posture, i.e., body statics, and, of course, movement patterns.

The aim of this chapter is to show that changes in body shape or statics (i.e., body contours) are so specific and relevant that often it is possible by mere inspection to identify the single muscle involved, movements affected, and related joint dysfunction. This proficiency speeds up the difficult and laborious diagnosis of dysfunction of the motor system. The importance of diagrammatic sketches and photographs is emphasized.

The focus of this discussion is on inspection, i.e., with visual characteristics. If used judiciously, inspection allows us to assess changes in individual muscles, their relative weakness or hyperactivity, and/or shortness. This information is important for the assessment of not only muscle function as such, but also body statics, kinematics, and joint function.

DIAGNOSIS BY VISUAL INSPECTION: AIMS AND POSSIBILITIES

Main concerns when assessing the motor system are as follows:

1. Identifying dysfunction
   a. By analysis of body contours; first, bony prominences and their relative position examined from in front, from the side, from the back, and from above
   b. By comparison of findings with "the norm" (or a model)
   c. By identifying the area of the most important asymmetry
   d. By drawing horizontal and vertical lines through the most important points to locate maximum distortion (see Figs. 7.1 to 7.4)
2. Visual criteria of dysfunction of individual muscles
   a. Attachment points are closer together if the muscle is shortened or hyperactive, or further apart if it is weak

b. Of particular importance if these points are connected by a single joint or belong to the same motor segment (Inspection alone, however, is not sufficient to make a complete diagnosis of dysfunction, e.g., joint movement restriction)[1]
3. Inspection is nevertheless most important in directing our attention to the most relevant lesion

The dysfunction that is most important tends to determine the asymmetry, i.e., deviation from midline, and should be distinguished from compensatory excursions.

Normal Body Statics

The main criterion of normal body statics is to maintain balance with minimum expenditure of energy.[2] The visual criteria must be assessed from the front, side, and back and from above. In all these views, vertical and horizontal reference lines connecting important points can be established for use in measurements and comparison. If body statics are normal, the lines should be parallel (horizontal or vertical).[3]

BACK VIEW (FIG 7.1)

The Spine
   a. The plumb line from the occipital protuberance passes through the spinous processes (at the cervicothoracic, thoracolumbar, and lumbosacral junctions) to the coccyx between the feet.
   The most important horizontal lines are:
   b. between the ear lobes (tips of the mastoid processes) (2)
   c. between the acromia (3)
   d. between the lower margin of the 12th (last) ribs (4)
   e. between the iliac crests (5)
   f. between the posterior superior iliac spines (6)
   g. between the ischial tuberosities (7)

The Upper Extremity
   h. The plumb line from the greater tubercle to the humerus passing through the olecranon and the middle of the wrist (8)
   i. The horizontal line between the major tubercles (the lateral angles of the scapula (9)
   j. between the olecrani (10)
   k. between the styloid processes of the radius and ulna (11)

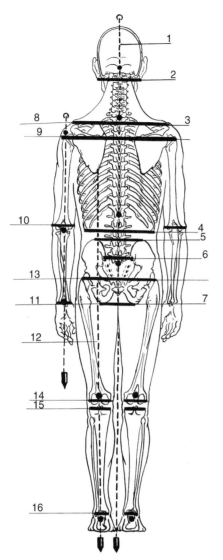

Fig. 7.1. Important reference lines for the assessment of body statics (back view).

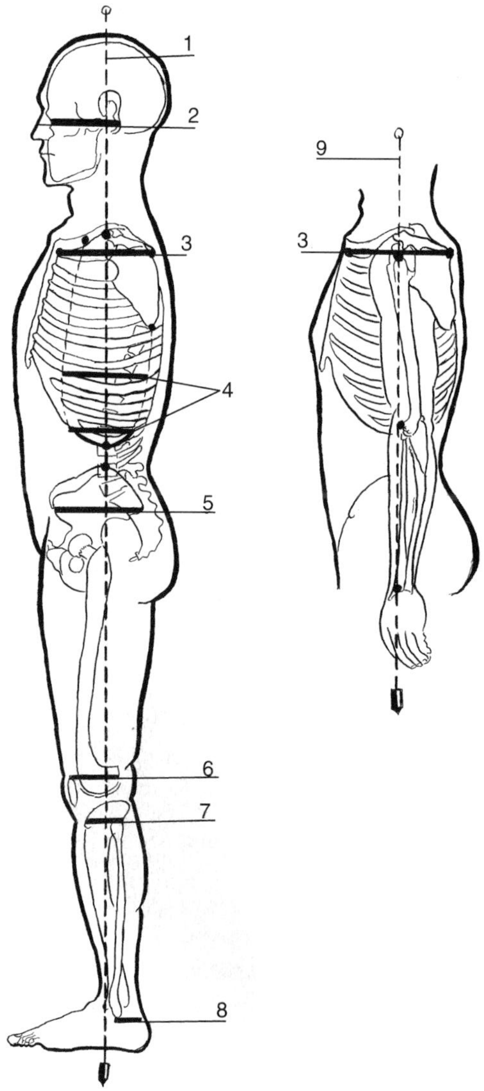

Fig. 7.2. Important reference lines for the assessment of body statics (side view).

The Lower Extremity

l.   The plumb line from the lower scapular angle through the midpoint of the iliac crest between the femoral condyles to the midpoint of the calcaneal tuberosity (12)

m. The horizontal line between the greater trochanters of the femora (13)

n.   between the femoral condyles (14)

o.   between the condyles of the tibia (15)

p.   between the malleoli of the tibia and fibula (16)

SIDE VIEW (FIG. 7.2)

a.   The plumb line from the external auditory canal to the acromion, following the axillar line to the midpoint of the iliac crest, the greater trochanter to the lateral

condyle of the femur, the tibia down to a point a finger's breadth in front of the lateral ankle (1)

b.   The horizontal between the occipital protuberance and the lower margin of the zygomatic arch (2)

c.   The line between the medial end of the spina scapulae through the head of the humerus to the medial end of the clavicula (3)

d.   The horizontal lines connecting two points in the course of each rib: one on the vertical below the midpoint of the clavicle, the other on the vertical from the lower angle of the scapula (4)

e.   The line from a point just below the anterior superior iliac spine to the prominence of the posterior superior iliac spine (5)

f.   The line from the upper edge of the patella to the lower edge of the lateral femoral condyle (6)

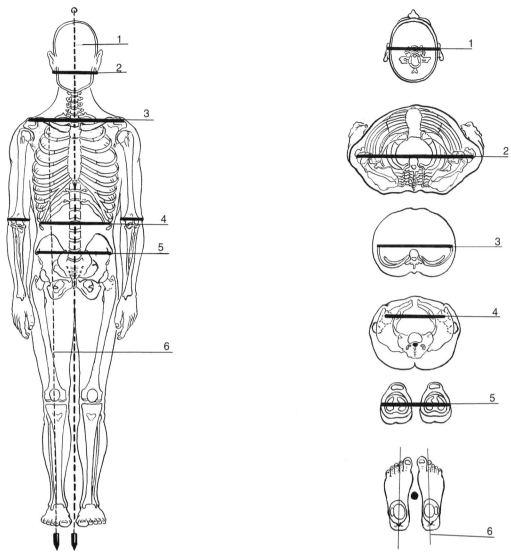

Fig. 7.3. Important reference lines for the assessment of body statics (front view).

Fig. 7.4. Important reference lines for the assessment of body statics (view from above).

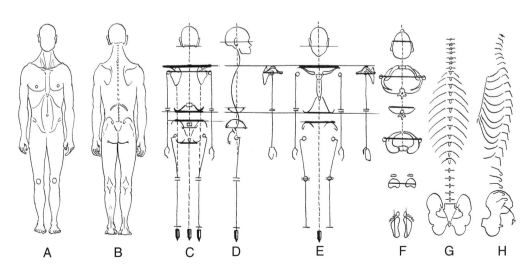

Fig. 7.5. Normal body statics (diagrams).

g. The line from the upper edge of the tuberositas tibiae to the upper surface of the fibular head (7)

h. From the lower edge of the outer malleolus to the attachment point of the Achilles tendon (8)

i. The plumb line from the external auditory canal through the head of the humerus, slightly in front of the ulnar epicondyle to the midpoint of the wrist or the slightly flexed first interphalangeal joint of the forefinger (9)

FRONT VIEW (FIG. 7.3)

a. The plumb line from the center of the forehead passes through the jugular notch of the sternum, the xiphoid, the navel, the pubic symphysis, to midpoint between the feet (1):

b. The first horizontal line passes through the lower edge of the auricles (or the lower edge of the zygomatic arches) (2)

c. The second line through the acromia (3)

d. The third through the lower margin of the last ribs (4)

e. The fourth through the anterior superior iliac spines (5)

f. The plumb line from the midpoint of the clavicula passes through the midpoint of the patella and of the talocrural joint (6)

VIEW FROM ABOVE (ASSESSMENT OF ROTATION) (FIG. 7.4)

a. The line connecting both auricles (1)

b. The line connecting both acromia (2)

c. The line connecting the anterior ends of the ribs (3)

d. The line connecting both greater trochanters (4)

e. The line connecting the outer condyles of the femora (5)

f. The line connecting the midpoint of the heel with the second toe (which ought to be symmetric in relation to the midline) (6)

Drawn on the basis of the data and illustrations described in this chapter, the diagram in Figure 7.5 represents normal conditions and is used for registration of muscular dysfunc-tion (Fig. 7.5). Typical changes from normal body statics are illustrated in Figure 7.6.

Disturbed Body Statics

The main criterion of static function is that muscles maintain balance with minimum activity. Therefore, visual evidence of increased tension or hypertonus is of great importance. Noticeable signs of muscular imbalance also imply asymmetry, and therefore visual signs of hypotonus and asymmetry of tonus are also significant. Direct signs of disturbed equilibrium, such as a forward-drawn posture or deviation to one side (see Fig. 7.6), illustrate clearly that the patient would indeed lose his or her balance if muscle activity did not prevent it.

Because muscular imbalance manifests in individual muscles and therefore (primarily) in certain regions, but is followed by compensatory reactions in other areas that restore balance, it is most important to determine which muscle (muscles) and which region are primarily affected and where compensation takes place. Unfortunately, pain related to overstrain may occur in both areas and is therefore a most unreliable symptom. It is logical to infer that the direction in which the body (with the center of gravity) deviates should be an important guide line. The horizontal lines in the illustrations serve as an additional guide to show the direction toward which equilibrium will deviate. If these lines are not parallel owing to spinal curvature, the side where these lines diverge, or in the case of several curvatures where the sum of divergence is greatest, corresponds to the direction toward which the patient would fall if muscular contraction did not prevent it.

Disturbed Statics in Dysfunction of Individual Muscles or Muscle Groups[4]

These criteria in a *shortened muscle* include attachment points that are closer together than normal and increased prominence of its contours owing to hypertonus. In a *weakened muscle,* criteria include increased distance between

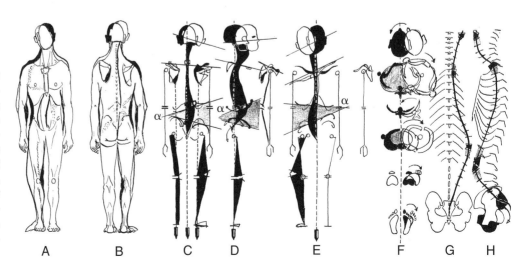

Fig. 7.6. Abnormal body statics (diagrams). a,b: Muscle dysfunction. Dotted lines stand for dysfunctional muscles. c–f: Disturbed body statics. Black, deviation from the vertical; gray, divergence of horizontal lines; angle α, open in the direction of body deviation. g, h: Joint dysfunction. Black, restriction; gray, hypermobility (see also Fig. 7.36).

A   B   C   D   E   F   G   H

attachment points and flattening of its contours owing to hypotonus.

The imbalance just described results in the asymmetric position of the salient parts of the bones to which the muscles attach. It also goes hand in hand with articular dysfunction.[1] Those cases in which the attachment points were closer together were associated with a preponderance of movement restriction. Hypermobility was found in neighboring segments of joints where movement restriction was found.

Diagnostic Criteria of Body Statics

These criteria include the following:

- The direction in which the body deviates from the norm
- Diagnosis of the region (muscles) primarily affected
- Diagnosis of the individual muscles affected
- Diagnosis of the individual joint dysfunction in the region of affected muscles and attachment points
- Diagnosis of hypermobility, in particular in the vicinity of movement restriction

Assessment of Disturbed Motor Patterns

NORMAL LOCAL MOTOR PATTERNS[6]

The criteria for normal local patterns, such as in one extremity joint or concerning one section of the spinal column, are as follows:

- Movement is carried out exactly in the desired direction
- Movement is smooth and of a constant speed
- Movement follows the shortest possible path
- Movement is carried out in its full range

- Direction of movement is determined mainly by the agonists and also by the synergists
- Precision of movement is guaranteed by the neutralizers
- Fixation of attachment points is guaranteed by fixator muscles, excluding motion in the vicinity
- Smoothness of movement is guaranteed by the eccentric contraction of the antagonists

DISTURBED LOCAL MOTOR PATTERNS BECAUSE OF SHORTENED MUSCLES

The shortened muscle is also hyperactive as a rule. Its irritation threshold is lowered and therefore it contracts sooner than normal; i.e., the order in which muscles contract in the normal pattern is altered. If, therefore, the agonist is shortened, the relationship to the synergists, neutralizers, fixators, and antagonists is out of balance and the local pattern, i.e., the direction, smoothness, speed, and range of motion, are disturbed in a characteristic way. (See subsequent section for discussion concerning visual assessment of individual muscles.)

If the synergists, neutralizers, and fixators are shortened, it is again the short synergists, neutralizer, or fixators that contract first and distort the pattern. If the antagonist is shortened, the entire pattern is altered and substitution occurs (see discussion concerning weak muscles in subsequent section).

DISTURBED LOCAL MOTOR PATTERNS BECAUSE OF A WEAKENED MUSCLE

The threshold of irritation in the weakened muscle is raised and therefore, as a rule, the muscle contracts later

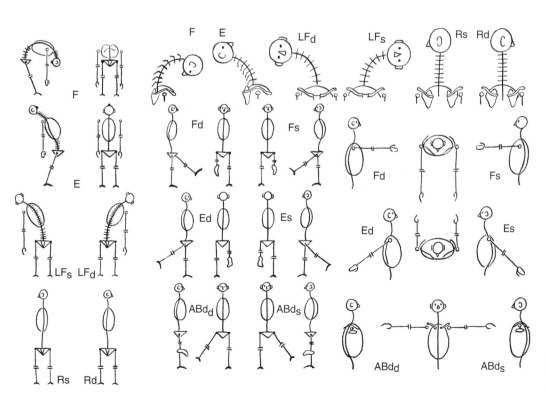

Fig. 7.7. Normal movement patterns (diagrams).

than normal or, in some cases, not at all. Hence, the order in which muscles contract is altered, as is coordination. The most characteristic feature, however, is substitution, altering the entire pattern. This change is particularly evident if the weak muscle is the agonist. If, however, the neutralizers and/or the fixators are weak, the basic pattern persists but there is accessory motion; if the antagonists are weak, the range of movement is increased.

COMPLEX MOTOR PATTERNS[7]

The criteria for complex motor patterns are as follows:

- Typical synkinesis in distant regions with primary movement in other parts of the motor system
- Smooth propagation of motion from one region to other parts of the body
- A constant (optimal) relationship between the speed of motion initiated in one region with the speed of synkinesis in other regions
- If local patterns are changed, synkinetic patterns remain intact, as long as substitution does not take place

The results of assessment of local motor patterns are given in Figure 7.7. Deviation from the normal patterns can be registered on the diagrams.

For the sake of clarity, the findings in the figures to follow are exaggerated. The most important probable objection to such exaggeration is that it is rare under clinical conditions that only one muscle is dysfunctional, although one muscle is usually the most affected and relevant. Hence, the results are artificial, in a way. We believe, however, that it is impossible to understand the complex clinical picture without knowledge of the significance of a single shortened or weakened muscle.

VISUAL CRITERIA OF DYSFUNCTION OF INDIVIDUAL MUSCLES

A key element in diagnosis is a set of tests that show weakness on the one hand and tightness on the other.[6] In this section, we show how both shortened muscles and weak muscles can change body posture and in particular the contours of the human body. We also provide the visual criteria of some muscles prone to such change that are noted frequently in clinical practice.

In this chapter, certain key muscles that are prone to shortening are addressed. They are the biceps femoris, the tensor fasciae latae, the piriformis, the quadratus lumborum, the upper trapezius, and the sternocleidomastoideus.[6] Muscles with a tendency to weakness that are discussed are the gluteus maximus and the rectus abdominis. A more complete list is given in Chapters 2 and 6.

In the following illustrations, the normal position is in black and the altered position, the result of dysfunction, is in white. Where the abnormal hides the normal, the normal is drawn by a dotted line. Again, for the sake of clarity, the changes have purposefully been exaggerated.

Gluteus Maximus

GENERAL CHARACTERISTICS

This muscle has a tendency to be inhibited or weak.

FUNCTIONAL ANATOMY

Points of attachment:	Origin	Insertion
	1. Upper part of the innominate	1. The superficial fibers cross over the greater trochanter and attach to the iliotibial tract.
	2. Lower part of the sacrum	
	3. Coccyx-lateral surface	
	4. Lumbodorsal aponeurosis	2. The lower part of the fibers attach at the gluteal tuberosity of the femur
	5. Sacrotuberous ligament	
	6. The fascia of the gluteus medius	

DISTURBED STATICS BECAUSE OF WEAKNESS (FIG. 7.8)

	Origin	Insertion
Direction of pull at the attachment points on contraction:	1. Upper part of the innominate dorsomediocaudally	1. Proximal part of the thigh dorsolateral
	2. Sacrum: lower part mediodorsocaudally	
	3. Coccyx: mediodorsocaudally	
Possible change in position of anatomic structures (owing to weakness):	1. Innominate: anteversion, external rotation	1. Flexion, adduction, rotation of the thigh at the hip joint
	2. Sacrum: anteversion, ipsilateral flexion, and rotation to the same side	2. Knee: flexion, adduction and internal rotation
	3. Lumbar spine: hyperlordosis with scoliosis toward the ipsilateral side	3. Hip joint: flexion adduction, internal rotation of the thigh
	4. Lower part of the sacrum and coccyx: contralateral deviation	
Joint mobility:	Sacroiliac joint: Ipsilateral movement	

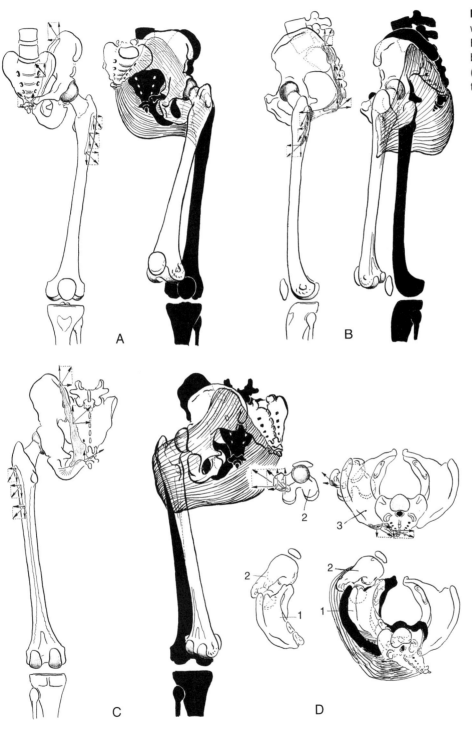

Fig. 7.8. Disturbed statics in a weakened gluteus maximus. Front view (a) side view (b), back view (c) view from above (d); 1, pelvis; 2, femur; 3, gluteus maximus.

A

B

C

D

CHANGES IN BODY OUTLINE BECAUSE OF WEAKNESS (FIG. 7.9)

	Origin	Insertion
Front view:	1. Increase in transverse diameter of pelvis, mainly in caudal portion	1. Increase in transverse diameter of hip.
	2. Upper margin of ilium is lowered, anterior superior iliac is depressed	2. Greater trochanter is displaced upward and protrudes
	3. Ramus sup. os pubis is lowered and protrudes anteriorly	3. Valgosity at knee; patella is shifted medially
Side view:	1. Buttocks protrude posteriorly and pelvis is flattened anteriorly	1. Anterior shift mainly of distal part of thigh, forward protrusion of knee
	2. Increased lumbosacral lordosis	2. Slight flexion of all major joints of extremity
Back view:	1. Increase in vertical diameter of ipsilateral buttock	
	2. Gluteal line is lowered	
	3. P.S.I.S. is closer to sacrum	

DISTURBED MOTOR PATTERNS BECAUSE OF WEAKNESS

If there is weakness of this muscle, the hamstrings and lumbar extensors become more active (see Fig. 7.12).

Biceps Femoris
GENERAL CHARACTERISTICS

This muscle has a tendency to become shortened and overactive.

FUNCTIONAL ANATOMY

Points of attachment:	Origin	Insertion
	1. Long head: posterior aspect of ischial tuberosity	1. Long head is joined by short head and together form a common tendon that runs along lateral condyle and establishes a tripartite anchor to lateral aspect of fibular head
	2. Short head: lateral lip of linea aspera of femur	

IMPAIRED BODY STATICS BECAUSE OF SHORTENING (FIG. 7.10)

Changes at the ipsilateral side:

	Origin	Insertion
Direction of pull at the attachment points on contraction:	1. Ischial tuberosity is pulled in caudal-lateral-dorsal direction	1. Fibular head is pulled in craniodorsal direction
Possible changes in position of anatomic structures:	1. Innominate retroflexion adduction and internal rotation	1. Flexion adduction and external rotation of leg below knee (ventromedial shift of distal end of thigh)
Joint mobility:	1. Hip extension (tightening of sacrotuberous ligament)	1. Knee joint: flexion, external rotation, and torsion in relation to thigh, fixation of tibiofibular joint; valgosity

Fig. 7.9. Changes in body outline because of weakness of the gluteus maximus. Front view (a), side view (b), back view (c).

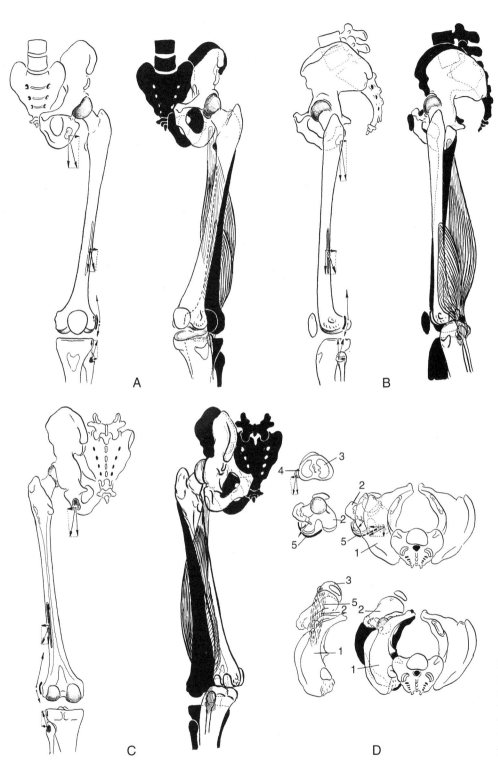

Fig. 7.10. Disturbed body statics because of a shortened biceps femoris. Front view (a), side view (b), back view (c) view from above (d); 1, pelvis; 2, femur; 3, tibia; 4, fibula; 5, biceps femoris.

CHANGES IN BODY OUTLINE BECAUSE OF SHORTENING
(FIG. 7.11)

	Origin	Insertion
Front View:	1. Decreased transverse diameter of upper part of hemipelvis 2. Innominate is lowered and concave; anterior superior iliac spine raised; upper edge of pubic bone is raised and less prominent	1. Increased transverse diameter of lower part of hemipelvis 2. Lateral contour of thigh at level of trochanter is more prominent 3. Knee lies more medial and so does patella; medial condyle protrudes
Side View:	1. Pelvis is drawn forward and its dorsal outline flattened	1. Distal end of thigh is thrust forward and patella protrudes
Back View:	1. Increased concavity of pelvic outline above buttocks and increased prominence of buttock and greater tuberosity	1. Protrusion of medial femoral condyle 2. Dorsal protrusion of fibular head and of biceps muscle tendon

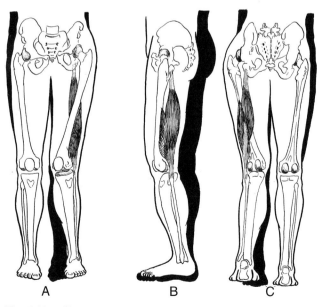

Fig. 7.11. Changes in body outlines because of a shortened biceps femoris. Back view (a), side view (b).

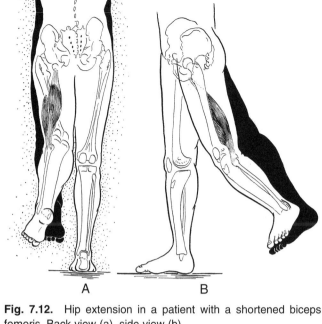

Fig. 7.12. Hip extension in a patient with a shortened biceps femoris. Back view (a), side view (b).

DISTURBED MOTOR PATTERNS BECAUSE OF SHORTENING AND OVERACTIVITY

This pattern may include an altered activation sequence of muscles during extension of the hip joint (Fig. 7.12).

The order of muscle contraction during hip extension is

1. Hamstrings
2. Gluteus maximus
3. Contralateral erector spinae
4. Ipsilateral erector spinae

Delayed activation of the gluteus maximus may occur when the biceps femoris is overactive.

Tensor Fasciae Latae
GENERAL CHARACTERISTICS

This muscle has a tendency to become shortened and overactive.

FUNCTIONAL ANATOMY

Points of attachment:	Origin	Insertion
	1. From anterior part of outer lip of iliac crest to anterior superior iliac spine	1. Anteromedial tendinous fibers terminate in lateral patellar retinaculum 2. Posterolateral half of muscle tendon attaches below knee onto lateral tubercle of tibia via iliotibial tract

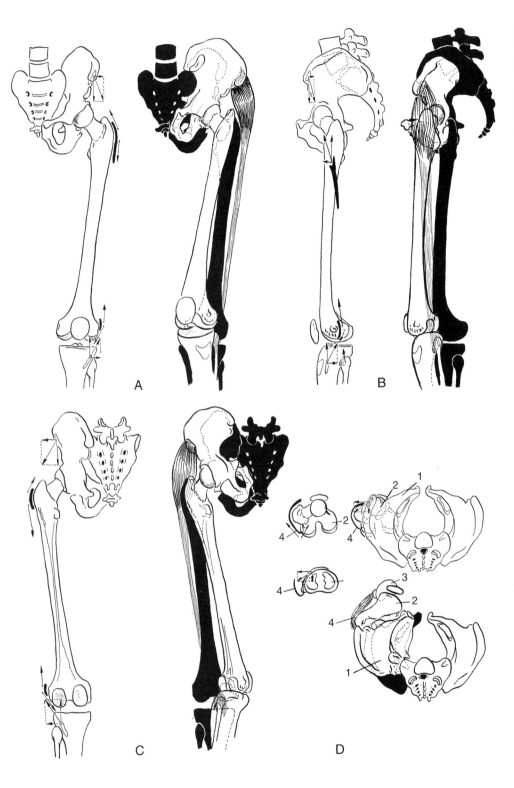

Fig. 7.13. Disturbed body statics because of a shortened tensor fasciae latae. Front view (a), side view (b), back view (c), view from above (d); 1, pelvis; 2, femur; 3, tibia; 4, tensor fasciae latae.

IMPAIRED BODY STATICS BECAUSE OF SHORTENING
(FIG. 7.13)

Changes at the ipsilateral side:

	Origin	Insertion
Direction of pull at the attachment points on contraction:	1. Caudolatero-dorsal pull at anterior superior spine	1. Craniolatero-dorsal pull at proximal end of tibia 2. Ventromedial deviation of thigh is result of muscle's tendency to approximate tibia toward pelvis
Possible changes in position of anatomic structures:	1. Innominate abduction, anteflexion, and external rotation 2. Flexion, adduction, and internal rotation of proximal end of thigh	1. Ventromedial deviation of distal end of thigh: abduction, flexion, and external rotation of proximal end of tibia
Joint mobility:	1. Hip joint: abduction, flexion, internal rotation	1. Knee joint: stabilization, flexion, rotation

CHANGES IN BODY OUTLINE BECAUSE OF SHORTENING
(FIG. 7.14)

	Origin	Insertion
Front view:	1. Increased transverse diameter of upper part of hemipelvis 2. Iliac crest is raised and protrudes anteriorly 3. In addition, tense muscle belly of tensor fasciae latae forms round protrusion	1. Increased transverse diameter in hemipelvis 2. Lateral contour of thigh forms straight line; tense fibers of iliotibial band visible 3. Lateral femoral condyle protrudes; patella deviates laterally.
Side view:	1. Pelvis deviates posteriorly; relative concavity at level of hip joint and increased convexity at level of coccyx 2. Increased lumbar lordosis	1. Knee slightly flexed and protrudes anteriorly
Back view:	1. Superior deviation of posterior superior iliac spine appears deeper and at greater distance from sacrum 2. Ischial tuberosity, however, approaches sacrum	1. Protrusion at level of contracted muscle: pelvis is inclined to the same side 2. Valgosity at knee and abduction of tibia

DISTURBED HIP FLEXION MOTOR PATTERN BECAUSE OF
SHORTENING (FIG. 7.15)

Direction of Movement	Visual Criteria
1. Hip joint: flexion, abduction, internal rotation 2. Knee joint: flexion, abduction	1. Ipsilateral innominate is lowered and rotates; pelvis shifts toward ipsilateral side 2. Lumbar spine extends and side bends 3. Hip flexion and abduction 4. Lateral deviation of patella and toes

Piriformis

GENERAL CHARACTERISTICS

This muscle has a tendency to become shortened and overactive.

FUNCTIONAL ANATOMY

Points of attachment:	Origin	Insertion
	1. Anterior lateral surface of sacrum between first and fourth sacral foramen 2. Part of fibers attach to margin of greater sciatic foramen at capsule of sacroiliac joint and sacrospinal ligament	1. Fibers run through greater sciatic foramen and attach to greater trochanter of femur on medial side of its superior surface

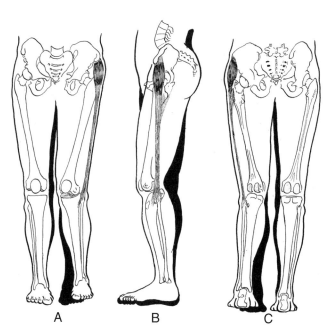

Fig. 7.14. Changes in body outline because of a shortened tensor fasciae latae. Front view (a), side view (b), back view (c).

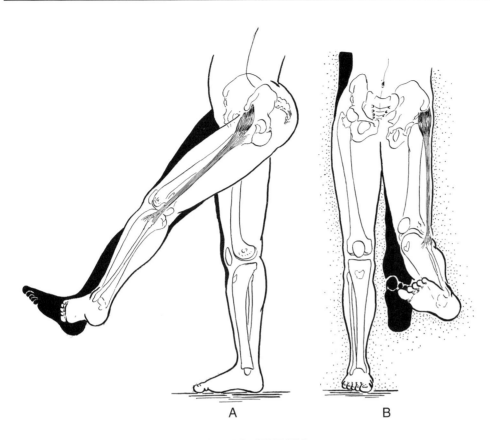

Fig. 7.15. Hip flexion in a patient with a shortened tensor fasciae latae. Side view (a), front view (b).

IMPAIRMENT OF BODY STATICS BECAUSE OF SHORTENING
(FIG. 7.16)

Changes at the ipsilateral side:

	Origin	Insertion
Direction of pull at attachment point on contraction:	1. Laterocaudo-ventral pull at lower part of sacrum	1. Craniomedio-dorsal pull at greater trochanter producing approximation of sacrum and greater trochanter, causing lateroventral deviation of caudal part of pelvis
Possible changes in position of anatomic structures:	1. Sacrum is tilted back and bent to opposite side, resulting in flexion of sacrum 2. Pelvis is thrust back; tendency to "fall" backward 3. To compensate, the patient stands on contralateral leg	1. Thigh: abduction, outward rotation and flexion; leg and knee deviate to side and forward with tendency to varosity at knee
Joint mobility:	1. Hip joint: outward rotation, abduction 2. Sacroiliac joint: compression	

CHANGES IN BODY OUTLINE BECAUSE OF SHORTENING
(FIG. 7.17)

	Origin	Insertion
Front View:	1. Anterior superior iliac spine lies higher and is less prominent 2. Upper edge of pubic bone deviates craniomedially	1. Lateral contour of greater trochanter is flattened 2. Leg is in abduction and external rotation 3. Patella and toes are deviated laterally 4. On changing weight toward ipsilateral leg, position of toes remains unchanged, but valgosity at knee becomes evident
Side View:	1. Pelvis is thrust backward and both sacral kyphosis and lumbar lordosis are reduced	1. Knee and talocrural joint are slightly flexed
Back View:	1. Transverse diameter of hemipelvis is reduced; posterior superior iliac spine lies nearer to sacrum and is more prominent	1. Knee deviates laterally; lateral edge of popliteal fossa in a more dorsal and medial in more ventral position

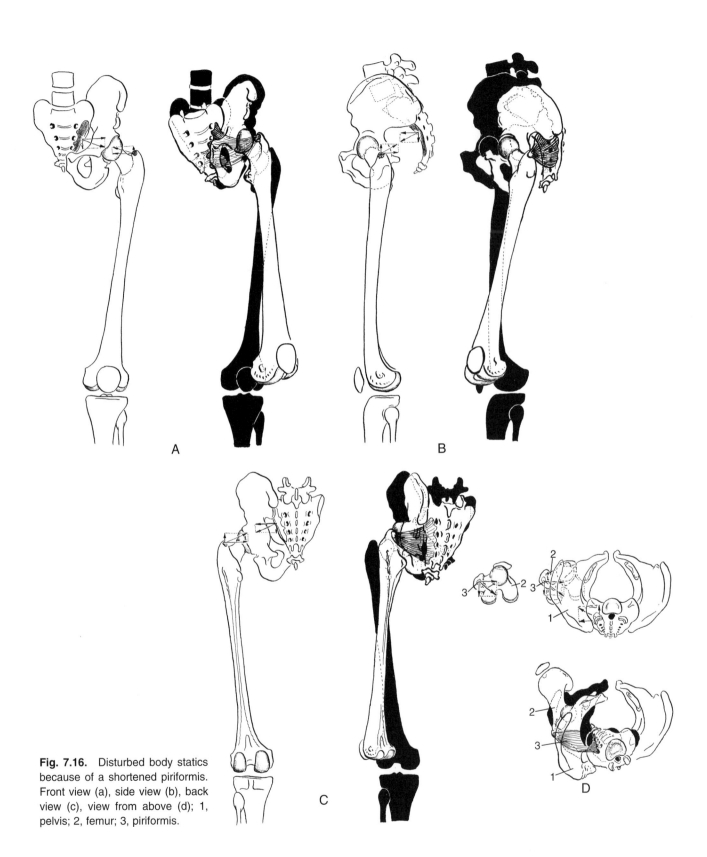

Fig. 7.16. Disturbed body statics because of a shortened piriformis. Front view (a), side view (b), back view (c), view from above (d); 1, pelvis; 2, femur; 3, piriformis.

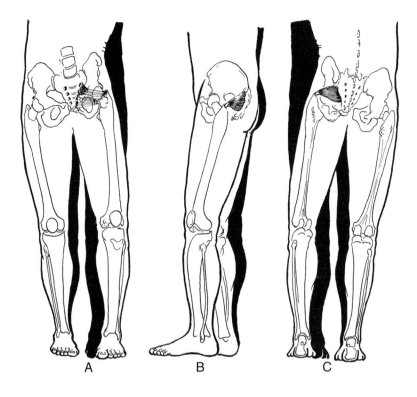

Fig. 7.17. Changes in body outline because of a shortened piriformis. Front view (a), side view (b), back view (c).

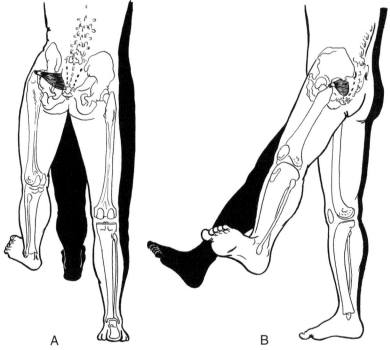

Fig. 7.18. Hip flexion in a patient with a shortened piriformis. Back view (a), side view (b).

DISTURBED HIP FLEXION MOTOR PATTERN BECAUSE OF
SHORTENING-HIP FLEXION (FIG. 7.18)

Direction of Movement	Visual Criteria
1. Shearing force at sacroiliac joint with compression 2. External rotation, abduction, flexion at hip joint	1. During gait, patient raises ipsilateral innominate with internal rotation 2. Flattened lateral outline at hip 3. Leg is flexed, abducted, and in outward rotation with foot and toes deviated laterally

Quadratus Lumborum

GENERAL CHARACTERISTICS

The quadratus lumborum has a tendency to become shortened
and overactive.

FUNCTIONAL ANATOMY

Points of attachment:	Origin	Insertion
	1. Vertical iliocostal fibers: medial half of 12th rib 2. Diagonal iliolumbar fibers: End of first three of four lumbar transverse processes 3. Diagonal lumbocostal fibers: 12th rib	1. Posterior part of iliac crest and iliolumbar ligament 2. Iliac crest and, frequently, iliolumbar ligament 3. All lumbar transverse processes

IMPAIRED BODY STATICS BECAUSE OF SHORTENING (FIG. 7.19)

Changes at the ipsilateral side:

	Origin	Insertion
Direction of pull at attachments on contraction:	1. 12th rib caudomedially; transverse processes laterally	1. Iliac crest: craniomediodorsally
Possible changes in position of anatomic structures:	1. Lowering of 12th rib, increased lumbar lordosis and thoracic kyphosis; lumbar scoliosis to same and thoracic scoliosis to opposite side	1. Raising, external rotation, and retroflexion of innominate
Joint mobility:	1. Fixation of the 12th rib, increased pressure on intervertebral and lumbosacral joints 2. Thoracolumbar hypermobility	1. Flexion and adduction position of hip joint

CHANGES IN BODY OUTLINE BECAUSE OF SHORTENING
(FIG. 7.20)

	Origin	Insertion
Front View:	1. Transverse diameter of ipsilateral lower part of thorax is diminished 2. Waist is narrower	1. Increased transverse diameter of hemipelvis, mainly lower part 2. Anterior superior iliac spine deviates laterally and is more prominent 3. Patient puts weight mainly on ipsilateral leg; contralateral leg is abducted and slightly flexed
Side View:	1. Increased lumbosacral lordosis	1. Decreased sagittal diameter of pelvis 2. Sacrum with coccyx tiled dorsally and protrudes; ventral contour of pelvis is flattened
Back View:	1. Lumbar spine deviates to side, resulting in scoliosis 2. 12th rib and innominate approach lumbar spine; transverse diameter of trunk at waist diminished on that side; lateral contour more concave 3. Frequent compensatory thoracic scoliosis to opposite side	1. Apex of sacrum with coccyx and ischial tuberosity approach thigh 2. Transverse diameter of buttock is diminished 3. Gluteal fold is raised 4. Posterior superior iliac spine closer to the sacrum

DISTURBED HIP EXTENSION MOTOR PATTERNS BECAUSE OF
SHORTENING (FIG. 7.21)

The quadratus lumborum contracts before the hamstrings and
the gluteus maximus.

Direction of Movement	Visual Criteria
1. Lumbar spine: extension, side bending 2. Pelvis: lateroflexion and anteflexion	1. When attempting to extend leg, patient first extends and side bends lumbar spine instead of hip joint 2. Innominate of same side is raised and thorax is lowered, approaching the pelvis; "S"-scoliosis results

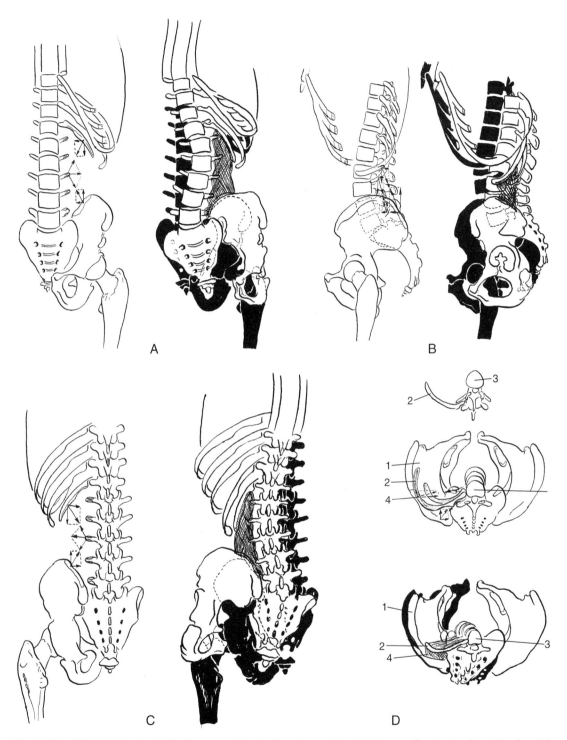

Fig. 7.19. Disturbed body statics because of a shortened quadratus lumborum. Front view (a), side view (b), back view (c), view from above (d); 1, pelvis; 2, lower rib; 3, lumbar spine; 4, quadratus lumborum.

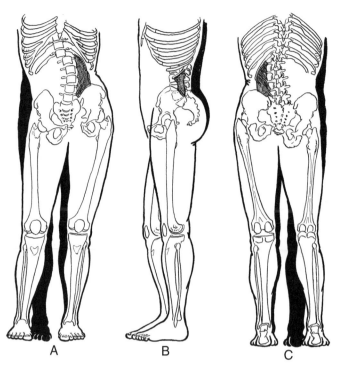

Fig. 7.20. Changes in body outline because of a shortened quadratus lumborum. Front view (a), side view (b) back view (c).

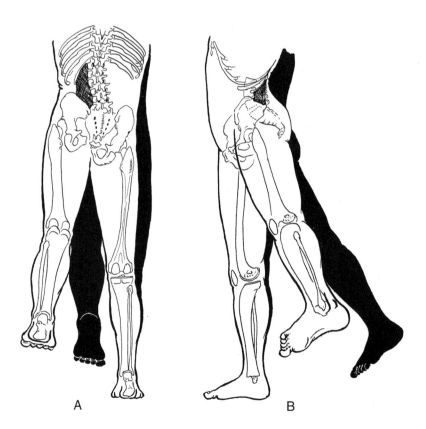

Fig. 7.21. Hip extension in a patient with a shortened quadratus lumborum. Back view (a), side view (b).

DISTURBED TRUNK FLEXION MOTOR PATTERN (IN THE STANDING POSITION) BECAUSE OF SHORTENING OR OVER-ACTIVITY (FIG. 7.22)

The quadratus lumborum contracts before the iliopsoas and rectus femoris.

<u>Direction of Movement</u>

1. Lumbar spine: extension, side bending (same side)
2. Thoracic spine: flexion, side bending (opposite side)
3. Hip joint: flexion

<u>Visual Criteria</u>

1. On trunk anteflexion, lumbar spine goes into extension and bends to same side; thoracic spine goes into flexion and bends to opposite side
2. Flexion takes place mainly in hip joint; entire body shifts forward

Rectus abdominus

GENERAL CHARACTERISTICS

The rectus abdominus has a tendency to become weak.

IMPAIRED BODY STATICS BECAUSE OF WEAKNESS (FIG. 7.23)

Changes at the ipsilateral side:

	<u>Origin</u>	<u>Insertion</u>
Direction of force at attachment points of contraction:	1. Cartilaginous end of 5th–7th ribs and xiphoid caudally	1. Pubic bone cranially
Possible change in position of anatomic structures:	1. Ribs and cartilages with xiphoid deviate cranially and contralaterally, resulting in extension and side bending of thoracic spine in opposite direction 2. Compensatory scoliosis and increased kyphosis in upper thoracic spine	1. Caudal shift of pubic bone produces anteflexion of innominate 2. Pelvis deviates dorsally and contralaterally resulting in increased lordosis of lumbar spine and in scoliosis towards ipsilateral side
Joint mobility:	1. Hypermobility at thoracolumbar and lumbosacral junctions	1. Hypermobility at symphysis; pelvic obliquity

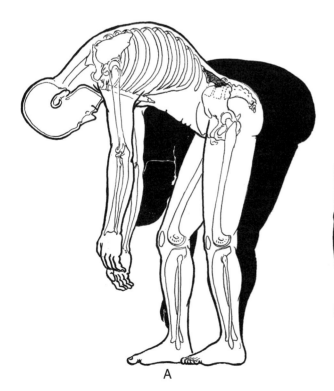 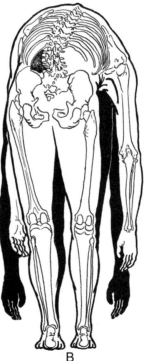

Fig. 7.22. Trunk flexion in a patient with a shortened quadratus lumborum. Side view (a), back view (b).

A B

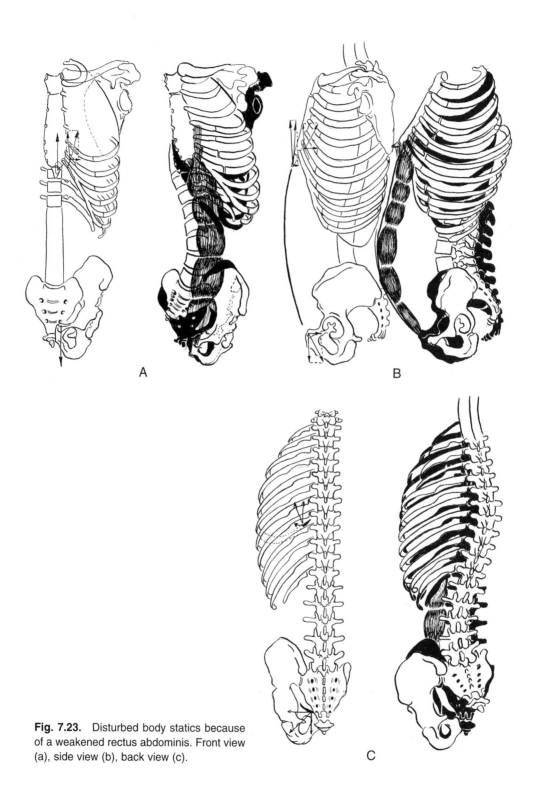

Fig. 7.23. Disturbed body statics because of a weakened rectus abdominis. Front view (a), side view (b), back view (c).

CHANGES IN BODY OUTLINE BECAUSE OF WEAKNESS
(FIG. 7.24)

	Origin	Insertion
Front View:	1. Increase in vertical diameter of abdomen 2. Trunk deviates to contralateral side	1. Increase in transverse diameter of lower part of pelvis 2. Pubic bone deviates down and to side
Side View:	1. Increased protrusion of abdominal wall; sternum is lifted and xiphoid is close to skin surface	1. Increased lumbar lordosis and prominence of end of sacrum
Back View:	1. Scoliosis toward ipsilateral side mainly in lumbar region	1. Innominate is lowered and waist is flattened; deeper on opposite side

DISTURBED MOTOR PATTERNS BECAUSE OF WEAKNESS

As a rule, the psoas substitutes for a weak rectus abdominis. The iliopsoas, erector spinae, quadratus lumborum, and rectus femoris may all become overactive when the rectus abdominus is weak or inhibited.

Direction of Movement	Visual Criteria
1. Lumbar spine: extension with lateroflexion to same side Thoracic spine: flexion with side bending to opposite side 2. Pelvis: lateroflexion to opposite side 3. Hip joint: flexion	1. While stooping, the patient's lumbar spine remains lordotic as the patient side bends to the same side; flexes thoracic spine, and side bends to the opposite side. 2. Also flexes hip and entire body is shifted back

Upper Trapezius

GENERAL CHARACTERISTICS

This muscle has a tendency to become shortened and overactive.

IMPAIRED BODY STATICS BECAUSE OF SHORTENING
(FIG. 7.25)

Changes at the ipsilateral side:

	Origin	Insertion
Direction of pull at attachment points on contraction:	1. Occipital bone: caudoventrally and slightly laterally 2. Upper cervical spine: mainly laterally and slightly caudoforward	1. Acromion: in craniomedial direction
Possible changes in position of anatomic structures:	1. Head deviates to side, forward, and into retroflexion with rotation to opposite side resulting in increased craniocervical lordosis 2. Lateral pull at spinous processes results in lateroflexion on upper cervical spine coupled with rotation in opposite direction owing to caudolateral pull 3. To compensate, some scoliosis at cervicothoracic junction to ipsilateral side with increased kyphosis	1. Clavicle with acromion deviate craniomedially 2. Medial pull produces compression of clavicle against sternum 3. To compensate, some side bending at shoulder girdle to opposite side with rotation to ipsilateral side
Joint mobility:	1. Fixation at cervical and upper thoracic spine; hypermobility at craniocervical and cervicothoracic junction	1. Fixation at sternoclavicular; hypermobility at acromioclavicular joint

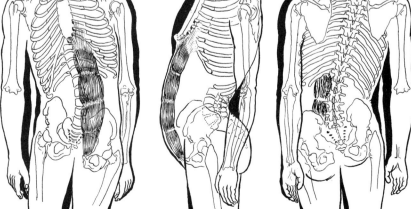

A B C

Fig. 7.24. Changes in body outlines because of a weakened rectus abdominis. Front view (a), side view (b), back view (c).

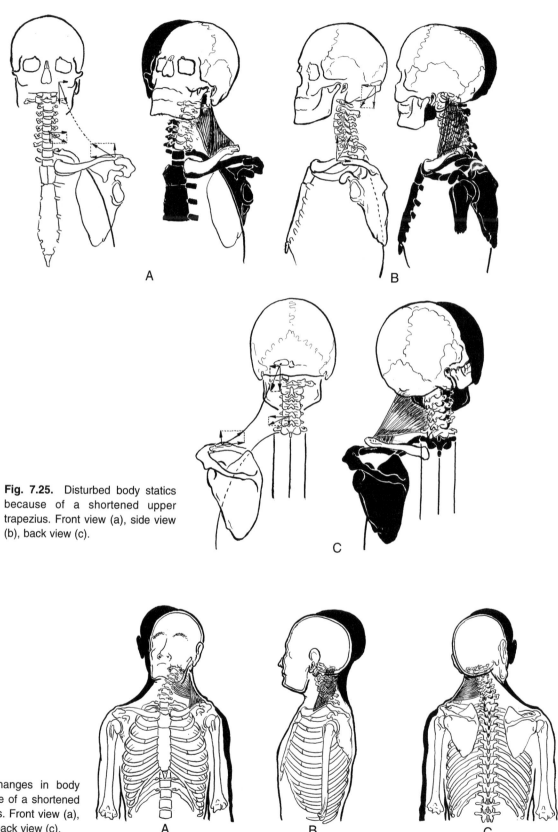

Fig. 7.25. Disturbed body statics because of a shortened upper trapezius. Front view (a), side view (b), back view (c).

Fig. 7.26. Changes in body outline because of a shortened upper trapezius. Front view (a), side view (b), back view (c).

CHANGES IN BODY OUTLINE BECAUSE OF SHORTENING
(FIG. 7.26)

	Origin	Insertion
Front View:	1. Head inclined to ipsilateral and rotated to opposite side; ear is seen and lowered; other ear is partly hidden and raised 2. Nose deviates contralaterally	1. Shoulder girdle rotates to ipsilateral side and is raised: decreased transverse diameter 2. Acromion deviates mediocranially 3. Prominent upper contour of shoulder; flattened outline of lateral part of clavicula
Side View:	1. Head is thrust forward and bent back; ipsilateral ear points antero-inferiorly	1. Acromion deviates cranially 2. Increased distance between acromion and humeral head 3. Flattened cervical lordosis and prominent cervicothoracic junction
Back View:	1. Head and neck inclined to ipsilateral side 2. Contralateral ear is raised and more visible 3. Horizontal fold (sign of extension) at craniocervical junction 4. "S" scoliosis noted–contralateral in cervical and ipsilateral cervicothoracic region	1. Shoulder girdle is raised; decreased transverse diameter 2. Flattened lateral contour of neck and shoulder 3. Lateral outline protrudes at level of acromion

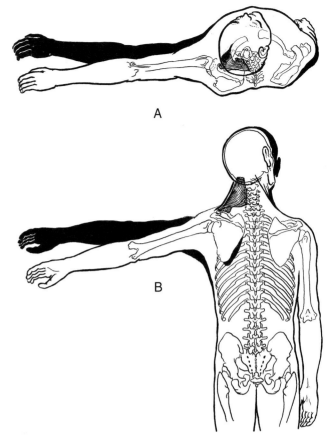

Fig. 7.27. Arm abduction in a patient with a shortened upper trapezius. View from above (a), back view (b).

DISTURBED MOTOR PATTERNS BECAUSE OF SHORTENING
ON SHOULDER ABDUCTION (FIG. 7.27)

The upper trapezius contracts before the deltoid (clavicular portion) or the supraspinatus, creating a dysfunctional scapulohumeral rhythm.

Direction of Movement	Visual Criteria
1. Acromioclavicular joint: movement of shear between clavicle and shoulder blade 2. Head: extension, ipsilateroflexion, contralateral rotation 3. Cervical spine: forward shift, ipsilateral flexion, contralateral rotation 4. Shoulder girdle: upward displacement	1. Elevation and outward rotation of shoulder and arm 2. Head is inclined to ipsilateral and rotated to contralateral side; head is thrust forward and in extension 3. "C" scoliosis of cervical and upper thoracic spine

DISTURBED MOTOR PATTERN DURING CERVICAL EXTENSION
(FIG. 7.28)

The upper trapezius bilaterally contracts before the spinal extensors.

Direction of Movement	Visual Criteria
1. Head extension: ipsilateroflexion, contralateral rotation 2. Cervical spine: forward shift, lateroflexion to the same, rotation to opposite side 3. Shoulder girdle: elevation	1. On back bending the head, patient side bends it to same side and rotates it to opposite side 2. Cervical spine drawn forward, inclined to same side and rotated to opposite side 3. "C" scoliosis of cervicothoracic spine 4. Shoulder raised and rotated with arm and scapula to same side

Sterncocleidomastoid

GENERAL CHARACTERISTICS

The sternocleidomastoid muscle has a tendency to become shortened and overactive.

FUNCTIONAL ANATOMY

Points of attachment:	Origin	Insertion
	1. Clavicular division: sternal end of clavicle	1. Both divisions attach to lateral surface of mastoid process and to lateral half of superior nuchal line of occiput
	2. Sternal division: anterior surface of manubrium sterni	

IMPAIRED BODY STATICS BECAUSE OF SHORTENING (FIG. 7.29)

Changes at the ipsilateral side:

	Origin	Insertion
Direction of pull at points of attachment:	1. Sternal end of clavicle: craniodorsolaterally	1. Mastoid process: caudoventromedially
	2. Medial surface of manubrium sterni: craniodorsolaterally	

	Origin	Insertion
Possible changes in position on contraction:	1. Clavicle: Sternal end raised, shoulder girdle pushed back (if head is fixed); slight rotation of shoulder girdle to same side; lowering of lateral end of clavicle with shoulder and arm	1. Head: deviates forward to opposite side and rotates also to opposite side
		2. Cervical spine: lordosis limited to craniocervical junction; cervical vertebrae are thrust forward and deviate to opposite side
Joint mobility:	1. Restriction at sternoclavicular and sternocostal joints on same side with hypermobility on opposite side	1. Restriction at craniocervical and cervicothoracic junction

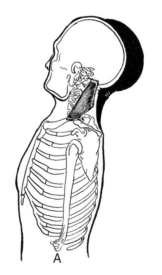
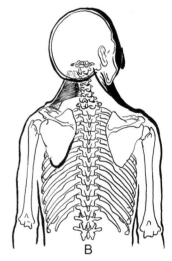

Fig. 7.28. Head extension in a patient with a shortened upper trapezius. Side view (a), back view (b).

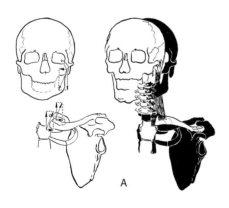
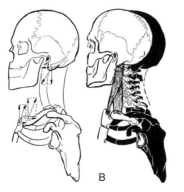
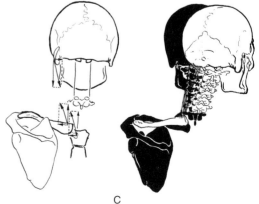

Fig. 7.29. Disturbed body statics because of a shortened sternocleidomastoideus. Front view (a), side view (b), back view (c) (the shoulder blade has been left out on purpose).

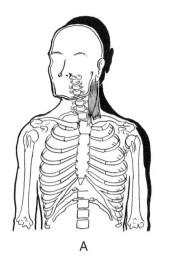
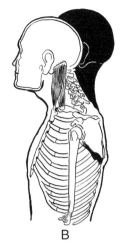
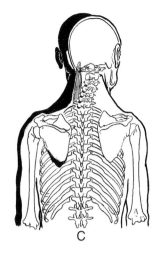

Fig. 7.30. Changed body outlines because of a shortened sternocleidomastoideus. Front view (a), side view (b), back view (c).

CHANGES IN BODY OUTLINE BECAUSE OF SHORTENING (FIG. 7.30)

	Origin	Insertion
Front View:	1. Decrease in transverse diameter of shoulder girdle, less prominent shoulder outline 2. Both heads of shortened muscle and upper and lower clavicular fossa clearly seen under skin 3. Shoulder girdle with thorax slightly rotated to same side	1. Head deviates to side and rotates to opposite side 2. Ear on that side is lowered, turned forward, well visualized 3. Lateral contour of neck on ipsilateral side flattened and at right angles with shoulders
Side View:	1. Sternal end of clavicle with manubrium sterni raised and tilted back, xiphoid process on other hand protrudes 2. Acromion with shoulder and arm lowered and thrust back	1. Head thrust forward, chin raised, occiput lowered 2. Ipsilateral ear rotated forward and lowered 3. Reduced cervical lordosis, but increased extension at craniocervical junction
Back View:	1. Lateral angle of scapula lowered, inferior angle raised, arm close to trunk	1. Occiput deviates to opposite side; ipsilateral mastoid process lower and anterior, contralateral raised and posterior 2. "C" scoliosis of cervical and upper thoracic spine

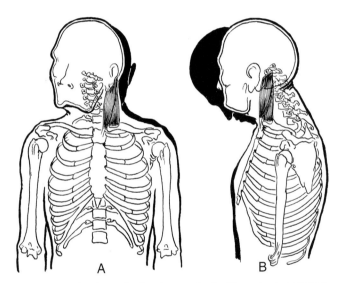

Fig. 7.31. Head anteflexion in a patient with a shortened sternocleidomastoideus. Front view (a), side view (b).

DISTURBED CERVICAL FLEXION MOTOR PATTERNS BECAUSE OF SHORTENING (FIG. 7.31)

The sternocleidomastoid and scalenes will substitute for the longus colli.

Direction of Movement	Visual Criteria
1. Extension at CO/1 and C1/2 ipsilateral inclination with rotation to contralateral side 2. Ante- and lateroflexion of neck	1. Head of patient is lowered, chin thrust forward and to opposite side 2. Ipsilateral ear lowered and deviates to opposite side 3. Extension of upper cervical and flexion of lower cervical spine

PRACTICAL APPLICATION

Case History

Patient K., male, complained of gnawing pain in his left shoulder that radiated over the anterior surface of the thorax.

ANAMNESIS

Six months previously, when patient K was lifting a small refrigerator, pain started in the right buttock and radiated down the posterior surface of his thigh. Pain disappeared within a fortnight without treatment. He then began to complain of shoulder pain, mainly while standing, which gradually worsened. Standing with feet apart lessened the pain, but pain intensified when he held his feet close together. Pain disappeared when lying on the nonpainful side.

ANALYSIS OF BODY STATICS (PAIN-PROVOKING POSITION)

Front View

The changes in body statics are illustrated in the diagrams in Figures 7.31b to 7.32b by vertical and horizontal lines. Figure 7.32c illustrates muscle dysfunction. The vertical line (1) de-

viates from the (ideal) midline to the left, with maximum deviation at the level of the navel, the point at which the (altered) vertical line between the legs and that from the head intersect. The horizontal line diverges toward the left to the right) with maximum divergence between the lower margin of the rib cage (4) and the greater trochanters (6).

Note, however, the divergence to the right of the line between the acromia and the lower margin of the rib cage. As deviation from the plumb line is clearly to the left and divergence of the mentioned lines is greater to the left than to the right (see angles α and β), it can be inferred that deviation of the pelvis to the left is primary and deviation of the shoulder girdle to the right is secondary (compensatory).

Side View

Figure 7.33b shows forward deviation of the patient's body from the plumb line, particularly noticeable at the legs. Note little deviation of the trunk, but, again, forward deviation of the neck. The horizontal lines diverge mainly in front, mostly between the lower margin of the rib cage and the crista iliaca (4,5). The horizontal lines between the spina scapulae and clavicle and the lower margin of the rib cage (3,4), corresponding to the mainly straight thoracolumbar spine,

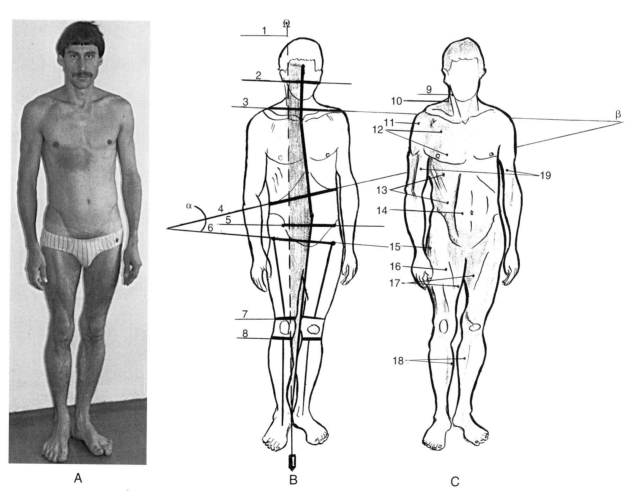

Fig. 7.32.   Front view of Patient K. in the pain-provoking position: photograph (a), diagram (b), and diagram of dysfunctional muscles (c).

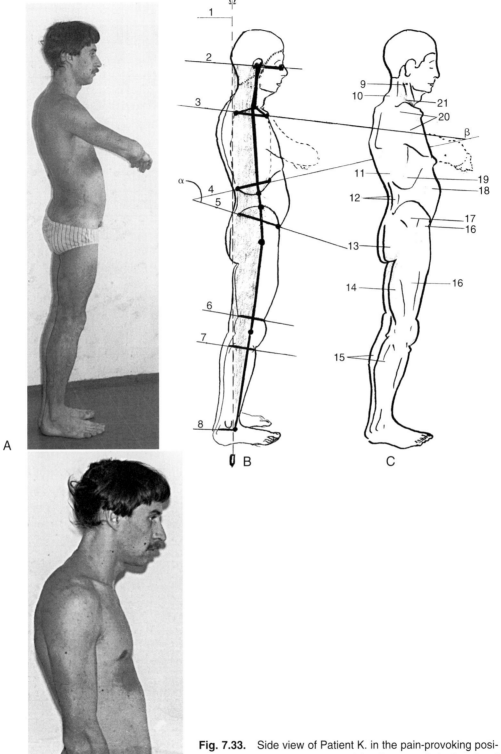

Fig. 7.33. Side view of Patient K. in the pain-provoking position: photograph (a), diagram (b), diagram of dysfunctional muscles (c), and (d) photograph of upper part of profile.

converge dorsally. It can be inferred that body statics (balance) are disturbed, with a tendency to fall forward. The angle between the lower margin of the rib cage and the crista iliaca is therefore primary and the shoulder is the secondary compensation.

Back View

In Figure 7.34b, the patient stands with his legs apart, i.e., in the relief position. Little deviation from the vertical is seen between the legs; deviation is limited mainly to the cervicothoracic spine, with a maximum at the level of the lower angles of the scapulae. Maximum divergence of the horizontal lines is between the biacromial line and the line connecting the lower margins of the rib cage (3,4). The line between the trochanters is now almost parallel to the lower margin of the rib cage (4,5) (compare Fig. 7.32b).

ANALYSIS OF MUSCLE FUNCTION (PAIN-PROVOKING POSITION)

Front View (Figs. 7.32c to 7.34c)

What can be seen on the body outlines is in keeping with the disturbance of statics (see Figs. 7.32b to 7.34b). The pelvis deviates to the left and the spina iliaca anterior superior appears higher; the trunk deviates to the right and the shoulder is lowered. The head is slightly inclined to the right with left rotation.

Closer inspection reveals outward rotation of the left leg, which is adducted; the right leg is flexed at the knee. Note the tension of the sartorius on the right and protrusion of the short adductors on the left. The shoulder is closer to the pelvis on the right and the thorax to the left, which is in keeping with increased tension of the obliquus externus on the right where its attachments to Poupart's ligament and the iliac crest are seen. The abdomen protrudes more on the left and hypertonus of the pectoral muscles is visible on the right side. Also on the right side, the nipple is lowered, the outline of the pectoralis major at the axilla is sharper, the shoulder is drawn forward and protrudes anteriorly, the supraclavicular fossa is deeper, and the outline of the sternocleidomastoid and trapezius muscles is clearer. The acromial end of the clavicle is raised on the right side, and there is a step between the acromion and the head of the humerus.

On the left side, the contours of both the trapezius and sternocleidomastoideus are vague. The head is not only inclined, but deviates to the right. The transverse diameter of the shoulder girdle appears smaller on the right. The head is rotated to the left, the right ear more visible on the right. The right arm is slightly flexed and the hand is pronated; the contour of the biceps is more prominent.

Side View (see diagram in Fig. 7.33c)

The main feature is the forward drawn position, particularly of the lower extremities and the neck. This posture results in tension in the triceps surae and the hamstrings, in the muscle belly of the tensor fasciae latae, and, to the lesser degree, in the lower iliotibial band. This tension contrasts with the hypotonus in the gluteus maximus, producing flattening of the buttocks and lowered gluteal lines. Also noted are lumbosacral hyperlordosis and increased thoracic kyphosis with some tension (prominence) of the erector spinae and a protruding, flabby contour of the upper part of the abdomen. The head and neck are thrust forward and tension is evident in the right sternocleidomastoideus and upper trapezius. Lordosis is present at the craniocervical junction. In Figure 7.33d, the contour of the acromion is clearly outlined when the arms are hanging down, and, again, note the step-like prominence of the acromion in relation to the head of the humerus. We also see better the cervicothoracic kyphosis with a raised lower angle of the shoulder blade. The lower cervical spinous processes are clearly visible (also a sign of low cervical kyphosis). The forward thrust position of the head of the humerus is also obvious. The elbow is flexed and deviates dorsally, and there is visible tension in the biceps brachii. The relative flattening of the thorax with a prominent xiphoid process is also clear.

Back View (see diagram in Fig. 7.34c)

The patient stands with his legs apart in the relief position. Outward rotation of the foot is more pronounced on the left and tension is greater at the Achilles tendon on the left. On the left side, prominence of the triceps surae is greater and the depression below the knee on the medial surface is deeper.

The popliteal fossa is deeper on the right (with the knee flexed) and the patella is rotated inward. The lateral outline of the biceps femoris is more prominent on the right, the contour of the semimembranosus and semitendinosus is more prominent on the left, and there is a concavity on the medial surface above the knee. Above this concavity is the prominence of the short adductors; the gluteal lines are lowered on both sides.

The pelvis deviates only slightly to the left, but rotation to the left is apparent. The transverse diameter of the hemipelvis is therefore greater on the left side, and the outline of the gluteus medius can be seen. Above the pelvis, tension is increased in the paravertebral muscles on the left; hypertonus, principally in the latissimus dorsi, is visible in the craniolateral direction. Below the axilla, note the prominence of the teres major. The convex outline of the infraspinatus below the spinae scapulae can be seen only on the left side. Here, too, the upper extremity is adducted and slightly flexed on the left side. The contour of the left shoulder forms almost an angle, i.e., hypotonus of the deltoid muscle is noted. On the right side, on the other hand, the waist line is deeper, and above it, tonus of the latissimus dorsi appears diminished. The lower angle of the scapula is more prominent on the right side and the shoulder is drawn forward. Increased kyphosis in addition to scoliosis are evident at the cervicothoracic junction. The head and neck are inclined and rotated to the left; the ear is clearly visible. There is also some hypertonus at the upper trapezius on the left side, but the lower fibers of that muscle as well as the middle trapezius are flattened.

ANALYSIS OF RESULTS

From the changes in body statics and comparison of the pain-provoking and relief positions, it follows that the main and primary disturbance is at the pelvis: the parallel lines (see Fig. 7.32b) show maximum divergence toward the left, and pelvic deviation is significant. In the relief position, on the other hand (see Fig. 7.34b), less deviation is noted, consistent with increased tension of the obliquus externus abdominis on the right side and of the quadratus lumborum on the left side (see also Fig. 7.20).

The other important change in body statics is the forward-drawn posture with lumbar hyperlordosis. It can be inferred that the straight abdominal muscles are not primarily weak, but are inhibited because of the shortened lumbar section of the back extensors (including the quadratus lumborum). Spasm of the external obliquus on the left side is clearly visible, and it is spasm of the abdominal muscles that is the most frequent cause of the forward-drawn posture.

The numerous asymmetries of muscular tonus described are mostly compensatory. In the legs, it involves the biceps femoris on the right, the adductors on the left, and the hamstrings and triceps surae on both sides. In the trunk, it involves the pectoralis on the right and the latissimus with the teres major on the left. Others include the sternocleidomastoideus on the right and the upper trapezius on both sides, but more so on the right. The asymmetric position of the arms goes along with increased tension of the biceps brachii on the right and adduction on the left. These findings are illustrated in Figure 7.35 (see also Figs. 7.5 and 7.6).

In a similar way, it is possible to examine movement, in particular gait, as shown in the preceding discussions concerning disturbed movement patterns for each muscle. It is even possible to infer from typical changes in body statics which movement pattern will be affected, and from the disturbed movement, which muscle is either shortened or weak.

Visual diagnosis is also useful when checking therapeutic results by comparing findings, such as in photographs,

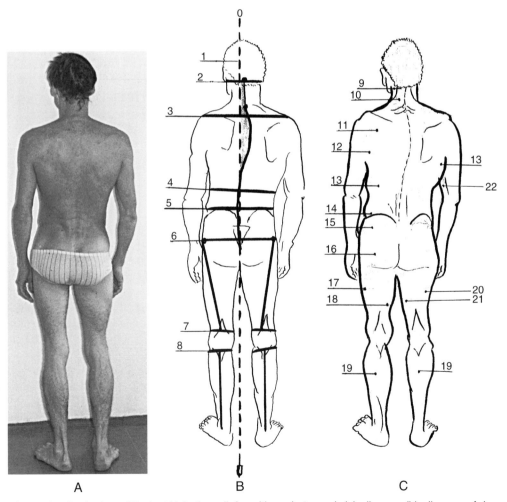

A   B   C

Fig. 7.34. Back view of Patient K. in the relief position: photograph (a), diagram (b), diagram of dysfunctional muscles (c).

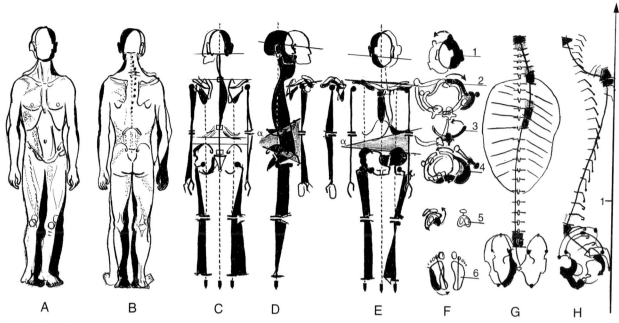

Fig. 7.35. Diagrams of patient K: (a) Dysfunctional muscles in the pain-provoking position (dotted lines, changed muscle contours); (b) Dysfunctional muscles in the relief position; (c) Disturbed statics in the relief position, back view (black, changes in vertical outlines); (d) Disturbed statics in the pain-provoking position, side view (gray, change of horizontal lines; angle α is open in the direction of body deviation); (e) Disturbed statics in the pain-provoking position, shown in the same way; (f) Disturbed statics from above, (1) head, (2) shoulders, (3) lower thorax aperture, (4) pelvis, (5) knees, (6) feet; (g) level of spinal dysfunction; (h) side view.

before and after treatment. Inspection works fast and at a distance. Its results, however, must be checked by using other methods of clinical examination; in particular, palpation, testing of active and passive mobility—the full range of physical examination.

REFERENCES

1. Lewit K: Manipulative Therapy in Rehabilitation of the Locomotor System. Oxford, Butterworth, Heineman, 1991, pp 23-25.
2. Rash PJ, Burke RK: Kinesiology and Applied Anatomy. Philadelphia, Lea & Febiger, 1971.
3. Kogan OG, Schmidt IR, Vasilyeva LF: Visualno-palpatornaya diagnostika patobiomeckanisticheskick ismeneniy posvonochnika (Diagnosis of pathobiomechanical spinal disorders by inspection and palpation). Manualnaya Medicina 3:10, 1991.
4. Janda V: (1990) Differential diagnosis of muscle tone in respect of inhibitory techniques. In Paterson JK, Burn L (eds): Back Pain, an International Review. Boston, Kluwer Dordrecht, 1990, p 196.
5. Vasilyeva LF, Kogan OG: Manual diagnosis and manual therapy of atypical motor patterns. Presented at the 10th International Congress of the Fédération Internationale de Médicine Manuelle (FIMM). Brussels, September 1992.
6. Janda V: Muscle Function Testing. London, Butterworth, 1993.
7. Kogan OG, Vasilyeva LF: Atipichniy lokomotorniy pattern, diagnostika i lecheniye. (Atypical locomotor patterns, diagnosis and treatment). Novokuznetsk, 1990.

Acknowledgments

I am grateful to my teachers for their contribution to the ideas of this publication, particularly concerning the role of the musculature, its functional anatomy, and biomechanics. I am grateful to Dr. Lewit, who first opened the door of manual medicine to Russia. I am indebted greatly to the work of Janet G. Travell and David G. Simons; to Vladimir Janda for his ideas of muscular patterns; and to O.G. Kogan and I.R. Schmidt for their help in analysis of static dysfunction.

I thank Karel Lewit and I. Lewitova for their painstaking and constructive criticism and active editing of the text. Last, but certainly not least, I thank I. Litvinov for the wonderful illustrations in this chapter.

Ludmila Vasilyeva

8 Evaluation of Lifting

LEONARD N. MATHESON

CHIROPRACTIC FUNCTIONAL CAPACITY EVALUATION

As the chiropractor assists the patient in restoring pre-injury functional capacity, periodic functional capacity evaluation is necessary. Functional capacity evaluation (FCE) denotes a form of work evaluation consisting of a battery of tests that focus on selected work tolerance areas. Matheson[1] defined work tolerances as the observed and measured physical capabilities of the evaluee that affect competence to perform the physical demands of work tasks. The term *functional* connotes purposeful, meaningful, or useful activity, implying a definable task that has a beginning and an end with a result that can be measured. The term *capacity* connotes the maximum ability of the individual, beyond the level of tolerance that is measured. Capacity is the evaluee's potential. The term *evaluation* is a systematic approach to monitoring and reporting performance that requires the evaluator to observe, measure, and interpret the evaluee's performance in a structured task. The information gathered in the FCE is descriptive and, when standards of performance are available, normative. Descriptive results are used to compare the evaluee's ability with the physical demands of work or with the evaluee at a previous point in time. Normative results are used to compare the evaluee to a reference population.

An FCE requires that the evaluee put forth maximum voluntary effort for the defined task. The defined task may require full strength, full velocity, endurance, a target number of repetitions, a maximum rate of responding, or some other "full effort" performance. When the measurement of function is less than maximum, the evaluator must be able to determine to what degree this deficiency is a function of the biochemical, cardiovascular, metabolic, or psychophysical limits inherent in the evaluee.

LIFT CAPACITY TESTING

For several reasons, the evaluation of lifting capacity is a key ingredient of most FCE. Lifting is an important component of many jobs, because of either the proportion of job activities that require lifting or the criticality of the lifting task as a component of the job. Lifting is important because it is a *central organizing variable* that provides an excellent estimate of general work capacity.[1] Additionally, lifting is an important variable because lifting tasks appear to be related to both increased frequency and increased severity of industrial injuries.[2-5]

LIFTING AND LOWERING

Lifting is defined as the vertical displacement of an object with mass that is accelerated vertically through the application of force along the direction of the lift. Lifting is generally considered movement of an object held by one or both hands in opposition to gravity, i.e., lifting upward.

Some FCE systems consider lifting separately from lowering. Lowering is a distinct task and is defined as the controlled movement of an object vertically downward. The force applied to initiate movement is gravity. The individual's maximum lowering ability is taken as his or her ability to resist this force so that the object remains under control or, at the least, is controlled at the termination of the vertical movement. By contrast, vertical movement downward of an object accelerated by gravity without resistance applied by the worker is considered a "drop" rather than a lower.

In practice, when lifting and lowering are evaluated jointly, the maximum lift-lower usually is the individual's lifting capacity. People generally are able to lift approximately 20% less than they are able to lower, although this percentage varies from person to person and depends on the starting height, the vertical displacement of the lift or lower, and the frequency of the task.

LIFTING CAPACITY FACTORS

Several factors inherent in the lifting task influence the maximum load that can be lifted.

Horizontal Displacement of Load

The distance between the center of gravity of the load held by the hand or hands and the center of gravity of the worker is a crucial determinant of maximum lifting capacity for several reasons:

1. The human biomechanical system exponentially multiplies the effect of the load on the human body so that it rapidly increases as horizontal displacement increases.

2. The stability of the worker-load system is maximized when horizontal displacement is minimized.
3. Risky lifting-lowering maneuvers are minimized or eliminated as horizontal displacement is minimized. Certain behaviors such as torquing of the spine when moving an object through a lateral arc of motion can be eliminated entirely if the horizontal displacement is sufficiently small so as to place the object against the worker's abdomen or pelvis.

Location of the Hands at the Origin of the Lift

The common reference point for lifting and lowering is the position of the hands on the object. This positioning is taken as the point of origin of the force and the center of resultant force vectors. Lifting is accomplished most easily through intermediate vertical ranges so that the biomechanical system can be used most efficiently. At the extremes of the range upward or downward, workers are less capable of full muscular exertion. Different muscle groups are called into play depending on the starting height of the lift, some of which are more inherently powerful or fatigue-resistant than others. In addition, secondary limitations occur that depend on the starting height of the lift-lower, including cardiovascular demands and effects of various strategies of trunk stabilization on the cardiorespiratory system.

Vertical Displacement of the Lift

The vertical range over which an object is lifted or lowered affects the workers's lifting capacity in the same way and for the same reasons that the starting height of the lift affects lifting capacity. In addition, however, the vertical displacement of the lift affects lifting capacity in terms of the amount of work that is required in the lift-lower. Work is a product of force applied over distance. Muscles have the capability to produce power, which is force per unit of time. The biomechanical system is limited in terms of both power and the ability of the system to sustain that power to produce work. The amount of work performed is directly related to the distance over which the object is lifted or lowered.

Frequency of the Lift-Lower

Because of the inherent power and endurance limitations in the worker's biomechanical system, the number of times a lift-lower task can be repeated is limited. This limitation is directly related to several factors that interact:

- Degree to which the load approximates the individual's maximum single lift capacity
- Duration of the individual task
- Rest period after each individual task
- Duration of the task set

Biomechanical Couplings

Both the maximum load and the consistency of the worker's ability to lift and lower are directly affected by the adequacy of his or her biomechanical couplings. A firm stance on a stable surface and a strong and comfortable grip on the object are the two most important issues with healthy workers. When the evaluation concerns an individual who has one or more impaired biomechanical components in the linkage, that linkage may become critically limiting, depending on the degree to which the task and/or the posture and movement of the worker stress this component. If the task and/or posture and movement of the worker do not stress the impaired component, the effect may be negligible. Conversely, if the component is stressed, it may be the primary limiting factor.

Aerobic Capacity

For tasks that are prolonged at loads that are significantly less than the worker's maximum lift capacity, the aerobic capacity of the worker becomes important if the frequency of the task is sufficiently high. Generally speaking, aerobic capacity becomes important if a light load is lifted once every 2 minutes or more often or a heavy load is lifted once every 5 minutes or more often. In regard to tasks that involve lifts more frequently than six to eight times per minute, aerobic capacity may begin to be important after the second or third minute of continuous activity.

Anaerobic Capacity

This capacity of the worker is important in high frequency tasks involving loads below the worker's maximum single lift load and in low frequency tasks involving loads near the worker's maximum load. Anaerobic capacity is a function of the load of the task relative to the worker's maximum and the mix of work to recovery time in the task.

Metabolic Capacity

This capacity of the worker is important in repetitive tasks with a frequency of once every 5 minutes or greater than are sustained for more than 1 hour. Tasks performed less frequently or of shorter duration generally are not affected by the worker's metabolic capacity, unless it is substantially impaired as a consequence of illness or severe dietary problems.

Test Instructions and Performance Target

The type of instructions provided to the evaluee significantly affect their subsequent performance. Coaching during the activity affects the evaluee's consequent performance. Although few studies have addressed this topic, the effects they have reported have been substantial.[6] As one component of the instructions given to the evaluee, the "cognitive target" provided in a maximum strength task is an important component of demonstrated lift-lower capacity. The difference between "your maximum possible lift" and "your maximum dependable lift that you can replicate several times per day" is substantial. Evaluators must provide a specific cognitive target so the evaluee does not select his or her own.

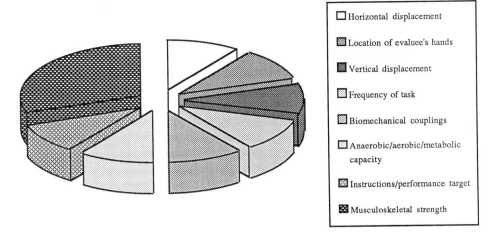

☐ Horizontal displacement

▨ Location of evaluee's hands

▨ Vertical displacement

▨ Frequency of task

▨ Biomechanical couplings

☐ Anaerobic/aerobic/metabolic
   capacity

▨ Instructions/performance target

▨ Musculoskeletal strength

Fig. 8.1. Factors that contribute to maximum performance in a lift capacity test.

Musculoskeletal Strength

The worker's strength is the largest single contributing factor to his or her ability to perform a maximum lift. Depending on the other factors listed, however, the contribution that musculoskeletal strength makes to the ability of the worker to perform to a particular level will be limited. In the simplest case, musculoskeletal strength is limited by the "weakest link" in the biomechanical chain that exists between the surface on which the evaluee is standing and the grip that the evaluee maintains on the load.[7,8] This factor, however, presents only a level of the potential performance that cannot be exceeded. This ceiling can be approximated in lifting tasks that are infrequent, or that are performed over a limited vertical range, involve holding the object close to the body, and with good biomechanical couplings and test instructions that are perfectly understood by the evaluee. Figure 8.1 is a graphic depiction of the author's estimation of the degree to which each of these factors contributes to the ability of the evaluee to perform a maximum lift in a work setting.

CLASSES OF STRENGTH TESTS

Lifting and lowering is a synthesis of the worker's biomechanical, cardiovascular, metabolic, and psychophysical capacity. The development of tests has been influenced by progress in hardware technology, so that the focus in this early phase of the development of the science of lift capacity testing has been on the biomechanical system. Any one of the four domains, however, may be the most limiting in any single test for any given evaluee. Usually, strength tests are limited primarily by the evaluee's psychophysical capacity. Psychophysical factors affect the worker's ability to lift in terms of the degree to which maximum voluntary effort approximates inherent biomechanical, cardiovascular, and metabolic capacities. Factors such as fear or anxiety about the task or confidence in his or her ability to perform it directly influence the level of effort that the worker is willing to put forth. Other attitudinal factors, such as the relative risk-to-reward ratio or work-to-value ratio as perceived by the worker also affects the level of effort and, thereby, the worker's performance.

Three general classes of strength testing have been identified. They are differentiated in terms of the effect of the test on muscular contraction, considered in terms of both the muscles' force of contraction and the rate of shortening.

1. Isometric. Under load, the muscle length does not change. Force is measured in one biomechanical position.
2. Isokinetic. The muscle lengthens or shortens at a fixed rate as a consequence of external control of the velocity of movement of the biomechanical unit. Force is measured throughout the range of movement.
3. Isoinertial. The muscle shortens at a variable rate in response to a constant external resistance. As the biomechanical trigonometry changes to accomplish movement, changes in muscle length occur at varying velocities. Constant resistance is inferred from the constancy of the mass that is moved. Acceleration is assumed to be negligble.

Various technologies have been developed to assess these general classes of strength tests and are identified by name in terms of the type of function that each *intends* to assess. Some confusion results in that, because of the complexity of the biomechanical system involved in lifting and lowering, the external system used to test the biomechanical system may not be able to control the test at the level of the individual muscle's function so that the intended mode of test is actually achieved. For example, although isokinetic testing intends to evaluate the strength of the biomechanical system at a set velocity, accelerative movement occurs early in the task up to the point at which the desired velocity is achieved. Even after that point, a rebound phenomenon may occur before stabilization at the desired velocity is achieved. As a result, each of the modes is inexactly sampled by the technologies that it is intended (and advertised) to test.

A lifting task usually involves a combination of types of muscle contractions, depending on the biomechanical segment that is considered. These types will change during the task. For example, a "squat lift" from floor to knuckle, whether accomplished in an isokinetic or isoinertial mode, usually involves the upper extremities in isometric activity if the worker's style of lift emphasizes lower extremity extension. Conversely, with a lifting style such as that used by competitive weight lifters, this same vertical range might be undertaken with the lower extremities performing isometric stabilization while the upper extremities provide an accelerative force to overcome the inertia imposed on the mass by gravity as it sits at rest. With these caveats in mind, the description of each test technology is grouped in terms of the type of function that each is intended to address.

Isometric Testing

This form of testing is the simplest type of technology and tends to be the most reliable in that, because the body is tested in a static posture, the geometry between the biomechanical linkages (termed "kinematics") can be controlled and, thus, replicated.

In terms of safety, however, isometric strength testing has prompted debate. On the one hand, Garg, Mital, and Asfour,[9] Chaffin,[10] and Caldwell, Chaffin, and Dukes-Dobos[11] reported that isometric strength tests are safe. Because it does not allow acceleration and, thus, the increased inertial loads that are a consequence of acceleration, isometric testing should place less stress on the body and inherently be more safe than other methods that allow acceleration. On the other hand, Kishino and co-workers,[12] describing their experience with isometric strength testing of individuals diagnosed as having spinal soft tissue injuries, found that most reports of muscle strain or prolonged soreness occurred as a consequence of isometric testing. They hypothesized that this result was attributable to the longer period of time that peak force must be maintained in an isometric test (typically 3 to 5 seconds), whereas the peak force in an isokinetic or isoinertial test is transitory. Battié et al[13] and Zeh et al[14] raised the same issues after finding problems with prolonged symptomatic responses and a small incidence of reported back injuries after testing nominally healthy people in an employment setting.

Three important issues with regard to the safety of isometric testing have not been fully explored on a scientific basis. The first issue relates to the value of psychophysical limits in terms of producing safe lifting performance. Psychophysical limits are developed throughout the individual's lifetime as he or she is involved with tasks that place demands on the biomechanical, cardiovascular, and metabolic systems. The learning proceeds through trial and error so that the individual develops internal controls, termed "work function themes," which in essence are rules that the individual follows to remain free of injury while involved in work tasks. These rules are applied unconsciously and require input from the individual's sensorium in terms of the degree to which a task places demand on the individual's functional capacity. This feedback is applied as a consequence of the worker's

perception of the difficulty of the task. Information about task difficulty is supplied through feedback loops that provide the individual with information concerning, initially, the biomechanical demand, and soon thereafter, the cardiovascular demand of the task. The biomechanical demand depends on sensors that function best when joints and muscles are in movement. These sensors are less functional and, thereby, less useful when the biomechanical system is static. Thus, isometric strength testing has proven useful for differentiating individuals who are putting forth various levels of maximum voluntary effort because it is difficult for the individual to gauge the degree to which he or she has put forth effort and, thus, maintain consistency with less than a full effort trial. It is precisely for this reason that isometric strength testing, unless used carefully, has the potential to place workers who have inherent defects in the biomechanical system at risk for stressing the defective segment to the point of strain.

A second issue concerns the unusual nature of the isometric task. Whereas isometric tasks with the fingers and hands are relatively common in everyday life, isometric whole body tasks are extremely unusual. Thus, the worker involved in an isometric "lifting" evaluation is performing a task that has little familiarity. Although posture is controlled, the psychophysical skill brought to the task in terms of achieving maximum performance efficiently and with safety is less than it would be in a task that is more familiar. For example, the first trial in a particular posture is often wasted because of problems with balance.

The third issue relates to the care and precision with which instructions are given. Because the technology is relatively simple, clinicians may tend to use less care in its application than otherwise would be appropriate. Rather than beginning the lifting task gradually with a "ramp up" to full effort, many evaluators allow the evaluee to increase explosively to full effort before the mechanical system's inherent elasticity has been entirely diminished. This situation results in inertial effects that greatly increase the force within the biomechanical system.

Isometric strength testing has been demonstrated to be highly reliable, with test-retest correlation coefficients exceeding $r = .90$.[5] Coefficients of variation have been in the neighborhood of 10 to 13%.[15] With regard to validity, one disadvantage of isometric strength testing is that force values are measured only at a specific segment in the arc of motion. Selection of the segment to replicate is an important consideration to allow results in an isometric strength test to predict performance in a dynamic task. Perhaps more importantly, it may be that the spine responds differently to an isometric task than to a dynamic task. Marras, King, and Joynt[16] found that electromyographic (EMG) activity was highest in the latissimus dorsi muscles during an isometric task, whereas the erector spinae group produced greater EMG activity during an isokinetic task.

In spite of concerns about safety and validity, isometric tests can be useful because they are brief and so are the least costly type of test to administer. The ARCON ST is an exam-

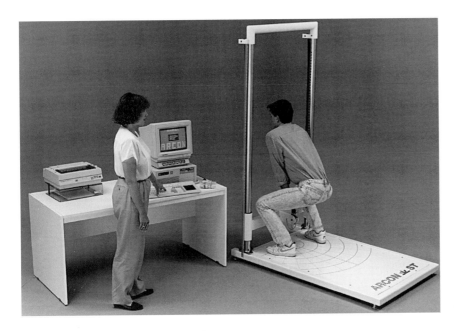

Fig. 8.2. ARCON ST (Advanced Rehabilitation Concepts, Irvine, CA).

ple of this type of test that is used widely. (Fig. 8.2). Additionally isometric test technology has been in existence for quite some time and thus is less expensive to manufacture and is widely available.

Because of the way in which isometric tests handle inertia, they have the *potential* to be quite safe. One method to improve safety is to provide performance feedback so that the evaluee is able to increase psychophysical input and, thereby, appropriately gauge his or her effort level. One method to improve reliability is to provide carefully developed instructions that are well understood by the evaluee. Both of these approaches have been used in the ERGOS Work Simulator (Fig. 8.3). The ERGOS is a multiple-task evaluation instrument that presents instructions to the evaluee in three ways, supplemented by input from an evaluator who is present during the evaluation. Primary instructions are presented auditorially through the use of a synthesized "voice" in combination with text presented on a color video display terminal. Secondary instructions are presented pictorially following the text presentation, using synthesized photographs that depict the posture to use with the evaluation task. Subsequently, during the isometric tasks, the evaluee is provided "real time" feedback concerning force generation through the use of a force curve that presents performance on the basis of a 24 cycles per second along a logarithmic scale. In the bimanual, isometric, whole body strength tasks, right hand performance is presented separately from left hand performance across the same scale, using two different colors for the force curve.

Isokinetic Testing

The concept of isokinetic exercise was first introduced by Hislop and Perrine.[17] The term isokinetic refers to dynamic shortening or lengthening of a muscle in contraction performed at a constant velocity regardless of the force generated

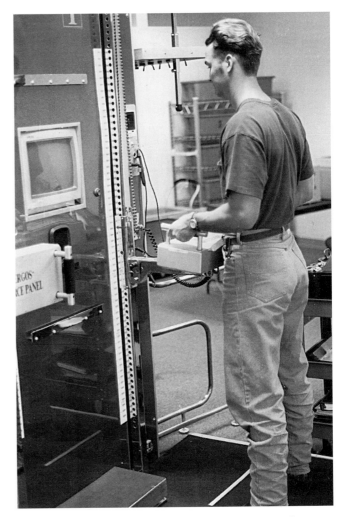

Fig. 8.3. ERGOS Work Simulator (Work Recovery Systems, Tucson, AZ).

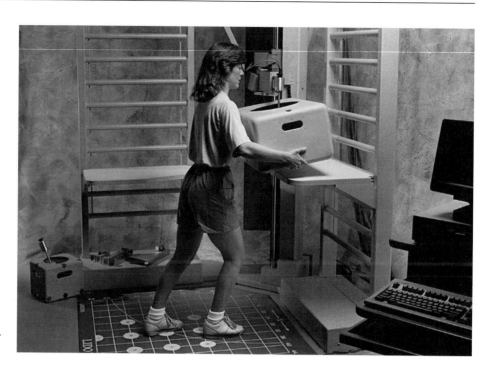

Fig. 8.4. LIDO Lift (Loredan Biomedical, West Sacramento, CA).

by the muscle. Acceleration is minimized so that the force exerted is equal to the force necessary to move the object at a constant velocity. Because the inertial effects of force application are controlled, maximum force can be measured throughout the entire range of elongation or shortening.

Isokinetic testing has been found reliable in several studies.[18–23] Isokinetic lifting simulation was shown to be reliable in studies done by Porterfield and colleagues,[24] Frykman, Harman, and Vogel,[25] and Alpert described the reliability of isokinetic lifting stimulation.[26] The latter researchers used the LIDO Lift, presented in Fig. 8.4.

Some critical issues have been raised regarding the use of isokinetic testing of lifting.[12,27] Although isokinetic testing is dynamic, it does not mimic functional activities because work is not usually performed with a fixed speed. Kishino et al[12] reported that although isokinetic equipment can be a useful tool in industry and rehabilitation, it had important equipment limitations that limited its ability to predict performance in an actual work setting. Timm[28] reported that lifting is composed of various combinations of isometric, isotonic, and isokinetic effort that isokinetic technology may not mimic sufficiently to be effective as an evaluative or rehabilitative tool. Mayer et al[29] compared isokinetic lifting on the Cybex Liftask with a Progressive Isoinertial Lifting Evaluation (PILE), and found the correlations between the two tests were low. They concluded that the tests do not evaluate the same parameters and cannot be substituted for each other. Alpert et al,[26] however, found isokinetic testing a valid predictor of subsequent progressive lift capacity testing.

Isoinertial Testing

Isoinertial denotes a dynamic test of lifting capacity in which the muscle is contracted in order to move a mass imparting

constant resistance along a vector. The constant-resistance assumption is violated in lifting and lowering because of the accelerative nature of gravity. Thus, the force imparted by the person performing the lift is accelerative. As a consequence, true isoinertial lift testing is not possible. Various testing strategies have been developed, however, to *constrain* the opportunity for the evaluee to use acceleration. One such strategy involves testing over limited vertical ranges that correspond to the range of motion available to the evaluee to use a single biomechanical segment (e.g., from floor to knuckle level or from knuckle level to shoulder level). This quasi-isoinertial strategy has been developed because it more closely replicates the actual demands of lifting than do either the isometric or isokinetic strategies.

Isoinertial lift capacity typically is tested using one of two similar approaches. Snook and Irvine,[30,31] Garg, Mital, and Asfour,[9] Kahlil and co-workers,[32] and Pytel and Kamon[33] advocate the "psychophysical" approach, which involves the concept of maximum acceptable weight (MAW). The maximum acceptable load is adjusted by the evaluee by adding or removing lead shot from a tote box that is lifted at a particular frequency to determine the acceptability of the load. The load is adjusted until the evaluee determines that the load reflects his or her MAW, given the frequency, size of the box, and both the starting height and vertical range over which the box is lifted. Karwowski[34] found this approach was reliable only for low and moderate lifting frequencies (not greater than six lifts per minute). Mital[35] reported that the psychophysical method tended to overestimate the MAW of lifting.

Matheson[36] described the WEST Standard Evaluation (WSE), a progressive lift-lowering test procedure in which load is increased incrementally while providing the evaluee an opportunity to decrease vertical range as he or she approximates maximum "range of motion under load." The WSE is the most widely used commercial test of lifting capacity, with approximately 1100 units in use in 1991 throughout North America and Australia. Matheson[37] reported that this approach has good intratest reliability with coefficients of variation of less than 5%. Jacobs, Bell, and Pope[38] used a similar progressive lifting capacity approach in the Operational Lift Task (OLT). In this test, weight in a crate is increased incrementally until the subject is unable to lift the load.

Another progressive lift capacity approach to isoinertial measurement of lifting performance developed by Kroemer[39] involves a progressive lifting capacity protocol in which the evaluee is presented with gradually increasing loads using a weight machine that captures the weight and maintains a fixed trajectory. The study reported a coefficient of variation of 3.2 to 3.9% in an overhead lift and 5.2 to 7.8% in a knuckle-height lift. The same subjects showed higher variability with static tests. The coefficient of variation with the static tests ranged from 11.6 to 15.4%.

Mayer et al[40] modified the progressive lift capacity approach to develop the Progressive Isoinertial Lift Evaluation (PILE), which requires four lift-lowers over a standard vertical range within a 20-second period before the evaluee is asked whether the load is equivalent to a MAW acceptable weight. If not, the load is changed incrementally. Different weight increments are used based on gender with 10-pound increments for men and 5-pound increments for women. The PILE also involves an age-based heart rate limitation and restricts the evaluee to loads of less than 55 to 60% of ideal body weight based on gender and height. This approach has been found reliable in a small sample. Test-retest reliability of the PILE showed a correlation coefficient of $r = .87$ for the lift from floor to 76 cm and $r = .93$ for the lift from 76 cm to 137 cm.

Matheson et al[41] provided further elaboration of this approach. Using the same four repetitions with a 30-second cycle and "masked weights," which limit the evaluee's knowledge of the amount of weight lifted to the actual experience of the lifting task itself, these researchers demonstrated good reliability on a test-retest basis: test-retest reliability of $r = .77$ for the lift from floor to 76 cm and $r = .81$ for the lift from 76 cm to 122 cm with a frequency of four lifts every 30 seconds. This basic protocol has been revised by other researchers. Alpert et al[26] used a frequency of one repetition per 30-second cycle and a starting point of 50% of the subject's isokinetic maximum; they reported test-retest reliability of $r = .91$. Using the one-repetition-per-cycle frequency over five vertical ranges, Golden demonstrated good test-retest and inter-rater reliability,[42] reporting test-retest reliability that depended on the test and ranged from $r = .62$ to $r = .87$.

Subsequent modifications to the PLC protocol have been undertaken by Matheson and colleagues[43,44] in the EPIC Lift Capacity Test (ELC). These changes include standardization of the load increments across genders, determination of the vertical lifting ranges based on the evaluee's height, and development of six subtests in the test battery, with later tests using information from the evaluee's performance on early

tests. The WEST-EPIC #1, which uses the ELC protocol, is presented in Figure 8.5. The ELC has become a "gold standard" against which to measure the validity of other more expensive types of lift test technology. The developers of the EPIC Lift Capacity test implemented a training and certification program for test users that provides certification of professionals and of technicians. Professionals are certified to perform the evaluation within their area of training and expertise. They may also supervise technicians. Technicians are certified to provide the evaluation under the supervision of the certified professional. The primary issue that distinguishes the professional from the technician is the professional's training, which provides the ability to make correct judgments concerning the appropriate response to symptoms that occur as the test progresses.

In the isoinertial approach, the objects used are similar to those found in real-world tasks. As a consequence, this approach is generally considered to have good validity. Some researchers, however, have raised concerns about the safety of this approach.[14] Others note that the practicality of the test is limited in that it typically requires 20 to 30 minutes to de-

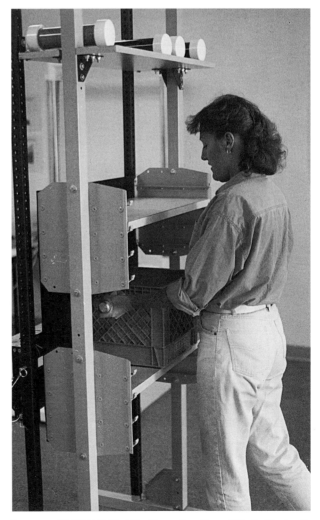

Fig. 8.5. WEST-EPIC Lift Capacity Test (Work Evaluation Systems Technology, Signal Hill, CA).

Factor	Isometric	Isokinetic	Isoinertial
Safety	Low > High	Moderate > High	Moderate
Reliability	High	Low > High	Low > Moderate
Validity	Low > Moderate	Low > Moderate	High
Cost Equipment	Moderate	High	Low
Cost Administration	Low	Moderate	High

Fig. 8.6. Comparison of lift capacity evaluation technologies using the National Institute of Occupational Safety and Health test selection criteria.

termine the MAW for any particular combination of frequency, starting height, and vertical displacement, and that both the time and effort expended by the worker is substantially more than is found using an isometric or isokinetic approach.[26]

The potential value of isoinertial strength testing with a disabled population depends on its reliability and validity. With this approach to testing, both test-retest and interrater reliability depend on the care with which the test is conducted. Within-test "reliability checks" in the ELC are available to confirm the evaluee's performance reliability through a comparison of performance at different frequencies or at different ranges of motion. These comparisons among individuals are dependable and provide a reasonable benchmark with which to compare an evaluee's performance to determine whether or not it represents a best effort.

The evaluation of lift capacity can be accomplished in many ways. Selection of the appropriate test depends on several factors. A hierarchy of factors has been established by the National Institute of Occupational Safety and Health.[45] The author has applied this hierarchy to the various types of technology that are available to evaluate lift capacity to produce a comparison of these approaches (Fig. 8.6). Figure 8.6 depicts a comparison of lift capacity evaluation systems that can be used to select the technology that the evaluator wishes to pursue. When a range of ratings is listed, the evaluator can improve the ratings through training and the application of diligence and a high degree of professional skill and acumen. In most cases, the range depends on the evaluator's training, experience, and skill.

The evaluation of lift capacity has developed beyond clinical art to have a firm base in science, aided by well-thought-out and appropriately designed technology. The intent of this chapter is to present an overview of the technology and applications to assist the clinician in using this technology more effectively.

REFERENCES

1. Matheson LN: Industrial Rehabilitation Resource Book. Santa Margarita, California: Performance Assessment & Capacity Testing, 1992.
2. Pheasant S: Ergonomics. Work and Health. Gaithersburg, MD, Aspen, 1991.
3. Magora A: Investigations of the relation between low back pain and occupation. Indust Med 39:31, 1970.
4. Magora, A: Investigations of the relation between low back pain and occupation. III. Physical requirements: sitting, standing and weight lifting. Indust Med 41:5, 1972.
5. Bigos SJ, Spengler DM, Martin NA, et al: Back injuries in industry: A retrospective study. II. Injury factors. Spine 11:252, 1986.
6. Matheson L, Mooney V, Caiozzo V, et al: Effect of instructions on isokinetic trunk strength variability, reliability, absolute value, and predictive validity. Spine 17:914, 1991.
7. Andersson GBJ, Chaffin DB, Pope MH: Occupational biomechanics of the lumbar spine. In Pope MH, Andersson GBJ, Frymoyer JW, (eds). Occupational Low Back Pain: Assessment, Treatment and Prevention. St. Louis, Mosby Year Book, 1991, pp 20–43.
8. Chaffin DB, Andersson GBJ: Occupational Biomechanics. New York, John Wiley & Sons, 1984.
9. Garg A, Mital A, Asfour SS: A comparison of isometric strength and dynamic lifting capability. Ergonomics 23:13, 1980.
10. Chaffin DB: Biomechanics of manual material handling and low back pain. In Occupational Medicine: Principles and Practical Applications. Chicago, Year Book, 1975, pp 443–467.
11. Caldwell LS, Chaffin DB, Dukes-Dobos FN, et al: A proposed standard procedure for static muscle strength testing. Am Ind Hyg Assoc J 35:201, 1974.
12. Kishino ND, Mayer TG, Gatchel RJ, et al: Quantification of lumbar function. Part 4: Isometric and isokinetic lifting simulation in normal subjects and low-back dysfunctional patients. Spine 10:921, 1985.
13. Battié MC, Bigos SJ, Fisher LD, et al: Isometric lifting strength as a predictor of industrial back pain reports. Spine 14:851, 1989.
14. Zeh J, Hansson T, Bigos S, et al: Isometric strength testing: Recommendations based on a statistical analysis of procedure. Spine 11:43, 1986.
15. Chaffin DB, Herrin GD, Keyserling WM: Preemployment strength testing. An updated position. J Occup Med 20:403, 1978.
16. Marras WS, King AI, Joynt RL: Measurements of loads on the lumbar spine under isometric and isokinetic conditions. Spine 9:176, 1984.
17. Hislop HJ, Perrine JJ: The isokinetic concept of exercise. Phys Ther 47:114, 1967.
18. Aitkens S, Lord J, Bernauer E, et al: Analysis of the validity of the Lido Digital Isokinetic System (research paper). Davis, California: University of California, Davis School of Medicine, 1987.
19. Burdett R, Van Swearingen J: Reliability of isokinetic muscle endurance tests. J Occup Sports Phys Ther 8:484, 1987.
20. Langrana NA, Lee CK, Alexander H, et al: Quantitative assessment of back strength using isokinetic testing. Spine 9:287, 1984.
21. McCrory MA, Aitkens, SG, Avery CM, et al: Reliability of concentric and eccentric measurements of the LIDO active isokinetic rehabilitation system. Med Sci Sports Exerc 21(Suppl):S52, 1989.
22. Rose S, Delitto A, Crandell C: Reliability of isokinetic trunk muscle performance, Phys Ther 68:824, 1988.
23. Smith SS, Mayer TG, Gatchel RJ, et al: Quantification of lumbar function. Part 1: Isometric and multispeed isokinetic trunk strength measures in sagittal and axial planes in normal subjects. Spine 10:757, 1985.
24. Porterfield JA, Mostardi RA, King S, et al: Simulated lift testing using computerized isokinetics. Spine 12:683, 1987.
25. Frykman PN, Harman EA, Vogel J: Using a new dynamometer to compare three lift styles (abstract). Med Sci Sports Exerc 20:87, 1988.

26. Alpert J, Matheson L, Beam W, et al: The reliability and validity of two new tests of maximum lifting capacity. J Occup Rehabil 1:13, 1991.

27. Rothstein JM, Lamb RL, Mayhew TP: Clinical uses of isokinetic measurements. Phys Ther 67:1840, 1987.

28. Timm KE: Isokinetic lifting simulation: A normative data study. J Occup Sports Phys Ther 10:156, 1988.

29. Mayer TG, Barnes D, Nichols G, et al: Progressive isoinertial lifting evaluation: II. A comparison with isokinetic lifting in a disabled chronic low-back pain industrial population. Spine 13:998, 1988.

30. Snook SH, Irvine CH: Maximum acceptable weight of lift. Am Ind Hyg Assoc J 28:322, 1967.

31. Snook SH: Psychophysical considerations in permissible loads. Ergonomic 28:327, 1985.

32. Khalil TM, Waly SM, Genaidy AM, et al: Determination of lifting abilities: A comparative study of four techniques. Am Ind Hyg Assoc J 48:951, 1987.

33. Pytel JL, Kamon E: Dynamic strength test as a predictor for maximal and acceptable lifting. Ergonomics 24:663, 1981.

34. Karwowski W: Maximum load lifting capacity of males and females in teamwork [Abstract]. Proceedings of the Human Factors Society, Louisville, Kentucky: University of Louisville, 1988, pp 680–699.

35. Mital A: The psychophysical approach in manual lifting: A verification study. Hum Factors 25:485, 1983.

36. Matheson LN: WEST 2 Examiner's Manual. Work Evaluation Systems Technology, 1982.

37. Matheson LN: Evaluation of lifting & lowering capacity. Vocational Evaluation and Work Adjustment Bulletin, 19:107, 1986.

38. Jacobs I, Bell DG, Pope J: Comparison of isokinetic and isoinertial lifting tests as predictors of maximal lifting capacity. Eur J Appl Physiol 57:146, 1988.

39. Kroemer KHE: An isoinertial technique to assess individual lifting capability. Hum Factors 25:493, 1983.

40. Mayer TG, Barnes D, Kishino ND, et al: Progressive isoinertial lifting evaluation. I. A standardized protocol and normative database. Spine 13:993, 1988.

41. Matheson L, Mooney V, Jarvis G, et al: Progressive lifting capacity with masked weights: Reliability study (abstract). PAR Research Foundation, Physical Assessment and Reactivation Center, Irvine Medical Center, Irvine California. Presented at the *International Society for the Study of the Lumbar Spine,* Boston, MA, June, 1990.

42. Golden NS: An assessment of interrater reliability and intertest correlation of a progressive psychophysical lifting evaluation which measures occasional lifting capacity (thesis). University of Iowa, August, 1990.

43. Matheson L: EPIC Lift Capacity Evaluation Manual. Santa Ana, CA, Employment Potential Improvement Corporation, 1992.

44. Matheson L, Mooney V, Grant J, et al: A test to measure lift capacity of physically impaired adults. Part I: Development and reliability testing. In press, Spine 1995.

45. National Institute for Occupational Safety and Health: Work Practices Guide for Manual Lifting [Technical Report 81-122]. Cincinnati, OH, Division of Biomedical and Behavioral Science, NIOSH, 1981.

9 Back School

PAUL D. HOOPER

NEW PERSPECTIVES IN BACK PAIN EDUCATION

Research over the past several decades has provided much new information about back pain. During this time, diagnostic procedures have improved considerably (e.g., magnetic resonance imaging, computed tomography, electromyography), as have methods of treatment. Likewise, our understanding of spinal anatomy, mechanics, and pathology has increased. Even so, certain aspects show no evidence of change. The overall prevalence of back pain remains around 80%, with an annual incidence of 5%. The number of people disabled by back pain between 1971 and 1981 increased by 168% (14 times faster than the population growth). The annual cost associated with back pain in the United States is estimated to be in excess of $50 billion.[1] Although the significance of past advancements cannot be ignored, no single procedure has been shown to alter the long-term outcome for patients with back pain. Even procedures, such as surgery, that positively affect the short-term course show little lasting benefit.[2]

As the problems and costs associated with back pain continue to increase, it is clear that we must approach back pain with a different attitude. Clinicians providing care for patients with back pain must accept the responsibility to promote self-reliance and resist the temptation to make patients dependent on care. Employers must assist the individual in obtaining care and make every effort to hasten the injured individuals' return to work. The third-party provider must promote prevention programs, in both the work place and the clinic. Finally, the patient must accept the responsibility for his or her own recovery. The single most important aspect is the motivation of the patient to get better.

The purpose of this chapter is to take a look at the use of education programs as one factor in reducing the incidence and severity of back pain. In this area, education programs have developed into a formal presentation commonly referred to as the "back school." The specific objectives of the following discussion are as follows:

- to describe the general purpose of the back school and the role it plays in the prevention of back pain
- to describe the historical development of the back school
- to review the literature regarding the effectiveness of the back school

- to describe some of the better known back school programs
- to discuss the various formats used in presenting a back school program
- to discuss the physical requirements for presenting a back school program
- to discuss the various applications of the back school in a private practice, as a public service, and in the workplace
- to discuss the most common problems and the limitations of the back school

PURPOSE

The back school is a particular method of teaching back pain prevention and self-care. It is a precisely directed presentation conducted in a setting designed and supplied for the sole purpose of educating the patient. This process of education may take many directions. The programs used by the author are directed at patients with back pain and at workers with back injuries. These programs include the following categories:

- Introductory back orientation program (Basic Training).[3] This type may be used as an introduction to back safety for patients and/or for employees as part of an industrial safety program.
- Back training and exercise program for all patients and employees with a history of back pain—the classic back school (Put Your Back Problems Behind You!!!)[4]
- Intensive back training and exercise program for patients and employees currently receiving some form of disability or compensation for back problems—back school plus specific rehabilitation procedures
- Back safety and injury response training for management and supervisory personnel. An extended program designed to acquaint those involved in work-related injuries with the realities of back pain.

The principal goals of the back school program are education and self-responsibility. A necessary step in decreasing the impact of any health problems involves improved understanding through patient education. In addition, to resolve the problem, patients must accept responsibility for their own health.

As a practicing chiropractor, I have treated many patients with back pain. Most recovered quickly, but as so often occurs, many had recurrences. Like many authors who have addressed the topic of back pain, my interest in prevention began after personally experiencing recurring back problems. As my interest grew, I successfully applied the principles that I learned to my own back. Pleased with the changes that I experienced, I implemented a back school in my private practice.

My initial attempts to educate patients in back pain prevention were based on existing programs described in the literature. Over the past decade, I have modified my ideas concerning the treatment and prevention of back pain. I firmly believe that treatment is virtually useless without the cooperation of everybody involved, including the patient, the clinician, the employer, and the provider. This cooperation may be attained only through proper education.

HISTORICAL PERSPECTIVES

Although often described as a disease of modern society, back pain is not a new problem. Man has been afflicted with back pain since ancient times. Work-related back injuries date back as far as 2780 BC.[5] Likewise, attempts to reduce the incidence of back pain through education programs date back several centuries.[6] In modern times, however, the emphasis on education has increased in an attempt to minimize the impact of back pain. This process began largely because of the observations of Fahrni in the late 1950s, who noted a significant difference in the incidence of back pain in a "ground-dwelling" population when compared to industrialized societies. He attributed this difference in part to postural or lifestyle variations. Fahrni claimed that ground-dwelling populations spent more time in a flexed posture, and that decreasing the lumbar lordosis would assist in preventing problems from developing. He was one of the first physicians to teach therapists in patient education techniques.[7]

At about the same time, Williams developed a series of back exercises (Williams flexion exercises) in an effort to reduce the incidence of back pain.[8] Williams thought that flexion of the lumbar spine would eliminate back pain, and he urged that every effort be made to reduce the lumbar lordosis. McKenzie also thought environmental factors contributed to the development of back pain, but he recommended an entirely different approach, one that incorporated extension exercises in an effort to increase the lumbar lordosis.[9]

The back school as a formal approach was first mentioned in the literature in the early 1970s with the work of Zachrisson-Forsell. What was known as the Swedish back school was developed in an automobile factory in response to an increasing problem with on-the-job back injuries.[10,11] This program was designed for a specific population group and was probably a response to the lack of effectiveness of the then current treatment approaches. Berquist-Ullman and Larson published the first statistical studies regarding the effectiveness of these education programs in 1977.[12] The next few years saw the development of several other back school programs, including the Canadian Back Education Units (CBEU) and the California

back school.[13,14] Thousands of back school programs have since developed; some are formal and involve the use of specific audiovisual aids and materials, whereas others are more informal and involve readily available props.

STATISTICS

The impact that patient education programs have on the outcome of any disease is difficult to gauge. Some evidence indicates that certain diseases, such as measles and typhoid, have been positively impacted by these programs. Objective evidence regarding the effectiveness of the back school, however, is mixed. Some studies have shown that the back school has a positive effect on patients with low back pain.[12,15-17] Other studies have shown that the back school makes little difference when compared to more common and traditional approaches.[18] In an extensive review of the literature, Linton and Kamwendo state support is limited for the idea that a low back school can influence factors such as sick leave, work status, pain intensity or duration, etc.[19] Berwick et al found no measurable impact in comfort or level of functional status.[20] On the other hand, Feldstein et al[21] demonstrated that back injury prevention programs were successful at changing behavior, at least in the short term.

One study by Brown et al[22] offers some encouraging support for the use of back school. The study investigated the cost effectiveness of a 6-week back school and rehabilitation program in terms of decreased lost work time and medical costs as compared to a control group. A key finding in this study was that back school participants had half as many reinjuries as nonparticipants. Data indicated that the back school was helpful in reducing the number of reinjuries in these workers for at least 6 months. The back school group had a savings in medical costs of $9,743 during the postintervention period. The authors concluded that the back school group had less lost work time, lost time cost, medical cost, and injury during the postintervention period.[22]

In contrast to the relatively scarce support for the back school in the literature, a number of studies in industry indicate that back pain prevention programs, including the use of a back school, have a significant impact on reducing back pain costs.[23] Some examples are as follows:[24]

- American Biltrite saw Workers' Compensation claims drop from $180,000 to $40,000 annually at the end of a back school program.
- Southern Pacific Transportation Company saw a 22% decrease in the incidence of on-the-job back injuries and a 43% reduction in lost work time. They calculated the savings at $1 million in a single year.
- Boeing Company participated in a controlled study of the effectiveness of back education on its workers in which 3424 workers were provided with a back school and 3500 were not. Although the overall incidence of back injuries was not statistically significant between the two groups, those in the back school group were demonstrated to have lower lost work times.

When one considers the staggering costs of back injuries on the work force, even a small reduction in injury rates or lost work time has a significant impact.

One aspect of the back school that appears to be consistent in the literature is the positive impact of this type of program on the patient's attitude. Dutro and Wheeler cite different studies that indicate that most individuals attending back school programs found them useful; in addition, most felt the program had indeed lowered their level of pain.[25] Because much evidence points to a variety of psychosocial factors, including motivation and lack of control, as key factors in the development of chronic back pain and/or disability, this effect on patient attitude may be the most important role for the back school. In fact, I contend that the back school is more useful in changing an individual's attitude about their back problems than it is in changing the way they lift.

PROGRAMS

Several programs have been established as major contributors to the evolution of the back school, including the Swedish Back School, the Canadian Back Education Units, and the California Back School. Although many other programs exist, including modifications of those listed, it is worthwhile to view the format of these programs.

The Swedish Back School

Developed by Zachrisson-Forsell, this program consists of four 45-minute sessions conducted over a 2-week interval. Each session includes a 15-minute sound-slide presentation followed by a 30-minute presentation provided by a physical therapist. Class size is relatively small (six to eight subjects).

Specific goals of the Swedish Back School are to (1) increase patient self-confidence; (2) understand the role treatment plays in the condition, and (3) reduce the costs of care. An outline of class content follows.

Class 1. The focus of the first session is on anatomy and biomechanics of the back, the development of back pain, and the types of treatment available. Emphasis is placed on resting positions and some treatment advice is given.

Class 2. This session focuses on the stresses imparted on the back from poor posture and improper daily activities. Exercises are demonstrated for strengthening the abdominal musculature.

Class 3. In this more practical session, participants are asked to apply information gained during the first two sessions. Various activities of daily living (ADL) are demonstrated and practiced.

Class 4. This session includes a review of the first three classes and patient is provided with a written summary of the information presented. Patients are encouraged to become physically active.

The Canadian Back Education Units[27]

This program, developed by Hall, consists of four 90-minute lectures held at weekly intervals. Class size is slightly larger (15 to 20 subjects) and a variety of professionals serve as the instructors, including an orthopedic surgeon, a psychologist, a psychiatrist, and a physical therapist.

Class 1. This session is taught by an orthopedic surgeon and focuses on anatomy, mechanics, and the aging process of the spine.

Class 2. In this session, a physical therapist teaches proper body mechanics. First aid methods for obtaining temporary relief from back pain are also included.

Class 3. This session addresses the psychiatric aspects of chronic pain and the influence of emotions on back pain. The instructor is a psychiatrist.

Class 4. The final class is team taught by a physical therapist, who teaches basic back exercises, and a psychologist, who demonstrates relaxation techniques and discusses stress management.

The California Back School[28]

This program, developed by White Matmiller, includes three 90-minute sessions held at weekly intervals. A fourth follow-up session is scheduled 1 month later. Class size is small (4) and most classes are taught by a physical therapist.

Class 1. The focus of this discussion is on basic anatomy and aging of the spine. In addition, the natural history of back pain is outlined. Information on pain relief and activities of daily living (ADL) is included. Each patient is evaluated using an obstacle course and an exercise tolerance test.

Class 2. This session concentrates on ADL and coordination exercises. The obstacle course is used to train patients in lifting techniques and other ADL. Participants learn back exercises and on-the-job safety procedures.

Class 3. This class includes a quiz on the information provided, along with a second text on the obstacle course. Instruction is given on more complex ADL, and individual problems are addressed. Patients are given a stress test, Personal Concerns Inventory (PCI), and instructed on its use.

Class 4. This session focuses primarily on problem solving. Patients are once again tested on the obstacle course. The PCI is reviewed and suggestions are made for reducing stress. Each of the programs discussed provides participants with essentially the same basic information, including anatomy, posture, body mechanics, first aid, exercise, stress reduction, nutrition, and lifestyle habits. Although the format varies slightly, each has similar goals. To be effective, a back school should be able to adapt to the particular environment (i.e., private practice, industrial, etc.) and to the needs of the participants.

THE BACK SCHOOL IN A CHIROPRACTIC PRACTICE

Although the back school should not be viewed as the solution to back pain, it is an essential component in the treatment and prevention of back pain. It should be an integral part of any encounter with patients with back pain. Because so many patients seen in a chiropractic office have a primary complaint of back pain, the back school should be a standard part of treatment. Arthur White stated, "Back school is the center of the fastest moving specialty in health care today . . . We will see chiropractors using back school in all of its forms and it may change the face of the chiropractic health delivery system. Chiropractors have traditionally delivered their treatments and moved quickly to their next patients. They have not, in general, spent time on education and prevention. If and when they do so, the public and other health care professionals will see them as the largest body of spine care specialists with the most tools with which to treat spinal disorders."[29]

In addition to reducing the impact of back pain on patients, the back school should play a role in preventing back problems. As costs for health care continues to escalate, the role of prevention is increasing in importance. As an example, the National Institute for Occupational Safety and Health (NIOSH) has set, as a priority, a national health objective for the year 2000 to implement back injury prevention and rehabilitation programs in at least 50% of worksites. As of 1985, only 28.6% of worksites with 50 or more employees offered back care activities.[30]

A description of the back school programs used by the author follows. Although the focus of attention is on the work-related back injury, each of the programs is readily adaptable for a general practice setting.

Introductory Back Safety Orientation for Industry

The purpose of this aspect of the back school program is to provide all newly hired employees with an orientation course in back safety. Topics to be addressed should include the following:

- Basic back anatomy and biomechanics. This section is structured to reduce the fear of the unknown. Anatomy is presented in such a way that those attending back school have an appreciation for the unique design and function of the human spine. The role of the muscles, bones, discs, and nerves is presented. The nature of injuries to each of these tissues and the type of treatment used for various injuries are discussed.
- Cost of injuries, both to industry and to the worker. Individuals should appreciate the impact of back pain on everyday life. Most estimates place the total costs of back pain at greater than $50 billion annually, but this number is unmanageable for most people. More practically, discussion should include the average cost of visits to the doctor, the loss of wages that often result from back injuries, and the costs on home and family life.
- Overview of how back injuries occur. Too often patients view the onset of back pain as rapid. In fact, many doctors also look at back pain in much the same manner. For example, when an individual bends to pick up a box and develops back pain, she or he tends to blame the box. The patient is often cautioned about picking up boxes in the future. In contrast, an individual who picks up a box and has a heart attack would not consider blaming the box for their heart problem. The patient understands that, although the episode may have been triggered by a particular activity, the activity did not create the problem. It is important to understand that back problems are like heart disease, they don't just happen . . . they develop.

- Causes of back pain. Back pain has no single cause. Rather, it is the result of an accumulation of stresses over a period of time. These factors include stress, poor posture, poor living and working habits, poor body mechanics, loss of flexibility, and an overall decline in health. To minimize the impact of future episodes of back pain, each of these areas must be addressed.
- First aid for back injuries. One of the most important aspects of any back school program is first aid. Because many people with back pain are likely to have future episodes, it is imperative that they know how to respond when problems do occur. The response may have a significant impact on the severity and duration of the episode. When a patient sprains an ankle, they typically apply ice. For some reason, however, when a back sprain occurs, patients often apply heat, many times at a doctors advice. In the event of back injury, patients should be instructed to: (1) stop whatever they are doing, (2) relax in a comfortable position, (3) perform some type of "first aid exercise" (i.e., press-up, knee-to-chest, or standing back bend), and (4) apply ice.
- Self-responsibility. Ultimately, the solution to back pain lies not in the doctor's hands, but in the patient's. Consequently, the primary goal of the back school should be to provide the individual with enough information to allow them to take an active role in their own back care and to encourage them to accept the responsibility to do so.

This orientation program may be presented in a classroom style format and should last approximately 30 minutes. It can be adapted to accommodate small, medium, and large groups.

Back Safety Program for Industry

The purpose of this component of the back school is to provide all employees with information necessary to avoid serious back injuries. Topics of discussion are similar to those covered in the orientation program (see previous section). The content is expanded and the format includes active participation on the part of the employees. It is suggested that two separate sessions be included in this section. Each should be approximately 30 to 45 minutes in length and scheduled within 2 weeks of each other. Class size should be limited to 20 to 25 participants to allow interaction.

Back Training and Exercise Program

Those individuals who have had back pain previously are at a high risk for future problems; in fact, a positive history of back pain is one of the most significant risk factors for future problems.[31,32] In addition to the increased risk, these individuals typically are more interested in prevention programs. For these reasons, this group requires more extensive training.

It is suggested that this group enroll in an extended back school program consisting of three 45-minute sessions. Class size should be limited to 10 to 12 individuals to allow individual attention to specific needs and problems.

Class 1. Topics discussed include the causes of back pain, anatomy and biomechanics, first aid for back injuries, and relaxation techniques.

Class 2. Topics include lifting techniques and instruction in ADL, safety tips, and specific flexibility exercises.

Class 3. Discussion includes the risk factors for back problems, good health tips, stress management, strengthening and coordination exercises, costs of back pain to industry and to the individual, and self-responsibility.

Intensive Back Training and Exercise Program

Those individuals currently receiving care for a back injury or those currently receiving some form of disability should enroll in an intensive program to address their condition and their problems. This type of training consists of three classes as described in the preceding section plus any follow-up exercise and ADL training as indicated by their condition. It is important to appreciate that those patients who may be disabled need to be in some form of rehabilitation or exercise program. In the case of an injured athlete, one would not expect full recovery without some form of directed activity. It is equally unlikely to expect an injured "industrial athlete" to recover unless they are active.

Back Safety and Injury Response Training

Until recently, the use of education and training programs to reduce the incidence of low back pain has focused on the injured worker. One of the most significant components of any back safety or injury prevention program, however, is the training provided to supervisory staff. The way in which the "company" responds to an injured employee has a great deal to do with the seriousness of the injury. With this in mind, one must look at a somewhat unique aspect of the back school. The purpose of this portion of the program is to provide the supervisory staff (e.g., management, store managers, union stewards, etc.) with the information necessary to deal effectively with the injured employee when an accident occurs. The class is designed to consist of one full day of 6 hours duration; class size is limited to 30 to 40 individuals. Topics to cover include the following:

- Risk factors, both occupational and personal
- Anatomy and biomechanics
- Costs of back injuries, to the individual and to industry
- Types of back pain
- Causes of back pain
- First aid for back injuries on the job

- Management issues, how to deal with the injured worker (e.g., referral process, light duty, company attitude, etc.)
- Legal considerations

Recent information indicates that management education and support may be one of the most effective ways of minimizing the costs of back injuries on the job. Fitzler and Berger describe an industrial program in which management was taught to accept low back pain and workers were encouraged to report all episodes. Treatment was immediately available and included worker education. Every effort was made to keep the worker on the job. Workers compensation costs were reduced tenfold in a 3-year period.[33,34] In another study, Wood described the effects of a personnel program designed to minimize the impact of back problems. The program stressed early access to care in addition to changing the attitude of management.[35]

Management should make every attempt to provide injured employees with reasonable access to care. Programs discouraging early return to work should be discontinued. Employers should explain fully the employee's rights under the Workers' Compensation guidelines and work to develop an atmosphere of cooperation. Prolonged disability from back problems is often associated with adversarial situations between the worker and the employer, litigation, and lack of follow-up and concern.[36] (This topic is discussed in greater detail later in this chapter.) Only through education, of both the injured worker and the employer, can we take the necessary steps to reduce this aspect of the back pain problem.

FORMATS

Over the years, I have taught back schools in a variety of formats, including lectures to large groups, small group sessions with 6 to 10 individuals, and one-on-one instruction. Each particular format has advantages and disadvantages and the design of any back school program should be adapted to the specific audience for which it is intended. As stated previously, many industrial back safety programs are best presented in a lecture format. A program intended for patients recovering from a recent back pain episode requires a more personal approach, such as small group sessions. Some patients with particularly difficult or chronic problems may need individual instruction.

Before addressing what is needed to implement a back school in private practice, it is important to take into account the requirements and demands of your particular situation. Many well-meaning individuals have attempted to establish some type of on-going patient education program only to find that the logistics were complicated and the demands impractical. As with any patient education program, the back school will change along with your time, energy, and experience.

Many different formats for the back school have been attempted. The most successful for patient care has been a series of three classes, each between 45 and 60 minutes in length. In our facility, classes are scheduled on Mondays and Thursdays and participants are scheduled on three consecutive nights (i.e., Monday, Thursday, Monday or Thursday, Monday, Thursday). Consequently, the entire series of classes is completed in a period of 8 days. Class size is limited to six to eight individuals to allow individual attention.

Group Versus Individual Training

At times, certain patients may require individual attention. As a general rule, however, small groups of patients are more productive. The advantages of teaching back school in small groups include that the friendly environment reduces intimidation; patients learn from each others' mistakes and experiences; the variety of experiences and questions is greater; those in the group provide psychological support for each other; in any state, it is encouraging to realize they are not alone; teaching several individuals at a single session is cost efficient.

Curriculum

Although the curriculum varies from one location and program to the next, certain basic elements are found in most back school programs. The information provided should include the following:

- Anatomy—basics of spinal anatomy. It is important to describe the anatomy in terms that are clear to the patient. Understanding the parts of the back enables the patient to better appreciate the role each part plays in their problems and in their recovery. In addition, the more an individual understands about the back, the less fearful they become.
- Posture. Many authors have suggested that poor posture plays an important role in the development of back pain. Although not everyone agrees on which posture is most detrimental or most helpful, it is clear that any posture that is sustained is, at the very least, a contributing factor to back pain. Patients should learn how to recognize both healthy and harmful postures. They should be able to identify positions and movements that alleviate their symptoms and be taught to modify their work habits to improve posture.
- Body mechanics. The relationship of activities of daily living to the development of back pain is an important aspect of the back school program. Patients should be encouraged to use their bodies in safe ways, which is accomplished by teaching safe lifting techniques and by demonstrating and practicing a variety of everyday movements and activities (e.g., lifting, pulling, etc.)
- First aid. This aspect of the back school is one of the most important. Even if patients understand how to use their back and establish good back habits, accidents and injuries still occur. When they do, the reaction to the injury has a great deal to do with the seriousness of the condition. Patients should learn to respond to any future problems by relaxing, assuming appropriate movements and positions, performing first aid exercises, and applying ice and support.
- Exercise. One goal of a back school program should be to teach exercises to minimize future back problems. These exercises will vary with the background and philosophy of the instructor, but they should include relaxation techniques, flexibility and stretching exercises, strengthening programs, balance and coordination procedures, and endurance exercises.
- Stress reduction. Many back school programs have included specific attempts to reduce stress in back pain patients. Efforts to reduce stress and tension are a most productive tool for the management of many musculoskeletal problems, including back pain, and should be a focus of the back school.
- Nutrition and lifestyle habits. The relationship between lifestyle and health is described to raise the level of patient awareness in this area. Topics covered include good nutritional habits, smoking, alcohol, regular exercise, and relaxation.

Needs

To determine the optimal back school program that is both effective and practical, the following warrant consideration: (1) patient population, (2) available space, (3) personnel, (4) available time, (5) available equipment, and (6) fees.

PATIENT POPULATION

One of the primary considerations in developing and designing a back school is the nature of the intended participants and the demographics of the community in which the program will function. Those participating in a back school may be current back pain patients, a general patient population, back-injured workers (Workers' Compensation), participants in an industrial safety program, management and safety personnel, school-age children, or pregnant patients. As stated previously, it may be helpful to develop several different formats aimed at reaching different groups.

AVAILABLE SPACE

The back school does not require a large amount of space in which to function. It is possible to use separate facilities specifically designed for patient education, or you may want to "double up" an area that is used for other activities. If space is a problem, teaching back school principles to small groups or even one-on-one is more practical. Scheduling back school sessions at a time when the office is not involved in patient treatment activities is another consideration. A back school that includes an obstacle course and an exercise area requires an open room with approximately 200 square feet of floor space. The only requirements are that the room be carpeted and clean. If the back school follows a large lecture format, you may want to consider renting a small meeting room in a local hotel, at the local public library, a nearby public school, church, or fitness center. In one instance, I found a nearby dance studio ideal for our purposes.

PERSONNEL

One of the most important aspects in developing a back school is determining who will provide the instruction. Some authorities believe that only experts in the field of back pain have significant success in the back school.[37] A great deal can be accomplished with existing office staff, however, particularly those who have a history of back pain. The next option is to look for help in the community. Every community has people with some health and/or education experience (physical therapists, licensed practical nurses, registered nurses, retired teachers, etc.) who are eager and willing to work a few hours a day and enjoy interacting with people. An advertisement in a local newspaper should provide a list of qualified people. It is also possible to find the right person from among your patients. Whoever is selected, she or he needs to be friendly, uninhibited, and willing to listen and learn. (Note: This search should not be viewed as an opportunity to recruit new patients. Being serious about finding the right person for the job increases the likelihood that the back school will be successful.)

AVAILABLE TIME

The time schedule for back school sessions will vary. Sessions that take place during the normal work day while patient care is being administered, necessitate both space and personnel dedicated solely to this purpose. Scheduling back school sessions during nonpeak office hours, during evenings, or on weekends places less of a burden on your facility and personnel.

AVAILABLE EQUIPMENT

One advantage of a back school is that no sophisticated or expensive equipment is required. Most items needed are found around the house or on the job, such as a vacuum cleaner, suitcase, floor mop, grocery sacks, etc. It is helpful, however, to have a slide projector, a cassette tape recorder, and/or a television with a video cassette recorder.

FEES

Perhaps one of the most practical questions concerns how much to charge and who is to pay. Fees vary from location to location, but a reasonable fee is the cost of an extended office visit. Many insurance companies pay for these services and sometimes the patient's employer is willing to pay. Whatever the cost, and whoever pays the bill, it has been stated that, for every one dollar spent on education and prevention, nine dollars are saved!

Useful billing codes are as follows:

- 97100—therapeutic exercise
- 97540—ADL and/or job-related activities training
- 97708—ADL evaluation

READY, FIRE, AIM!

In planning a back school, consider the options that are most practical for your situation and BEGIN! Anticipate changes as you gain experience. Many questions will remain unanswered and the chances of success may be uncertain. If you wait until all questions are answered and the best possible facility, staff, and format are secured, chances are you will never start. Certainly, the chances of success are much better once you begin!

Promoting the Program

To be successful, the back school must reach the intended audience. Depending on the type of program developed, this connection may take place in a variety of ways. If the back school is intended as a resource for your back pain patients, they simply need to enroll in back school. If the program is intended as a public service, making the necessary contacts with local service organizations or groups is required. Any interest in presenting this information to industry necessitates active "marketing" of these services. The following information is provided to assist in the latter endeavor.

Note: The back school will be an effective public relations program for your practice. Most people contacted, and certainly most participants in the back school, will have a positive feeling about the program and about you. The back school, however, is not intended to be a marketing tool for your practice or a way to attract new patients. It is a service to those individuals with back pain and this fact must remain the primary focus.

Use in industry remains one of the primary functions of this type of educational program. The chiropractor is widely recognized as an expert in the area of back pain, and the back school allows the professional to positively impact the industrial community. To introduce a back school into local industries, the chiropractor must first make contact with the necessary individuals. She or he must establish themselves as an expert and be able to convince management that this program will be useful. This relationship between the chiropractor and industry, often develops gradually over a period of time; once established, however, it should prove to be of benefit to everybody concerned.

An initial contact is made with a representative from the company or industry. This first contact will hopefully lead to a most important step, the interview, which is used to establish what type of services are needed.

The Interview

After arranging an appointment with the appropriate company representative, the real work begins. This first meeting is an opportunity to leave a lasting impression with the company and that impression should be first class. It is important to know as much as possible about the company before this meeting. The following information is helpful.

- What is the nature of the company, i.e., manufacturing, heavy construction, material handling, high-tech, etc.
- How many employees does the company have locally
- Does the company have other facilities or branches
- How long has the company been in existence and at this location
- What is the future market for the products or services of this company

This information is available through a variety of sources. The local library has demographic information on most industries, as does the local chapter of the Chamber of Commerce. In addition, a receptionist or some other contact at the company will often provide a great deal of information.

It is useful to view this first meeting in much the same way as we look at an initial patient interview. This first encounter is the time to identify the primary problems and to establish if there is a need for prevention services and, if so, what type of assistance is needed. For example, if a company has a large number of repetitive stress claims for wrist and hand injuries but no significant problems with back pain, it may not help them much to provide a back school. Another company may have a real problem with noise pollution or with exposure to toxic chemicals. It is helpful to have a list of individuals in the vicinity who deal with other work-related problems. If you are unable to help directly, perhaps you can refer the company to someone who can.

In addition to identifying problem areas, it is important to establish the attitude of the company in health-related areas. This information is crucial in developing a clear understanding of the health-related problems faced by the company and the role that a prevention program may play.

INDUSTRIAL CASE HISTORY

The Industrial Case History is designed to provide information about the demographics of the company, the nature of injuries and problems that are common in their work environment, and the manner in which they view health issues. It is a most useful resource for this first meeting. It is unlikely that any company representative will have the answers to all of the questions on this form; they will need to do some homework to provide all of the information required. This situation affords an opportunity to schedule a second meeting and also helps to establish the first way in which one can function as a consultant to the company, i.e., to review their Workers' Compensation claims.

One of the first steps in developing a prevention program with a company is evaluating their past on-the-job injuries. Review of the workers compensation claims for the past 2 years provides information on the type of injuries common

to the company, the location or job description where the injuries occurred, and the manner in which the claims were handled.

Once this evaluation is accomplished, it may be helpful to do an on-site evaluation or analysis of any problem areas that arise in the records review. Of particular interest are areas that have had a high incidence of injury, especially back injuries. Other areas of interest include slips and falls, knee injuries, arm and shoulder injuries, and wrist and hand problems.

As with patient care, once problems have been clearly identified through a thorough case history and examination, the clinician is in a position to offer suggestions to address the problems identified. This advice may include the use of back school programs.

NEW PERSPECTIVES

The significance of past advancements cannot be ignored, yet no single procedure has been shown to alter the long-term outcome for patients with back pain. As stated previously, even procedures such as surgery, show little lasting benefit.[38] Similarly, the back school has not been shown to provide any long-term changes in persons suffering with back pain.[39,40] Consequently, our approach to the back pain problem needs to change.

One of the newest areas of back pain prevention programs is education of management and supervisory staff. This type of program involves addressing methods of prevention and worker training and, perhaps more importantly, developing appropriate management skills for supporting the injured employee. The emphasis of most industrial back safety programs is on preventing injuries. Here, the emphasis is on minimizing the impact of the injury on the injured worker and on preventing drawn out litigated cases that often end in disability.

Several studies have shown that the manner in which a supervisor, company doctor, or employer responds to the injured workers has a significant impact on the seriousness of the injury.[41,42] Chronic back pain and disability are not solely a result of physical injury, but are associated with a complex interaction of factors, including psychosocial issues. Management and the clinician must make every effort to understand the impact of injury on the individual.

Industry can facilitate worker recovery by providing early return-to-work policies, maintaining contact with the injured worker, and accepting his or her injury as real. Efforts should be made to reduce the likelihood of litigation. One study by the California Workers' Compensation Institute showed that the most critical element in reducing litigation was information. Most injured workers went to an attorney because they felt they did not properly understand the Workers' Compensation system.[43] Other studies clearly demonstrate that the presence of an attorney delays the "healing" time.[44,45]

With these factors in mind, an innovative educational program was established that was designed to teach the management team how to deal effectively with the injured worker. Topics covered include the following:

- Costs of back injuries—to industry and to the individual
- Causes of back pain/types of back pain
- Risk factors, both occupational and personal
- Anatomy and biomechanics of the back
- First aid for back injuries on the job
- Management issues—how to deal with the injured worker (e.g., referral process, light duty, company attitude, etc.)
- Legal considerations

THE "10%" FACTOR

One of the predominant statistics in the literature pertaining to back pain is that approximately 10% of workers account for 80% of the costs.[46] To gain control of the back pain problem in industry, we must take a close look at this small group of individuals to try to determine why their situations are so different.

The Injured Worker

To understand better the back-injured worker who becomes chronically disabled, we must take a look at the situation from a new and different perspective. No longer is it adequate to equate the impact of the injury with the "seriousness" of the physical ailment. We must instead differentiate between the *disease* of low back pain and the *illness* associated with low back pain.[47]

The process of disease is defined solely as a biologic disturbance. The illness is the subjective experience of the disease by the person in his or her environment. As such, understanding the behavior of an individual with a disease or a disorder in the context of that environment becomes crucial. Two individuals with similar *diseases* often respond totally different ways. One patient may be totally disabled, whereas the other may be merely inconvenienced. In spite of the numbers provided previously, there is some thought that the *disease* of low back pain has not increased in incidence during the past several decades, whereas that of the *illness* has increased dramatically.

Part of our efforts in preventing or managing industrial back pain should be directed at identifying individuals at risk.[48]

RISK FOR INJURY

In the general uninjured population, certain factors *(injury predictors)* may serve to differentiate the group at risk for a back injury:

- History of back pain is the single most important predictor[49]
- Trunk strength deficits. The probability of injury is three times greater when the job lifting requirements approach or exceed the individuals' functional capacity[50]
- Individuals involved in heavy manual labor, vibration and driving, heavy lifting, and prolonged sitting[1]

- Short length of time on the job[51,52]
- Lack of job satisfaction/poor supervisory rating[53,54]
- High stress levels at work[55]
- Poor general health[56]/smoking[57]

RISK FOR DEVELOPING CHRONIC BACK PAIN

Other factors *(chronicity predictors)* may have relevance in evaluating a group of patients with acute low back pain to delineate those 5 or 10% who will develop a chronic problem:

- Clinical presentation of a patient over the initial weeks after injury may be a valuable guide in determining chronicity. Factors include:
  - Leg pain, particularly the presence of root tension signs[58,59]
  - Nonorganic signs, which may be associated with symptom magnification syndrome, hypochondriasis, and/or malingering[60]
  - Pain self-report. A pain complaint that does not conform to known physiologic patterns, particularly when coupled with an abnormal pain drawing[61]
  - Nonspecific diagnosis. The lack of a specific pathoanatomic diagnosis is associated with a less favorable outcome[62]
- Age. Individuals younger than age 25 years are at greater risk of injury but usually return to work sooner.[63] Those injured workers between the age of 30 and 55 tend to have higher incidences of chronicity and disability[66]
- Sex. Eighty percent of back injury compensation claims are filed by men,[65] although an occupationally injured woman is more likely to remain disabled.[66]
- Education. An inverse relationship exists between educational level and low back pain and disability, with the most pronounced incidence in the least educated.[67,68]
- Context of the injury. An acute event related to lifting, bending, or twisting or an accident such as a slip or fall, has a predictive value for chronicity.[45]
- Inconsistency of medical care[69]
- Lack of availability of interim light duty work[45]

RISK FOR BECOMING DISABLED

In addition to the factors just mentioned, another set of predictors *(chronic outcome predictors)* might be helpful in identifying those individuals for whom treatment or intervention is likely to fail. It is this patient who most contributes to the "high cost" of industrial back problems. These factors include:

- Compensation and litigation[70]
- Lag time. The longer it takes for an injured worker to receive care, the longer it takes for a referral to a specialist to occur, and the longer she or he must wait for procedures such as surgery. A chronic outcome is more likely in this situation.

- When surgery is suggested but not performed
- Lack of available work upon return[45]

Total Management of the Back-Injured Worker

Success in this task includes an understanding of the following:

- The injured worker—what type of worker is injured
- The injury—how does the injury occur, what types of activities are associated with back injuries
- The response to injury—what happens at the time of injury, to whom does she or he report, who does she or he see, what help does the company offer
- Return-to-work factors—what is the company policy, what is the employee attitude and experience, modified work program, who are the stake holders
- What makes an injury serious

SUMMARY

Patients must take a more active role in their recovery. Clinicians are being asked to abandon passive treatment in favor of methods that encourage patient activity and participation. After three decades of interest, however, controversy surrounds the effectiveness of the back school as a means of combatting back pain. The back school is treated by some as an important part of the solution to the growing problem of back pain. By others, it is considered unnecessary and unproductive.

After 17 years of active involvement in back school programs, I have seen interest in this topic increase and decrease. The substantial commitment of time, effort, and energy needed to establish and continue a successful back school program in a chiropractic practice or any other clinic may account for the current decline. It is clear, however, that efforts to decrease the incidence and impact of back pain have failed, and I am convinced that the back school is a vital and necessary step toward recovery for all patients with back pain.

Appropriate management of back injuries, particularly those sustained on the job, *must* include a cooperative effort involving the injured worker, the company, the clinician, and the insurer. This cooperation is achieved only through proper education. The individual who provides this information is in a unique position in the industrial arena and in the treatment of back pain.

REFERENCES

1. Haldeman S: Presidential address, North American Spine Society: Failure of the pathology model to predict back pain. Spine 15:718, 1990.
2. Weber H: Lumbar disc herniation: A controlled prospective study with ten years of observatoin. Spine 8:131, 1983.
3. Hooper PD: Basic Training. Diamond Bar, CA, Injury Prevention Technologies, 1992.
4. Hooper PD: Put Your Back Problems Behind You!!!, Diamond Bar, CA, Injury Prevention Technologies, 1992.
5. Brandt-Rauf PW, Brandt-Fauf SI: History of occupational medicine: Relevance of Imhotep and Edwin Smith papyrus. Br J Ind Med 44:68, 1987.
6. Peltier L: The back school of Delpech in Montpelier. Clin Orthop 179:4, 1983.
7. Fahrni WH: Backache and Primal Posture. Vancouver, Musqueam Pub., Ltd., 1976.
8. Williams PC: Low Back and Neck Pain: Causes and Conservative Treatment. Springfield, Charles C Thomas, 1974.
9. McKenzie R: The Lumbar Spine: Mechanical Diagnosis and Therapy. Wellington, New Zealand, Spinal Publications, 1985.
10. Zachrisson M: The Low Back School, Danderyd, Sweden, Danderyd's Hospital sound the slide program, 1972.
11. Zachrisson-Forsell M: The Swedish Back school. Physiotherapy 66, April, 1980.
12. Berquist-Ullman M, Larson U: Acute low back pain in industry. Acta Ortho Scand (Suppl):170, 1977.
13. Hall H: The Canadian Back Education Units. Physiotherapy 66:118, 1980.
14. Matmiller AW: The California Back school. Physiotherapy 66:115, 1980.
15. Hall H, Iceton JA: Back school: An overview with specific reference to the Canadian Back Education Units. Clin Orthop 179:10, 1983.
16. Klaber-Moffett JA, Chase SM, Portek I, et al: A controlled perspective study to evaluate the effectiveness of a back school in the relief of chronic low back pain. Spine 11:120, 1986.
17. Matmiller AW: The California Back school. Physiotherapy 66:115, 1980.
18. Kvien TK, Nilsen H, Vik P: Education and self-care of patients with low back pain. Scand J Rheumatol 10:320, 1981.
19. Linton SJ, Kamwendo K: Low back schools: A critical review. Phys Ther 67:1375, 1987.
20. Berwick DM, Budman S, Feldstein M: No clinical effect of back schools in an HMO: A randomized prospective trial. Spine 14:338, 1989.
21. Feldstein A, Balanis B, Vollmer W et al: The Back Injury Prevention Project Pilot Study. J Occup Med 35:114, 1993.
22. Brown KC, Sirles AT, Hilyer JC, et al: Cost-effectiveness of a back school intervention for municipal employees. Spine 17:1224, 1992.
23. Hooper PD: Preventing Low Back Pain. Baltimore, Williams & Wilkins, 1992.
24. Dutro CL, Wheeler L: Back school and chiropractic practice. J Manipulative Physiol Ther 9:209, 1986.
25. Dutro CL, Wheeler L: Back school and chiropractic practice. J Manipulative Physiol Ther 9:209, 1986.
26. Zachrisson-Forsell M: The Back school. Spine 6:104, 1981.
27. Hall H: The Canadian Back Education Units. Physiotherapy 66:118, 1980.
28. White AH: Back School and Other Conservative Approaches to Low Back Pain. St. Louis, C.V. Mosby, 1983.
29. White A: The Back school of the Future. In White L (ed): Back School. Philadelphia, Hanley and Belfus, 1992.
30. Department of Health and Human Resources: Draft Objectives for the Year 2000. Washington, DC, U.S. Public Health Service, 1989.
31. Pedersen PA: Prognostic indicators in low back pain. J R Coll Gen Pract 5:99, 1981.
32. Lloyd DCEF, Troup JDG: Recurrent back pain and its prediction. J Soc Occup Med 33:66, 1983.
33. Fitzler SL, Berger RA: The Chelsea back program: One year later. Occup Health Saf 7:52, 1982.
34. Fitzler SL, Berger RA: Attitudinal change: The Chelsea back program. Occup Health Saf 3:24, 1983.
35. Wood DJ: Design and evaluation of a back injury prevention program within a geriatric hospital. Spine 12:77, 1987.
36. Nordin M, Crites-Battie M, Pope MH, et al: Education and training. In Pope MH, Andersson GBJ, Frymoyer JW, et al (eds) Occupational Low Back Pain: Assessment, Treatment and Prevention. St. Louis, Mosby Year Book, 1991.
37. Saunders HD, Isernhagen SJ: Back Schools. In Isernhagen SJ (ed): Work Injury. Rockville, MD, Aspen, 1988, p 27.
38. Weber H: Lumbar disc herniation: A controlled prospective study with ten years of observation. Spine 8:131, 1983.

39. Hall H, Iceton JA. Back school: An overview with specific reference to the Canadian back education units. Clin Orthop 179:10, 1983.

40. Klaber-Moffett JA, Chase SM, Portek BS, et al: A controlled, prospective study to evaluate the effectiveness of a back school in the relief of chronic lbp. Spine 11:120, 1986.

41. Barnes D, Smith D, Gatchel R, et al: Psychosocioeconomic predictors of treatment success/failure in chronic low-back pain patients. Spine 14:427, 1989.

42. Frymoyer J, Cats-Baril W: Predictors of low back disability. Clin Orthop 221:89, 1987.

43. Tebb A: Litigation in Workers' Compensation. Presented at the State Workmen's Compensation Advisory Committee, San Diego, CA, October, 1974.

44. Block AR, Kremer E, Gaylor M: Behavioral treatment of chronic pain variables affecting treatment efficacy. Pain 8:367, 1980.

45. White AWM: Low back pain in men receiving workmens' compensation. Can Med Assoc J 95:50, 1966.

46. Frymoyer JW, Pope MH, Rosen J, et al: Epidemiologic studies of low back pain. Spine 5:419, 1980.

47. Vernon H: Chiropractic: A model of incorporating the illness behavior model in the management of low back pain patients. J Manipulative Physiol Ther 14:379, 1991.

48. Polatin PB: Predictors of low back pain disability. In White AH, Anderson R (eds): Conservative Care of Low Back Pain. Baltimore, Williams & Wilkins, 1991.

49. Bigos SJ, et al: A prospective evaluation of commonly used pre-employment screening tools for acute industrial back pain. Spine 17:922, 1992.

50. Chaffin DB, Park KS: A longitudinal study of low-back pain associated with occupational weight lifting factors. Am Ind Hyg Assoc J 34:513, 1973.

51. Bigos SJ, Spengler DM, Martin NA, et al. Back injuries in industry: A retrospective study. III. Employee-related factors. Spine 11:252, 1986.

52. Astrand NE: Medical, psychological, and social factors associated with back abnormalities and self-reported back pain. Br J Ind Med 44:327, 1987.

53. Magora A: Investigation of the relationship between low back pain and occupation. Scand J Rehab Med 5:191, 1973.

54. Westrin C, Hirsch C, Lindegard B: The personality of the back patient. Clin Orthop 87:209, 1972.

55. Niemcryk S, Jenkins CD, Rose RM, et al: The prospective impact of psychosocial variables on rates of illness and injury in professional employees. J Occup Med 29:645, 1987.

56. Spengler DM, Bigos SJ, Martin MA, et al: Back injuries in industry: A retrospective study. I. Overview and cost analysis. Spine 11:241, 1986.

57. Frymoyer JW, Pope MH, Clements JH, et al: Risk factors in low back pain. J Bone Joint Surg [Am] 65:184, 1983.

58. Biering-Sorensen F: A prospective study of low back pain in a general population. Scand J Rehab Med 15:81, 1983.

59. Troup JDG: Straight-leg-raising (SLR) and the qualifying tests for increased root tension: Their predictive value after back and sciatic pain. Spine 6:526, 1981.

60. Waddell G, McCullough JA, Kummel EG, et al: Nonorganic physical signs in low back pain. Spine 3:117, 1980.

61. Kirkaldy-Willis WH: The clinical picture—introduction. IN Kirkaldy-Willis WH (ed): Managing Low Back Pain. 2nd Ed. New York, Churchill-Livingstone, 1988.

62. Frymoyer JW, Cats-Baril W: Predictors of low back pain disability. Clin Orthop 221:89, 1987.

63. Bigos SJ, Spengler DM, Martin NA, et al: Back injuries in industry: A retrospective study. III. Employee-related factors. Spine 11:252, 1986.

64. Frymoyer JW: Back pain and sciatica. N Engl J Med 318:291, 1988.

65. Klein BP, Jensen RC, Sanderson LM: Assessment of workers' compensation claims for back strains/sprains. J Occup Med 26:443, 1984.

66. Dzioba RB, Doxey NC: A prospective investigation into the orthopedic and psychological predictors of outcome of first lumbar surgery following industiral injury. Spine 9:614, 1984.

67. Deyo RA, Tsui-Wu Y: Descriptive epidemiology of low back pain and its related medical care in the U.S. Spine 12:264, 1987.

68. Astrand NE: Medical, psychological, and social factors associated with back abnormalities and self-reported back pain. Br J Ind Med 44:327, 1987.

69. Weisel SW, Feffer HL, Rothman RH: Industrial low back pain—a prospective evaluation of a standarized diagnostic and treatment protocol. Spine 9:199, 1984.

70. Robertson LS, Keeve JP: Worker injuries: The effects of workers' compensation and OSHA inspections. J Health Polit Policy Law 8:581, 1983.

10 Patient Education

CRAIG LIEBENSON and JEFF OSLANCE

Patient education is as essential to successful rehabilitation as are exercise or other treatment strategies. Sometimes education, advice, and training are all that a person needs. Improving a patient's sitting posture or recommending a headset for prolonged telephone work are just two examples. Patient education is preferred over exercise because once a person learns how to reduce strain, that knowledge is with them forever, whereas exercises must be performed over and over again.

Traditional subjects for patient education include spinal anatomy, pain sources, first aid for acute recurrences, body mechanics, and preventive exercises. We place the most important areas to cover into four categories. First, reassurance that the natural history of most pain syndromes is toward a speedy resolution. Second, body mechanics that are universally applicable (i.e., workstation ergonomics, lifting advice). Third, the importance of focusing on function in addition to pain relief as a goal of care for the subacute, chronic, and high risk patient. Finally, explaining the difference between hurt and harm so the patient is less likely to immobilize themselves and become deconditioned in their attempt to achieve pain relief.

NATURAL HISTORY

Close to 90% of back pain episodes resolve within 6 weeks.[1-10] This excellent prognosis should not, however, lead to a negligent approach to managing this problem. A review of 1989 Workers' Compensation low back pain claims revealed that, "cases that go on to have prolonged disability are the primary contributors to the expense of low back pain."[9] It was determined that "25% of low back pain cases accounted for 96% of the costs." Persons who are still suffering after 6 weeks are at considerably higher risk for lasting disability and chronic pain. According to Nordin, ". . . there is a very small window of time in low back pain care; we must act quickly within 4-6 weeks to bring patients into an active reconditioning program if we expect to return them to productive lives and prevent recurrence."[11] With recurrence rates around 50% and the high costs associated with chronic disabling pain, aggressive conservative care focusing on restoration of function and patient education should be the standard of care.

Unfortunately, because of the excellent prognosis for most patients, many health care providers are misled into be-lieving that early aggressive conservative care is not necessary for patients with low back pain. Experts and emerging consensus-based guidelines disagree vehemently with this traditional approach, stating that the typical management approach of bed rest with medication is responsible for fostering disability in those prone to it. Troup, an esteemed British orthopedic surgeon, stated that, "The first attack is the ideal time for active and perhaps aggressive treatment but if it is tacitly assumed that the vast majority of patients recover from back pain whether or not they are treated then the opportunity may be missed."[10] It is essential to pursue rapid resolution of symptoms aggressively to minimize the likelihood of recurrent symptoms as well as the development of a chronic, disabling pain syndrome. The Quebec Task Force on low back pain disorders said, "Management strategies should be directed at maximizing the number of workers returning to work before 1 month and minimizing the number whose spinal disorders keeps them idle for longer than 6 months."[6] Prolonged disability or pain will lead to both physical and psychologic deconditioning, which we should strive to prevent through appropriate care of acute episodes.

In the early management of back pain episodes, manipulation is the single most effective treatment strategy.[12] Rehabilitation with exercise has also been shown to hasten return to work and reduce the rate of recurrences.[13,14] Radicular syndromes are associated with a less favorable outcome. Nonetheless, over 90% of individuals with pain below the knee and nerve root tension signs recover without surgical intervention.[15,16] The length of time prescribed for bed rest may be longer (up to 1 week), the value of manipulation less certain, and the overall length of time required to achieve symptom resolution more than 6 weeks, but the prognosis for recovery is still good.

The prognosis is poorer for chronic pain syndromes. Patients may benefit from a trial of manipulative therapy, but a biopsychosocial approach is definitely indicated. Exercise, education, and encouragement are the mainstays of successful care. Psychologic intervention may be needed as well. Focusing on function and reducing the patient's fear about movement are critical to success. Carefully explaining that hurt does not equal harm and that we do not follow a "no pain-no gain" philosophy is an important prelude to rehabilitation. Functional goals must be clearly established and objective outcomes used to monitor and demonstrate progress.

In chronic pain management, it is essential to focus on control and not cure and to place yourself in the role of helper rather than healer.[17]

Rarely is back pain the presenting symptom of a serious disease. A thorough history and clinical examination should be obtained, however, to rule out infections, tumors, and other serious diseases that can manifest with spinal pain. Reassuring patients that their problem is mechanical and not a sign of internal disease is an important step in patient education.

Standard of Care and Identification of High Risk Patients

Over 80% of the population will experience back pain during their lifetime. Only 5 to 15% of these individuals, however, will become chronic suffers. Because of the disproportionately high cost associated with chronic cases, much attention has been placed on finding better treatment and prevention strategies for this minority. The authors of a large review of worker's compensation low back claims concluded that, "the primary goal of low back pain management should be the prevention or reduction of prolonged disability."[9]

A question posed by guidelines panels is, How many treatments are appropriate and for how long? The Mercy Guidelines concluded that 6 weeks of care is usually sufficient for "uncomplicated" cases.[5] Three to five sessions per week for 1 to 2 weeks is appropriate, followed by "Progressively declining frequency is expected to discharge of the patient . . ."[5] Spinal manipulative therapy has been shown to lead to a 34% better rate of recovery (at the 3-week mark) when compared to other traditional forms of therapy.[12] Between 1 and 19 sessions with manipulation have been proven effective over a 2-month period.[12] Shekelle said, "an appropriate trial of therapy is 12 manipulations lasting up to a month."[12]

Risk Factors

The various factors that may lead to a slower course of recovery are presented in Table 10.1. The factors associated predictively with chronic or recurrent episodes are listed in Table 10.2.

According to the British Guidelines, low educational attainment and heavy physical occupation are lesser risk factors, but will interfere significantly with successful rehabilitation.[8]

Table 10.1. Factors That May Predict a Longer Recovery

Past history of >4 episodes
>1 week of symptoms before presenting to doctor
Severe pain intensity
Pre-existing structural pathology or skeletal anomaly (i.e., spondylolisthesis) directly related to new injury or condition

(From Haldeman S. Chapman-Smith D. Petersen DM: Frequency and duration of care. In Guidelines for Chiropractic Quality Assurance and Practice Parameters. Gaithersburg, Aspen, 1993, pp 115, 130.)

Table 10.2. Risk Factors for Chronicity (British Management Guidelines for Back Pain)

- Previous history of low back pain
- Total work loss (because of low back pain) in past 12 months
- Radiating leg pain
- Reduced straight leg raising
- Signs of nerve root involvement
- Reduced trunk strength and endurance
- Poor physical fitness
- Self-rated health poor
- Heavy smoking
- Psychologic distress and depressive symptoms
- Disproportionate illness behavior
- Low job satisfaction
- Personal problems—alcohol, marital, financial
- Adversarial medicolegal proceedings

(From Waddell G: The Low Back Pain Guidelines (British). Clinical Standards Advisory Group: Back Pain. London, HMSO, 1994.)

BODY MECHANICS

Reducing strain is essential to preventing recurrences. Teaching office workers to take frequent "microbreaks" every 20 to 30 minutes can help immeasurably. Studies have shown that tissue creep occurs after just 15 minutes.[18] Also, if just 4% overload is encountered, a negative metabolic state is established.[19,20] Proper chairs and workstations are a must for patients with low back and neck pain as well as those suffering from upper extremity repetitive strain disorders (i.e., carpal tunnel syndrome).

Work station ergonomics is a practical place to get started when looking for sources of mechanical overstrain. Go through the workstation checklist with your patients (see Appendix 10.1).

Lifting Technique

Lifting technique is often debated; typically, squatting is recommended over stooping. Unfortunately, most workers fail to follow this advice if repetitive lifts are required. Garg and Herrin noted the increased energy expenditure associated with squatting versus stooping.[21] What appears to be an attainable goal is maintaining the lordosis, independent of thigh and trunk angles.[22] Adams and Hutton reported that less compressive load on a fully flexed lumbar disk (i.e., stooped posture) is needed to cause posterior herniation of nuclear material than would cause end plate fracture in the upright position.[23] According to McGill, "Because ligaments are not recruited when lordosis is preserved, nor is the disk bent, it appears that the annulus is at low risk for failure."[22] This statement was supported by the work of Hickey and Hukins.[24] Lifting while maintaining lordosis allows the further benefit of activating the musculature and thus providing for neuromuscular control to protect ligamentous tissues.

Lifting technique is important, but when you lift may be even more significant. As a result of the increased fluid content in the disk after lying down at night, disk bending stresses are increased by 300% and stress to ligaments is increased by

80% in the morning.[25] Thus, the risk of injury during forward bending activities is increased in the early morning.

Prolonged flexion, such as in sitting, can render the back vulnerable to lifting. McGill and Brown found that after just 3 minutes of full flexion, subjects lost half their stiffness.[26] Adams and Hutton believe that prolonged full flexion may cause ligamentous creep and render the spine susceptible to flexion overload during lifting.[23] According to McGill, a brief course of extension exercises before lifting may prevent injury.[22]

Co-contraction of the lumbar erector spinae muscles during lifting appears to redistribute compressive forces on the spine by adding guide wires to a flexible rod, like rigging on a ship's mast.[22] The increase in compressive loading on the spine is substantial if even a small amount of torsion is required during lifting.[22] To prevent injury, objects should not be lifted if they were awkwardly placed. To reduce the extensor moment, the load should be held as close as possible and lifted smoothly.[22] A jerk lift is only appropriate for highly trained individuals who must lift light, awkwardly placed objects. The purpose of this lift is to avoid loading the spine in flexion for any longer than is absolutely necessary.[22] Table 10.3 summarizes current advice about lifting.

Ergonomic Factors

One of the most deleterious activities people engage in is sitting. Erect sitting involves disk pressures significantly higher than that of normal standing. Sitting slumped forward (anterior sitting) increases disk pressure even more, and the greatest increase in pressure is associated with slumping backwards (posterior sitting).[27,28] Using a lumbar support or back rest reduces disk pressures.[29] A seat-backrest angle of 95–105° reduces both erector spinae EMG activity and disk pressure.[29,30]

The chair seat should provide a stable base and yet not be too constraining.[31] The height of the chair is important. A seat height that is too low places too much strain on the ischial tuberosities. Too high a seat increases pressure on the thighs. Chairs lacking variable height adjustments may need to be complemented by a footrest. The seat edge should not touch the popliteal fossa; this situation leads to too rigid a sitting posture. A slight depression for the buttocks is beneficial for stability. A concave seat increases weight bearing through the greater trochanters and internally rotates the femur, again restricting movement of the legs. Seat angle is controversial, although it is apparent that a forward sloping seat increases lumbar lordosis during sitting and maintains the erect sitting position.

Table 10.3. McGill's Rules for Lifting[22]

Maintain normal lordosis
Do not lift immediately after prolonged flexion or rising from bed
Lightly co-contract the back muscles before and during lifting
Keep the load as close as possible as long as lordosis is maintained
Avoid twisting

The proper desk height is normally about 27 to 30 cm above the seat.[32] The shoulders should be able to relax with the elbows bent 90° and the hands relaxed on the desk surface. A slanted desk (10 to 20°) may also be helpful for reducing neck strain.

FOCUSING ON FUNCTION

Functional restoration gets to the heart of a recurrent disorder more effectively than searching for the technique to "fix" the problem. Pain relief is enough of a goal for many first-time pain patients. When pain is recurrent or chronic, however, or the individual is at high risk for a chronic, disabling condition, enabling the patient to focus on function becomes a high priority for the treating physician. We should help the patient to understand that a more fit back is less likely to become injured; whatever the cause of their pain (disk, facet, myofascial, etc.), they will be more stable if function is restored. In fact, 80% of the time, an exact cause cannot be identified, but clusters of functional changes can address their symptoms.[33]

A deconditioned individual has two options for achieving lasting pain relief. First, they can avoid all strenuous activities. Second, they can increase their functional capacity (Fig. 10.1). These options are really the only means available to prevent spinal problems. Either the load is reduced or the capacity to handle that load is increased. Convincing a patient to reduce external strain is optimal, because once they change their workstation or learn better biomechanics, they have that knowledge forever. If, however, only limited reductions in external strain are possible, improving their intrinsic functional capacity or performance is the only remaining option. Exercise is always more difficult to accomplish than education because of problems associated with motivation and compliance.

PATIENT MOTIVATION

Achieving compliance in patients asked to share responsibility for management of their pain rests on convincing them that body mechanics and functional improvement are essential for long-term success. No amount of persuasion is adequate, however, unless their fears and anxieties are also addressed. Most chronic patients fear that activity will cause them more pain. Explaining the difference between hurt and harm will help considerably (see Chapter 2).

Exercises that stretch stiff, shortened tissues may in fact cause pain or discomfort but are not injurious. In fact, patients will learn how to stretch safely and to feel a comfortable "good hurt." Also, strengthening exercises are best performed in a pain-less range, with pain only felt the following day (see Chapter 14). This postexercise soreness should involve only the trained muscles and not be felt in any symptomatic spinal or postural areas. Occasionally, "McKenzie" exercises cause some discomfort, but this pain should be local. These exercises are avoided if any radiating pain is perceived. Learning that they can control their symp-

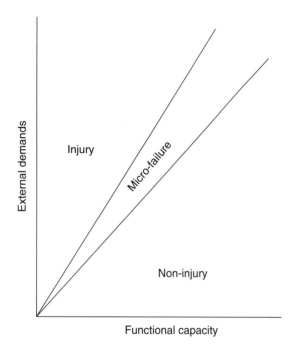

Fig. 10.1. Relationship between external demand and functional capacity.

toms becomes a liberating experience for most patients. As stated previously, the rehabilitation specialist should teach patients how to control their symptoms and not promise to "cure" or "fix" the problem.

Patients need to know the exact goals of exercise. For instance, a goal might be to strengthen the "big muscles" (i.e., abdominals, gluteals, and quadriceps) to take strain off the lumbar spine. When proper goal setting is accomplished and those goals are mutually acceptable, patient adherence and compliance are easier to achieve. If excessive fear and anxiety persist, then referral to a pain psychologist may be needed. A psychologist may be able to teach better coping strategies or relaxation techniques and can uncover hidden obstacles, such as drug or alcohol dependency, job dissatisfaction, or family stress.

REFERENCES

1. Benn RT, Wood PH: Pain in the back: An attempt to estimate the size of the problem. Rheumatol Rehabil 14:121, 1975.
2. Horal J: The clinical appearance of low back pain disorders in the city of Gothenburg, Sweden. Acta Orthop Scand Suppl 18:1, 1969.
3. Rowe ML: Low back pain in industry. J Occup Med 11:161, 1969.
4. Berquist-Ullman M, Larsson U: Acute low back pain in industry. Acta Orthop Scand Suppl 170:1, 1977.
5. Haldeman S, Chapman-Smith D, Petersen DM: Frequency and duration of care. In Guidelines for Chiropractic Quality Assurance and Practice Parameters. Gaithersberg, Aspen, 1993, pp 115, 130.
6. Spitzer WO, Le Blanc FE, Dupuis M, et al: Scientific approach to the assessment and management of activity-related spinal disorders: A mono-graph for clinicians. Report of the Quebec Task Force on Spinal Disorders. Spine 12(suppl 7):S1, 1987.
7. Bigos S, Bowyer O, Braen G, et al: Acute Low Back Problems in Adults. Clinical Practice Guideline, Quick Reference Guide Number 14. Rockville MD, U.S. Department of Health and Human Services, Publish Health Service, Agency for Health Care Policy and Research Pub. No. 95-0643, December 1994.
8. Clinical Standards Advisory Group (CSAG): Back Pain. London, HMSO, 1994.
9. Webster BS, Snook SH: The cost of 1989 Workers' Compensation low back pain claims. Spine 19:1111, 1994.
10. Troup JDG: The perception of musculoskeletal pain and incapacity for work: Prevention and early treatment. Physiotherapy 74:435, 1988.
11. Nordin M: Early findings of NIOSH-CDC model back clinic reveal surprising observations on work-related low back pain predictors. Spine Lett 1:4,5, 1994.
12. Shekelle PG: Spine update spinal manipulation. Spine 19:858, 1994.
13. Linton SJ, Hellsing AL, Andersson D: A controlled study of the effects of an early intervention on acute musculoskeletal pain problems. Pain 54:353, 1993.
14. Lindstrom A, Ohlund C, Eek C, et al: The effect of graded activity on patients with subacute low back pain. Phys Ther 72:279, 1992.
15. Saal JA, Saal JS: Nonoperative treatment of lumbar herniated disc with radiculopathy. Spine 14:431, 1989.
16. Bush K, Cowan N, Katz DE, et al: The natural history of sciatica associated with disc pathology: A prospective study with clinical and independent radiologic follow-up. Spine 17:1205, 1992.
17. Fordyce WE: Pain history musings. APS J 3:140, 1994.
18. Bogduk N, Twomney LT: Clinical Anatomy of the Lumbar Spine, 2nd Ed. Melbourne, Churchill Livingstone, 1991.
19. Andersson GBJ: Occupational biomechanics. In Wienstein JN, Wiesel SW (eds): the Lumbar Spine: the International Society for the Study of the Lumbar Spine. Philadelphia, WB Saunders, 1990, p 213.
20. Sato H, Ohashi J, Owanga K, et al: Endurance time and fatigue in static contractions. J Hum Ergol (Tokyo) 3:147, 1984.
21. Garg A, Herrin G: Stoop or squat: A biomechanical and metabolic evaluation. Am Inst Indus Eng Trans 11:293, 1979.
22. McGill SM, Norman RW: Low back biomechanics in industry: The prevention of injury through safer lifting. In Grabiner M (ed): Current Issues in Biomechanics. Champaign, IL, Human Kinetics, 1993.
23. Adams MA, Hutton WC: Mechanics of the intervertebral disc. In P Ghosh (ed): The Biology of the Intervertebral Disc. Boca Raton, FL, CRC Press, 1988, pp 39-71.
24. Hickey DS, Hukins DWL: Relation between the structure of the annulus fibrosis and the function and failure of the intervertebral disc. Spine 5:106, 1980.
25. Adams MA, Dolan P, Hutton WC: Dirurnal variations in the stresses on the lumbar spine. Spine 12:130, 1987.
26. McGill SM, Brown S: Creep response of the lumbar spine to prolonged flexion. Clin Biomech 7:43, 1992.
27. Andersson GB, Murphy RW, Ortengren R, et al: The influence of back rest inclination and lumbar support on lumbar lordosis. Spine 4:52, 1979.
28. Andersson GB, Jonsson B, Ortengren R: Myoelectric activity in individual lumbar erector spinae muscles in sitting. A study with surface and wire electrodes. Scand J Rehabil Med 3(suppl):19, 1974.
29. Schuldt K, Ekholm J, Harms-Ringdahl K, et al: Effects of changes in sitting work posture on static neck and shoulder muscle activity. Ergonomics 29:1525, 1986.
30. Andersson GB, Ortengren R, Nachemson AL, et al: The sitting posture: An electromyographic and discometric study. Orthop Clin North Am 6:105, 1975.
31. Ortiz D, Smith R: Ergonomic Considerations. In Basmajian JV, Nyberg R (eds): Rational Manual Therapies. Baltimore, Williams & Wilkins, 1993, pp 441-450.

32. Grandjean E: Fitting the Task to the Man. 4th Ed. London, Taylor and Francis, 1988.

33. Moffroid MT, Haugh LD, Henry SM, et al: Distinguishable groups of musculoskeletal low back pain patients and asymptomatic control subjects based on physical measures of the NIOSH low back atlas. Spine 19:1350, 1994.

APPENDIX 10.1. How to Care For Your Back and Neck: A Section Addressed to the Patient

Who is at Risk?

Everyone. But, those who sit, bend, or twist a lot are at higher risk. Not liking one's job or having problems at home also places one at higher risk. Finally, not being in good shape, especially in your back and abdominal muscles, is an additional factor.

What Can Be Done?

Surgery is necessary for back pain less than 1% of the time. Most back or neck pain is what we call "mechanical" pain. One of the great myths is that arthritis and disk syndromes are responsible for most people's pain. In fact, one third of all people without back pain have herniated disks. It is now frequently considered a coincidental finding. Most spinal disorders can be treated with simple conservative care involving manipulation, self-care advice, and exercise.

If you are in acute pain, the initial goal is to stabilize the painful area. We want to protect your back or neck by teaching you how to find relief positions that take strain off the painful area. For instance, you will be advised to avoid certain strenuous positions or movements, such as sitting or bending and twisting. This advice typically consists of prescribing limited activities and the use of pain-relieving methods (ice, heat, ultrasound, electrical muscle stimulation, manipulation, massage, traction, etc.). A support may be given and bed rest recommended, but this regimen is used for the minimum time possible to decrease the danger of deconditioning (becoming excessively weak or stiff).

Perhaps most important is the reassurance that you will receive that your condition has been evaluated thoroughly and that you do not have any serious medical conditions. If you do have a disk syn-

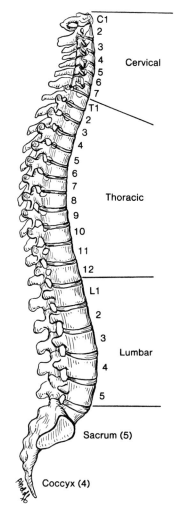

Fig. 10A.1. Spinal column (side view). (From Basmajian JV: Primary Anatomy. 8th Ed. Baltimore, Williams & Wilkins, 1982.)

drome, which is resulting in pressure on a nerve, a diagnosis will be made and appropriate treatment will be initiated.

The second goal of care is to get you active again. This process is called remobilization, which is accomplished by relaxing tense muscles and loosening stiff joints. Gradually and safely, you will be increasing the activities you perform with less and less fear of reinjury. Stretching and light cardiovascular exercises, along with manipula-

Table 10A.1. Stages of Care

Stages:	Stabilization	Remobilization	Reconditioning
Goals:	Pain Relief, Reassurance, Protection	Restore Mobility	Improve Strength and Flexibility
Treatment Strategies:	Find relief positions Limited bed rest Supports/braces Physical agents (ice, heat, ultrasound, electrical muscle stimulation, etc.) Manual therapy (manipulation, massage, traction) Analgesics or anti-inflammatories	Manipulation Stretching Ergonomic advice (i.e., how to sit) Cardiovascular exercise	Strengthen "big muscles" (abds, buttocks, thighs) Stretch postural areas (calves, back) Biomechanical advice (i.e., how to lift)

tion, are the primary modes of care in this stage. Fewer physical therapy techniques are used and you will receive advice about how to prevent or reduce strain in daily activities, e.g., how to sit without causing strain.

The third and final goal of care is to achieve reconditioning of your "weak link." Typically, after a painful episode, movements are guarded and weakness develops. Unless addressed, this condition predisposes you to future recurrences. You will learn a combination of stretching and strengthening exercises designed to improve the function of your back or neck. At this time, advice about lifting and bending usually is given.

The stages of care are shown in Table 10A.1.

What Does the Spine Look Like?

The spine is one of the most remarkable organs of the body. It's job is to protect the spinal cord and serve as a mobile rod for bending the trunk, thus allowing us great mobility. These two opposing functions of stability and mobility are both accomplished by this single amazing structure.

The spinal column has three curves when viewed from the side (Fig. 10A.1). Each vertebra forms a number of joints with its neighboring vertebral segments (above and below) (Fig. 10A.2). One of the most important spinal structures is the disk. It is a cartilaginous structure that serves as a shock absorber between each vertebrae. It has a tough criss-crossing network of ligaments (annulus fibrosis) forming a protective ring around its gel-like fluid interior (nucleus pulposus) (Fig. 10A.3). Viewed from above, you can see the spinal canal, which houses the spinal cord, and thus the relationship between the disk and nerve roots (Fig. 10A.4).

Where Can the Pain Come From?

Nearly all the structures of the back and neck can cause pain. Most commonly, muscles, tendons, ligaments, or joints become sources of pain when they are irritated or overloaded. Sciatic (leg) pain comes from irritated nerve roots.

Certain movements are particularly likely to cause problems. Bending over to lift something places tremendous strain on our backs. The combination of bending and twisting can cause damage

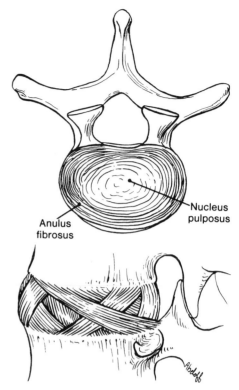

Fig. 10A.3. The disk. (From Basmajian JV: Primary Anatomy. 8th Ed. Baltimore, Williams & Wilkins, 1982.)

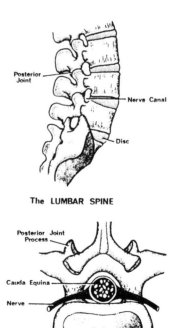

Fig. 10A.4. Relationship of the disk and spinal nerve roots. (From Kirkaldy-Willis WH: Management of Low Back Pain. 3rd Ed. New York, Churchill Livingstone, 1994.)

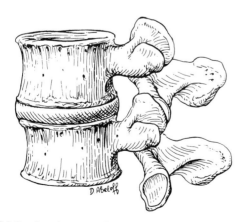

Fig. 10A.2. Lumbar vertebral joints. (From Basmajian JV: Primary Anatomy. 8th Ed. Baltimore, Williams & Wilkins, 1982.)

even if we don't lift anything in that position (Fig. 10A.5). Prolonged sitting, even in a good chair, places a great deal of strain on the muscles and disks of the back. Being on the telephone or working at a computer for long periods of time can strain the neck, upper back, shoulders, elbows, or wrists.

It is common for joints or muscles to be the source of pain referred to the low back, buttocks, thighs, between the shoulder blades, neck, head, face, or arms. Figures 10A.6 to 10A.13 show classic representations of pain referred from certain key muscles.

Joints and ligaments are also able to cause local and referred (some distance from its origin) pain. Figures 10A.14 and 10A.15 show typical referred pain patterns from irritated vertebral facet joints in the cervical and lumbar spines, respectively.

The most famous culprit of severe pain is the "herniated disk" which can pinch on a nerve root, sending pain or numbness down the leg, even to the foot (Fig. 10A.16). If strained too much, the disk can bulge or possibly tear, causing gel (nucleus pulposus) to herniate into the area containing the spinal nerves (Fig. 10A.17). A bulge is common and often does not cause pain. Herniations can pinch on nerves or irritate them, causing "sciatica" (leg pain). The fascinating thing is that disk disorders occur in one third of all people who have no symptoms; thus, such a finding in a patient may be coincidental. A thorough examination is necessary to determine if a disk problem is actually causing your symptoms.

Another structural problem occurs when arthritic spurs (degenerative joint disease) jut out from the vertebral joints and either pinch nerves (stenosis) or restrict our normal mobility. Here too, it is common for degenerative joint changes to occur in the spine and be painless. In fact, arthritis increases with age, as does graying of the hair and wrinkling of the skin, yet back pain peaks between ages 28 and 50 years.

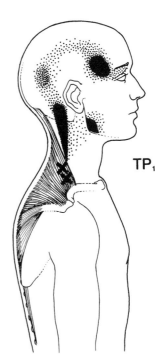

Fig. 10A.6. Referred pain from the upper trapezius muscle. (From Travell JG, Simons DG: Myofascial Pain and Dysfunction: The Trigger Point Manual. Vol. 1. Baltimore, Williams & Wilkins, 1983.)

What Can I Do?

Back and neck pain are interwoven into our lives. They are normal yet unpleasant experiences that, if mismanaged, can become chronically disabling. In the past, doctors believed bed rest, pain relievers, and perhaps some physical therapy (heat, ultrasound, etc.) were all that was needed to tide someone over until the problem receded. Most of the time, such an approach succeeded in alleviating the pain. But, all too often (up to 20% of the time), it failed. According to recent independent, government studies from Canada, the United States, and Great Britain concerning the back pain problem, consensus has emerged that this poor report card is largely related to the overprescription of bed rest and medication and failure to focus care on quickly restoring functional integrity to your muscles and joints.

What is the solution? Today, we know that manipulation (i.e., chiropractic adjustments) is the most effective treatment for quick pain relief. The Rand Corporation, British Low Back Pain Guidelines, and the U.S. Agency for Health Care Policy and Research have concluded that manipulation is one of the most effective forms of early intervention for back pain. Manipulation in combination with exercise and simple education have proven to be far superior to traditional prescriptions of prolonged bed rest and medication.

When you are in pain, the first rule of pain relief is to avoid additional strain. Figures 10A.18 and 10A.19, show the different amounts of muscular effort required to stabilize different postures. You should minimize assuming strenuous postures all the time, but they should be avoided completely when you are suffering an acute episode.

If we are involved in high risk activities, such as repetitive lifting or prolonged sitting, it is important to learn how to modify our

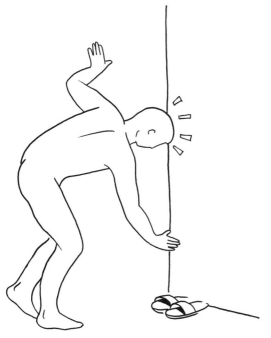

Fig. 10A.5. Dangerous bending and twisting position.

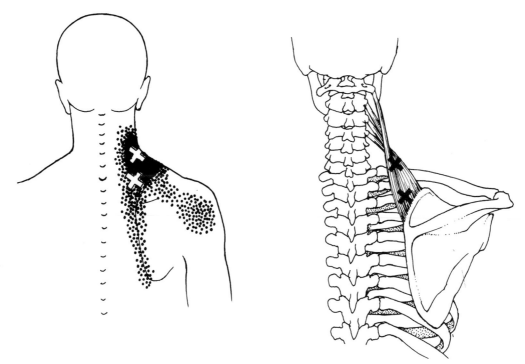

Fig. 10A.7. Referred pain from the levator scapulae muscle. (From Travell JG, Simons DG: Myofascial Pain and Dysfunction: The Trigger Point Manual. Vol. 1. Baltimore, Williams & Wilkins, 1983.)

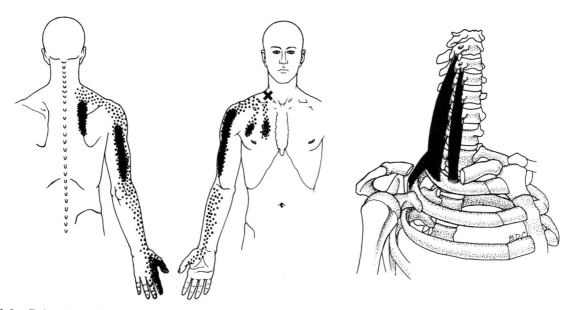

Fig. 10A.8. Referred pain from the scalene muscles. (From Travell JG, Simons DG: Myofascial Pain and Dysfunction. The Trigger Point Manual. Vol. 1. Baltimore, Williams & Wilkins, 1983.)

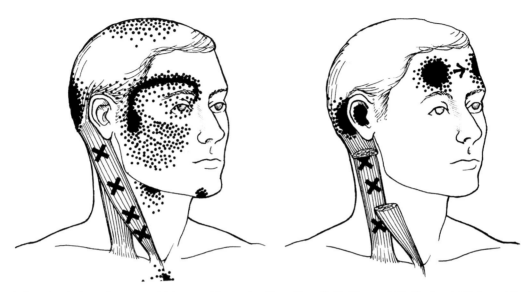

Fig. 10A.9.   Referred pain from the sternocleidomastoid muscle. (From Travell JG, Simons DG: Myofascial Pain and Dysfunction: The Trigger Point Manual. Vol. 1. Baltimore, Williams & Wilkins, 1983.)

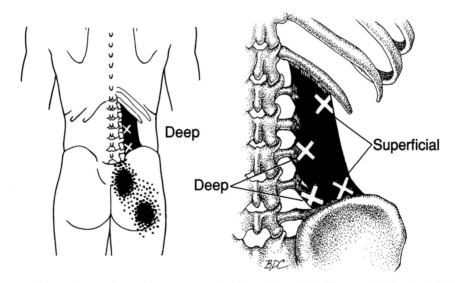

Fig. 10A.10.   Referred pain from the quadratus lumborum muscle. (From Travell JG, SImons DG: Myofascial Pain and Dysfunction: The Trigger Point Manual. Vol. 2. Baltimore, Williams & Wilkins, 1992.)

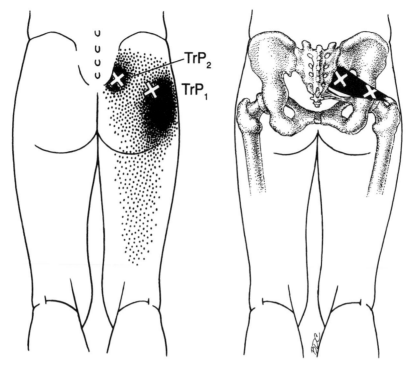

Fig. 10A.11. Referred pain from the piriformis muscle. (From Travell JG, Simons DG: Myofascial Pain and Dysfunction: The Trigger Point Manual. Vol. 2. Baltimore, Williams & Wilkins, 1992.)

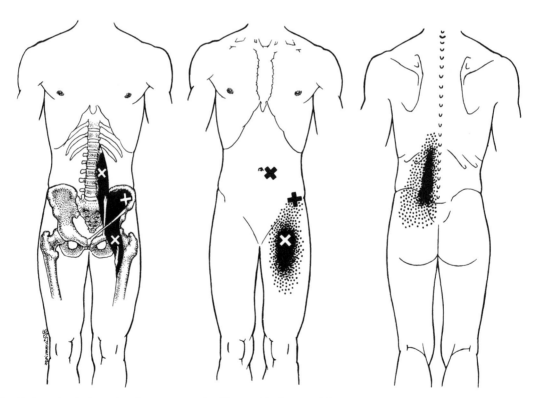

Fig. 10A.12. Referred pain from the iliopsoas muscle. (Travell JG, Simons DG: Myofascial Pain and Dysfunction: The Trigger Point Manual. Vol. 2. Baltimore, Williams & Wilkins, 1992.)

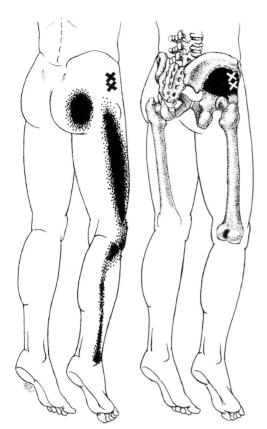

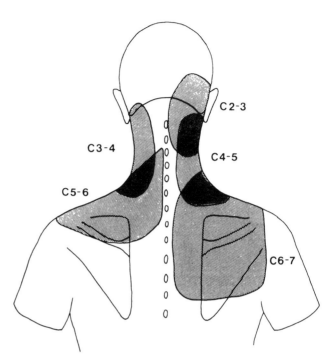

Fig. 10A.13. Referred pain from the gluteus minimus muscle. (From Travell JG, Simons DG: Myofascial Pain and Dysfunction: The Trigger Point Manual. Vol. 2. Baltimore, Williams & Wilkins, 1992.)

Fig. 10A.14. Referred pain from the cervical spine joints. (From Dwyer A, April C, Bogduk N: Cervical zygapophyseal joint pain patterns: A study in normal volunteers. Spine 15:453, 1990.)

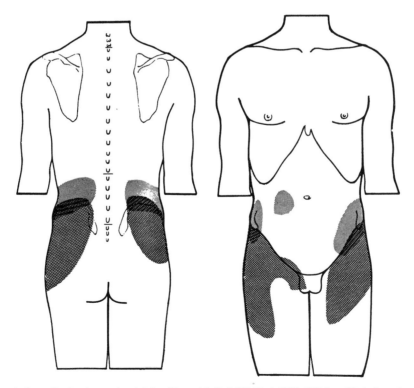

Fig. 10A.15. Referred pain from the lumbar spine joints. (From McCall IW, Park WM, O'Brien JP: Induced pain referral from posterior lumbar elements in normal subjects. Spine 4:441, 1979.)

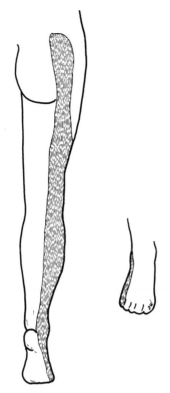

activities so we use better biomechanics and posture. It may also be necessary to perform stretches during breaks to allow muscles and ligaments that have fatigued to regain their strength. Finally, strengthening exercises for our abdomen, buttocks, legs, and back may be needed to help us avoid fatigue in our neck and lower back. A customized program of manipulation, exercise, and education will be devised to meet your needs.

Body Mechanics and Posture

Normal spinal posture helps reduce potential strain. Unfortunately, our modern lifestyles, in concert with the forces of gravity, conspire to ruin our healthy upright posture. The elderly are often slumped because of bad posture or sometimes from osteoporosis (Fig. 10A.20). This habit of slumping begins in childhood when we sit in front of televisions, sit in school, sit in cars, etc. Sitting and inactiv-

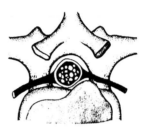

Fig. 10A.16. Referred pain from an irritated or "pinched" sciatic nerve root. (From Cox JM: Low Back Pain: Mechanism, Diagnosis, and Treatment. 5th Ed. Baltimore, Williams & Wilkins, 1990.)

Fig. 10A.17. Herniated disk. (From Kirkaldy-Willis WH: Management of Low Back Pain. 2nd Ed. Edinburgh, Churchill Livingstone, 1992.)

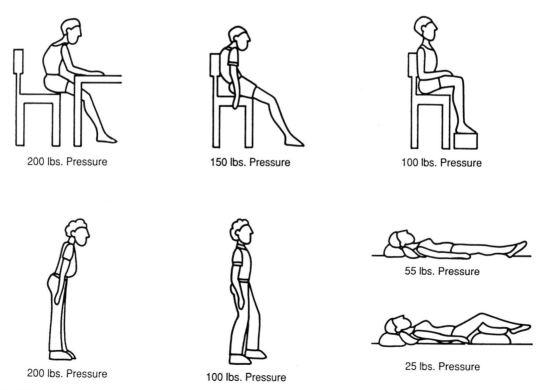

200 lbs. Pressure

150 lbs. Pressure

100 lbs. Pressure

200 lbs. Pressure

100 lbs. Pressure

55 lbs. Pressure

25 lbs. Pressure

Fig. 10A.18. Effects of posture on lumbar disk pressure. (Adapted from Dutro S and Wheeler L: Pregnancy and exercise. In White A, Anderson R (eds): Conservative Management of Low Back Pain. Baltimore, Williams & Wilkins, 1991.)

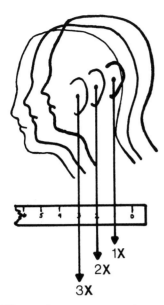

Fig. 10A.19. Effects of posture on neck muscle activity. For every inch that the head moves forward of its normal posture, the compressive forces on the lower neck increase by the additional weight of the entire head. (From Curl D: Head Pain. Baltimore, Williams and Wilkins, 1994.)

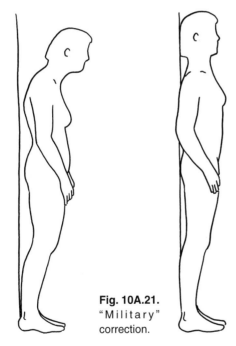

Fig. 10A.20. Slumped posture.

Fig. 10A.21. "Military" correction.

ity automatically invite poor posture, thus overstraining our spinal muscles, ligaments, and joints.

The Slumped or Forward Drawn Posture

We are born in the fetal position with our spines rounded forward. As we grow, our spine extends in both our lower back and neck, which allows us to look straight ahead, walk upright, and use our hands. Unfortunately, modern occupations and lifestyles, by overusing the sitting position in cars, while eating, watching television, and working at desks and computer workstations, have imbalanced our nor-

mal upright posture. The resulting forward drawn or slumped posture is reinforced by gravity, which makes it even harder to maintain a normal upright posture. The signs of poor posture include the following (Figure 10A.20):

–weight over the balls of our feet
–sway back
–increased roundness of mid-upper back
–shoulders rounded forward
–head forward
–chin poked

To correct poor posture, it is helpful to attempt the "military position," which will move you back in the right direction. A good rule of thumb is to assume the "military position" and then back off about 10% (Fig. 10A.21). It is a good idea to move in this direction about every 20 minutes as a way of "fine tuning" our posture until it improves automatically. After just a few months, our new posture will become a habit. The military repositioning involves:

–flattening your low back against a chair or wall
–rolling your shoulders back and down
–tucking your chin in while you glide your head backward

The sitting posture is fatiguing because of the pressure it places on the disks of our low back and the amount of muscular effort required to keep both our back and neck upright. The most important thing to remember about sitting is to keep the low back straight or slightly arched. This positioning will prevent us from slumping, thus preventing both lower back and neck strain (Fig. 10A.22). Driving or sitting in a car is one of the situations encountered most frequently. The best way to sit in a car is with your low back well supported and the seat back slightly reclined. The seat should be at a height such that your hips are level with or slightly higher than your knees (Fig. 10A.23). It is important to have the seat far

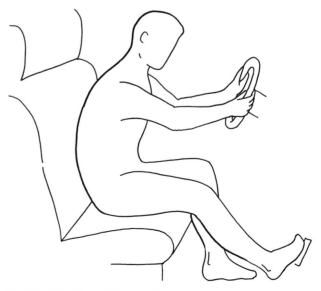

Fig. 10A.22. Poor driving posture.

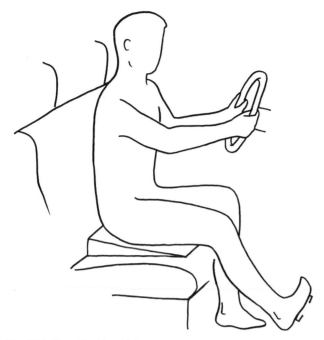

Fig. 10A.23.   Healthy driving posture.

that the back is higher than the front (or use a foam wedge) (see Fig. 10A.23).

A desk that is too low will promote a slumped posture. Any reading or writing, even on a desk of proper height, may cause neck and shoulder overstrain (Fig. 10A.25). In such cases, students and desk workers will benefit from a writing wedge or book support (Fig. 10A.26).

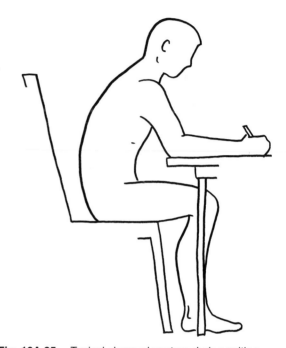

Fig. 10A.25.   Typical slumped posture during writing.

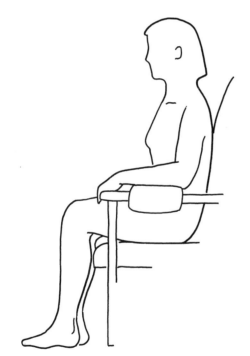

Fig. 10A.24.   Good sitting posture with arm rests.

enough forward so you do not have to elevate (shrug) your shoulders to reach the steering wheel. You should not feel the need to slump forward.

When sitting in a chair, the same basic rules apply. Make sure your feet rest comfortably on the floor and use armrests if they are available (Fig. 10A.24). When you perform work at a desk or computer, you may want to experiment with the tilt of your seat. It is often more comfortable for your back and neck if the seat is tilted so

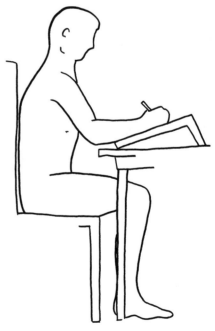

Fig. 10A.26.   Use of a writing wedge to improve posture.

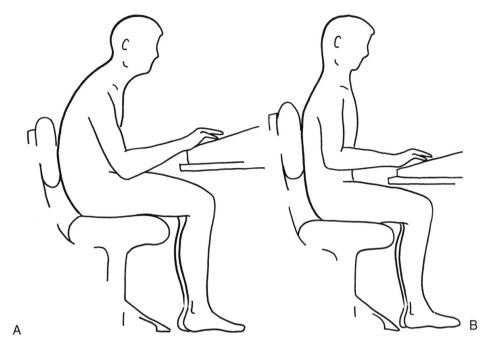

Fig. 10A.27. Improper sitting posture **(a)** and proper sitting posture for reducing finger, wrist, elbow, shoulder, neck, and back strain **(b)**.

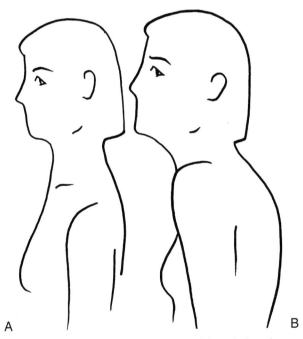

Fig. 10A.28. Proper head/neck posture **(a)** and slumping and the dowager's hump **(b)**.

When typing or imputing on a computer keyboard, your hands should rest on the keyboard without your wrists bent, your elbows should be bent at a right angle (90°), and your shoulders should be completely relaxed (not shrugged) (Fig. 10A.27). Table 10A.2 is a

checklist of the important points to review with regard to your work-stations.

When you sit or stand, it is important that your shoulders are relaxed back and down. This positioning will help prevent the slumped posture and, with it, the head-forward posture. Slumping eventually leads to a permanent rounding of the upper back (dowager's hump) (Fig. 10A.28). Additionally, with the head in a forward position, the muscles in the back of the neck and between the shoulder blades are easily fatigued and become strained. Many headaches, neck, shoulder, arm, and shoulder blade pains result from this posture. A simple

Table 10A.2. Workstation Ergonomic Checklist

Chair	Y/N
Seat height adjustable	
Feet should be on floor and knees no higher than hips	
Arm rests	
Good lumbar support	
Seat back should be able to recline (95 to 105°)	
Tiltable seat pan	
Tilt seat forward for desk work	
Tilt seat backward for reclining work	
Computer	
Center of monitor nose level	
No glare on monitor	
Keyboard height so that wrists are not bent, elbows at a 90° angle, and shoulders relaxed (not shrugged)	
Other	
Document holder	
Head set	

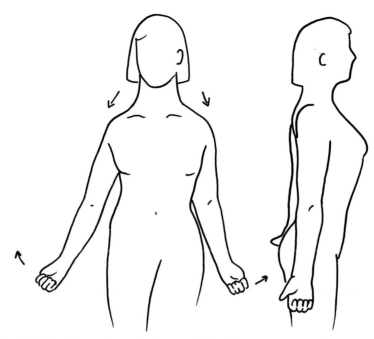

Fig. 10A.29. Postural exercise for round shoulders and head forward posture.

exercise can be performed frequently throughout the day for just 20 to 30 seconds each time to prevent these ill effects of the slumped posture. As shown in Figure 10A.29, you can roll your shoulders back and down (by squeezing your shoulder blades together), rotate your hands outward, and tuck your chin. This same exercise can also be performed at home while lying on your abdomen. Hand weights can even be added for a greater strengthening effect. If your lower back arches too much, you can try placing a pillow under your abdomen.

Your posture for sleeping is also important. The ideal sleep posture is one in which all the normal spinal curves are maintained with minimum strain. The fetal position achieves this goal (Fig. 10A.30). Our lumbar spine and pelvis should not twist too much and a pillow between the knees or thighs may be all that is required to avoid the common half tummy/half fetal sleep position (Fig. 10A.31). When sleeping on our backs, a pillow under the knees will keep the low back relaxed to that it does not overarch (Fig. 10A.32).

Sleeping is often a difficult adventure for individuals with neck pain. Finding just the right pillow can be a "nightmare." The ideal pillow will cradle and support your neck without distorting its normal alignment (Fig. 10A.33a). If your pillow is not supporting you properly, you might wind up with recurrent "stiff necks," headaches, or even referred pain to the shoulder, arm, or hand. It is important to avoid using too little or no pillow, which places the unsupported neck under strain all night long (Fig. 10A.33b). It is equally unwise to use too many pillows or too firm of a pillow, which pushes the neck up and pinches the joints together (Fig. 10A.33c). Whether you lie on your side or your back, your pillow must be soft enough to mold to your head and yet still fill in the space between your bed and your neck. Remember, your head is bigger than your neck, so accommodating both without distorting the position of your neck is the key. Sometimes, a bolster or special orthopedic pillow is helpful to fill in this space. If you are a side sleeper and have broad shoulders, you will need a larger pillow than someone with narrower shoulders. Finally, it is important to place your pillow between your neck and shoulder, not under your shoulder.

Lifting is probably the area of greatest concern for all back doctors. The most important rule is to "keep your back straight."

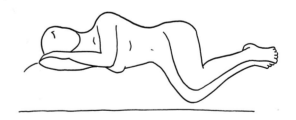

Fig. 10A.30. Fetal position.

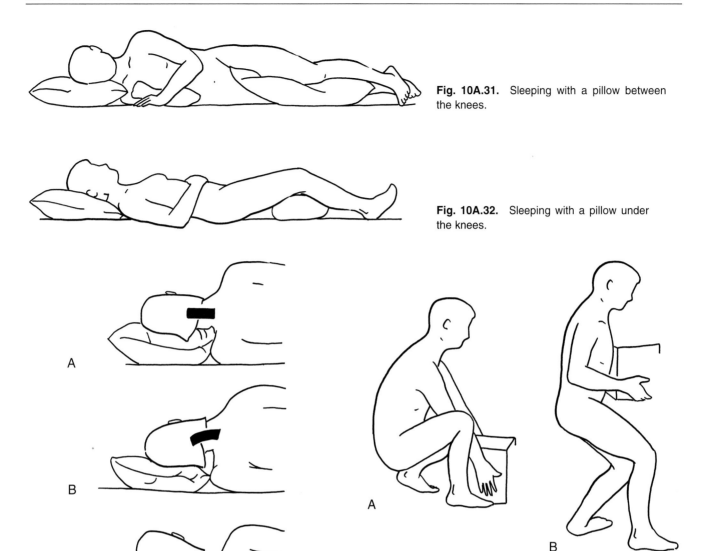

Fig. 10A.31.   Sleeping with a pillow between the knees.

Fig. 10A.32.   Sleeping with a pillow under the knees.

Fig. 10A.33.   **a,** healthy neck/pillow relationship; **b,** too small of a pillow; **c,** too large of a pillow.

Fig. 10A.34.   Proper lifting technique from the ground.

Second, avoid twisting when you lift. The combination of bending and twisting is the death knell for your lumbar disks. It is also important to try to lift objects as close to your chest as possible; the farther the object is from you, the greater is its "mass." Another recent discovery documents that the back is especially vulnerable immediately after sitting for a prolonged period (just 15 minutes will do it) or after a night's sleep. Remember to use good lifting habits, especially immediately after getting up from a chair or after a night's sleep. Whenever possible, try to avoid lifting from the floor; place things at knee, waist, or chest height. Lifting children can be especially difficult because they obviously do not sit still like boxes do. Nonetheless, because we will do lots of bending and lifting if we have kids, the sooner we learn to do it right, the less likely we are to have recurrences of disabling back pain. Figure 10A.34 shows the proper technique for lifting an object on the ground. Figure 10A.35 shows poor technique in lifting with the back bent instead of straight. Table 10A.3 summarizes the key components of proper lifting technique.

Reaching for things above shoulder level is another strenuous activity for your back. Use of a foot stool is an excellent way to reduce the strain (Fig. 10A.36). If a stool is unavailable, then a trick is to tighten your abdominal and buttocks muscles so you flatten your back (Fig. 10A.37). This maneuver will prevent the tendency to stick out your buttocks and overarch your back.

Carrying suitcases, groceries, or a baby are all challenges for a person with a bad back. When packing for a vacation, it is better to

Table 10A.3. Proper Lifting Technique

Lift with your back straight
Never bend and twist while lifting
Keep the object as close to your chest as possible
Keep things that need to be moved at waist level whenever possible

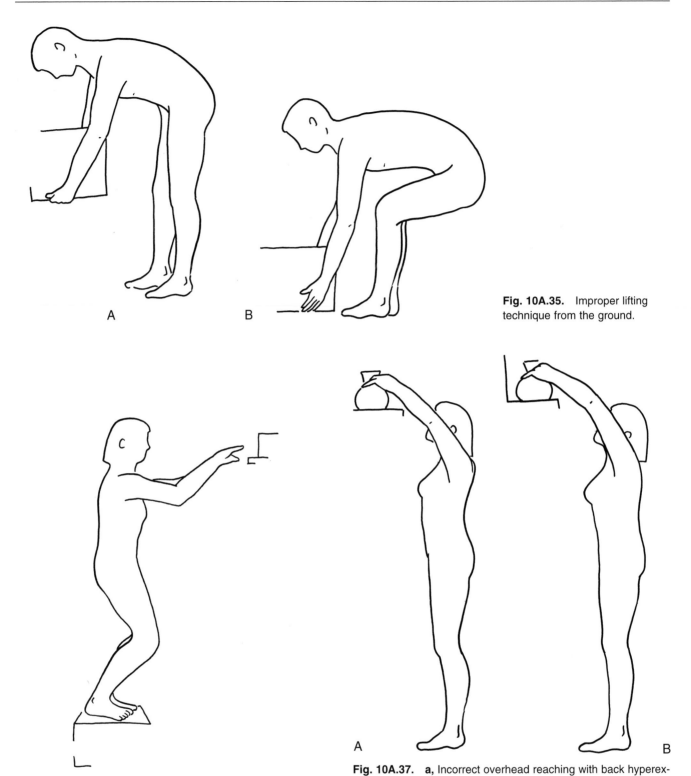

Fig. 10A.35. Improper lifting technique from the ground.

Fig. 10A.36. Use of a stool for overhead activities.

Fig. 10A.37. **a,** Incorrect overhead reaching with back hyperextended; **b,** Correct overhead reaching with back flat.

pack two smaller suitcases than one oversized one; you can then balance the loads and avoid straining your back (Fig. 10A.38). Avoid carrying a baby or any other object with outstretched arms. By holding the weight close to your chest, you greatly reduce the potential strain (Fig. 10A.39). This advice is particularly important when putting a baby in a car seat. By holding the

baby close to you, you are less likely to injure your back (Fig. 10A.40).

Pushing and pulling can be yet another source of lumbar strain. Given a choice between the two, pushing is preferred because the legs can be used more effectively (Fig. 10A.41). When buying a carriage for your baby, try to find one that is fitted to your height.

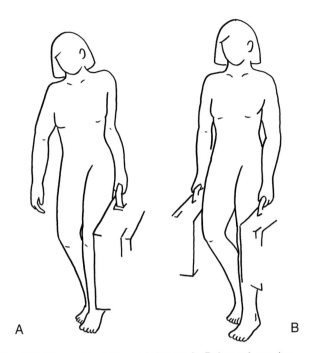

Fig. 10A.38. **a,** Too heavy a suitcase; **b,** Balanced carrying.

If you are tall, the carriage will need longer arms (Fig. 10A.42). In any case, try to keep your back straight and avoid slumping when you stroll a baby. The same is generally true when selecting a vacuum cleaner—a taller unit will help you to keep your back straight.

Changing your baby is another opportunity for back strain. The rule is to have a changing station of appropriate height so that you do not have to bend too far forward (Fig. 10A.43). Sometimes, a foot stool can be used to reduce back strain.

The foot stool is a handy aid for much counter top work. Ironing, cutting vegetables, folding laundry, and brushing your teeth are just a few examples of situations in which a low counter top can cause overstrain (Fig. 10A.44). If a foot stool is not available, it is sometimes possible to bend your knees and lean them against the cupboard (Fig. 10A.45).

First aid for an acute episode of back pain

One of those acute, disabling episodes of back pain can easily provoke anxiety and even anger. Fortunately, such episodes typically are transient and usually begin to calm down after just 2 to 3 days of rest (or up to 1 week if they are accompanied by pain/numbness below the knee). Proper care of the acute episode leads to dramatic improvement quickly.

Much can and should be done to ensure that an acute episode does not mushroom into a severe, disabling episode. Try to reduce any source of external strain on your back. Assuming proper rest positions is of vital importance. Lying on your back with your knees bent is one of the best "relief" positions for the spine (Fig. 10A.46) in that it reduces pressure on the disks and relaxes the muscles. Applying ice for 20 minutes four to six times per day normally is advisable.

Heat is generally avoided in the acute stage because it can actually increase swelling or inflammation in the back. Anti-inflammatories may be helpful for the first few days to reduce the swelling quickly. Your chiropractor or other specialist may fit you for a lumbar brace and give you specific therapeutic exercises to try. Some of the safest exercises are simple stretches or lumbar extension exercises (Figs. 10A.47 to 10A.50). Walking may also be suggested. Gentle treatments may be applied that will also speed the process along. As soon as your acute pain begins to ease, more aggressive conservative treatments will follow that will get your back functioning again as quickly as possible.

In order for your back to calm down, you must learn ways to perform normal activities without placing any undue strain on the back. Sitting should be minimized and sometimes avoided altogether. The

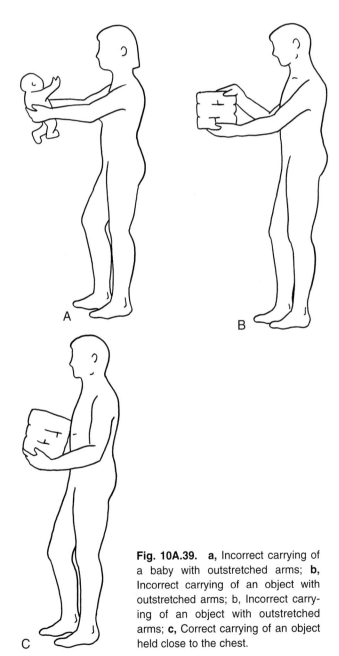

Fig. 10A.39. **a,** Incorrect carrying of a baby with outstretched arms; **b,** Incorrect carrying of an object with outstretched arms; b, Incorrect carrying of an object with outstretched arms; **c,** Correct carrying of an object held close to the chest.

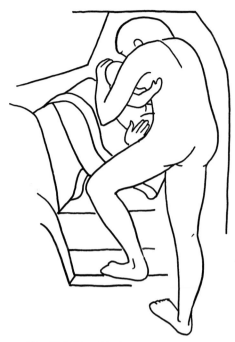

Fig. 10A.40. Placing a baby in a car.

early morning is always a critical time. Not only are we usually stiffest then, but also our disks are swollen from not being compressed by gravity. Getting out of bed safely by avoiding doing a sit-up is absolutely crucial. It is best to get up on our side and try to avoid twisting or bending at the waist (Fig. 10A.51). The next

danger comes when leaning forward over the sink. In this situation, it is prudent to bend your knees or use a foot stool so that when you bend forward, all the pressure does not go into your back (see Fig. 10A.45). Getting in and out of the car is another challenge. Avoid pivoting at your waist; instead, keep your torso rigid as you turn your entire body to get in and out of the car.

Until your back "goes out," you do not realize just how many activities place strain on your back. Just putting on pants, socks, stockings, etc. usually entails stressful bending. Two options exist for avoiding this stress. Try either dressing on your back or standing against a wall (Fig. 10A.52). Getting up out of a chair is another simple activity that seems like "murder" when your back is "out." If you are in a chair, scoot to the edge of the chair before rising and use arm rests if available to push yourself up (Fig. 10A.53). Avoid bending forward if possible. Lovemaking is another activity that can seem daunting if you have a bad back. It may be easier if you are on your back with your knees bent. Another possibility is making love while lying on your side. It is important that a bad back not interfere with family life, if you can help it.

Exercise

A sedentary lifestyle is a recipe for back and neck pain. Exercise nourishes all the tissues of the spine and increases flexibility and strength. When recovering from an acute episode of pain, exercises actually help the tissues to heal faster. Unfortunately, not all exercises are appropriate for the back and neck. Some exercises that actually can cause harm are as follows:

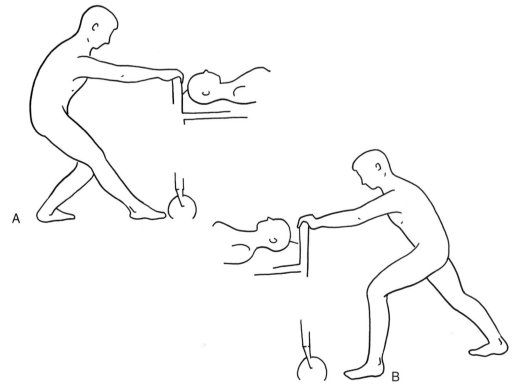

Fig. 10A.41. a, Unsafe pulling; **b,** Safe pushing.

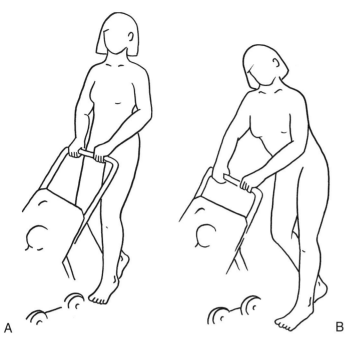

Fig. 10A.42. **a,** Stroller arms of proper height; **b,** Slumping because stroller arms are too low.

Toe touches. They stretch the back and hamstrings simultaneously, which is too dangerous (Fig. 10A.54).

Sit-ups. Never come up all the way because the disk pressure is too high. Also, they can be bad for the neck if you pull on your neck or poke your chin forward as you come up (Fig. 10A.55).

Hamstring curls. The tendency is to overarch (hyperextend) the lumbar spine during this exercise (Fig. 10A.56).

Lat Pull Downs. A great exercise, but not the way it is commonly performed. You should not have to crane your head forward to avoid the weight stack nor should you hyperextend the low back (Fig. 10A.57). Have your back to the machine and place a stool far enough forward so that the weight can be lowered without having to move your head out of the weights way. Also perform a slight posterior pelvic tilt by contracting both your abdominals and gluteals to protect your lower back.

Once your pain is stabilized and your back and neck is beginning to "loosen up" again, it is important to focus on improving the function of your back. Reconditioning involving stretching and strengthening is every bit as important as learning how to sit or lift. Before you go out and join a gym or get back into that workout routine, however, you should be aware of some of the more dangerous exercises commonly performed today. The four most common errors made in the gym are hyperextending the low back, slumping at the waist, poking the chin forward, and excessive shrugging of the shoulders. The exercises in which improper form is seen most commonly include the following:

1. Hyperextending the low back
   –sitting leg extensions
   –hamstring curls
   –lat pull downs
   –supine flys
   –overhead press
   –lunges
   –squats
   –trunk curls on an incline board*
   –sit-ups
   –Roman Chair

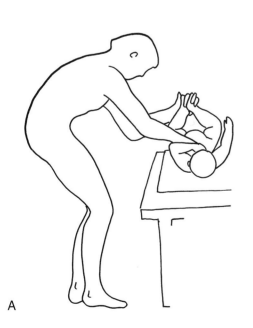

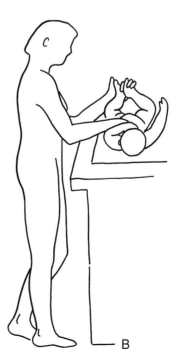

Fig. 10A.43. **a,** Changing station height too low; **b,** Correct changing station height.

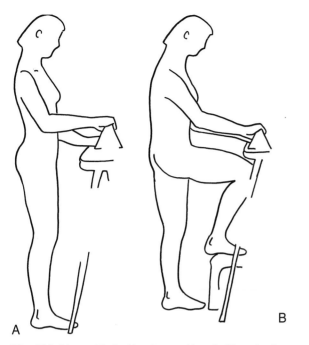
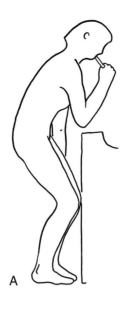
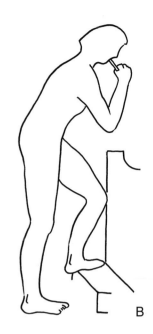

Fig. 10A.44. **a,** Typical ironing position; **b,** Use of a footstool to reduce a low back strain.

Fig. 10A.45. **a,** Brushing teeth with both knees bent; **b,** Use of a footstool to reduce low back strain.

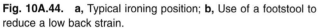
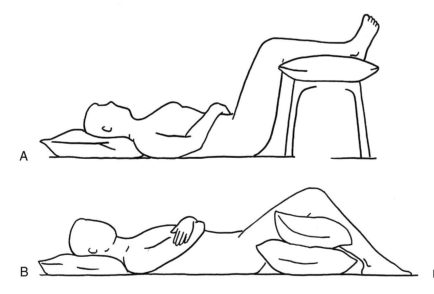

Fig. 10A.46. Back relief positions.

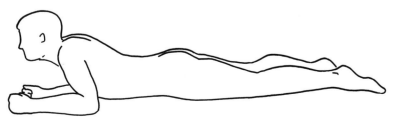

Fig. 10A.47. Back extension "sphinx" exercise.

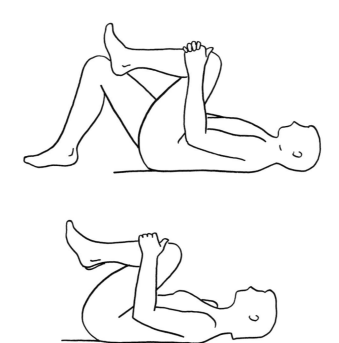

Fig. 10A.48. Single and double knee(s) to chest exercise.

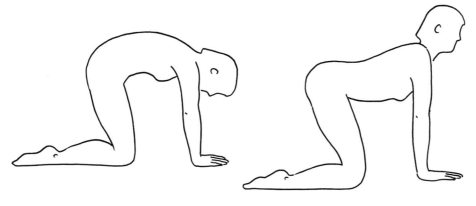

Fig. 10A.49. Cat exercise.

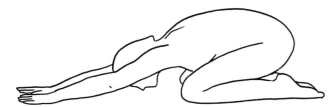

Fig. 10A.50. Prayer stretch.

–stairclimber
–push-ups
2. Slumping at the waist
  –sitting leg extensions
  –sitting chest press
  –stairclimber

  –exercise bicycle
  –hamstring stretches (toe touch or on floor)
  –stiff-legged dead lift*
  –bent forward rowing*
3. Head forward posture with chin poked forward
  –sit-ups
  –stairmaster
  –exercise bicycle
  –lat pull downs
  –push-ups
4. Hiking or shrugging of the shoulders
  –rowing machine
  –bent over rows
  –lateral arm raises
  –overhead press
  –push-ups

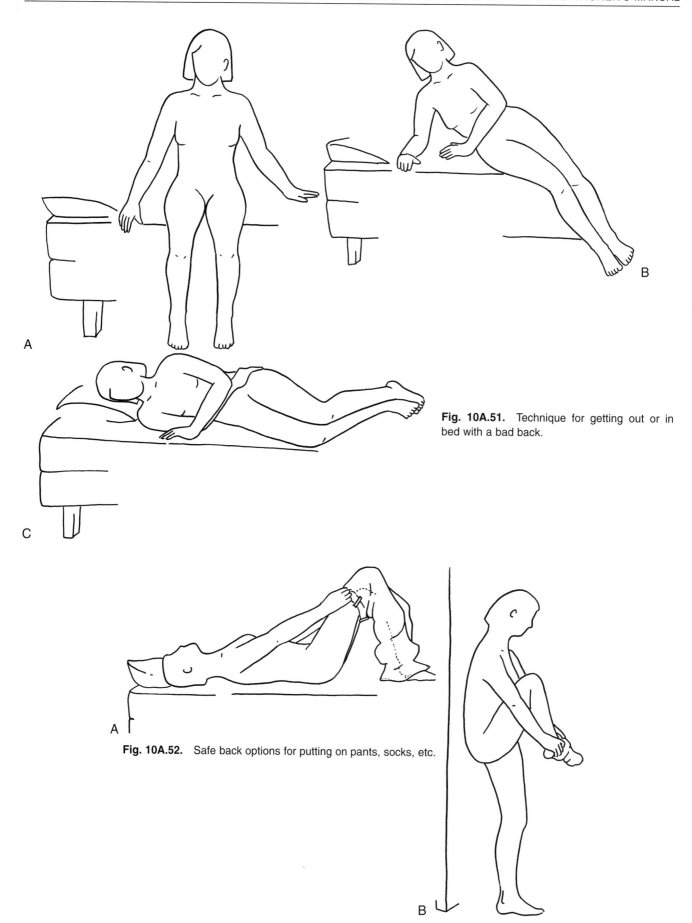

Fig. 10A.51. Technique for getting out or in bed with a bad back.

Fig. 10A.52. Safe back options for putting on pants, socks, etc.

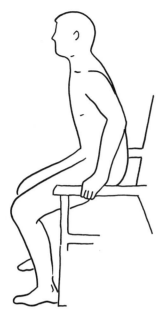

Fig. 10A.53. Safe technique for rising from a chair.

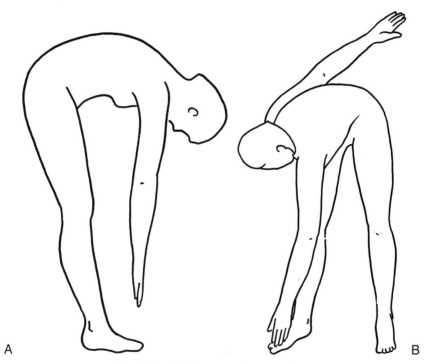

A   B

Fig. 10A.54. Dangerous toe touches.

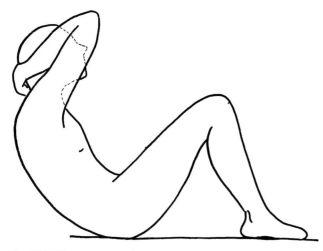

Fig. 10A.55. Improper sit-up.

spire against maintaining a relaxed shoulder posture. Desks or workstations that are too high or poorly placed (or absent) arm rests contribute to elevation of the shoulders. Again, proper posture and form during exercise is necessary to prevent adding further fuel to this fire. A good rule of thumb is that the shoulders should be relaxed back and down. It is never a good idea during an exercise to either roll the shoulders forward or hike them up toward the ears.

Summary

If you have suffered a severe episode of back or neck pain or you experience chronic pain in these areas, there is a proven way to control these symptoms. The long-term solution involves learning how to reduce strain and improve posture. The advice you receive from your rehabilitation specialist and that is included in this handout is designed to help you to help yourself. Back

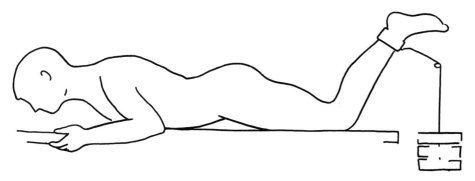

Fig. 10A.56. Harmful hamstring (back of thigh) exercise.

These four cardinal errors can often be corrected by paying attention to proper posture and form. The lumbar spine should normally be kept in a "mid-range" position, often called the "neutral position" or "functional range." This position varies for everybody. Some people are most vulnerable when they slump, others when they hyperextend. A gentle co-contraction of your abdominals and your buttocks is usually sufficient to isometrically hold your spine in a stable position or range so that many of the exercises just mentioned can be performed safely. Certain exercises (*), however, should just be eliminated completely from our routines. Your back specialist will show you alternatives.

When your head is forward of your torso, it is vulnerable to injury. This position fatigues your neck muscles and places the cervical spine under great strain. Poking your chin further irritates the joint between the back of your head (occiput) and the first vertebrae of the neck (atlas). It also creates a "guillotine"-like effect between the transition of the lower part of your neck and the upper part of your thoracic spine. By simply making sure you are not slumping at your waist and keeping your shoulders back to prevent them from rolling forward, your head position will often correct itself.

Excessive shoulder shrugging is a common problem. Emotional tension leads to shoulder and neck tension, which results in "having the weight of the world on your shoulders." Frequent sighing is a tip off to this occurrence. Also, most desks and chairs con-

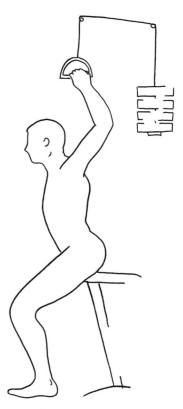

Fig. 10A.57. Improper form during "lat pull-down" exercise.

or neck pain arises from exposure to mechanical strain that gradually accumulates throughout your lifetime. If you learn to sit, lift, bend, carry, and sleep smarter, the likelihood of discomfort and risk of re-injury is reduced. If you have deconditioned as a result of leading a sedentary lifestyle or from restricting your activities as a consequence of pain, then you may also need to start a therapeutic stretching and strengthening program. Learning how to perform typical activities of daily life without increasing strain, and also training muscles to be more fit, will enable you to control your symptoms and prevent the likelihood of more serious problems in the future.

IV

FUNCTIONAL RESTORATION

11 Role of Manipulation in Spinal Rehabilitation

KAREL LEWIT

Rehabilitation is defined as the restoration of function in the motor system. This definition implies recuperation of active voluntary motion. To place emphasis on active exercise is therefore justified to achieve normal active control of movement. Structures that move passively, however, such as joints, ligaments, fasciae, and tendons, frequently play a key role in this recovery, and passive treatment of these structures can be effective, even for severe muscle spasm. In fact, the use of passive manipulative therapy by a qualified individual may enable a patient to carry out active motion, whereas omitting these methods would result in frustration and loss of time.

Manipulative treatment is an important factor in the restoration of passive motion, particularly now that up-to-date techniques affect not only joints but also the soft tissues, in particular fasciae, as well as muscles in spasm and with trigger points (TrP). Many of these techniques also make use of the patient's muscles and therefore may be considered semi-active. Such methods are perhaps a link between passive and active treatment.[1–3]

Even more important is the diagnostic value of the techniques described by professionals who use manipulation for the assessment of changes or lesions in the tissues and structures that constitute the locomotor system. These assessment techniques are useful not only for joints, but also for soft tissues, including muscles and fasciae. No less important is the contribution of these professionals to the diagnosis of disturbances in spinal statics (e.g., short leg, poor posture).[4–6]

CHANGES IN FUNCTION

The condition affecting the motor system that most often requires treatment, including rehabilitation, is not the obvious loss of motor control or motor function, but *pain,* also termed *myofascial pain* (MP). Use of this descriptive term seems justified in so far as this pain, whatever its true origin, is expressed or felt mainly in muscles and their attachment points. Despite its enormous incidence, this affliction is poorly understood; no pathologic structural changes have so far been confirmed as relevant, and it is the secret hope of many researchers that discovery of such changes is just round the corner.

One of the features of manipulation and other techniques used to treat MP is that they act immediately. This feature is also true of other methods of what may be called "reflex therapy," e.g., acupuncture or local anesthesia. Such immediate effects would hardly be possible if the underlying cause were a pathologic change of structure that requires healing and could not be *reversed* immediately. This concept is easily understood, however, if the existence or reality of changes in function is recognized. For structure in the living organism in general, and in the locomotor system in particular, is no more real than is function: muscles in spasm (with TrP), incapable of lengthening; restricted joints (perhaps because of meniscoid entrapment and/or spasm); and short muscles or fasciae requiring stretching (shifting).[7–10]

An example of an even more elementary situation is tension and muscle pain that accompanies an uncomfortable position; discomfort improves immediately with a change of position. As observed by Brugger, if a person sitting in a round-shouldered position is examined, the muscles of the shoulder girdle, arms, and even of the legs are tense and tender on palpation. The moment the person changes into an erect (lordotic) relief position (Fig. 11.1), the same muscles are soft and painless. Nothing has changed except body statics, but relief has been obtained.

A strong reluctance remains, however, within the medical profession to accept altered function as an important cause of disease and suffering. In fact, the term "functional" is widely used as a euphemism for psychologic or even imaginary problems. In internal medicine, some changes in function apparently are accepted, e.g., cardiac arrhythmia or endocrine dysfunction, but such acceptance remains an insurmountable obstacle in the motor system, where function is paramount. Anatomic verification at autopsy has become the obsession, as though physiology was of little importance, it being, indeed, unverifiable post mortem. I therefore like to use a simple example from engineering.

If an automobile stops functioning, the cause may be a broken cylinder or ballbearing. Alternatively, the problem may result from maladjusted combustion or ignition. In the first case, there is gross pathology. Because a machine cannot heal, we must replace the damaged part. In the second case, the structure is intact, we have only to adjust the ignition or combustion (i.e., *function*) and the machine performs again.

An important warning is appropriate at this point: just as it may take equal effort to adjust a complicated engine as to change some spare parts, treatment of changes in locomotor

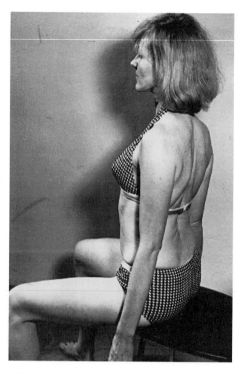

Fig. 11.1. Brugger's relief (lordotic) position.

function is sometimes quite involved. Unfortunately, physiology is no less complicated than anatomy. As, however, changes of function are by definition reversible, treating functional pathology of the locomotor system is a rewarding challenge.

The fact that some changes in function are immediately reversible provides a rational explanation for some "miracle cures" after treatment by manipulation and other "reflex therapy" methods. Unfortunately, locomotor dysfunction has remained a medical no man's land, lost between such specialties as rheumatology, orthopedics, neurology, and rehabilitation medicine. In view of its importance, a clear distinction between structural and "functional" pathology (dysfunction) is fundamental, for diagnosis and management as well as for classification. It can be compared only to the distinction between hardware and software.

If we accept changes in function as relevant in MP, then we should be able to explain why and how dysfunction can truly cause it. This explanation seems relatively easy: whatever the type of dysfunction we treat—a muscular TrP, a restricted joint, a change in soft tissues, or altered body statics or movement patterns, we invariably meet increased tension. In fact, impaired function of the motor system is associated less with inability to move than with pain resulting from increased tension. If we move in the direction of a restricted joint, overstrain, assume unfavorable positions, or perform strenuous work, the common denominator is increased tension (strain).

The link between strain and pain should be readily understandable. Pain is, in the first place, a warning sign of impending danger and, in the locomotor system, is an indicator of the need to protect against overstrain. The role of pain in this setting is all the more important in that the motor system carries out voluntary movement and thus has no other means to protect itself against our whims. Pain receptors, therefore, are found precisely where tension is most prominent in the motor system, i.e., in muscles with their attachment points, joint capsules, ligaments, meningeal sheaths, and the outer layers of the annulus fibrosus.[11,12]

From what has been said, it can well be understood that MP is the most frequent type of pain experienced by the human organism. As disturbed function plays the main role in causing this type of complaint, it is necessary to explain some basic approaches in dealing with it. The question is where and how to apply treatment. If we have a painful structural lesion, e.g., inflammation, we know where to apply treatment. Function, on the other hand, implies correlation and interplay of many structures. Therefore, "he who applies treatment to the site of pain is usually lost." This fundamental change in approach threatens the clinician with the loss of firm ground; in fact, many who are involved in treating dysfunction tend to apply these methods (e.g., manipulation) mainly to the painful area and not to the real source of dysfunction.

Chain Reaction in Functional Pathology

Experience has shown that changes in function follow certain patterns; as a rule, if we find one change, there is another connected with it, i.e., we observe certain *chain reactions*. At first, this observation was purely the outcome of clinical experience. On closer scrutiny, however, it was possible to show that these chain reactions follow certain rules that correspond to the basic functions of the locomotor system:[13] (1) gait, involving mainly the lower extremities and the pelvis with the lumbar spine; (2) body statics, involving mainly the trunk and neck; (3) respiration, involving mainly the thorax; (4) prehension, involving mainly the upper extremities, the shoulder girdle, and the neck: and (5) food intake, involving mainly the orofacial system and the neck. The first of these chains is presented with a detailed commentary, the rest in Tables 11.1 to 11.5 that the reader will understand by analogy.

These chains not only illustrate a different approach in the diagnosis of what we call functional pathology of the motor system, but also are important in therapy. The point is to determine the most *relevant* link in the chain and to choose the most appropriate method of treatment. When successful, treating the key link should improve the chain as a whole.

The cause of disturbed function is frequently in the motor system itself; it may, however, lie outside, in particular in the viscera, triggering characteristic patterns or chains.

The chains presented in the tables do not claim to be complete, constant, or fixed. In addition, reflex changes in the skin and (if chronic) changes in fasciae and periosteal pain points must be considered, but their inclusion in the tables would make them too involved to be useful. It is worth noting, however, that these chains are characteristically formed on one side of the body.

Table 11.1. Gait: Stance Phase and Swing Phase*

Stance Phase

1. Increased tension:	Toe and plantar flexors, triceps surae, glutei, piriformis, levator ani, erector spinae
2. Tender attachment points (referred pain):	Calcaneus (plantar aponeurosis and Achilles tendon), fibular head (biceps femoris), ischial tuberosity (hamstrings), coccyx (gluteus maximus, levator ani), iliac crest (gluteus medius, lumbar erector spinae), greater trochanter (gluteus medius, piriformis), and spinous processes L4-S1 (erector spinae).
3. Joint dysfunction (blockage):	Midfoot joints, ankle, tibiofibular joint, sacroiliac joint, low lumbar spine

Swing Phase-flexion and internal rotation

1. Increased tension:	Extensors of the toes and foot, tibialis anterior, hip flexors, adductors, recti abdominous, thoracolumbar erector spinae (upper extensors)
2. Tender attachment points (referred pain):	Pes anserinus (adductors), patellae (rectus femoris, tensor fasciae latae), minor trochanter, symphysis (upper and lateral aspect), xiphoid
3. Joint dysfunction (blockage):	Knee, hip, sacroiliac joint, upper lumbar spine and thoracolumbar junction, (atlantooccipital joint)

^aChain reactions are related to the stance phase of gait concerning first the physiologic extensors and external rotators of the lower limb. Group 1 lists the functional sequence of muscles to become involved. Group 2 lists attachment points (or referred pain) of the above muscles that are likely to become tender if the muscles are hyperactive or tensed. Group 3 lists joints likely to develop dysfunction (blockage) in this chain reaction. Joints are not related to single muscles, their dysfunction is the result of changed static and dynamic function as a result of (mainly) muscular dysfunction.

Table 11.2. Body Statics

Tension in muscle parts
  Sternocleidomastoid: short craniocervical extensors
  Scaleni and deep neck flexors: levator scapulae, upper trapezius
  Iliopsoas and recti abdominous: erector spinae and quadratus lumborum
Tender attachment points (points of referred pain)
  Posterior atlas arch, transverse process of atlas, spinous process of C2, linea nuchae, medial aspect of collar bone, upper and vertebral margin of scapula, xiphoid, symphysis, lowest ribs, iliac crests
Joint dysfunction (blockage)
  Craniocervical junction, cervicothoracic junction, upper ribs, thoracolumbar junction, lumbosacral and sacroiliac junction

Table 11.3. Lifting the Thorax at Respiration (Typical Respiratory Dysfunction)

1. Increased tension:	Upper section of abdominal muscles, pectorales, scaleni, sternocleidomastoids, short extensors of craniocervical junction, levator and trapezius
2. Tender attachment point (referred pain):	Posterior atlas arch and transverse process, spinous process of C2, linea nuchae, medial end of clavicle, upper margin of scapula, sternocostal junction (referred from scaleni) and upper ribs
3. Joint dysfunction (blockage):	Craniocervical junction, cervicothoracic junction, upper ribs, thoracic spine

Table 11.4. Upper Extremity Prehension

Extension

1. Increased tension:	Finger and wrist extensors, thenar, supinators and biceps, deltoideus, supra and infraspinatus, upper fixators of shoulder blade, interscapular muscles
2. Tender attachment points (points of referred pain):	Proc. styloideus radii and lateral epicondyle, attachment points of supra- and infraspinatus, attachment points of levator scapulae, and spinous process of C2 (referred pain)
3. Joint dysfunction (blockage):	Elbow, acromioclavicular joint, midcervical spine, cervicothoracic junction, upper ribs

Flexion

1. Increased tension:	Finger and wrist flexors, pronators subscapularis and pectoralis, sternocleidomastoids scaleni
2. Tender attachment points (points of referred pain):	Medial epicondyle, medial end of clavicle, sternocostal junction, Erb's point, transverse process of atlas
3. Joint dysfunction (blockage):	Carpal bones (carpal tunnel syndrome), elbow, glenohumeral joint, cervicothoracic and craniocervical junctions

Table 11.5. Head and Neck: Food Intake, Mastication, and Speech

1. Increased tension:	Masticatory muscles, digastricus, sternocleidomastoids, short extensors of craniocervical junction, trapezius and levator scapulae, deep neck flexors, pectorales
2. Tender attachment points (points of referred pain):	Hyoid, posterior atlas arch and transverse processes, spinous process of C2, linea nuchae, medial end of collar bone, upper margin of scapula, and angle of upper ribs
3. Joint dysfunction (blockage):	Temporomandibular joint, craniocervical junction, cervicothoracic junction, upper ribs

Structural Versus Functional Pathology

A short survey of the main characteristics of dysfunction as contrasted with structural pathology may be useful to demonstrate the fundamental difference in approach.

1. The first step is to decide whether the problem described by the patient results mainly from dysfunction or from structural pathology.
2. A structural lesion frequently causes dysfunction that then produces the clinical manifestations; on the other hand, dysfunction by itself may cause clinical manifestations.
3. The reversibility of dysfunction makes immediate cure a possibility, whereas structural pathologic change requires healing.
4. The aim of structural diagnosis is to localize and determine the nature of the lesion; in dysfunction, it is essential to investigate correlations and interplay, i.e., the chain reactions.

5. Structural diagnosis aims at the organ at fault, functional diagnosis at the organism as a whole.

6. In cases of dysfunction, structural diagnosis gives negative results, whereas with functional diagnosis, we typically find more than we expect from the patient's history.

7. The aim of therapy of pathologic change involving a structure is healing or excision; in dysfunction, it is to treat the relevant link of the chain.

8. In structural pathology, modern technology plays an ever-increasing role, whereas in functional pathology, clinical methods remain unchallenged.

9. In structural pathology, the relationship between cause and effect is unambiguous, whereas in dysfunction, cause and effect are frequently interchangeable.

10. Methods and techniques of "alternative" or "complementary" medicine are relevant mainly in disturbance of function.

DIAGNOSTIC UTILITY OF PALPATION AND THE BARRIER PHENOMENON

As stated previously, dysfunction causes increased tension in various structures (tissues) of the motor system, and this tension relates to pain. The main tool in the diagnosis of changes in tension is *palpation.* Palpation is an art that was once important in medicine. Together with inspection and auscultation, it was the basis of clinical medicine; regrettably, it is now largely neglected. For this reason, it is necessary to give a concise analysis of palpation in relation to manipulation.[14–17]

Palpation

The first step is to apply our fingers to the body surface and to concentrate on what we want to investigate: resistance to pressure, temperature, moisture, smoothness or roughness of skin, and tissue mobility. If we intend to proceed from one tissue layer to the next, we never simply increase the pressure, but shift our attention and apply small movements, i.e., we change both intensity and direction of pressure, using discreet motion (Fig. 11.2). We may want to palpate the shape of a structure, the transition of muscle to tendon, or where the tendon is attached. Then, we want to palpate the relative mobility of soft tissue structures one against the other: skin against muscle, muscles and fasciae against bone, not forgetting the important task of movement palpation in joints and mobile segments of the spinal column. In this effort, we use not only our *sense of touch* but also *proprioception.*

One of the most elegant methods of diagnosing superficial hyperalgesic zones (HAZ) is skin drag: we move over the skin, and in areas with more moisture (sweat), resistance (drag) is increased. Most of these methods have one thing in common: during palpation, we move our fingers or hands.

The diagnosis of a TrP, which is discussed in another section, has another important feature, which is more pronounced in this case yet common to other methods of palpation: provoking a twitch response, i.e., we establish *interaction* with the patient. In this way, a most important feedback relationship between doctor and patient is established, providing a wealth of information and at the same time providing the basis for effective therapy. This relationship develops when applying all types of massage, and the good therapist, whether consciously or not, profits by this feedback, sensing the reaction of the patient's tissues and correcting his or her moves accordingly.

Barrier Phenomenon

To make both palpatory diagnosis and treatment more effective and better understood, we must be aware of the barrier phenomenon. It seems to be common to most structures and tissues of the motor system, and thus plays a key role in manipulative therapy. It was first described by osteopaths in joints, but it is relevant wherever manipulation is applied.[18]

Moving a joint from a neutral position involves first a range of motion in which resistance is uniform and negligible. As we approach the end of the range, however, we meet resistance, which gradually increases. The moment resistance *starts* to increase, i.e., when we meet the slightest resistance, we have reached the barrier. In other words: the sooner we sense the barrier, for diagnosis as well as for therapy, the better our sense of palpation and our technique. It follows that the normal barrier is soft and resilient and can be easily sprung. On the other hand, a pathologic or restrictive barrier is one that is met too soon and feels abrupt (Fig. 11.3). In the diagram in Figure 11.3, we see that the anatomic barrier is never reached under normal conditions; the physiologic barrier corresponds to the normal range of movement. The pathologic barrier signifies movement restriction. The neutral point (N_0) may shift to the normal side (N_1), if there is such a patho-

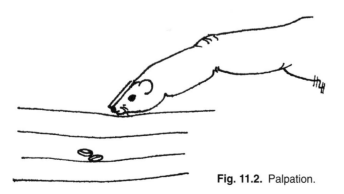

Fig. 11.2. Palpation.

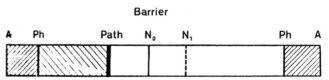

Fig. 11.3. Barrier phenomenon: anatomic, physiologic, and pathologic barriers.

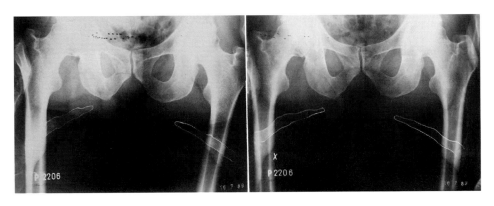

Fig. 11.4. Palpatory changes pre- and post-treatment.

logic barrier. Barriers are found not only in joints, but also in tissues that can be stretched or shifted against each other.

However useful the barrier phenomenon may be for diagnosis and treatment, it also has an important protective function. This role is most obvious in joints: resistance increases before full range is reached; however fast we may stretch our arm, the antagonist stops the movement in time to prevent damage. Other protective mechanisms come into play when we stretch connective tissue or cause shifting between different tissue layers, e.g., fascia against bone. The stretch reflex is part of this protective mechanism.

To use the barrier phenomenon for diagnosis and treatment of pain and dysfunction, take the following steps. By engaging the barrier (taking up the slack), we determine the range of movement (shift or stretch) and recognize the location and quality of the barrier. After engaging the (pathologic) barrier, we *wait;* after a few seconds, the barrier "gives" and myofascial release is obtained. Release may last from a few seconds to half a minute (or even more); this release must be *sensed,* making sure we have normalized the barrier, i.e., normalized tension and thereby obtained relief of pain. As shown subsequently in discussion of specific techniques, this release is as true for joint mobilization or muscle relaxation as for skin stretch or shifting fasciae or subperiosteal tissues, using the barrier phenomenon as common denominator.

The clinical importance of release lies in the relief of pain originating in the structures treated. Palpation thus provides an invaluable criterion of painful lesions without structural pathology, i.e., in cases of dysfunction. In fact, if we have obtained release, we know that the structure treated will be less painful.

Unfortunately, the evidence for these statements is only clinical, based on palpation, and the charge of subjectivity cannot be ruled out. As the palpating finger (hand) is constantly moving, changing both intensity and direction, meaningful measurements are difficult to conceive. This situation is complicated further by the feedback relationship between therapist and patient.

The problem of palpatory diagnosis has been further underlined by the discovery of palpatory illusion. On palpation of the pubic symphysis, and even more so of the ischial tuberosities in the recumbent patient, shifts as great as 2 cm can be noted. After simple "reposition maneuvers" or using

soft tissue techniques, symmetry is readily restored, and yet radiographic examination shows no change has occurred. If, however, the radiographic image includes the palpating fingers, it is clear that the position of the fingers has changed (Fig. 11.4). Hence, the change has occurred in the soft tissues or "media" through which the bony landmarks were palpated. This observation provides evidence that most "adjustments" noted by chiropractors or osteopaths after manipulation to restore "symmetry," as indeed they sense, are in the soft tissues, because joint realignment is not evident radiographically.[19]

Meaningful research in palpation has rarely been undertaken, in part because of the complexity of the task. Interpersonal reliability studies have so far been frustrating, because no one person knows exactly what the other is doing. Nevertheless, palpation yields invaluable information that is essential for diagnosis and therapy, in the same way the blind rely on the information gained from palpation all through life (Figs. 11.5 and 11.6).[20–25]

DIAGNOSIS AND TREATMENT OF SOFT TISSUE LESIONS

In a simple outline of the most useful techniques, the barrier phenomenon offers the most useful basis. The simplest model with which to start involves the soft tissues, beginning with the skin.

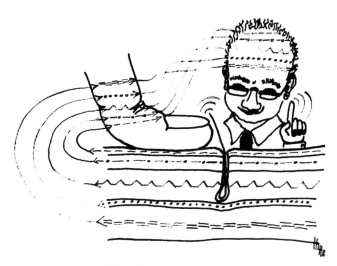

Fig. 11.5. "Low-tech" medicine.

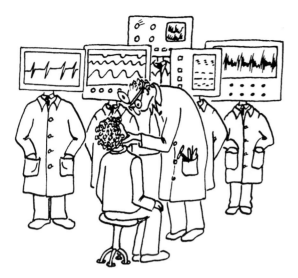

Fig. 11.6. "High-tech" medicine.

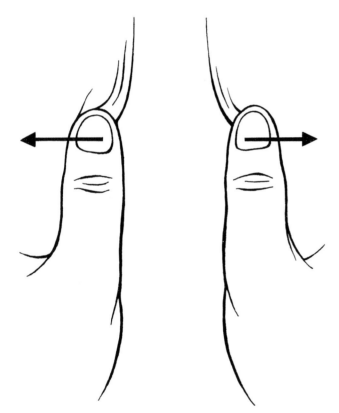

Fig. 11.7. Palpation of skin drag.

Skin (Fig. 11.7)

Hyperalgesic skin zones (HAZ) are found most conveniently by using skin drag, which consists of moving the cushions of the finger tips over the surface of the skin, sensing resistance or drag. Drag is increased in HAZ owing to increased moisture (hyperactivity of sweat glands). In the same areas, the skin fold is thicker, and if we stretch the skin in this region, we meet resistance sooner than on the normal side (stretching

in the same direction); no springing (hard "end feel") is noted on engaging the barrier. If we hold on after engaging the barrier without increasing stretch, the barrier gives after a latency period of a few seconds and release takes place. Release may last from about 10 seconds to half a minute. We then find a normal barrier (like on the normal side) and skin drag is restored to normal. This reaction is found regularly; if there is an underlying cause of the HAZ, it soon recurs.

Connective Tissue (Fig. 11.8)

The most useful diagnostic technique is to create a fold and to *stretch* it (never squeeze!). Again, when creating a fold, we reach a barrier where resistance is first sensed, a resistance that differs from normal if there is a restrictive lesion. After engaging the barrier and holding it, release takes place after a few seconds and continues up to a half a minute, until the barrier is normalized.

Such connective tissue is found most characteristically in hypersensitive scars with tender spots where tissue tension is increased and pain is easily elicited. Such scars are usually surrounded by a HAZ with increased skin drag. They are a source of increased nociceptive input, comparable in some ways to a diseased, painful visceral organ or joint. Release can be obtained by stretching the skin overlying such a scar along with the deeper connective tissues.[26,27]

Shortness of the connective tissue is most characteristic for short (taut) muscles, usually in overactive muscles. Producing a tissue fold and stretching it is the most effective way to obtain lengthening because the stretch reflex can be avoided. Such a fold is useful wherever it can be produced: in the m. trapezius, pectoralis, the quadratus lumborum, the sternocleidomastoid, and most of the muscles of the extremities. This method is not suitable for muscles with TrP; in such cases, postisometric relaxation should first be used.

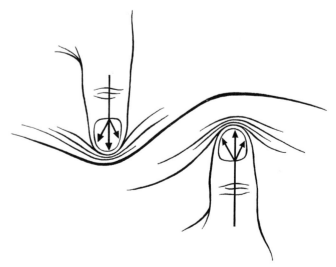

Fig. 11.8. Palpation of connective tissue changes.

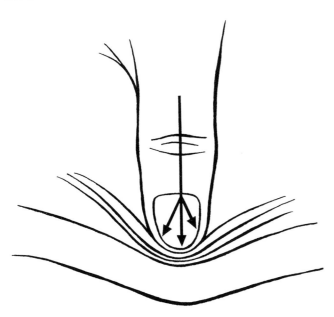

Fig. 11.9. Pressing deep soft tissue.

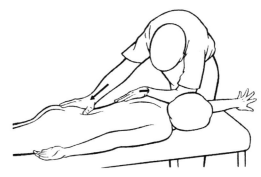

Fig. 11.10. Stretching (shifting) the gluteal fascia.

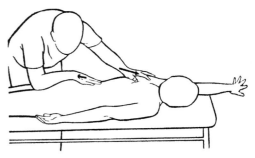

Fig. 11.11. Stretching (shifting) the dorsal fascia over the shoulder blade.

Pressure (Fig. 11.9)

Even if pressure is used, it is most important to engage the barrier with a minimum of force: after waiting for a few seconds, the finger will spontaneously sink deeper into the tissue. This method is most effective in muscles with superficial TrP, where it can replace postisometric relaxation (PIR). When the finger sinks into the muscle, it will reach the normal barrier after approximately 10 to 30 seconds, but if the direction of pressure is slightly changed, further release may be obtained. Such change in direction is important in large muscles, e.g., the gluteus maximus.

Shifting and Stretching Fascia (Fig. 11.10–11.12)[28,29]

When using this important technique, the most characteristic finding is that muscles (or all the soft tissues) on one side do not move as easily on the underlying bone as those on the other side if moved in the same direction, i.e., the barrier is reached sooner on one side and does not spring. It is important to note that the restricted side is not necessarily the painful side. A "tight and loose complex," i.e., one side is restricted and the other side is hypotonic, is frequently noted. Shifting is examined and treated in a craniocaudal or caudocranial direction on the back, but it should be assessed and treated in a circular manner around the axis of the neck and the extremities (see Figs. 11.10–11.12).

Because the fibers of most fascia are intertwined with muscle fibers, free mobility of fascia is essential for normal muscle and joint function. It is in chronic pain patients that mobility of fascia is frequently impaired; in such cases, joint (spinal) mobility is as a rule restored by moving the fascia. It also follows that unless we restore normal mobility of the fascia, muscle and joint dysfunction will recur. This principle is particularly important in fasciae that are common to a great number of muscles, like the lumbodorsal.

Sites of restricted fascial mobility also occur on the chest (characteristically in mastodynia); on the buttocks, frequently in a cranial direction; in the groin; around the elbow and knee; and around the ankles and wrists. In addition, some structures behave like fascia; the scalp should move easily in all directions in relation to the skull. Restriction in any direction is frequently linked with headache, and treatment methods that follow the same principles as for fascia can be most rewarding. Therefore, examination of scalp mobility is warranted for patients with headache and/or vertigo. Another such structure is the soft tissue pad at the heel, which should shift easily in all directions on the calcaneal bone. Restriction is characteristic of a painful calcaneal spur and should be treated.

The metatarsal and metacarpal bones can be shifted each against its neighbor; they are connected only by soft tissue, and resistance to this shift is characteristically increased in nerve root syndromes radiating to the toes (fingers). Not only is exact localization of the involved root possible, but also, by engaging the barrier and obtaining release (in a dorsoplantar or palmar direction), we can obtain striking therapeutic results. This restriction is usually linked with a HAZ of the skinfold between the toes (fingers) in the corresponding segment. This finding, too, can be diagnostic and can be treated with skin stretch accordingly.

Shifting Periosteal Tissue

Restrictive barriers are also found at painful periosteal points. By palpating such tender points, we can shift the surrounding tissues close to the bone and compare mobility with that of

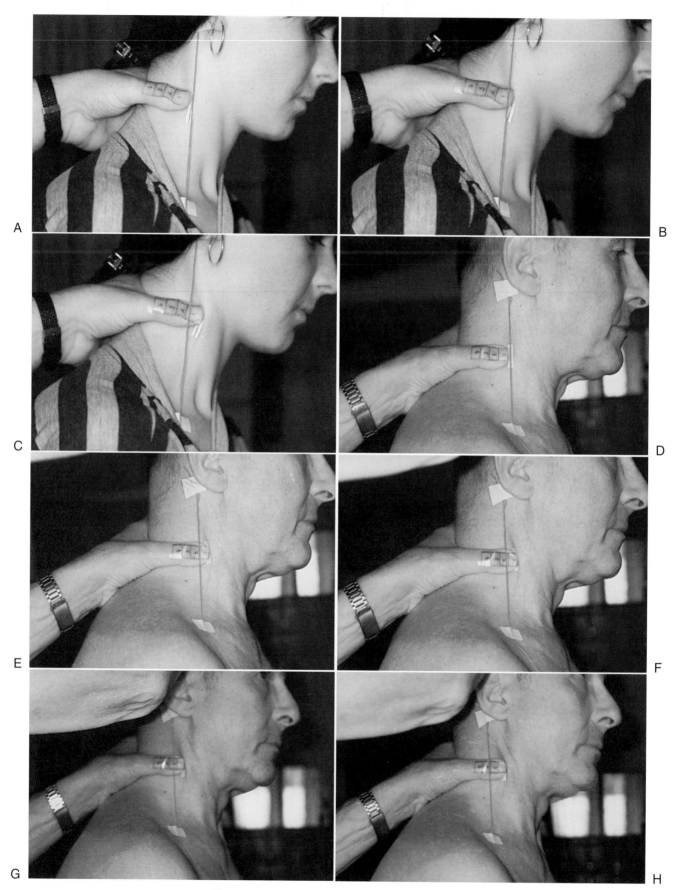

Fig. 11.12. Stretching (shifting) the cervical fascia.

the periosteal point on the normal side. Where we find restriction, usually in a tangential direction to the pain point, we take up the slack first for diagnosis and then to obtain release. Unlike periosteal massage or "deep friction," these soft tissue techniques are gentle; pressure is not directed to the pain point, but rather tangentially moves the periosteal tissue away from the point of pain. Painful spinous processes in the lumbar spine offer a good example. They are palpated in midline; however, if the palpating finger moves sideways, we find that only one side of the spinous process is really tender. On that side, we meet resistance if we try to exert deep pressure parallel to the spinous process. At this point, the slack is taken up and release follows, producing relief.

Soft Tissue Syndromes

Two "soft tissue syndromes" are of great practical importance. The first goes hand in hand with an apparent shift at the pubic symphysis and the ischial tuberosity, caused by increased tension (TrP) of the straight abdominal muscles and their attachment at the symphysis, and in the gluteal muscles, causing restriction of the cranial shift of the buttocks on one or both sides. Typically, the most prominent sign is a forward-drawn posture, which may be noted at the pelvis in relation to the feet, at the shoulder girdle in relation to the pelvis, and with the head thrust forward when looking at an object at eye level. We then also find increased tension in the back musculature with the patient standing, as well as in the neck muscles. Tension in the neck (and back) muscles subsides, however, when the patient is seated. If we engage the barrier by shifting the buttocks (m. glutei maximi) in a cranial direction and then obtain release, or if we use pressure where we sense hypertonus in the buttocks and obtain release, we normalize mobility at the buttocks as well as tension in the abdominal muscles and at the attachment points at the symphysis, and symmetry is restored. The tuberosities then appear symmetric on palpation. The forward-drawn position also disappears and, therefore, tension in the neck and back muscles reverts to normal. However striking this effect may be, the condition tends to recur if the abdominal and gluteal muscles are weak (Fig. 11.13) (see Chapter 14).[30]

The second soft tissue syndrome, described by Silverstolpe and Helsing,[31,32] can be detected because of a tender TrP in the midthoracic region, more frequently on the left side. On mechanical stimulation, this TrP causes a twitch response in the low lumbar area of the spinal erector and may even cause contraction of the hamstrings, producing sharp dorsiflexion. Typical findings include a tender point in the lateral gluteal area at the height of the upper end of the intergluteal fold and an even more tender point at the sacrotuberous ligament. When the index finger reaches this point (slightly ventral and craniad on the lateral edge of the tip of the sacrum), resistance is met. After taking up the slack, we obtain release after a latency of several seconds. Both the TrP in the thoracic spinal erector spinae and the lateral gluteal tender point (TeP) are gone.

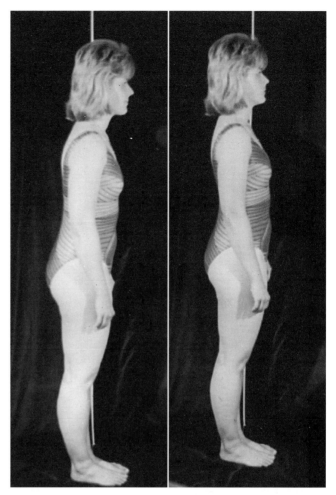

Fig. 11.13. Forward-drawn posture (left); after soft tissue treatment (right).

Both these syndromes affect most of the postural musculature, and therefore symptoms may arise in any part of the motor system, including headache with restriction in the craniocervical junction, and even tension in the masticatory muscles, backache, and pain in the area of the coccyx. Sacroiliac involvement typically is not part of these syndromes, but it may occur. The pathologic barrier at the sacrotuberous ligament is probably attributable to a TrP in the m. coccygeus.

POSTISOMETRIC RELAXATION (PIR) IN THE TREATMENT OF MUSCLE SPASM (TRP)[1,3,33–35]

Postisometric relaxation produces release in muscles in spasm, the most frequent type of spasm in myofascial pain (MP) being the trigger point (TrP). This technique was introduced by Mitchell for joint mobilization, and it is in its essence a type of soft tissue manipulation. Just as in the techniques described previously, the first step of PIR is to engage the barrier by lengthening the muscle to the point at which the first, slight resistance is met. After this point, however, the patient is told to exert slight resistance in the opposite direction, holding it isometrically for about 10 seconds, followed by the order to relax (let go). After a few seconds (waiting at the barrier), release takes place and the muscle lengthens (decontracts) for anything from a few seconds to half a minute. Clearly, a subtle, yet important difference exists in the mechanism of release in PIR relative to other techniques of manipulation: whereas connective tissue must be passively stretched during release, although with little force, muscle decontraction is an *active* process, just as is muscle contraction, and is only *monitored* by the therapist. "You cannot relax the patient's muscles for him, he has to do it himself." The moment the therapist tries to stretch the muscle, the patient produces the stretch reflex, which is counterproductive. If PIR is not satisfactory at the first attempt, we repeat the procedure (from the barrier reached after the first attempt) and prolong the isometric phase.

Postisometric relaxation is highly specific, and it is important during the isometric phase to contract precisely those muscle fibers that are in spasm, especially fan-shaped muscles such as the pectoralis major. It is also essential to use minimum force, because we then increase the likelihood of stimulating selectively those fibers with a low threshold of stimulation, i.e., those harboring TrP. Relaxation of the muscles brings about relief not only of the painful TrP, but also of the painful attachment point, as well as regions of referred pain (Fig. 11.14).[36]

As stated for the techniques described so far, accurate diagnosis is essential to the success of PIR. In some types of muscle spasm or cramps, the diagnosis may be obvious. Some TrP, however, may be excessively painful on palpation and yet are not felt spontaneously by the patient; these must be sought and identified. Clinically, they manifest themselves by referred pain, which can be far from its source, and it is important to know the sites of pain referral. Palpation technique must also be mastered. Usually, slight hypertonus is noted above a muscular TrP, but it is frequently so discreet as to avoid detection and diagnosis. By making the muscle harboring a TrP slip under our fingers, however, we produce a reaction in precisely those fibers that are perceived as a "taut band." The TrP lies within this band, and at this point, we should be able to evoke referred pain and the twitch reaction (Fig. 11.15). Interestingly, the more superficial a TrP, perhaps in the forearm or the erector spinae, where the patient is more likely to be aware of it, the better he or she tolerates examination. The hidden TrP, such as in the m. psoas or subscapularis, are most painful on palpation or when merely touched.

In its basic form, as just described, PIR has some serious drawbacks. Many patients, even when instructed, have difficulty putting up minimal resistance only and show their eagerness to cooperate by a display of strength. Others have difficulty relaxing, although prolonging the isometric phase to 20 seconds and more proves effective. Finally, many practitioners find it difficult to distinguish the patient's relaxation from "gentle stretch."

Using Eye Movements, Respiratory Synkinesis, and Gravity with PIR

For these reasons, combining the use of PIR with other "neuromuscular techniques" has improved our results and is particularly of value in promoting self-treatment. The first such combination is with eye movements. If the patient looks to the

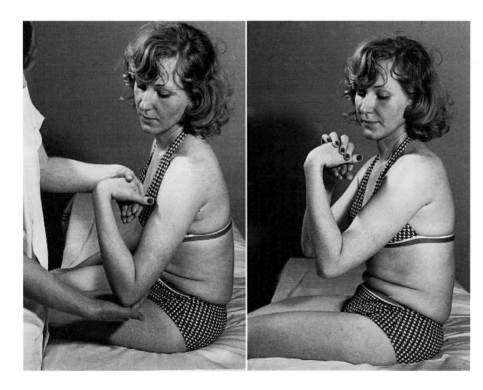

Fig. 11.14. Postisometric relaxation of wrist extensors (left); self-PIR of the wrist extensors (right).

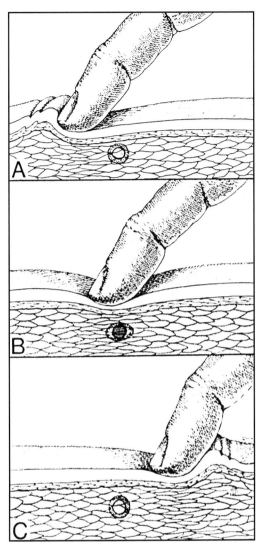

Fig. 11.15. Palpation of a trigger point by identifying the taut band. (From Travell JG, Simons DG: Myofascial Pain and Dysfunction: The Trigger Point Manual. Baltimore, Williams & Wilkins, 1983, p 61.)

right, he or she facilitates rotator muscles that can be resisted during the isometric phase; if the patient looks in the opposite direction, these muscles will relax. If he or she looks up, the muscles in the back and neck contract and can be resisted; when looking down, they will relax (Fig. 11.16). Here, too, the patient must first sense the barrier.[37]

Respiration plays an important role in PIR, inhalation having a facilitative and exhalation an inhibitory effect, particularly as it affects structures in the head, neck, and trunk and less so the extremities. The effect of respiration is particularly evident in *respiratory synkinesis.* This term describes when movement in one direction is coupled with inhalation, whereas movement in the opposite direction is coupled with exhalation. As an example, straightening up is linked with inhalation whereas bending down is linked with exhalation, indeed because it is difficult to exhale while straightening up

and to inhale while stooping. This principle is equally true for side bending, and even during backbending, *maximum* exhalation is required to obtain synkinetic contraction of the thoracic erector spinae (producing mobilization into trunk extension, Fig. 11.17).

Exhalation is coupled with forward flexion in a neutral erect position, whereas in a lordotic or prone position, the reverse holds true. This fact is borne out by isometric manual traction with the patient prone; owing to lumbar lordosis, the erector spinae contracts during exhalation, moving the buttocks upward. This movement is resisted during the isometric phase. During inhalation, the erector spinae relaxes and the buttocks move caudally (Fig. 11.18). In the cervical area, the opposite occurs: on inhalation, the neck muscles contract (isometric phase); on exhalation, relaxation takes place. For traction treatment (Fig. 11.19), it is sufficient to cradle the patient's head during the isometric phase, followed by relaxation during exhalation. This traction technique is apparently the most gentle and the most effective, particularly in acute wry neck, because no active pull is required (it can also be applied with the patient seated).

Respiratory synkinesis applies in particular to respiratory muscles (the scaleni, the sternocleidomastoids, the pectorales, and quadratus lumborum), which contract during inhalation and decontract during exhalation. The reverse holds for the abdominal and in particular for the masticatory muscles, which are activated during exhalation and inhibited during inhalation. In contrast, the digastricus and mylohyoideus are facilitated during inhalation and relax during exhalation. This action is best monitored with the thumb in contact with the lateral process of the hyoid, where it is possible to sense resistance at inhalation and relaxation at exhalation—when the thumb sinks toward the midline—without exerting pressure(!) (Figs. 11.20 to 11.22).

Respiratory synkinesis is also noted in regard to eye movement: looking up is coupled with breathing in and looking down with breathing out. This correlation is easily explained, because under natural conditions, looking up is followed by straightening up (the body follows the eyes), and looking down by stooping. In fact, it is difficult to exhale while looking up and to inhale while gazing downward. Therefore, combining looking up with inhalation (double facilitation) would be effective for treatment, whereas combining looking down with inhalation would be counterproductive.

Whenever possible, the force of *gravity* is used for both isometric resistance and relaxation. Gravity is used for resistance when the patient isometrically contracts the muscle harboring a TrP, and again for assistance as the patient relaxes the tense muscle. According to Zbojan, when gravity-induced relaxation is used alone, the contraction and relaxation phases should each last for at least 20 seconds.[37] If this technique is combined with respiration, however, the timing of contraction and relaxation should coincide with that of the respiratory phase. Therefore, respiration must be *slow.* The patient is told to hold his or her breath after inhalation and, if necessary,

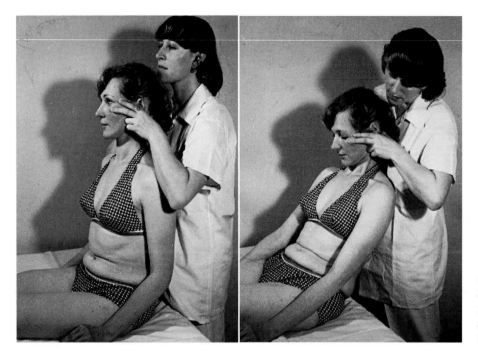

Fig. 11.16. PIR of the short cervical extensors using facilitative eye movements during resistance phase (left) and inhibitory eye movements during relaxation phase (right).

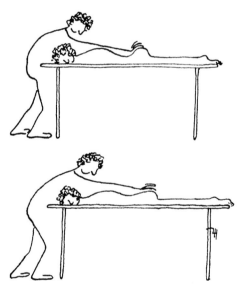

Fig. 11.18. Isometric manual traction of the pelvis.

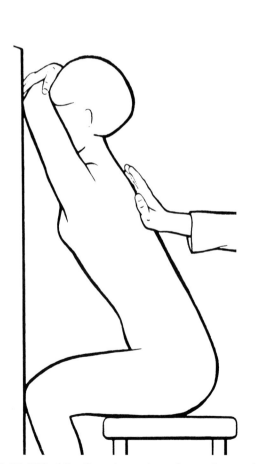

Fig. 11.17. PIR of the thoracic erector spinae using respiratory synkinesis.

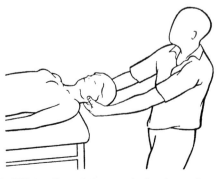

Fig. 11.19. PIR traction of the cervical spine using respiration only.

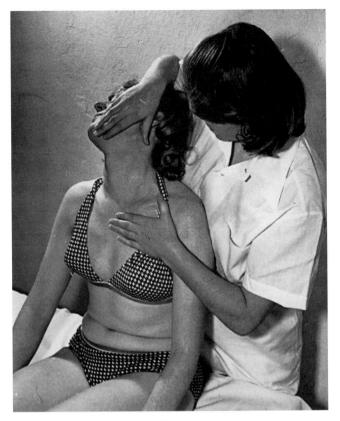

Fig. 11.20. PIR of the scalenes.

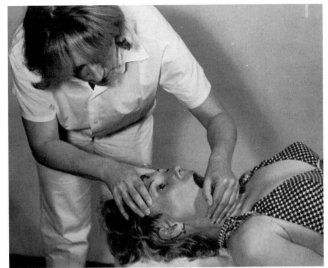

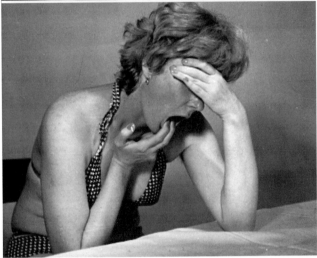

Fig. 11.21. PIR of the masticatory muscles; self-PIR of the masticatory muscles.

even after exhalation. Gravity-induced PIR lends itself naturally to self-treatment (Fig. 11.23 to 11.28).[37]

All of the neuromuscular methods described to this point can be combined to obtain the best possible effect. This combination is accomplished by a summation of physiologic stimuli, making the entire procedure automatic, so the patient can apply treatment even more than once a day.

However advantageous and effective the combination of methods may be, it requires careful thinking to identify the most effective method and to avoid incompatible or useless combinations. An ideal combination to obtain relaxation of the sternocleidomastoid (also self-mobilization of occiput/atlas) follows. The patient is supine, with the head rotated over the end of the table acting as a fulcrum. The patient is instructed to look toward the forehead and to breathe in; at a certain stage of inhalation, the sternocleidomastoid contracts, slightly lifting the head. When the patient looks down (toward the chin) and breathes out, the muscle relaxes and the head is lowered (see Fig. 11.27). Another example is gravity-induced PIR of the m. quadratus lumborum. The patient stands with legs apart and leans to the opposite side until the slack has been taken up. The patient then looks up and breathes in slowly until the quadratus lumborum automatically contracts, slightly straightening the trunk. The patient then holds his or her breath, looks down, and slowly breathes out; during exhalation, side bending increases automatically while he or she

relaxes (see Fig. 11.28). In both cases, looking up facilitates inhalation, which in turn facilitates the muscles in question and lifts the head and straightens the trunk. The force of gravity is adequate for resistance and for obtaining release during relaxation.

Whenever the combination of eye movement and respiration is used, the eyes should be directed first. In this way, the direction of muscle pull is determined and there should be time for the isometric and the relaxation phases. Holding the breath is helpful for the same reason.

An illustration of how to avoid mistakes in combination involves the upper trapezius muscle. The head is first side-bent away from the involved muscle to take up the slack. The patient is then instructed to look toward the affected side and to breathe in (see Fig. 11.29) while the operator resists his or her automatic attempt to exert pressure toward the affected side. During the relaxation phase, however, the therapist must not tell the patient to look to the other side, because the response would be to *rotate* the head and no relaxation of the

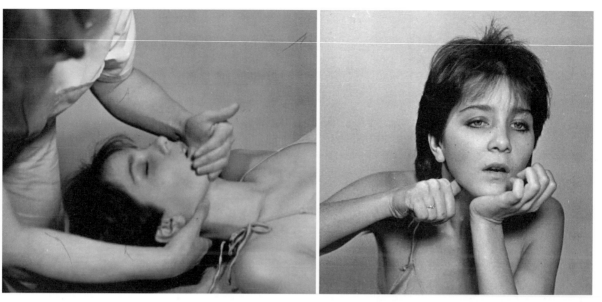

Fig. 11.22. PIR of the digastricus and mylohyoideus; self-PIR of the digastricus and mylohyoideus.

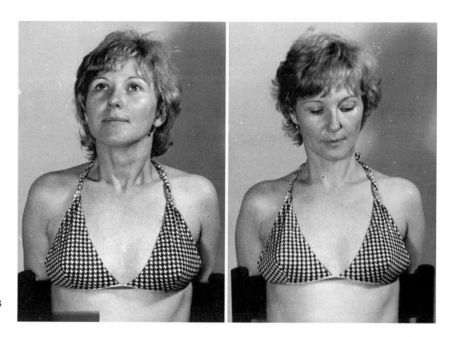

Fig. 11.23. Self-PIR of the upper trapezius using gravity.

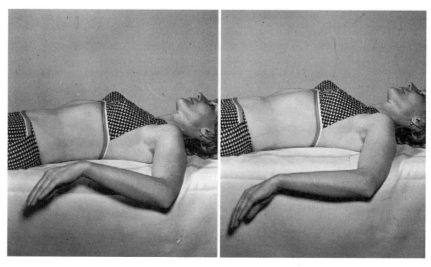

Fig. 11.24. Self-PIR of the infraspinatus using gravity.

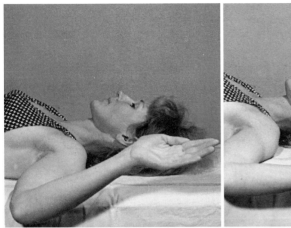

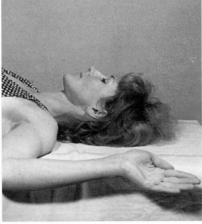

Fig. 11.25. Self-PIR of the subscapularis using gravity.

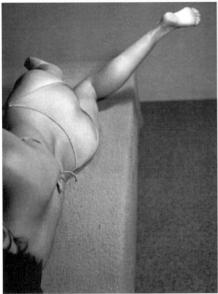

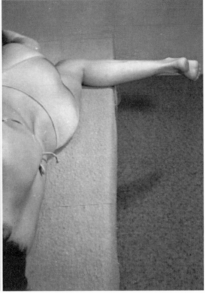

Fig. 11.26. Self-PIR of the piriformis using gravity.

trapezius would occur. Therefore, the correct command for the relaxation phase is: "let go and breathe out."

For mobilization in the cervicothoracic or thoracic region into side bending, the operator instructs the patient to look up and to breathe in (after taking up the slack into side bending), followed by "hold your breath" and then "relax and breathe out." The order to look down would make the patient bend forward, which would be incompatible with effective mobilization in the cervicothoracic and thoracic regions.

For gravity-induced PIR in trunk muscles, we make use of the facilitative effect of inhalation during the isometric phase and of the inhibitory effect of exhalation during the relaxation phase, beginning by telling the patient to look up, to facilitate inhalation, and then (with a few exceptions) to look down before breathing out and relaxation. To make the rhythm as slow as possible, the patient holds his or her breath after inhalation and possibly after exhalation. In muscles in the extremities, however, the effect of breathing in or out is doubtful, and so we rely on the patient to hold the extremity (or part of it) slightly raised for about 20 seconds (or more) followed

by relaxation for at least an additional 20 seconds (see Figs. 11.23 to 11.26).

JOINT MOBILIZATION (MANIPULATION WITHOUT THRUSTING)

Joint mobilization without thrusting makes use of the same principles that apply to all the manipulative techniques so far described, namely, engaging the barrier (taking up the slack) and obtaining release. This goal can be achieved by simply waiting and applying slight pressure or by repetitive springing of the barrier. Many practitioners find these techniques time consuming and in the end less effective than thrusting (from the barrier!); it has been the merit of osteopaths to continue with their use. This situation has changed greatly since the introduction of neuromuscular techniques into manipulation, making mobilization more effective and working within the barrier gentler, safer, and less time consuming. The reason for this result is that in a restricted joint, it is muscle spasm that is first met at the barrier, making slow

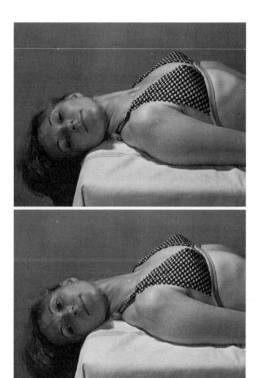

Fig. 11.27. Self-PIR of the sternocleidomastoid or self-mobilization of C0-C1 using a combination of methods.

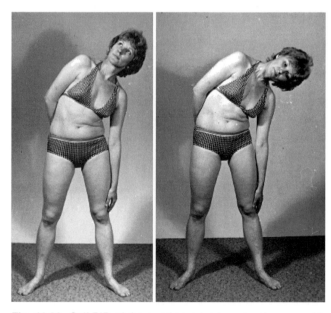

Fig. 11.28. Self-PIR of the quadratus lumborum using a combination of methods.

mobilization less successful. With the aid of neuromuscular techniques, this muscle spasm is overcome and, in some cases, the patient's muscles may even help in mobilization, i.e., we make use of the most physiologic means—the inherent forces of the patient's organism. Exceptions have

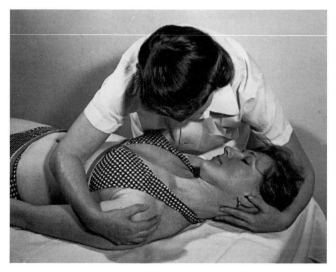

Fig. 11.29. PIR of the upper trapezius using a combination of methods.

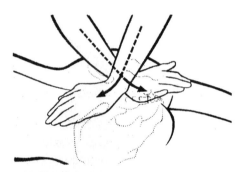

Fig. 11.30. Mobilization of the sacroiliac joint.

been noted, however. For joints that are not moved by muscles and therefore cannot be restricted by muscle spasm, such as the sacroiliac, acromioclavicular, and tibiofibular joints, simple passive mobilization is still most effective (Figs. 11.30 to 11.33 and 11.43 to 11.45).

Most of what has been said about neuromuscular techniques in the treatment of muscle spasm (TrP) is equally true for joint mobilization; indeed, wherever muscles are relaxed, the range of movement also increases in joints.[7] Some authors maintain that movement restriction is mostly attributable to muscle spasm; in my view, this conclusion cannot be drawn in every case, as explained in the previous discussion of the sacroiliac and other joints.[38,39]

A particularly effective neuromuscular technique for mobilization was described by Gaymans for side bending of the cervical and thoracic spine.[40] During inhalation, there is alternating increased resistance against side bending in the *even segments,* such as C1 (movement between occiput and atlas), C2 (movement between C2 and C3), C4, etc., which *relax with exhalation.* Resistance increases, on the other hand, against side bending at exhalation in the *odd segments* (C1,

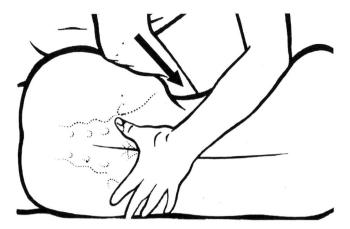

Fig. 11.31. Mobilization of the upper part of the sacroiliac joint.

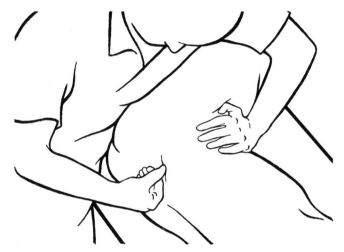

Fig. 11.32. Mobilization of the upper part of the sacroiliac joint.

C3, C5), which *relax during inhalation,* making mobilization easy. Resistance in all segments of the cervicothoracic junction (from C6 to T2) increases during inhalation, and relaxation occurs during exhalation. From T2 onward, increased resistance during inhalation is again noted in the even segments (T2, T4, T6, T8, and T10) followed by relaxation during exhalation; conversely, during exhalation, resistance increases against side-bending in the odd segments and relaxation (i.e., mobilization) takes place during inhalation (T3, T5, T7, T9).[40]

The most effective command for mobilization into side bending in the even segments is: "look up and breathe in," followed in the cervical region by "look down and breathe out." In the cervicothoracic and thoracic regions, the command again is: "look up and breathe in," followed by "relax and breathe out," to avoid increased flexion of the cervicothoracic junction and the thoracic spine, which is most unfavorable for mobilization. In the odd segments, however, combination with eye movements is unsuitable, because looking down would not increase resistance against side bending and looking up would not help mobilization into side bending

(Fig. 11.34). This effect is strongest in the upper cervical region and decreases in the lower thoracic region, in particular in the odd segments.

The strongest effect of inhalation and exhalation is in the segment C0/1; it is felt in all directions. The first order is "look up (toward your forehead) and breathe in," followed by "look down (toward your chin) and breathe out," except into retroflexion, in which eye movements would be at variance with the direction of mobilization (Figs. 11.35 to 11.37). In C2/3, postisometric traction seems as specific as side bending. So strong is the release effect of exhalation in these segments that usually no or only one repetition is required.

In rotary mobilization, we combine inhalation with the isometric phase and exhalation with the relaxation phase. In the cervical region, however, it is usually more appropriate to give the order "look up" during the isometric phase and "look

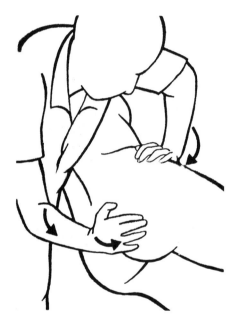

Fig. 11.33. Mobilization of the lower part of the sacroiliac joint.

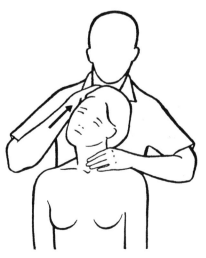

Fig. 11.34. Side-bending mobilization of the cervical spine.

down" during the relaxation phase instead of "look to the right" if movement restriction is to the left, followed by "look to the left," as is required in the cervicothoracic or thoracic region (Figs. 11.38 to 11.40).

Just as in PIR for muscle spasm, it is essential in the mobilization of joints to *wait* for the release effect. Release usually occurs late during exhalation (or inhalation), and it is best to avoid useless attempts to force it—it must be sensed and be free of interference, even by the order to breathe out, as long as relaxation continues. Once release has set in, it goes on, even if the patient continues to breathe normally.

Postisometric relaxation is not the only neuromuscular technique. We may inhibit antagonists by active motion, e.g., into rotation (Fig. 11.41). In some cases, we may use rhythmic contraction of a muscle for mobilization, e.g., of the scaleni for mobilization of the first two ribs (Fig. 11.42).

The original Muscle Energy Technique (MET) as described by Mitchell, Greenman, and others is similar to PIR, but more complicated in that it tries to reach the barrier in three planes at the same time and to apply resistance accord-

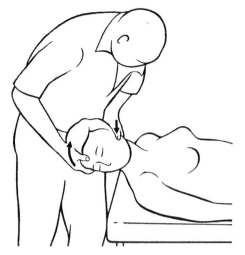

Fig. 11.37. Mobilization of C0-C1 lateral flexion.

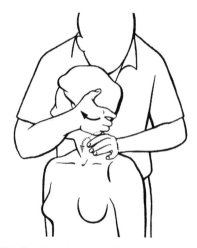

Fig. 11.38. Mobilization of restricted rotation in the cervical spine. Arrow, fixation by the thumb from behind.

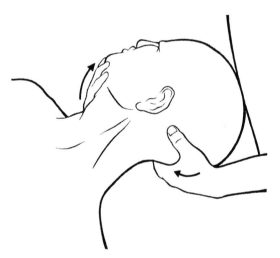

Fig. 11.35. Mobilization of C0-C1 retroflexion.

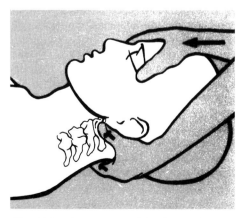

Fig. 11.36. Mobilization of C0-C1 anteflexion.

ingly. "Functional" and "counterstrain" techniques achieve release by moving the patient to a relief position in which spasm subsides, and then carefully bringing the patient back into neutral position, finally making sure that the full range of motion is well tolerated without recurrence of spasm. Such techniques can be useful in the acute stage, being gentle and well tolerated by the patient.[41,42]

As described in this chapter, PIR has the advantages of simplicity and the possibility of combination with eye movement, gravity, and respiration—making many of these techniques automatic and therefore well suited for self-treatment, one of the requirements of the rehabilitation process.

In joints that cannot be moved by their own muscles, it is important to remember the absence of spasm that could interfere with passive mobilization when the barrier is engaged. Simple passive mobilization can be obtained by a minimum of force just by springing those joints. The importance of minimum force lies in that the joint has to spring back into neutral after applying a springing force, and the intrinsic forces of

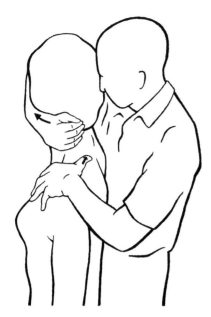

Fig. 11.39. Mobilization of rotation at the cervicothoracic junction.

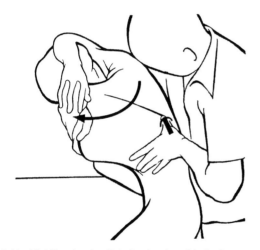

Fig. 11.40. Mobilization in slight kyphosis, with the lower vertebra fixed by the therapist's hand and thumb.

such joints are small. Examples include the sacroiliac joints (see Fig. 11.30 to 11.33) as well as the acromioclavicular, sternoclavicular, and tibiofibular joints (Figs. 11.43 to 11.45).

In all techniques producing release, the operator is constantly in a diagnostic situation, making correction possible and knowing when and where release has been achieved.

THRUST MANIPULATION

For many if not the majority of practitioners, the term manipulation is synonymous with thrust techniques. To this point, our main criterion has been the barrier and release phenomenon dealing not only with joints but also with most structures of the motor system. In this respect, thrust manipulation of

joints has an exceptional position. Here, the barrier is engaged in a similar way, but then a fast impulse of (relatively) little force and small amplitude is applied, separating the joint facets when a click is usually heard. At this moment, the resistance of the barrier suddenly breaks down (Figs. 11.46 to 11.48) as it is "taken by surprise." In other words, whereas all methods described so far only normalize the barrier, the thrust suspends it, and with it, its protective effect. As a result, *hypermobility* is produced, which is assumed to be only temporary.[43,44]

It is easily understood that most complications ascribed to manipulation and related to thrust techniques and that repeated thrusts at short intervals produce permanent hypermobility, a condition every experienced clinician views with apprehension. Complications are, in fact, most frequently the result of repeated (unsuccessful) thrust manipulation at short intervals. It is clear that the question of contraindication for manipulation mainly concerns thrusting. Proper technique is of vital importance when using a thrust. We should never thrust until the slack has been properly taken out and the patient has relaxed; therefore, we should never thrust in a painful direction. Nor should thrusts be applied where movement restriction is pronounced; in fact, if there is severe restriction in all directions, this is in itself a contraindication for a thrust manipulation. Because most serious complications after manipulation are caused by vertebral artery injury, the combina-

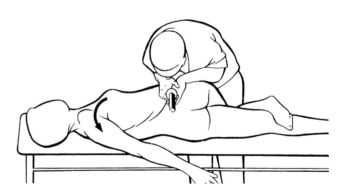

Fig. 11.41. Active repetitive mobilization of the lumbar spine with the patient lying on a side.

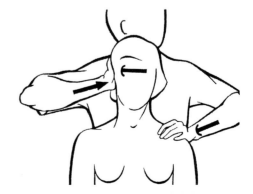

Fig. 11.42. Repetitive mobilization of the first and second ribs by isometric rhythmic contraction of the scalenus.

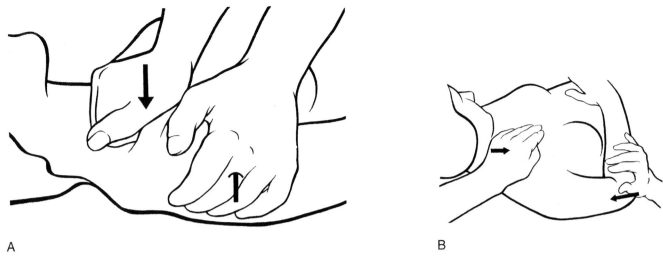

A   B

Fig. 11.43. Mobilization of the acromioclavicular joint by shifting the clavicle against the acromion ventrodorsally **(a)** and craniocaudally **(b).**

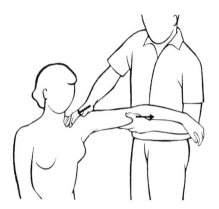

Fig. 11.44. Traction-mobilization of the acromioclavicular joint.

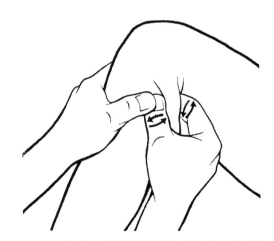

Fig. 11.45. Mobilization of the fibular head against the tibia.

tion of rotation, retroflexion, and traction should be excluded from our techniques on principle, because for the most part such complications do not arise with signs of clinical involvement of the vertebral arteries.

Thrust manipulation should be carried out with little force; if a "little tug" is not effective, we should change to neuromuscular techniques, the thrust (tug) serving as a test to see whether the joint or mobile segment is prepared to accept it, but never as a forced procedure to achieve the click. Our aim is not a click, but rather release and normal function, obtained by the most appropriate means.[45–52]

The usual list of "contraindications" involving tumor, acute inflammation, fracture, etc. is out of place because no competent practitioner would knowingly use manipulation in such cases as those. No one is infallible, however, and diagnostic errors are a possibility, particularly in the early stages of disease. Even in such cases, however, neuromuscular techniques are usually harmless and may even give temporary relief.

Clearly, to rely mainly or exclusively on thrust techniques is bad practice, the more so as it deprives the practitioner of such effective manipulative methods as soft tissue treatment and PIR. Nonetheless, a successful thrust gives intense, immediate relief and therefore remains a popular and useful procedure. When thrusting is properly administered and judiciously used, the rate of complications remains small, and therefore it is important to know when thrust manipulation is particularly useful. The most frequent situation is when symptoms persist and release and relief is not fully achieved after application of neuromuscular techniques. In this situation, the patient has also been well prepared (by these other methods) to receive a thrust.

The utility of thrusts if joint restriction is the cause of nerve entrapment is understandable, as the irritated nerve may

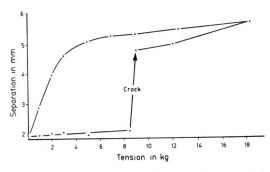

Fig. 11.46. Relationship between distraction force and joint surface separation for a joint that cracked when a distraction force was applied. (From Roston JB, Haines RW: Cracking in the metacarpo-phalangeal joints. J Anat 81:165, 1947.)

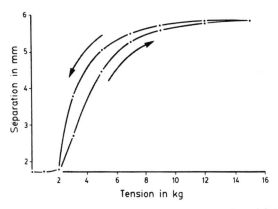

Fig. 11.47. Comparison graph to that in Fig. 11.46 for a joint that did not crack when distraction force was applied. (From Roston JB, Haines RW: Cracking in the metacarpo-phalangeal joints. J Anat 81:165, 1947.)

be edematous and therefore profit from the extra freedom given by temporary hypermobility. Its value is evident when the carpal bones are thrust into traction (Fig. 11.49) in a carpal tunnel syndrome, and in the cervicothoracic outlet syndrome (Fig. 11.50). It can be equally successful in root syndromes, by judicious use of a technique by which the intervertebral foramina are widened and little or no rotation takes place, and in simple traction techniques in the cervical and cervicothoracic area and in flexion techniques in the lumbar region (Fig. 11.51). Again, however, even if successful, a thrust should not be repeated at short intervals; likewise, it should never be repeated if the first thrust did not succeed with little force. Thrusts are useful for areas with minimal pain and spasm, so that only minimal resistance is met. Sometimes thrusting is the only possible technique to use in small children who do not cooperate and where fast action is required, but only experienced practitioners with faultless technique should venture into this arena. This caution applies particularly to the use of traction manipulation in the upper cervical spine.

TRACTION THERAPY

The object of manipulation is to rectify mechanical problems. The same is true of traction; in our opinion, the best form of traction is *manual traction.* Curiously, manipulators show remarkably little interest in traction and, more frequently than not, are not well acquainted with the technique of manual traction.

The most effective technique for therapy in the cervical area is postisometric traction, which has already been described. It is indicated for individuals with acute wry neck and root syndromes, and is specific in the treatment of C2/3 restriction (see Fig. 11.19).

For anatomic reasons, traction in the lumbar spine affect joints only minimally, but it is specific in the treatment of disk lesions. In fact, clinical improvement after traction is potentially diagnostic of a disk lesion.

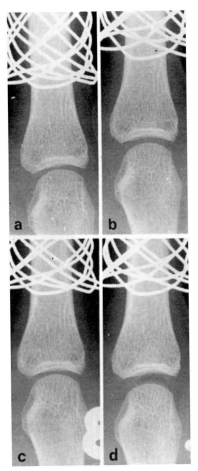

Fig. 11.48. Radiographs of the third metacarpophalangeal joint during the resting phase and distraction phase, before and after manipulation. **a,** Pretreatment, nondistracted joint space; **b,** Pretreatment, distracted joint space; **c,** Post-treatment, nondistracted joint space; **d,** Post-treatment, distracted joint space and gas arthrogram.

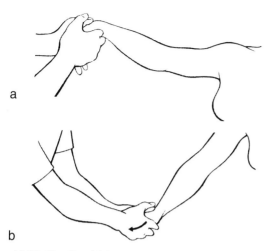

Fig. 11.49. Traction high-velocity thrust on the os capitum: **a,** Finding the os capitum and making contact; **b,** Taking up the slack and making the thrust.

The following techniques are most useful. In rhythmic traction prone (Fig. 11.52), the patient holds the end of the table while the operator pulls rhythmically with his or her hands around the patient's ankles (which should not be squeezed!), after first making sure that the patient is relaxed. The operator must then establish the correct rhythm to localize the effect in the low back. If the rhythm is too slow, the patient's whole body will move up and down on the table. By quickening the rhythm, the therapist will find out when only the leg and pelvis move while the rest of the back remains still, the low back being like a nodal point in a standing wave. Rhythmic traction prone can also be carried out by pulling only one leg, which also produces a slight side-bending effect at the same time.

If the prone position is poorly tolerated because of forced lordosis, traction is carried out in kyphosis with the patient supine. The therapist stands at the side of the table (which must be lowered) and places his or her foot on the table, the thigh and knee should be horizontal. The therapist then places the back of the patient's knee over his or her thigh and uses the patient's leg as a lever, rhythmically lifting the patient's pelvis and low back from the table and rocking it (Fig. 11.53).

As mentioned previously, postisometric traction in the lumbar region makes use of respiratory synkinesis: the therapist resists the buttocks moving upward during exhalation and makes use of relaxation during inhalation (see Fig. 11.18). While prone, with the legs hanging over the end of a high table, the patient may carry out self-treatment, lifting the buttocks on exhalation and dropping them, relaxing, during inhalation.

As with other manipulative techniques, traction must be adapted to the patient in such a way as to be painless and, if possible, to give immediate relief. If the patient experiences pain we must change the technique or desist altogether.

THEORETIC CONSIDERATIONS

All manipulative techniques deal with mechanical problems. The barrier phenomenon, with all its reflex implications, is also a mechanical problem, yet its nature is not sufficiently understood. However important muscle spasm and TrP may be, they cannot explain restriction in such joints as the sacroiliac and others, let alone barriers in connective tissue structures. One fact pertaining to joint and spinal manipulation that is well established, however, is that manipulation restores motion and that its object is reversible movement restriction. The implication of this statement is that the importance of the relative position of bones or vertebrae should not be overrated. This has practical relevance, because asymmetry, particularly in the pelvis, may appear considerable, but asymmetry without dysfunction does not require manipulation.

Recent experience and research have shed some light on this question. First, it has been shown that typical pelvic distortion with clear asymmetry of the anterior and posterior iliac spines is not regularly related to sacroiliac dysfunction and can, as a rule, be treated successfully by manipulation of structures outside the pelvis, most frequently those of the craniocervical junction. Second, findings show that the neu-

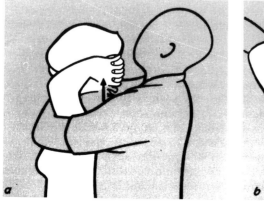
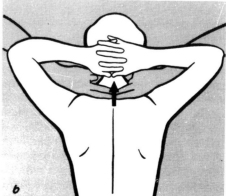

Fig. 11.50. Traction high-velocity thrust on the cervicothoracic junction.

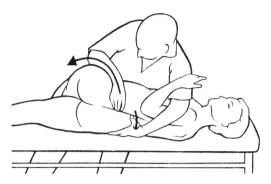

Fig. 11.51. Thrust manipulation of the lumbar spine with the patient on her side, in kyphosis, the lower leg bent and upper hanging down over the edge of the table.

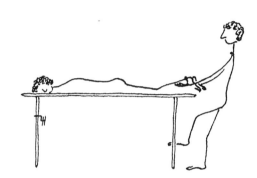

Fig. 11.52. Rhythmic traction prone of the lumbar spine.

tral position in the spinal column is not absolutely constant; after maximum side bending of the cervical spine or rotation, the vertebrae do not return to exactly the same position (Fig. 11.54).[53] Finally, we have learned that static loads can change the positon of vertebrae.

If we restore normal mobility of the spinal column and the pelvis, it will adopt the optimum individual position required for the prevailing conditions, which are by no means constant. If, for example, ventral and dorsal flexion is restricted, we are fully justified in mobilizing in both directions without regard to the position of the adjacent structures. For the sacroiliac joint, for example, it is adequate to restore springing at its upper and lower end, i.e., in what seems "opposite directions" (see Fig. 11.30 to 11.33), as long as mobility is fully restored.

DISTURBANCE OF BODY STATICS

Gutmann and Vele summed up the importance of static function: "The dominating principle of the spinal column is body statics. All other functions are subordinated to the requirements of the upright posture on two legs. Loss of mobility and painful impingement of nerve roots is preferred to sacrifice of the erect posture."[5,54,55]

Static function of the spinal column is a specific characteristic of the bipedal human race. Its importance increases in our technical civilization in which static loads are preponderant (sitting and standing). The clinical manifestation of static

dysfunction is pain with sitting or standing, especially when bending forward.

Under normal conditions, static equilibrium should be maintained without excessive muscular activity. Rash and Burke further specify that, "in stationary posture the center of gravity of each body segment should be vertically above the area of its supporting base, preferably near its center. If persistent gravitational torques are being borne by ligaments, or if excessive nuscular contraction is required to maintain balance, this principle is being violated."[56]

For the static function of the trunk and the spinal column, the position (tilt, inclination) of the base plays a decisive role, but assessment by purely clinical means is impossible. The exact position of the promontorium, of L5 and even of L4, can only be revealed radiographically under standard conditions—standing. The ideal method is radiographic examination of the entire spine. If this study is not available, a plumb line can show the position of the external occipital protuberance in the anteroposterior view and of the outer meatus acusticus in the side view. The position of the feet must be held constant; in the anteroposterior view, they should be symmetric to a line of the floor corresponding to the center of the x-ray screen. In the side view, the feet should be placed on the same line at the site of the outer ankle (Fig. 11.55).

The mechanism of balance differs in the coronal and the sagittal planes. This difference is readily understood if the effect of a heelpad is considered. An artificial difference of more than 1 cm in leg length is felt immediately (and resented) in the coronal plane, whereas raising (or lowering) of

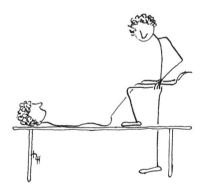

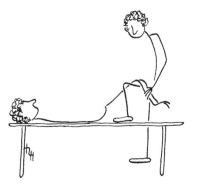

Fig. 11.53. Rhythmic traction supine of the lumbar region.

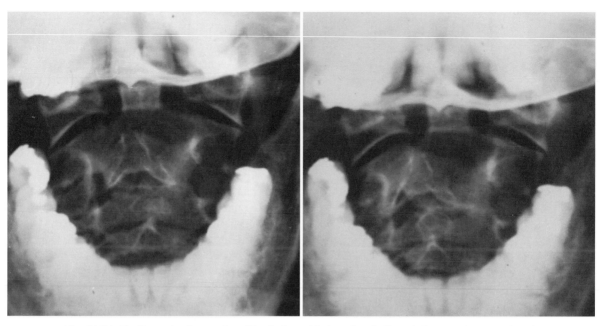

Fig. 11.54. Radiograph of neutral position before side bending (left) and after side bending (right).

both feet is hardly noticed. The responses differ because, in the coronal plane, the line of gravity passes between the two hip joints (stable equilibrium), and one can effectively correct pelvic obliquity by lifting one foot.

The physiologic reaction to pelvic obliquity—obliquity of the sacrum (!)—is scoliosis to the lower side, rotation to the side of the scoliosis, and pelvic shift to the higher side. The summit of the scoliotic curve is in the midlumbar region, and the thoracolumbar junction should be above the lumbosacral junction.[5]

With the most frequent type of abnormality, the thoracolumbar junction does not stand above the lumbosacral junction but is deviated to one side, more frequently to the side of scoliosis. Rotation depends on the degree of lordosis. If the lumbar spine shows no lordosis or even kyphosis, there may be no rotation or even rotation to the side of inclination (not scoliosis).[57]

The most important point, however, is that obliquity must concern the *base* of the spinal column, not the pelvis as such. Unfortunately, neither difference in leg length nor pelvic obliquity necessarily correlate with obliquity of the sacrum or L5 or even L4. Therefore, we may easily create an oblique base of the spinal column by correcting pelvic obliquity and/or leg length inequality. In other words, we correct the morphologic appearance of the legs and pelvis, but seriously disturb static function or balance of the spinal column (Fig. 11.56). Because this most relevant obliquity cannot be seen or palpated, radiographs are essential for correct assessment.

Radiographic evaluation is equally essential for the assessment of spinal statics at the base of the spinal column as for the assessment of correction. Unfortunately, the spinal column does not always "accept" our correction (heelpad),

in which case our intended correction may make things even worse. This circumstance, too, can only be revealed radiographically (Fig. 11.57). This failure often occurs if the pelvic obliquity is compensatory, as is the case in idiopathic scoliosis.

The criteria of improvement after static correction are as follows: the thoracolumbar junction returns to stand directly above the lumbosacral junction; scoliotic curvature decreases; and the pelvis and head (plumb line) return to midline (Fig. 11.58).

The same static disturbance can be caused by obliquity at the base of the spinal column, thus *creating* pelvic obliquity, but normalizing spinal statics (Fig. 11.59). In this case, obliquity is caused by asymmetry *inside* the pelvis. This obliquity, unlike that caused by leg length inequality, persists when the subject is seated and should be corrected by a board under the ischial tuberosity on the lower side of obliquity.

If correction is to involve a heelpad, it is essential to consider whether the spinal column can react clinically to mechanical correction. Such a response is not possible in the acute stage of lumbago or a root syndrome with obvious antalgesic posture. Unfortunately, the same is true in the event of movement restriction, especially in a key region. A good example is pelvic distortion related to a restriction (blockage) at the craniocervical junction (Fig. 11.60). It is therefore recommended to examine a patient for segmental dysfunction and to treat this problem first, before radiographic re-examination with a view to static correction.

If static correction is likely to be useful, we first test the patient's reaction to raising the foot with the aid of a board less than 1 cm high. If the patient finds it pleasant or is indifferent to it, it is probable that the measure will be well toler-

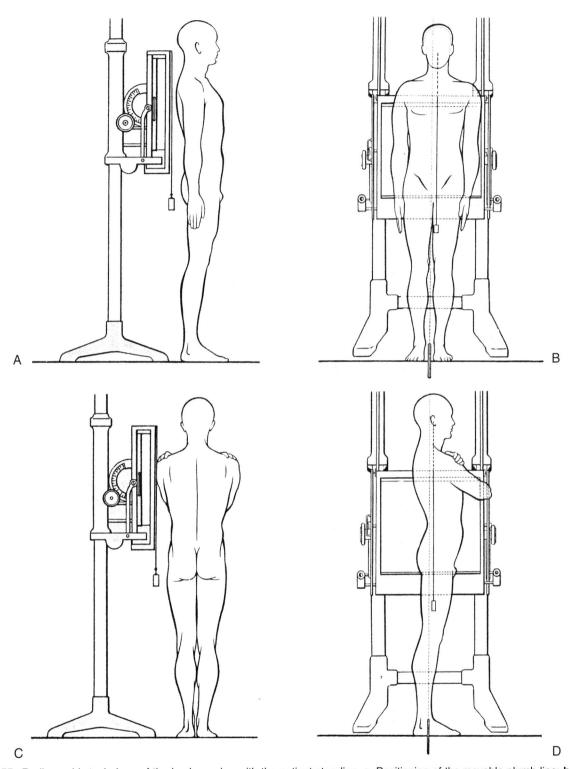

Fig. 11.55. Radiographic technique of the lumbar spine with the patient standing. **a,** Positioning of the movable plumb line; **b,** Device prepared for radiographic examination, anteroposterior view; **c,** Positioning of the plumb line; **d,** Device prepared for radiographic examination, lateral view. (After Gutmann G.: Klinisch–roentgenologishe Untersuchungen zur Statik der Wribelsule. In Wolff HD (ed): Manuelle Medizin und ihr wissenschaftlihen Grundlagen. Heidelberg, Physikalishe Medezin, 1970, pp 109–127.)

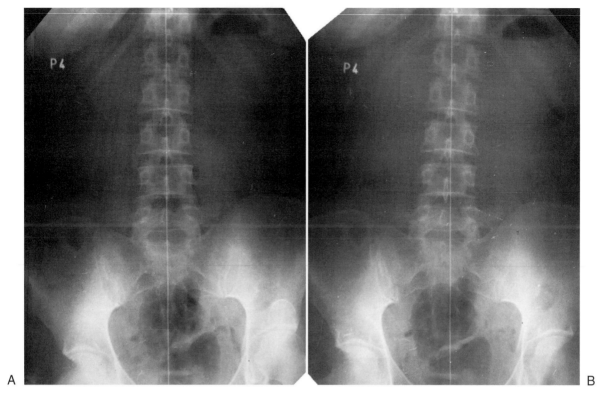

Fig. 11.56. Pelvic obliquity. **a,** Pelvis lower on the right (short right leg) with a horizontal sacrum, the lumbar spine is straight; **b,** With a right heelpad, sacral obliquity appears, with a deviation of the lumbar spine to the left and slight dextroscoliosis.

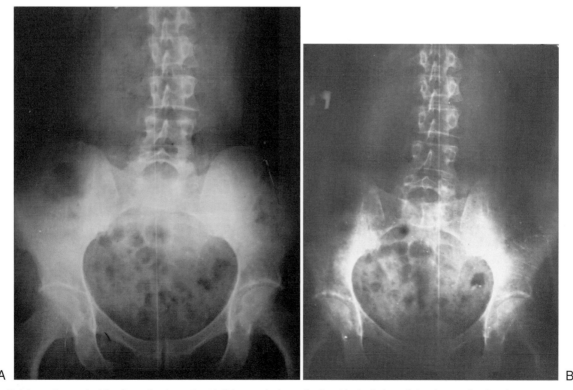

Fig. 11.57. Pelvic and sacral obliquity owing to a short left leg. **a,** Left scoliosis with deviation of the thoracolumbar junction to the left; **b,** Less pelvic obliquity after application of a left heelpad, but no improvement in lumbar statics.

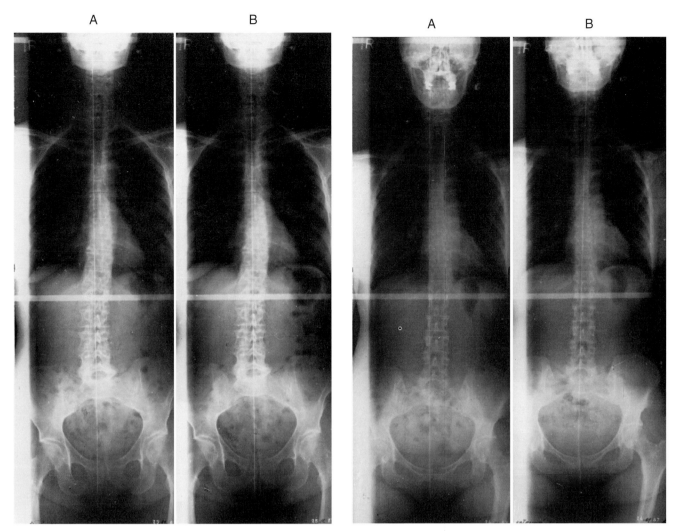

Fig. 11.58. Pelvic and sacral obliquity owing to a short leg. **a,** Before correction; **b,** After correction.

Fig. 11.59. Sacral obliquity without pelvic obliquity. **a,** Before correction; **b,** After correction.

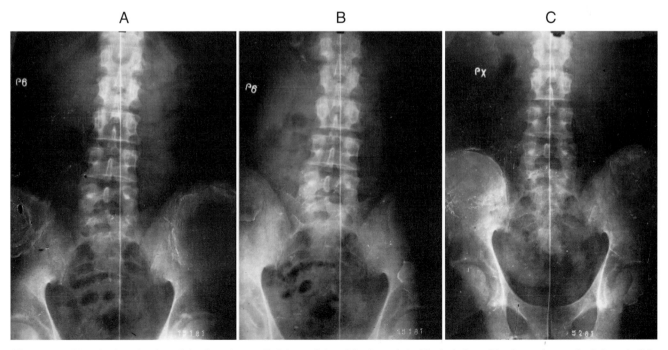

Fig. 11.60. Disturbed statics in pelvic distortion. **a,** Pelvis straight, obliquity at L4 with deviation of lumbar spine to the left and slight sinistroscoliosis. **b,** No improvement after applying a left heelpad. **c,** After treatment of a blocked atlanto-occipital joint, normal statics and no pelvic distortion.

ated and helpful. If, however, it is resented, but radiographic findings show marked improvement, then the patient is advised to try to get used to it if possible, i.e., to wear a heelpad only temporarily, so long as it does not cause discomfort or pain.

Once the patient has adapted, it is better to raise the heel of the shoe on one side or lower it on the other side; if, however, the difference is more than 1 cm, it is best to recommend a thicker sole on one side, so as not to spoil the shoe.

In the sagittal plane, the pelvis and spinal column are positioned above the perfectly circular femoral heads, and balance is maintained largely by muscular action, which should be kept at a minimum. Spinal curvature is largely a result of sacrum inclination; if this is considerable, lordosis will be considerable. Under normal conditions, the thoracolumbar junction is somewhat behind the lumbosacral junction, so that T12 lies 4 cm behind L5 on average.[58] If the thoracolumbar junction is in front of the lumbosacral junction, a forward-drawn position results, because of acute disk protrusion or muscular incoordination (see Fig. 11.13). This forward-drawn position is also important in the cervical spine and goes hand in hand with increased activity of the m. erector spinae representing an increased load for the spinal column (Fig. 11.61). Hence, static imbalance (overloading) in the sagittal plane is the result of muscular imbalance and must be treated as such, not by mechanical correction.

In both the frontal and the sagittal planes, however, spinal curvature is an expression of static function. If the spinal column is in good balance, i.e., if only a minimum force is required to assure static function, then spinal curvature fulfills its task. The same is true for scoliosis (if not excessive) as for lordosis or kyphosis. In the author's opinion, no other physiologic criterion is applicable for the assessment of spinal curvature.

One more important aspect warrants mention. The less curvature, the greater mobility, i.e., the less stability. On the other hand, the more curvature, the less mobility and greater stability.

MANIPULATIVE THERAPY AND ALTERNATIVE METHODS

From a method of treating mainly articular dysfunction, manipulative therapy has developed into a method that is used to treat dysfunction of any structure and tissue in the motor system, and it is possible that some visceral dysfunction may be influenced by manipulative techniques as well. The prerequisite for all this application, is the *art of palpation*. Palpation is however, first and foremost a diagnostic procedure, and so manual functional *diagnosis* has become the most important clinical contribution of manipulation, enabling us to make pertinent diagnosis of all tissues and structures in the motor system.

Precisely because of these diagnostic possibilities, we have learned that important tissue changes lie far from the site where the patient feels pain, and that, in fact, such changes usually are more numerous than those recognized by the patient because of pain. Not only are these changes frequently numerous, but also they form patterns or chain reactions that are the expression of dysfunction, concerning not one, but many structures, forming characteristic patterns. Only when we understand these patterns, are we able to get more than temporary results by our treatment.

Having made the diagnosis, we have many methods of treatment from which to choose. In most of the soft tissues, methods of physical medicine can be applied, from massage to the various forms of electrotherapy, to applications of heat or cold, to the magnet as well as the laser. In fact, technical progress is constantly providing us with new methods. It is, however, neither the scope nor the purpose of this publication to discuss the merits or disadvantages of these alternatives or of needle and local anesthesia.

Manipulative techniques have one great advantage over other methods: feedback resulting from palpation, which places the operator constantly in a situation of therapy and diagnosis. It is in this case that the barrier phenomenon is particularly useful, given its greater precision borne out by the close correlation of the pathologic barrier, increased tension, and pain. Similarly, relief of pain is associated with the palpable sensation of release so we *know* when a painful structure stops being painful, which is why the focus of this discussion is on those techniques based on the barrier phenomenon. In this connection, it can be said that whereas most methods of "complementary (alternative)" medicine treat mainly dysfunction, manipulative techniques provide the rational clinical diagnosis.

CLINICAL IMPLICATIONS

The importance of the diagnostic side of manipulative techniques has been stressed. It is the clinical implications that illustrate this point. The most frequent symptom of our patients is *pain*, which is, in itself, a diagnostic problem for most practitioners. We have consistently shown that with our methods, we are able to detect well-defined changes in almost all structures of the motor system and beyond: in skin, the connective tissues, muscles, fasciae, and joints in both the extremities and the spinal column.

Consider headache in a patient with "negative" neurologic, orthopedic, otorhinolaryngologic, stomatologic, or rheumatologic findings. We may find tension in the masticatory and submandibular muscles, with deviation of the hyoid; a scalp that does not freely move on the skull in some places (and in some direction); hyperalgesic skin zones in the cervical region; TrP in most of the neck muscles and in the cervicothoracic area; movement restriction in the temporomandibular joint; dysfunction of joints in the cervical spine and the cervicothoracic region, including the acromioclavicular and the sternoclavicular joints; and painful periosteal points with restricted mobility of subperiosteal tissue in some direction. We may observe a forward-drawn position of the head owing to increased tension in the abdominal muscles

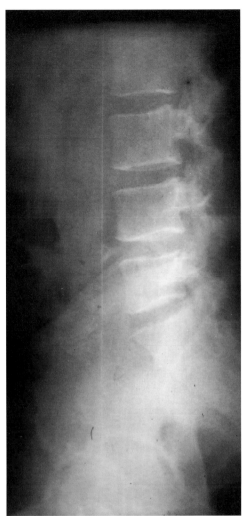

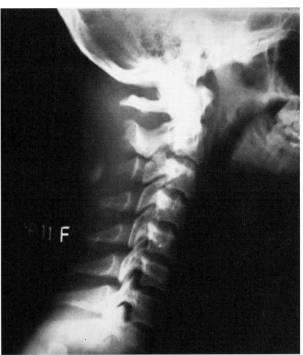

Fig. 11.61. Forward-drawn posture with thoracolumbar junction in front of the lumbosacral **(a)** and with straightening of a cervical curve **(b).**

with hypertonus of the glutei, and faulty motor patterns owing to muscular imbalance, faulty respiration, and/or exogenic reasons, e.g., at the workplace. This account of the possible findings is certainly not complete, but what is true for headache is as true for shoulder pain, low back pain, etc. in regard to "negative findings." The clinical implication of functional pathology—not a question of a single method but of a different clinical approach in which dysfunction is as real as structural pathologic change and therefore must be adequately diagnosed. Manipulative techniques have thus opened the way to what is now widely called "myoskeletal" or "musculoskeletal" medicine, dealing with the most frequent affections of the motor system and everyday ailments.

REFERENCES

1. Greenman PE: Principles of Manual Medicine. Baltimore, Williams & Wilkins, 1989, pp 88–93.
2. Lewit K: Manipulative Therapy in Rehabilitation of the Locomotor System. 2nd Ed. Oxford, Butterworth-Heinemann, 1991, pp 1–4, 79–82.
3. Mitchell PL, Moran PS, Pruzzo NA: An Evaluation and Treatment Manual of Osteopathic Muscle Energy Procedures. Valley Park, Mitchell, Moran, and Pruzzo Ass., 1979, pp 343–344.
4. Greenman PE: Verkrzungsausgleich, Nutz and Unnutz. In: Neumann HD and Wolff HD (eds): Theoretische Fortschritte und praktische Erfahrungen der manuellen Medizin. Bhl, Konkordia GmbH Druck und Verlage, 1979, pp 333–341.
5. Lewit K: Rntgenologische Kriterien statischer Strungen der Wirbelsule. Manuelle Med, 1982, pp 20–35.
6. Logan, HB: Textbook of Logan Basic Methods. St. Louis, Logan FM, 1950.
7. Schneider W, Dvorak J, Dvorak V, et al: Manuelle Medizin, Therapie. Stuttgart, Thieme, 1986, pp 8–13.
8. Burgger, A: Die Funktionskrankheiten des Bewegungsapparates. Funktionskrnakheiten des Bewegungsapparates 1:7, 1986.
9. Travell JG, Simons DG: Myofascial Pain and Dysfunction: The Trigger Point Manual. Vol 2. Baltimore, Williams & Wilkins, 1992.
10. Haldemann, S: Presidential address, North American Spine Society: Failure of the pathological model to predict back pain. Spine 15:718, 1990.
11. Malinsky J: The ontogenetic development of nerve terminations in the intervertebral disc of man. Acta Anat (Basel) 38:96, 1959.
12. Bogduk N, Tynan W, Wilson AS: The nerve supply of the human lumbar intervertebral disks. J Anat 132:39, 1981.
13. Lewit K: Chain reactions in disturbed function of the motor system. J Manual Med 3:27, 1987.
14. Beal MC: Louise Burns memorial lecture: Perception through palpation. J Am Osteopath Assoc 89:1334.

15. Chaitow L: Palpatory Literacy. London, Thorsons, 1991.

16. Greenman PE: Shichtweise Palpation. Manuelle Med 22:46, 1984.

17. Travell JG, Simons DG: Myofascial Pain and Dysfunction: The Trigger Point Manual. Vol 1. Baltimore, Williams & Wilkins, 1983.

18. Bourdillon JF, Day EA: Spinal Manipulation. 4th Ed. London, Heinemann, 1987, pp 38–40.

19. Lewit K: Pelvic dysfunction. In Paterson JK, Burn L: Back Pain, An International Review. Dordrecht, Kluwer, 1990, pp 271–284.

20. Keating JC, Bergmann TF, Jacobs GE, et al: Interexaminer reliability of eight evaluative dimensions of lumbar segmental abnormality. J Manipulative Physiol Ther 13:463, 1990.

21. Boline PD, Keating JC, Brist J: Interexaminer reliability of palpatory evaluation of the lumbar spine. Am J Chiroprac Med 1:5, 1988.

22. DeBoer KF, Harmon R, Tuttle CD, et al: Reliability study of detection of somatic dysfunction in the cervical spine. J Manipulative Physiol Ther 8:9, 1985.

23. Carmichael JP: Inter- and intraexaminer reliability of palpation for sacroiliac joint dysfunction. J Manipulative Physiol Ther 10:154, 1987.

24. Herzog W, Read LJ, Comway PJW: Reliability of motion palpation procedures to detect sacoiliac joint fixations. J Manipulative Physiol Ther 12:86, 1989.

25. Zachman Z, Traina AD, Keating JC: Interexaminer reliability and concurrent validity of the instruments for the measurement of cervical ranges of motion. J Manipulative Physiol Ther 12:205, 1989.

26. Huneke F: Herdgeschehen im Lichte der Heilansthesie. Schriftenreihe fr Ganzheitsmedizin. Stuttgart, Hippokrates, 1950.

27. Dosch P: Lehrbuch der Neuraltherapie nach Huneke. Ulm, Haug, 1964.

28. Ward R: Personal communication, 1990.

29. Greenman PE: Principles of Manual Medicine. Baltimore, Williams & Wilkins, 1990, pp 106–112.

30. Lewit K: Verspannungen der Bauch und Gessmuskulatur mit Auswirkung auf die Krperstatik. Manuelle Med 30:75, 1992.

31. Silverstolpe L: A pathological erector spinae reflex—a new sign of mechanical pelvis dysfunction. J Manual Med 4:28, 1989.

32. Silverstolpe L, Helsing G: Cranial visceral symptoms in mechanical pelvis dysfunction In Paterson JK, Burn L (eds): Back Pain, An International Review. Dordrecht, Kluwer, 1990.

33. Goodridge JP: Muscle energy technique: Definition, explanation, methods of procedure. J Am Osteopath Assoc 81:249, 1981.

34. Stiles EG: Muskelenergietechnik (MET). Therapeutische Grundstze und praktische Anwendung. In Frisch H (ed): Manuelle Medizin Heute. Berlin, Springer, 1985, pp 150–156.

35. Travell JG, Simons DG: Myofascial Pain and Dysfunction: The Trigger Point Manual. Baltimore, Williams & Wilkins, 1983, pp 4, 5–44.

36. Lewit K: Postisometric relaxation in combination with other methods of muscular facilitation and inhibition. J Manual Med 2:101, 1986.

37. Zbojan L: Antigravit cna relax cia, jej podstata a pouaeitie (gravity induced relaxation, its principles and practice application). Practick lka 68:147, 1988.

38. Korr IM: Proprioceptors and somatic dysfunction. J Am Osteopath Assoc 74:638, 1975.

39. The muscular and articular factor in movement restriction. J Manual Med 1:83, 1985.

40. Gaymans, F: Die Bedeutung der Atemtypen fr die Mobilisation der Wirbelsule. Manuelle Med 18:96, 1980.

41. Jones LH: Strain and Counterstrain. Newark, OH, The Academy of Osteopathy, 1981.

42. Greenman PE: Principles of Manual Medicine. Baltimore, Williams & Wilkins, 1989, pp 101–105.

43. Roston JB, Haines RW: Cracking in the metacarpophalangeal joints. J Anat 81:165, 1947.

44. Mierau D, Cassidy JD, Wowen V: Manipulation and mobilization of the third metacarpo–phapangeal joint. A quantitative radiographic range of motion study. J Manual Med 3:135, 1988.

45. Dvorak J, Orelli F: Wie gefhrlih ist die Manipulation der Halswirbelsule. Manuelle Med 20:44, 1982.

46. Grossiord A: Les accidents neurologiques des manipulations cervicales. Ann Med Phys 9:283, 1966.

47. Gutmann G: Verletzungen der Arteria vertebralis durch manuelle Therapie. Manuelle Med 21:2, 1983.

48. Memorandum of the German Association of Manual Medicine. Zur Verhtung von Zwischenfllen bei gezielter Handgriff-Therapie an der Halswirbelsule. Manuelle Med 17:53, 1979.

49. Smith RA, Estridge MV: Neurologic complications of head and neck manipulation. JAMA 182:5, 1962.

50. Fossgreen J: Editorial: Complications in manual medicine. J Manual Med 6:83, 1991.

51. Dvorak J: Inappropriate indications and contraindications of manual therapy. J Manual Med 6:85, 1991.

52. Patijn J: Complications in manual medicine: A review of the literature. J Manual Med 6:89, 1991.

53. Kirout J: Persistence orynkinetic patterns of the cervical spine. Neuroradiology 18:167, 1979.

54. Gutmann G: Klinisch-roentgenologishe Untersuchungen zur Statik der Wribelsule. In Wolff HD (ed): Manuelle Medizin und ihre wissenschaftlihen Grundlagen. Heidelberg, Physikalishe Medizin, 1970, pp 109–127.

55. Gutmann G, Vele F: Das aufrechte Stehn. Westdeutscher Verlage, Forschungsberichte des Landes Nordrhein-Westfahlan No 2796, Fachgruppe Medizin, 1978.

56. Rash PJ, Burke RK: Kinesiology and Applied Anatomy. Philadelphia, Lea & Febiger, 1971.

57. Lovett R: Lateral curvature of the spine and shoulders. Philadelphia, Blakiston, 1907.

58. Cramer A: Funktionelle Merkmale der Wirbelsulenstatik. In Wirbelsule in Forschung und Praxis,. Stuttgart, Hippokrates, 1958, pp 84–93.

12 Spinal Therapeutics Based on Responses to Loading

GARY JACOB and ROBIN McKENZIE

In this chapter, we explore the clinical reasoning for spinal assessment and therapy, variously referred to as the McKenzie approach, protocols, or system. Our purpose is to explicate the underlying philosophic and practical perspectives of the McKenzie approach, as it accounts for phenomena related to spinal loading and its unique manner of satisfying the "demands" of rehabilitation. This chapter is not intended to impart clinical competency regarding the skills necessary to use the McKenzie protocols in practice. Such competency requires study of "The Lumbar Spine"[1] and "The Cervical and Thoracic Spine"[2] by McKenzie, as well as the formal instruction that applies the clinical reasoning found within these texts to assessment and therapy of patients on a day-to-day basis. The material presented here can only hope to supplement such study and instruction.

APPROACH TO CLINICAL REASONING

In the following attempt to expand an understanding of the McKenzie system, new terminology is introduced. Hopefully what such terminology distinguishes will stimulate established and future students of the McKenzie approach to further appreciate its intrinsic principles.

Relation of the McKenzie Approach to Manipulation and Rehabilitation

Both manipulation and rehabilitation use movement as therapy. In manipulation, movement is used as therapy when the clinician moves the patient's spinal joint structures to end range. The rehabilitation tradition also uses movement as therapy, but with a preference for "activity as therapy," i.e., patients performing the movements themselves.

As with manipulation, the McKenzie approach uses spinal movements to end range. As with the rehabilitation tradition, the preference is for patient self-generated movements. The significant difference between the McKenzie approach and that of traditional manipulative therapy, however, is *not* that of rejecting manipulation in favor of patient-generated movements, although the latter is always preferred. Manipulation is actually an option according to McKenzie protocols, when patient-generated movements prove only partially successful.

The most significant difference between the McKenzie approach and other methods of treating the spine is the *crite-*

ria on which assessments and therapeutics of the spine are predicated. The issue of when and how criteria dictate the direction and type of force applied to the spine is critical to the understanding of the McKenzie approach.

QUESTION OF CRITERIA

The criteria according to which any inquiry is conducted for the purpose of resolving a problem profoundly affect how the solution is conceived. In other words, the answers you get depend on the questions you ask. The McKenzie approach predicates spinal assessment and therapeutics on asking questions about the mechanical and symptomatic responses to loading the spine.

Patients present with a variety of mechanical and/or symptomatic spinal complaints, and their responses to movements and positionings of the spine are variable. Sitting may exacerbate spine-related complaints in some individuals, whereas others find relief while seated. Standing, walking, or reclining may similarly evoke disparate responses in the same or different individual. It is noted, therefore, that patients have different stories to tell about how movement and positioning affect their spine-related complaints.

Concerns regarding specific spine-related complaints, which are essentially mechanical and symptomatic responses to movement and positioning, motivate patients to seek professional care. The details of how spine-related mechanics and symptoms are affected by movement and positioning, however, are seldom of specific concern to the clinician for purposes of assessment or therapeutics.

Standard range of motion examinations and orthopedic tests do not adequately explore how the particular patient's spinal mechanics and symptoms are affected by specific movements and/or positionings. Perhaps the greatest limitation of these examinations and tests is the supposition that each test movement need be performed only once to fathom how the patient's complaints respond. The effects of repetitive movements, or positions maintained for prolonged periods of time, are not explored, even though such loading strategies might better approximate what occurs in the "real world."

The mechanical or symptomatic response to a movement performed once might be radically different from what would occur if that movement were performed five or ten times,

225

thereby revealing an entirely different clinical picture. Similarly, the mechanical or symptomatic response to assuming a particular position for a few moments might be radically different from what would occur after assuming that identical position for a few minutes.

Just as mechanical and symptomatic responses are rarely considered regarding their relationship to repetitive movements and/or sustained positioning, little inquiry is directed to how mechanical and symptomatic responses relate *to each other;* i.e., how they respond in tandem to movement and positioning.

The possibility of mechanical and symptomatic responses serving as meaningful criteria on which to predicate treatment is precluded if cognition of such is wanting. Unfortunately, many spinal examinations are all too often only cursory formalities, serving as preludes to predetermined treatment plans, independent of specific assessment findings.

Treatment Without Specific Criteria

Treatment for spine-related complaints is often routinely and ceremoniously applied in the exact same manner for each patient, even though distinguishing mechanical and symptomatic presentations are potentially discernible between individuals. More often than not, the criteria that motivate the patient to seek care are *not* intimately connected with the criteria used by the clinician to assess the patient, to determine appropriate case management, or to monitor the effectiveness of care. Identical care applied to all patients with common spinal complaints is often the result of criteria that routinely conceive of a universal problem underlying all particular complaints.

A Priori Versus A Posteriori Approaches

Preconceived, *a priori* notions about common spinal disorders can blind clinicians to meaningful and individuating phenomena. *A priori* knowledge argues "from what is before" (i.e., from causes to effects) and attempts to be independent of particular experience. On the other hand, *a posteriori* knowledge argues "from what is after" (i.e., from effects to causes) and uses empiric knowledge derived from experience.

Implicit in the McKenzie approach is an a posteriori, empiric study of phenomena related to spinal loading, after which pathoanatomic explanations are proposed. A careful description of clinically presenting phenomena is possible independent of the pathoanatomic interpretation of the day, and this description should remain accurate if that interpretation changes tomorrow. With this approach, a priori judgments are less likely to prejudice the perception of the clinically presenting phenomena. It is acknowledged that one can only *attempt* this goal, as no one can truly be free of all pre-conceived notions.

Putting Pathoanatomic Criteria in Their Place

Predicating treatment on a priori constructs rooted in the pathology model has led to what has been called the "failure of the pathology model."[3] These a priori constructs, based on hypothesized pathoanatomy, have generated treatments that may be tangential to the patient's needs and obscure the clinical perception of phenomena specific to the individual patient's situation.

For example, if all spine-related complaints are perceived, a priori, to be the result of inflammation, this preconception limits the clinician's ability to appreciate the possibility of mechanical strategies for patient care. It conceptually promotes treatment strategies of rest and anti-inflammatory medication, which may not be efficacious if, indeed, mechanics and not chemistry is the relevant component in that patient's case.

Pathoanatomy and the McKenzie Approach

The McKenzie approach recognizes patterns of mechanical and symptomatic phenomena that are labeled "syndromes." Although the McKenzie approach names syndromes according to certain pathoanatomic suppositions, these syndromes refer primarily to phenomenologic patterns that can be discerned apart from any particular pathoanatomic interpretation. The assertion that the syndrome patterns detailed in the McKenzie approach accurately describe the phenomena related to spinal loading *independent* of the pathoanatomic interpretation of the day applies, as well, to those interpretations forwarded as part of the McKenzie approach.

By first describing presenting empiric phenomena before making pathoanatomic interpretations, we hope to afford the reader a fresh perspective without putting the "pathoanatomic cart before the empiric horse." The alternative method of first presenting the pathoanatomic conclusions of the McKenzie approach runs the risk of diminishing an appreciation for the clinical utility of the approach, the basis of which is therapeutic intervention and management made possible by careful observations of spine-related responses to movements and positionings, and not by the ability to ascribe meanings to these responses via dogmatic diagnostic conclusions based on pathoanatomic models.

Objective Signs Alone Are Not Adequate Criteria

Some clinicians maintain the a priori notion that concentrating on mechanical or other objective signs alone (and therefore ignoring symptoms) is a more scientific approach, because signs are more amenable to measurement. Mechanical or other objective signs, however, such as range of motion measurements or spinal imaging, do not adequately account for the phenomena of spine-related complaints.

What might at first seem to be indistinguishable objective measurements between two patients, may, on closer inspection, prove to be part of different clinical pictures when judged in the broader context within which they occur. The identical mechanical sign may be associated with different symptoms, or even different *other* mechanical signs, from patient to patient. In addition, the *apparently* same mechanical sign may respond differently to identical movement and/or positioning stimuli from patient to patient.

Orthodox Versus Alternative Health Care Signs

In orthodox medicine, the focus on signs and the a priori assumptions of a pathoanatomic model is the result of, or leads to, an inability or unwillingness to rationally appreciate spine-related symptomatology. This same approach taken by the so-called "alternatives" to orthodox medicine entails the use of "alternative" signs, which also avoids the recognition of symptoms as meaningful. In this regard, no alternative is really being offered.

Alternative approaches, often described as "holistic," frequently make the a priori claim to "treat *causes* not symptoms." This predilection often leads the patient and practitioner to *alternative signs* so removed from the phenomena at hand that both common signs *and* symptoms related to the patient's complaints are ignored. The signs sought may be so removed from the patient's complaints that they better resemble signs of "divination" (omens, portents, etc.) than any serious, rational diagnostic endeavor. Common, mundane signs and symptoms are ignored in the search for the miraculous.

The alternative health care complaint that symptoms *themselves* cannot be treated is appreciated as a valid objection to the pharmacologic suppression of symptoms via analgesics as a means of therapy. This concern, however, does not justify the total rejection of appraising symptoms as relevant phenomena.

Subjective Symptoms As Potentially Valid Criteria

Symptoms are an important key to the puzzle of spinal complaints. Signs and symptoms are important diagnostic components in most health care specialties. Unfortunately, when the specialty concerns common spinal complaints, symptoms are usually denigrated to the status of epiphenomena, principally because of the confusion that has resulted from the inability to appreciate rationally the symptomatic responses to spinal loading stimuli.

Because health care disciplines have been unable to make sense of spine-related symptoms, these symptoms have been relegated to the realm of nonsense. This lack of appreciation not only denies patients a certain dignity and respect (the absence of a concerned audience regarding their symptomatic story), but it also denies health care practitioners the clinical utility of that story.

Subjective Symptoms Alone Are Not Adequate Criteria

As with mechanical signs, symptoms taken by themselves do not account adequately for the clinical presentation of spine-related complaints. *Both* the symptomatic *and* the mechanical responses to spinal loading must be considered to best appreciate common spinal disorders.

Responses of Mechanical Signs and Subjective Symptoms to Loading As Criteria

The McKenzie approach is a system of assessment and therapeutics based on the recognition of patterns concerning the mechanical and symptomatic responses to the stimuli of loading (applying forces to) the spine. This recognition is derived from historical information related by the patient as well as clinical findings that compare mechanical and symptomatic responses before, during, and after (1) singular movements, (2) repetitive movements, and (3) sustained positionings.

Common Connecting Criteria

Spine-related complaints and the means for their resolution become intimately connected at each stage of the McKenzie approach because of the common connecting criteria, which is the mechanical and symptomatic response to loading strategies. These criteria, on which the approach is predicated, provide a rational thread connecting:

- Complaints
- Assessment
- Therapeutic prescription
- Monitoring the course of therapy
- Prophylaxis

SPINAL LOADING

Spinal loading refers to the administration of a force to the spine. No matter what position the spine is in, at least the force of gravity is loading the spine in that position and *internal forces* (within the disk) are at play. Although it is understood that the *unloaded* spine refers to the reclined position, it can also be viewed as a *different kind* of loading. Unloading the spine, as it is commonly understood, may diminish external axial forces to a motor segment while increasing internal forces as a result of the inhibition of fluid. These distinctions may have some importance considering the conventional a priori notion that any *unloading* action is of benefit to the spine. This is not necessarily true. For example, for a significant number of patients, low back and leg pain is worse in the morning, and others respond poorly to traction.

Loading can be viewed as a mechanical stimulus to which mechanical and symptomatic responses occur. Loading may be considered the independent variable, with the resulting mechanical and symptomatic responses the dependent variables.

LOADING TACTICS

Loading tactics refer to individual loading stimuli, procedures or methods that are components contributing to an overall loading strategy. They include the following:

- Dynamic loading
- Static loading
- Loading intensity
  - Loading frequency
  - Loading amplitude (overpressure, mobilization, manipulation)
- Loading within a specific movement plane direction
- Loading within a specific range of a movement plane
- Loading at a specific point of a movement plane

- Loading posture
- Loading source (source of force)
  - Patient-generated tactics
  - Patient use of appliance or machine
  - Clinician-generated tactics
  - Clinician use of tool, appliance, or machine

Dynamic Loading

This term refers to a system of forces on the spine *in motion,* or undergoing *movement,* under specific conditions.

Static Loading

Static loading refers to a system of forces on the spine at rest, or during *positioning,* under specific conditions. Static loading of the spine in a specific position for a prolonged period of time may be referred to as *sustained positioning.*

Loading Intensity

Intensity is defined as tension, activity, or energy. Curiously, the word intensity is derived, in part, from the Latin verb, *tendere,* to stretch. *Intensity* refers to the frequency and/or the amplitude accompanying loading. To increase the intensity of loading, the frequency and/or the amplitude can be increased.

LOADING FREQUENCY

Loading frequency refers to the number of loadings per unit time (cycles). In dynamic loading, loading frequency refers to the number of movements performed per unit time. In static loading, loading frequency refers to sustained positioning per unit time.

LOADING AMPLITUDE (OVERPRESSURE, MOBILIZATION, MANIPULATION)

Loading amplitude refers to the amount of force applied during each cycle. For the purpose of the McKenzie approach, loading amplitude usually refers to the amount of force applied to promote movement of the spine toward a more *complete* end range position. This movement is accomplished by the application of overpressure or manipulation.

Overpressure applied during dynamic loading permits further movement into end range with every cycle. Overpressure applied during static loading at end range permits positioning even further into that end range. It may be accomplished strategically by the patient's own means or with the use of a device or an appliance. It may also be accomplished by the application of a force by the clinician, using a "hands on" technique, with or without, alone or in combination with a device or appliance. When the clinician's hands perform the overpressure in a cyclic fashion, this practice is called *mobilization.* The chiropractic concept of "taking the slack out" corresponds to moving a joint to end range. The cyclic performance of this movement is mobilization.

The greatest loading amplitude is applied by means of spinal *manipulation.* Overpressure and mobilization are thought to bring spinal joint structures beyond voluntary end range, toward physiologic end range. Manipulation is thought to bring spinal joint structures beyond physiologic end range, just short of anatomic end range.

For the McKenzie approach, the mechanical and symptomatic responses to overpressure and/or mobilization are carefully noted in order to predict what the mechanical and symptomatic responses would be to manipulation. In other words, the responses to loading at physiologic end range serve as a criteria on which to predicate loading toward anatomic end range. Only therapeutically beneficial responses noted with the former permit performance of the latter. Complete recovery by means of the former obviates the latter. Manipulation is appropriate when loading of lesser intensity evidences beneficial responses that are not complete.

Loading Within a Specific Movement Plane Direction

Movement planes are derived from dimensions in space. Movement planes contain two opposite potential directions in which loading can occur, referred to as *movement plane directions.*

SAGITTAL MOVEMENT PLANE

In this plane, also called the anterior-posterior movement plane, movement occurs about the coronal axis. The opposite movement plane directions are referred to as flexion and extension.

Special features regarding this movement plane are noted for the cervical spine. Protrusion of the head in the sagittal plane involves extension of the upper cervical spine and flexion of the lower cervical spine. Retraction of the head in the sagittal plane involves flexion of the upper cervical spine and extension of the lower cervical spine. These movements may be referred to as *translation* through the sagittal plane.

TRANSVERSE MOVEMENT PLANE

Movement occurs about the longitudinal axis. The opposite movement plane directions within this plane are referred to as rotation right and rotation left.

CORONAL MOVEMENT PLANE

In this plane, also called the frontal or lateral movement plane, movement occurs about the sagittal axis. The opposite movement plane directions used by the McKenzie approach within the coronal movement plane are different for the cervical and lumbar spine. For the cervical spine, right lateral flexion and left lateral flexion are noted. For the lumbar spine, right and left side-gliding are noted.

Side-gliding refers to a superior anatomic part moving through the coronal plane in the opposite direction relative to an inferior anatomic part. It also refers to the trunk moving in the relative opposite direction, through the coronal plane, above the pelvis. This movement may be referred to as *translation* through the coronal plane.

Positioning within this movement plane results in the clinical presentation of the "antalgic list." This antalgic deformity, constituting an acute lumbar scoliosis, is a result of translation through the coronal plane. The antalgic list is referred to as a *lateral shift,* and is named according to the direction (right or left) by which the superior anatomic part is positioned relative the inferior anatomic part.

Loading Within a Specific Range of a Movement Plane

When dynamic loading occurs, it may involve movement to end range or only to within mid-range of a movement plane. During dynamic loading, each point in the movement plane has a "directional component" defined by the intended movement plane direction.

Loading at a Specific Point of a Movement Plane

Sustained positioning (static loading) may be at mid-range or end range. Sustained positioning in mid-range may have a directional component relative to a previously assumed sustained positioning. Static loading at end range is usually referred to as having the movement plane direction of which that end range is the culmination.

Loading Posture

This term refers to the orientation of the body (standing, sitting, etc.).

Consider the cervical spine loaded in the movement plane direction of extension. The patient may be standing, sitting erect, sitting slouched, lying prone, or lying supine with the head and neck off the end of a treatment table—all examples of different ways to position the body (loading postures) while extending the cervical spine.

Loading Source (Source of Force)

Loading tactics may be generated or modified by patients themselves, appliances or machines, as well as by the clinician's intervention. Certain appliances or machines are readily used by patients themselves, whereas other devices (because of expense, mechanics, or expertise required) may be used only in a clinical setting.

PATIENT-GENERATED TACTICS

Movements or positions may be accomplished by patients themselves. Patients may perform movements actively by recruiting muscular structures that specifically move or maintain positions of spinal joint structures concerned. They are also able to strategically perform "passive" movements of the spine. For example, patients may rotate the cervical spine by using the pressure of the hand against the cheek without recruiting the intrinsic neck musculature. Similarly, passive extension of the low back may be accomplished by performing a "press-up" from the prone position with the pelvis remaining on the exercise surface, thus recruiting only elbow extensors and not the extensors of the back.

PATIENT USE OF APPLIANCE OR MACHINE

Various devices that affect spinal loading and do not require the assistance of the clinician or presence in the clinical setting are available to patients. These appliances range from mattress and chair types to braces, traction devices, and exercise equipment.

CLINICIAN-GENERATED TACTICS

Force introduced by the clinician may be combined with, or apart from, patient-generated forces. Clinician-introduced forces range from mobilization to manipulation. Mobilization has been characterized as forces that do not bring joint structures beyond physiologic end range, whereas manipulation has been characterized as bringing joint structures beyond physiologic end range, but short of anatomic end range.

CLINICIAN USE OF TOOL, APPLIANCE, OR MACHINE

This category includes certain appliances or machines unavailable to patients because of expense, mechanics involved, or the need of a clinician's expertise. Examples include sophisticated traction units, "drop tables" that enhance manipulative procedures, treatment tables permitting various spinal positionings, and continuous passive motion units designed for the spine (Fig. 12.1). Surgical intervention is certainly a mechanical intervention that represents a loading tactic.

PREFERRED LOADING STRATEGY

Strategy refers to a plan devised to attain a goal. *Loading strategy* refers to the choice or rejection of particular loading tactics and the order in which those chosen loading tactics are employed. A *preferred loading strategy* is framed by deciding which:

- Loading tactics to avoid
- Loading tactics to pursue simultaneously
- Loading tactics to pursue sequentially
  - Immediate sequence
  - Delayed sequence: introduction of previously avoided loading tactic

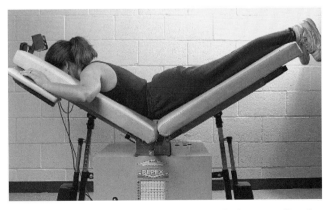

Fig. 12.1. McKenzie Repex (Repeated End range Passive Exercise) unit.

Tactics to Avoid

Specific loading tactics deemed therapeutically detrimental are to be avoided as constituents of the preferred loading strategy. The practitioner must take into account the effects of avoiding specific loading tactics as much as he or she considers the effects of pursuing specific loading tactics. Avoidance can be of equal, if not greater, importance in resolving an individual's spine-related complaints than which tactics to pursue.

Tactics to Pursue Simultaneously

The preferred loading strategy always involves the simultaneous performance of loading tactics; for example, it may concurrently load the cervical spine dynamically, in the movement plane direction of extension, while sitting, with overpressure, and a certain frequency of repetition.

Tactics to Pursue Sequentially

Loading tactics applied one after the other.

IMMEDIATE SEQUENCE

This term refers to loading tactics applied immediately, one after the other, e.g., loading the cervical spine in the movement plane direction of left lateral flexion, immediately followed by loading in the movement plane direction of extension.

DELAYED SEQUENCE

This term is used to describe the application of loading tactics separated by a significant length of time. It usually refers to the timely re-introduction of previously avoided loading tactics. Loading tactics once considered therapeutically detrimental, may, after the appropriate delay, prove to be of significant therapeutic benefit. For example, on Day 1, it is determined that right side-gliding (Fig. 12.2) is the most therapeutically beneficial movement plane direction for the lumbar spine, and loading in all other movement plane directions is considered detrimental. On Day 2, it is determined that the previously avoided loading tactic of extension is now therapeutically beneficial, and in fact, necessary for further resolution of complaints. On Day 5, it is determined that the previously avoided loading tactic of flexion is of benefit for the patient so that full function may be recovered.

PROPERTIES COMMON TO MECHANICAL *AND* SYMPTOMATIC RESPONSES TO LOADING

Although mechanical versus symptomatic responses to loading have unique features or perspectives, they have certain common response properties or *parameters,* described here as *response value, response temporal factors, point of response elicitation, movement plane-specific responses,* and *mechanically impeded end range.*

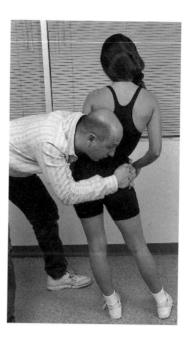

Fig. 12.2. Right lateral shift as a result of clinician overpressure during right side-gliding.

Response Value

Mechanical and symptomatic responses may be considered the same, better, or worse after a particular loading strategy is pursued. Considering before and after possiblities, responses may be:

- Normal before and remain normal afterwards
- Normal before and remain abnormal afterwards
- Abnormal before and remains abnormal afterwards with
  - Equal magnitude
  - Greater magnitude
  - Lesser magnitude
- Abnormal before and remains normal afterwards

Response Temporal Factors

These factors include *frequency of complaints, time required to elicit a response,* and *response persistence after loading cessation.*

FREQUENCY OF COMPLAINTS (RESPONSES)

The frequency with which mechanical or symptomatic responses to loading occur during a specified time period may be characterized as one of the following:

- Total absence of the response (no complaints)
- Intermittent frequency of the response (intermittent complaints)
- Constant frequency of the response (constant complaints).

A patient may have no symptoms, experience symptoms intermittently, or experience symptoms constantly during a specified period of time. Similarly, a patient may have no restricted ranges of motion, experience a restricted range of motion intermittently, or experience a restricted range of motion constantly during a specified period of time.

TIME REQUIRED TO ELICIT A RESPONSE

This parameter refers to the number or duration of dynamic or static loading cycles required to elicit a mechanical or symptomatic response as well as the *delay,* if any, for the response to occur after loading ceases.

The *number of loading* cycles refers to the frequency of a movement or sustained positioning per unit time; these may be relatively few or many. *Duration* refers to the amount of time a sustained positioning is held. An *immediate response* to dynamic loading or sustained positioning occurs on the initiation of the loading tactic. A *delayed response* occurs some time after loading ceases.

The range of possibilities are:

- No response elicited, regardless of the number and/or duration of loading cycles
- Response elicited on initiation of loading cycle (immediate response)
- Response elicited after relatively few and/or short duration of loading cycles
- Response elicited after relatively many and/or long duration of loading cycles
- Response elicited after cessation of loading cycle (delayed response)

Consider the following scenarios.

Responses elicited on initiation of the loading cycle (immediate response), for example, would be the patient who, during the performance of one dynamic extension or on initiating static extension, experiences symptoms or deviation from the intended movement plane direction. Another patient's response could be the relief of symptoms and aberrant movement.

Responses elicited after "relatively few" or "short duration" of loading cycles, for example, would be the patients for whom 10 spinal extensions or 5 minutes of static loading result in the onset or resolution mechanical and symptomatic responses.

Responses elicited after "relatively many" or "long duration" of loading cycles, for example, would be the patients for whom 50 dynamic spinal extensions or sustained extension end-range positioning for 30 minutes is required to experience the onset or resolution mechanical and symptomatic responses.

Responses elicited after cessation of the loading cycle (delayed response) are, by definition, responses that occur after the responsible dynamic or static loading stimuli ceases. Medicolegal issues arise concerning the meaning and the credibility of delayed responses, proportional to the delay.

RESPONSE PERSISTENCE AFTER LOADING CESSATION

Mechanical and symptomatic responses may demonstrate a varying degree of persistence after cessation of the loading strategy responsible for generating the responses. The possibilities are as follows:

- Responses do not persist after loading cessation
- Responses persist for a short period of time after loading cessation
- Responses remain after loading cessation

Consider a patient who has low back symptoms that, at the end range of flexion, radiate to the calf. If the radiation resolves immediately, every time the patient returns to the neutral standing position, this individual experiences a symptomatic response that does not persist.

If calf symptoms remain for a couple of minutes after returning, from flexion, to the neutral posture, this person has a response that persisted for a short period of time without remaining.

A response that persists is evident if dynamic flexion causes calf symptoms that remain for days after flexion loading ceases.

Mechanically, consider a patient with 50% flexion loss. Dynamic extensions result in a 25% flexion loss. Dynamic flexion results in a 75% flexion loss. After resting for a moment, however, after either dynamic tactic, the 50% flexion loss returns regardless of the movement plane direction pursued. These scenarios are examples of mechanical responses that did not persist after loading cessation.

If the patient has 0% flexion loss for 30 minutes as a result of performing 10 extensions, after which 50% flexion loss returns, this individual offers an example of a response that persists for a short period of time after loading cessation.

A response that persists is evident if dynamic extensions result in 0% flexion loss and remains so.

Point of Response Elicitation

Mechanical and/or symptomatic responses may occur as a result of loading at end range or between the two end ranges (mid-range) of a particular movement plane.

Movement Plane-Specific Responses

Loading within a particular movement plane direction may have mechanical and/or symptomatic responses that are movement plane (or even movement plane direction) *specific;* spinal loading in one movement plane direction may affect a response in the same or another movement plane. The possibilities include one or more of the following:

- No responses within the same or any other movement plane
- Responses in the same movement plane direction as loading occured
- Responses in the movement plane direction opposite to the loading direction
- Responses in a movement plane different from the loading movement plane

Responses in the same movement plane direction in which loading occurs are first and foremost in the minds of most clinicians. The patient who extends the spine and experiences a limited, symptomatic end range exhibits a mechanical and symptomatic response in the movement plane direction of extension. Repeated extensions cause further extension loss and symptoms. If no other movements are affected, these responses are occurring in the same movement plane direction in which loading occurred.

Consider two cases in which responses occur in the movement plane direction opposite to the loading direction. Two patients have flexion limited by 50%. One patient, after performing dynamic extensions, can achieve full flexion. The other, after performing dynamic extensions, is unable to perform any flexion at all. These cases are examples of loading in one movement plane direction that affects mechanical and symptomatic responses in the opposite direction of the same movement plane.

Responses in a movement plane different from the loading movement are noted in the following example. A patient with flexion limited by 50% due to symptoms can achieve full flexion after performing dynamic right side-gliding, but is in too much pain to perform any flexion after left side-gliding. In this case, loading within one movement plane (coronal) affects the mechanical and symptomatic responses in an entirely different movement plane (saggital). In fact, loading in the opposite direction of the coronal movement plane (side gliding) had opposite effects on mechanical and symptomatic responses in the saggital movement plane.

Mechanically Impeded End Range:
The Mechanical-Symptomatic Interface

"Mechanically impeded end range" is a significant phenomenon that can be perceived by both the clinician and the patient. That it is recognized from both perspectives makes mechanically impeded end range an "interface," in a sense, between "objective," clinically assessed mechanical and "subjectively" perceived symptomatic phenomena.

Consider patients who have restricted range of motion, but no significant discomfort; i.e., symptoms do not interfere with the progression of movement. These patients report that further movement is not possible. Not only is this limitation observed clinically, but also, if the clinician attempts to move the spinal area passively, an early end range is detected by the clinician. It may be stated that further motion is "mechanically impeded." This abnormal early end range resulting in mechanically impeded movement is referred to as a *"mechanically impeded end range,"* with loss of global motion of which both the clinician and the patient are aware.

Mechanically impeded end range does not refer to motion palpation of vertebral segments wherein the clinician often detects restrictions or fixations unknown to the patient, and in fact, full global range of motion may be present.

PROPERTIES UNIQUE TO MECHANICAL RESPONSES TO LOADING

Mechanical responses or objective signs constitute clinical evidence (signs) perceptible to the examining clinician. The signs include observed angulation, list, fixed deformities, range of motion phenomena, and mechanically impeded end range. The last term refers to mechanical interference with the progress of motion to normal, full end range. The signs need not be associated with symptoms.

Normal End Range and Curve Reversal

Curve reversal refers to the ability to move the spine from the extreme of one movement plane direction to that of the opposite movement plane direction. Curve reversal includes both the ability to reverse the "normal" anatomic curves in the sagittal plane and the ability to introduce curves in the opposite directions of the coronal movement plane.

Flexion in the sagittal plane *reverses* the cervical lordosis, increases the thoracic kyphosis, and *reverses* the lumbar lordosis. Extension in the sagittal plane increases the cervical lordosis, *reverses* the thoracic kyphosis, and increases the lumbar lordosis.

Lateral flexion or side gliding in the coronal plane promotes a convexity in the direction opposite that of the movement performed. The "normal" neutral spine has no curves in the coronal plane. These curves are introduced or created when movement in this plane is performed. Under normal circumstances, full range of motion from one extreme of the coronal movement plane to the other is accompanied by the ability to *reverse* curves that were introduced by movement and are not present in a neutral, resting anatomic position.

OBSTRUCTION TO CURVE REVERSAL

An *obstruction to curve reversal* is a significant mechanically impeded end range that prevents spinal motion from progressing past the neutral position into the opposite movement plane direction. Loss of the ability to reverse spinal curves results in such clinical conditions as torticollis, acute scoliosis, and fixed kyphotic or lordotic deformities.

MECHANICALLY IMPEDED END RANGE

Although loss of range of motion may result from factors other than mechanically impeded end range, only this factor is considered in this discussion.

The degree to which curve reversal and normal end range may be accomplished *mechanically,* when compared before and after loading, is listed in the order of diminishing success:

- Reversible curve achieving full, mechanically unimpeded end range
- Reversible curve with mechanically impeded end range
- Obstruction to curve reversal with mechanically impeded end range

A reversible curve achieving full end range would indicate that no mechanically impeded end range is present. A mechanically impeded end range may be present, but curve reversal is permitted nonetheless, i.e., the progression of movement is mechanically impeded after curve reversal is accomplished.

If the progression of movement is mechanically impeded before curve reversal is accomplished, the result is a substantial loss of movement and an extremely early mechanically impeded end range, referred to as a deformity, antalgia, list, or shift.

Movement Quality

Movement quality refers to the ability to remain within the course of the intended motion plane direction. It is assessed as:

• No deviation from movement plane direction
• Deviation from the intended movement plane direction

Value of Mechanical Responses

It is generally considered beneficial to effect mechanical responses to permit curve reversal with a full range of motion, as well as the ability to accomplish, without deviation, the intended movement plane direction.

PROPERTIES UNIQUE TO SYMPTOMATIC RESPONSES TO LOADING

The symptomatic responses related to spinal disorders commonly considered amenable to mechanical care are pain, paresthesias, and similar symptoms of discomfort. Other symptomatic (subjective) phenomena, however, are equally important. Symptomatic (subjective) phenomena refer to:

• Symptoms of discomfort
    – topography of symptomatic responses (centralization or peripheralization)
• Judgment of fear
• Subjective perception of mechanically impeded end range
    – with or without symptoms of discomfort at end range

Symptoms of Discomfort

These symptoms include pain, numbness, paresthesias, burning, and the like. They may be experienced during motion or at the end range of motion. Not only do the symptoms of discomfort have different qualities, but also their location may change in response to spinal loading. The location or topography of symptoms is a key feature of the McKenzie approach.

Topography of Symptomatic Responses

Symptoms may be *central,* which means they are experienced about the midline of the spine. Symptoms may be *symmetric,* meaning they are equally positioned on opposite sides of the spine. *Unilateral symptoms* affect one side of the spine only. The further from the spine symptoms are experienced, the more *peripheral* are the symptoms. When the topography of symptoms changes in response to loading, they may become more central or peripheral, referred to as the *centralization response* or the *peripheralization response,* respectively.

CENTRALIZATION RESPONSE

In this symptomatic response to loading, more peripheral symptoms diminish or resolve and more central symptoms remain, appear, and/or increase in severity.

PERIPHERALIZATION RESPONSE

This symptomatic response to loading, whereby more peripheral symptoms increase or appear, may or may not be associated with changes in central symptomatology.

Judgment of Fear

Fear of symptoms of discomfort, or fear that they might worsen if experienced, is also an important subjective phenomenon because it may affect an individual's willingness to pursue a specific loading strategy. When possible, it is important to distinguish between an individual's willingness and the individual's *ability* to perform spinal motion.

Subjective Perception of Mechanically Impeded End Range

Patients often report the inability to perform a spinal motion past a certain point because of a sense of being "blocked." They may report that, "Something is in there," "It feels like there is a rock or ball in there," "A wedge is in there," or the like. This subjective perception prevents further movement. Often, it is the perception of a mechanically impeded end range, without any symptoms of discomfort, that is reported by the patient as the reason for failure of further movement. The patient's subjective perception resembles what is felt at the end range of normal, unrestricted spinal range of motion. At other times, symptoms of discomfort occur at the same time the subjective perception of the "early" mechanically impeded end range occurs.

Value of Subjective Phenomena Responses

It is therapeutically beneficial to diminish the subjective perception of mechanically impeded end range, because the typical result is improved mechanics. It is also therapeutically beneficial to diminish a patient's fear because fear prevents the resumption of activities of daily living.

It is not always therapeutically beneficial to avoid symptoms of discomfort, however. The McKenzie approach puts into perspective which symptoms are therapeutically beneficial and which are therapeutically detrimental to pursue. It is beneficial to elicit the centralization response, even though the severity of central symptoms may increase. This increase is usually followed by improved mechanics and the ultimate reduction of central symptoms.

Peripheralization responses are therapeutically detrimental if they remain after cessation of the responsible loading action. In special circumstances, peripheralization that does not persist after end range loading ceases is considered beneficial.

The McKenzie approach demonstrates it is therapeutically beneficial to pursue certain symptoms and to avoid certain symptoms. This principle becomes clearer subsequently when the syndrome patterns themselves are discussed.

Putting symptoms into a perspective patients and clinicians can understand, rather than fear and avoid, provides a handle by which activity may control symptoms. The more common practice is actively avoiding all symptoms, which results in symptoms controlling activity.

LOSS OF RANGE OF MOTION

Loss of range of motion plays a considerable role in the evaluation of impairment and disability. It is curious, therefore, that the mechanical and symptomatic responses associated with range of motion loss do not ordinarily merit much attention.

Ostensibly, range of motion loss is an objectively measured, mechanical entity. Symptoms that the patient experiences with range of motion loss are recorded, if at all, without discriminating as to whether they occur during motion or at the end range of motion. As stated previously, range of motion loss may not be associated with any significant symptoms. The patient's only subjective experience may be that of perceiving the abnormally early end range, which may be perceived in the same manner as the "normal" proprioceptive cue to halt movement.

Range of motion studies usually have the patient perform only a single motion in each movement plane direction. The effects of repetitive movement or sustained positioning on range of motion loss in the same or in a different movement plane direction, are rarely assessed.

"Reasons" for Loss

Loss of range of motion does not result solely from mechanical factors that can be observed clinically or solely from subjective factors that can only be reported by the patient. Understanding range of motion loss requires integrating both of these perspectives. In summary, range of motion loss may be attributed to symptoms of discomfort, judgment of fear, and mechanically impeded end range, which were described previously. This underlines the importance of appreciating the patient's symptomatic experience in order to account fully for mechanical disorders of the spine.

The clinician, however, continues to play a key role. The clinical decision regarding the value of symptoms based on their topography, and not just on their intensity, is critically important. The way the clinician educates the patient dramatically affects that patient's judgment as to whether or not fear is appropriate. Lastly, regarding mechanically impeded end range, patients often perceive this early end range as "normal" because their subjective perception of the impeded end range may be identical to how "normal" end range feels. The clinician's assessment of mechanically impeded range as a mechanical sign plays an important role in those cases in which patients do not realize any motion has been lost at all.

MECHANICALLY IMPEDED END RANGE

The term *mechanically impeded end range* refers to an abnormally early end range that interferes with the progress of motion and may or may not be accompanied by symptoms. Patients may perceive the same proprioceptive cues (to halt motion) at the mechanically impeded end range as they do at normal and full end range.

The clinician and the patient both, in their own ways, may perceive mechanically impeded end range. The patient subjectively perceives a mechanically impeded end range preventing further movement, while the clinician may deduce its existence by observing the manner in which motion is impeded, or may "feel" it by passively moving the patient's spine until the mechanically impeded end range is detected.

Increasing Loading Intensity to Differentiate Restricted from Obstructed End Ranges

If loading of sufficient intensity (cycles or overpressure) is not applied, the mechanically impeded end range may be unaccompanied by symptoms. Overpressure is important in order to load joint structures further at the mechanically impeded end range, thereby "overstating" typical end range responses that occur there. The mechanical and symptomatic responses to loading mechanically impeded end ranges with a greater intensity differentiate mechanically impeded end ranges into two types, *restricted end range* and *obstructed end range*.

RESTRICTED END RANGE

This mechanically impeded end range behaves as if the progress of motion is limited, restrained, or "held back." It is slow to develop or resolve, with no mechanical or symptomatic responses during motion. Any mechanical response (e.g., deviation from the intended movement plane direction) occurs at the restricted end range only. If no symptoms are reported at the restricted end range, increasing the intensity of loading at the restricted end range will elicit mechanical and symptomatic responses in a characteristic fashion. Central or peripheral symptoms are experienced immediately and only at the restricted end range, and they do not persist long after loading at the restricted end range ceases. The centralization response never occurs. The peripheralization response, when it does occur, does not persist. Overpressure simply exaggerates the symptomatic response at end range, whereas increasing the frequency of restricted end range loading does not change the characteristic response. During the initial examination, no change in how mechanics or symptoms respond to dynamic or static loading at the restricted end range is appreciable.

OBSTRUCTED END RANGE

This mechanically impeded end range behaves as if an "obstacle" or "blockage" is interfering with the progress of motion. It may be quick to develop or resolve. Mechanical and symptomatic responses may occur at any point of the involved movement plane direction, as well as at the obstructed end range. Mechanical and/or symptomatic responses may develop immediately or after a delay in response to a particular loading strategy. If no symptoms occur at the obstructed end range, increasing the intensity of the loading will elicit mechanical and symptomatic responses in a characteristic fashion.

The centralization response or the peripheralization response may be noted during motion or at an obstructed end range. Elicitation of, or changes in, mechanical and/or symptomatic responses to loading may persist after cessation of loading. Overpressure or increased frequency of loading at the obstructed end range may radically change the mechanical and/or symptomatic responses during motion or at the obstructed end range. Overpressure at the obstructed end range may result in the centralization response, the peripheralization response, or the resolution of mechanically impeded end range, or it may cause its occurrence earlier during the range of motion. During the initial examination, an appreciable change in how mechanics or symptoms respond to dynamic or static loading at the obstructed end range is usually noted.

Differentiating Obstructed End Range Symptoms from Symptoms During Motion. Mechanically impeded end ranges have been described as exhibiting two different responses, one typical of a restricted end range, the other of an obstructed end range. Loading at the restricted end range shows no significant change during the initial examination, and may show no significant changes for quite some time. Loading at an obstructed end range, on the other hand, may demonstrate rapid changes concerning mechanical and symptomatic responses.

Ordinarily, differentiating symptoms during motion from symptoms at an obstructed end range is not difficult. When an obstructed end range resolves rapidly, however, symptoms occurring at a mechanically impeded end range may be mistakenly construed as symptoms occurring during motion. Confusion in this regard may muddle the proper choice of therapeutic measures.

Assume a case in which a mechanically impeded end range interferes with the progression of movement to full extension. Dynamic loading to the mechanically impeded end range of extension resolves the mechanically impeded end range within a minute or two—a typical response of an obstructed end range.

Assume that with repetitive dynamic loading to the obstructed end range, every cycle of movement results in a lesser degree of mechanically impeded end range, i.e., permitting more and more extension range of motion with each cycle of movement. If discomfort was associated with loading at the obstructed end range, the discomfort would occur further and further into the range of motion with each cycle as the stepwise pattern of improvement occurs.

Regarding static loading, assume again that the spine is mechanically impeded in extension. Loading is performed in a static manner at the obstructed end range. The patient then assumes a neutral posture and again performs sustained extension at the obstructed end range that is now encountered after a greater range of motion. With each cycle, any discomfort at the obstructed end range would occur further and further into the range of motion as the obstructed end range moves along, again in a stepwise pattern.

On occasion, obstructed end ranges resolve rapidly and almost spontaneously without any special effort needed. In other cases, an increase of loading intensity (cycles or overpressure) may be necessary, after which the obstructed end range rapidly "gives way." The stepwise pattern just described may not occur if the obstructed end range "retreats" so rapidly that it appears to "melt away." If loading at an obstructed end range causes its rapid retreat, *accompanied by a symptomatic marker,* the phenomenon may be construed mistakenly to represent symptoms during mechanically unimpeded motion. It should be recalled in these cases, however, that initial examination revealed a mechanically impeded end range before aggressive loading tactics were pursued.

McKENZIE ASSESSMENT OF MECHANICAL AND SYMPTOMATIC RESPONSES TO LOADING

The McKenzie approach is that of assessing the responses, reactions, or effects of spinal loading. During the initial encounter with the patient, this assessment is performed by evaluating the history, posture, and quality of movement of the patient, and by using dynamic and static testing procedures.

History

In addition to the usual history taken regarding neck and back complaints, the McKenzie assessment makes particular inquiries regarding the following:

- Are symptoms constant or intermittent?
- What is the topography of symptoms?
- Are symptoms better or worse with any of the following?
  - Bending
  - Sitting
  - Rising from sitting
  - Standing
  - Walking
  - Lying

– Rising from lying
– When still
– On the move

Inquiries regarding whether patients are better or worse with activities of daily living yield clues regarding the loading effects that movements and positionings have on mechanical and symptomatic responses. Certain activities load the spine within the movement plane direction of flexion (bending, sitting), whereas other activities have the relative effect of loading the spine in the movement plane direction of extension (standing).

Posture

On initial examination, the patient's sitting and standing postures are noted. This information reveals how the spine is habitually subjected to static loading by the patient. An inquiry may also be made as to what posture the patient assumes at home or at work.

Quantity and Quality of Movement

The patient is asked to perform a single movement for each movement plane direction examined. The examiner concentrates on mechanics (quantity and quality of movement), not on symptoms. At this point, the examiner also does not concentrate on mechanical responses to loading. Quantity and quality of movement refers to the ability to achieve end range with curve reversal and without deviating from the intended movement plane.

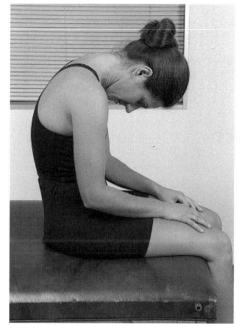

Fig. 12.4. Cervical flexion.

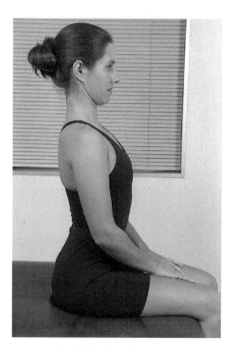

Fig. 12.5. Cervical retraction.

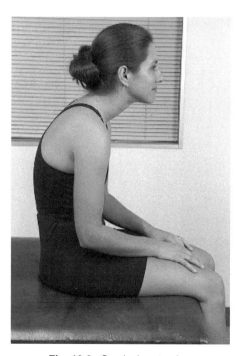

Fig. 12.3. Cervical protrusion.

Modifications from typical range of motion studies include adding protraction and retraction to the cervical spine examination and replacing rotation and lateral flexion with side gliding movements to the lumbar spine examination.

CERVICAL SPINE STUDIES

• Protrusion (Fig. 12.3)
• Flexion (Fig. 12.4)

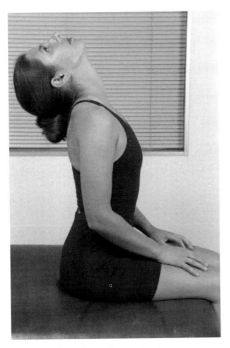

Fig. 12.6. Cervical extension.

- Retraction (Fig. 12.5)
- Extension (Fig. 12.6)
- Side-bending right
- Side-bending left
- Rotation right
- Rotation left

LUMBAR SPINE STUDIES

- Flexion (Fig. 12.7)
- Extension (Fig. 12.8)
- Side-gliding right (see Fig. 12.2)
- Side-gliding left (Fig. 12.9)

The movement plane directions evaluated for both the cervical and lumbar spines are those within which the clinically presenting antalgic postures occur. The movements required to achieve these antalgic postures are thought to be of value for both assessment and therapeutics of the respective spinal areas. Complaints, assessment, and therapeutics are, therefore, connected by similar mechanical considerations.

Dynamic and Static Tests

After quantity and quality of movement is assessed by the performance of single movements in each movement plane direction, dynamic and static tests are performed. These tests load the spine in a more aggressive manner than the single repetitions used to evaluate quality of movement. The patient is monitored closely concerning the mechanical and symptomatic responses to dynamic and/or static loading, especially concerning the most peripheral symptomatic complaints.

The mechanical and symptomatic responses that occur as a result of one or two movements may change significantly after further repetition of the same movement. The effects of loading in a certain movement plane direction are revealed best by repetition or sustained static loading. Dynamic loading or sustained positioning (static loading) better demonstrates mechanical and symptomatic responses to loading than does one movement or a moment's positioning, which may give a false first impression.

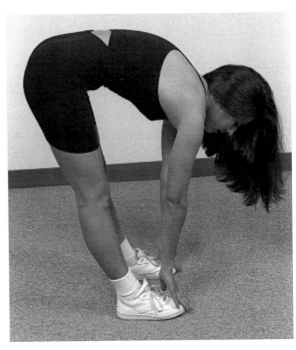

Fig. 12.7. Lumbar flexion.

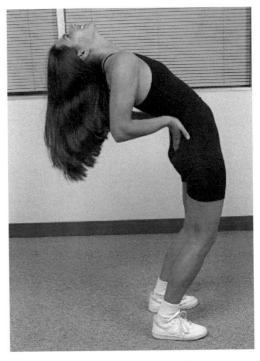

Fig. 12.8. Lumbar extension.

Fig. 12.9. Left lateral shift as a result of side-gliding left.

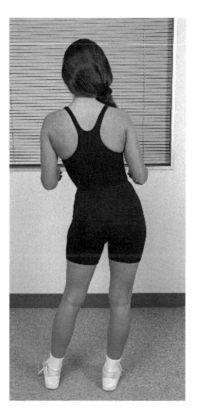

loading in the movement plane direction of concern ceases. The usual progression of dynamic tests for the cervical and lumbar spine follows:

Cervical Spine
- Flexion sitting
- Retraction sitting
- Retraction-then-extension sitting
- Retraction lying (head off edge of treatment table) (Figs. 12.10 and 12.11)
- Retraction extension lying (head off edge of treatment table) (Fig. 12.12 and 12.13)

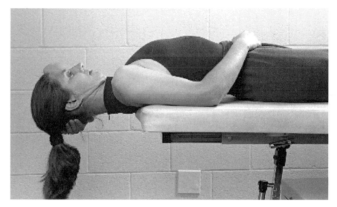

Fig. 12.10. Retraction lying.

Dynamic loading in sagittal movement plane directions is typically explored first, unless the patient has significant antalgia in a coronal movement plane direction, in which case, the coronal movement plane is explored first. If the patient appears amenable to therapeutic spinal loading strategies in the sagittal movement plane, dynamic or static loadings tests in other movement planes are usually not pursued.

If a clear clinical picture is not revealed, dynamic loading in the coronal plane is explored, which entails lateral flexion for testing the cervical spine, and side-gliding movements for the lumbar spine.

Should loading in the coronal plane not provide satisfactory answers, the transverse movement plane is explored. For the cervical spine, this process entails rotation, whereas for the lumbar spine, rotation is performed side-lying combined with flexion. This lumbar movement is typically loaded at end range and is a static test.

Static loading tests generally are used when dynamic tests do not provide a clear preferred loading strategy. As with dynamic testing, the sagittal plane is explored first. Other movement planes and static tests are secondary considerations to sagittal dynamic testing.

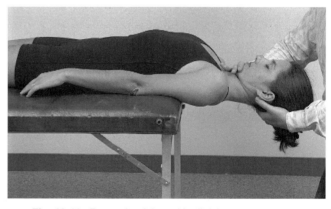

Fig. 12.11. Retraction lying with clinician overpressure.

DYNAMIC TESTS

Dynamic testing proceeds by performing a single motion within the movement plane direction being studied, followed by repetitive motion in the same movement plane direction. The clinician closely monitors how mechanics and symptoms respond during motion, at end range, and after the dynamic

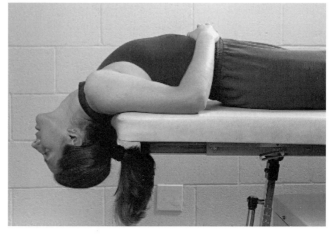

Fig. 12.12. Retraction-then-extension lying.

if required:
- Protrusion sitting
- Retracted side-bending right sitting (Fig.12.14)
- Retracted side-bending left sitting
- Retracted rotation right sitting (Fig. 12.15)
- Retracted rotation left sitting

Lumbar Spine
- Flexion standing
- Extension standing
- Flexion in lying (supine knee to chest) (Fig. 12.16)
- Extension in lying (prone "McKenzie" press up) (Fig. 2.17)

if required:
- Side-gliding right standing or prone extension with right lateral shift (Fig. 12.18)

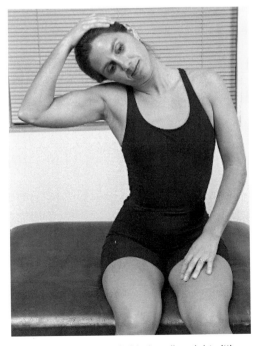

Fig. 12.13. Clinician traction-retraction-extension lying.

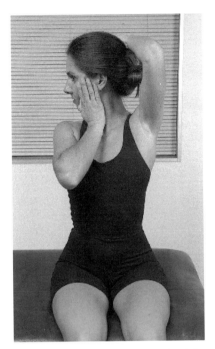

Fig. 12.15. Retracted rotation right sitting.

- Side-gliding left standing (see Fig. 12.9) or prone extension with left lateral shift

STATIC TESTS

Static loading is often used as an *ancillary* test to confirm dynamic testing or to further explore the effects of loading when dynamic testing yields no definitive conclusion. In particular, headaches of cervical origin often require sustained static loading to diagnose or treat the syndrome pattern involved. Choices for static testing follow.

Cervical Spine
- Protrusion
- Flexion
- Retraction (sitting or supine)
- Retraction then extension (sitting, prone, or supine)
- Retracted side-bending right or left
- Retracted rotation right or left

Lumbar Spine
- Sitting slouched (Fig. 12.19)
- Sitting erect (Fig. 12.20)
- Standing slouched
- Standing erect
- Lying prone in extension
- Long sitting
- Lateral shift right or left
- Rotation in flexion

USE OF OVERPRESSURE

Overpressure may be used in combination with dynamic and/or static testing, permitting further end range positioning.

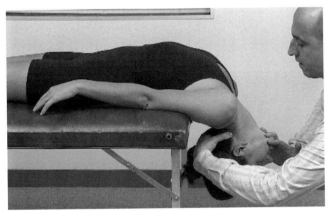

Fig. 12.14. Retracted side-bending right sitting.

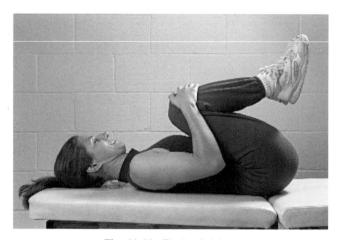

Fig. 12.16. Flexion in lying.

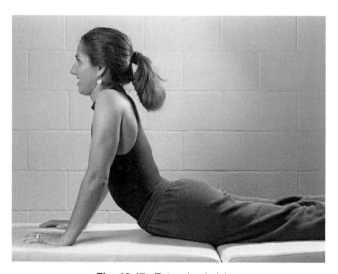

Fig. 12.17. Extension in lying.

A loading tactic may be considered a loading stimulus. A loading strategy is considered the sum of stimuli. A response is a reaction to loading stimuli (tactic or strategy), whereas behavior refers to the sum of responses.

The McKenzie approach recognizes behavior patterns as syndromes amenable to mechanical loading strategies.

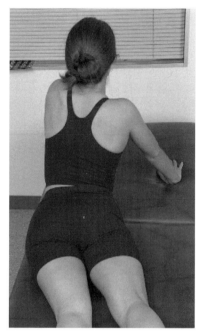

Fig. 12.18. Prone extension with right lateral shift.

Such overpressure may be patient generated or clinician generated (Figs. 12.21 to 12.23).

Spine-Related Responses Versus Behaviors

A response may be defined as the reaction elicited by a stimulus. In the McKenzie approach, the stimulus is mechanical (spinal loading), and the response is the mechanical or symptomatic reaction.

The McKenzie approach distinguishes between conditions that demonstrate beneficial responses to mechanical loading stimuli and those that either do not respond or demonstrate detrimental responses. Needless to say, it may not be fruitful to pursue mechanical therapies in cases that show no or detrimental responses to spinal loading strategies.

Regarding terminology used to describe mechanical and symptomatic responses to spinal loading, *behavior* is often used interchangeably with *response*. Behavior, however, is considered a broad term used to connote all the mechanical and symptomatic responses to a particular loading strategy.

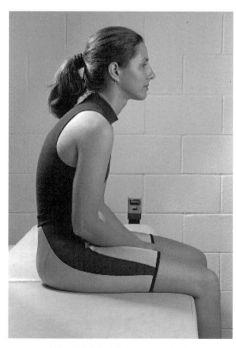

Fig. 12.19. Sitting slouched.

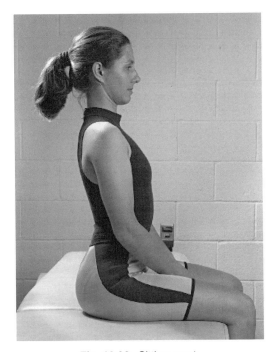

Fig. 12.20. Sitting erect.

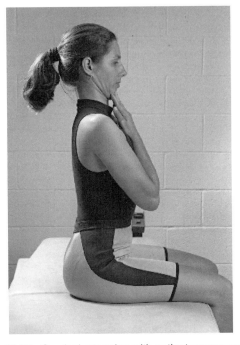

Fig. 12.21. Cervical retraction with patient overpressure.

respond to the mechanical influence of loading strategies in a predictable manner. Retrospectively, these conditions are considered mechanical spinal disorders after they prove amenable to mechanical methods. Spinal complaints that do not respond to, or are made worse by, the mechanical influence of loading strategies are screened out, including those conditions that may represent mechanical disorders not amenable to loading, psychogenic entities, inflammatory conditions, or those of even more pernicious causation. In these conditions, responses to mechanical loading strategies are atypical, lacking, or detrimental.

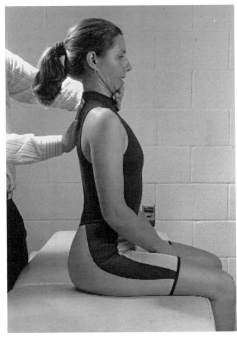

Fig. 12.22. Cervical retraction with clinician overpressure.

THREE SYNDROME PATTERNS

The clinical reasoning intrinsic to the McKenzie approach organizes mechanical and symptomatic responses to loading into three syndrome patterns. These patterns describe a discrete set of mechanical spinal conditions that respond to loading strategies in a specific manner.

Clinical Reasoning and Utility

The syndrome patterns do not encompass all spinal complaints and conditions, but rather define spinal conditions that

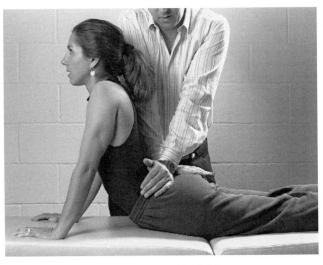

Fig. 12.23. Extension in lying with clinician overpressure.

Table 12.1 Summary of the Three Syndrome Patterns

	Mechanical or Symptomatic Responses	Frequency of Complaints (Responses)	Point of Response Elicitation	Rate of Response Elicitation	Response Persistence after Loading Cessation	Rate of Syndrome Resolution	Responses During Motion	Responses at Mechanically Unimpeded End Range	Responses at Mechanically Impeded End Range	Movement Plane Specific Responses	Preferred Loading Strategies	Reasons for Patient Failure
Postural	Symptomatic only	Intermittent	Sustained end range	Delayed onset after sustained end range positioning	None	Weeks	None	Symptomatic	None exist	Movement plane direction specific	Avoid symptoms	Ignorance, fatigue, self-conscious
Dysfunction	Symptomatic and mechanical	Intermittent	Restricted end range	Immediate at restricted end range	None	Months	None	None	Mechanical and symptomatic	Movement plane direction specific	Pursue symptoms	Avoiding symptoms
Derangement	Symptomatic and mechanical	Intermittent or Constant	During motion, obstructed or unobstructed end range	Immediate or delayed, during motion, at obstructed or unobstructed end range	Often persists	Days	Yes	Mechanical and symptomatic	Mechanical and symptomatic	Loading in one movement plane direction may affect another	Pursue centralization, avoid peripheralization	Avoiding symptoms of centralization

Pathoanatomic Syndrome Nomenclature

The syndrome patterns are identified by recognizing groupings or categories of mechanical and symptomatic responses to loading, not the pathoanatomic basis for them. Nonetheless, the syndromes have been named according to the hypothesized pathoanatomic basis for their behaviors. While these hypotheses are the McKenzie system's "best guess," it is important to remember two salient points regarding the pathoanatomic titles for these syndromes. The first is that the syndromes are grouped according to responses and *not* pathoanatomy. If research proves the McKenzie pathoanatomic hypotheses erroneous, the observed grouping of responses will remain as empiric fact. The second point is that the pathoanatomic titles of the syndromes help the clinician remember the configuration of complaints so named. It also helps *both* the clinician and the patient to remember the rules surrounding treatment of the syndromes.

Because the utility of the system rests in its ability to organize, classify, and predict associated mechanical and symptomatic responses to loading strategies, it may be granted that the pathoanatomic conclusions are *as if* conclusions.

The pathoanatomic titles for the syndromes are the postural, dysfunction, and derangement syndromes. These syndrome patterns are summarized in Table 12.1.

Postural Syndrome

P.S. MECHANICAL AND SYMPTOMATIC RESPONSES

Symptomatic responses characterize this syndrome. No mechanical responses are noted.

P.S. FREQUENCY OF RESPONSES (COMPLAINTS)

The frequency of responses is intermittent.

P.S. POINT OF RESPONSE ELICITATION

Responses are elicited at a mechanically unimpeded end range, usually in one movement plane direction only.

P.S. RATE OF RESPONSE ELICITATION

This syndrome exhibits delayed onset of symptoms in response to sustained static loading at end range. Sustained positioning at end range must be assumed for a relatively long period of time (e.g., 20 minutes) before symptoms are elicited. The delayed onset of symptoms in response to sustained static loading may not be evident during the initial examination because of failure to provide adequate static loading time for the delayed onset response to occur.

P.S. RESPONSE PERSISTENCE AFTER LOADING CESSATION

Symptomatic responses elicited after sustained static loading at end range resolve once that loading tactic is terminated. This behavior is typical of the Postural Syndrome and contributes to the intermittent nature of complaints.

P.S. RATE OF SYNDROME RESOLUTION

The characteristic responses of the Postural Syndrome may take weeks to change with proper therapy. This period of time may be required before it is possible to sustain positioning at the culpable end range absent a symptomatic response. Changes in the end-range symptomatic response, characteristic of this syndrome, cannot be accomplished during the initial evaluation.

P.S. RESPONSES DURING MOTION

Curve reversal and the ability to achieve mechanically unimpeded end range without deviation from the intended movement plane direction are fully preserved. No symptoms occur during motion. The centralization or peripheralization responses are never noted during motion.

P.S. RESPONSES AT MECHANICALLY UNIMPEDED END RANGES

There is no deviation from the intended movement plane directions. The symptomatic responses occur only after sustained loading at the culpable mechanically unimpeded end range. Over-pressure does not change symptoms significantly. Symptoms are central, bilateral, or unilateral, depending on the nature of the sustained end range positioning. The centralization or peripheralization responses are never noted. Responses that do occur do not persist after loading ceases.

P.S. RESPONSES AT MECHANICALLY IMPEDED END RANGES

Mechanically impeded end ranges do not exist in the Postural Syndrome.

P.S. MOVEMENT PLANE-SPECIFIC RESPONSES

Loading in the symptomatic movement plane direction does not result in mechanical or symptomatic responses within the opposite or within other movement plane directions. Loading in the opposite direction of the symptomatic movement plane direction, or in another movement plane, does not *directly affect* the mechanical or symptomatic responses of the symptomatic movement plane direction.

Avoiding loading at the symptomatic end range is therapeutic in and of itself. Loading in all other movement plane directions is equally therapeutic, inasmuch as they all avoid the symptomatic end range, although they have no *direct* therapeutic benefit.

P.S. PREFERRED LOADING STRATEGY

In the Postural Syndrome, avoiding the symptomatic end range is of paramount importance. Pursuing symptoms at the culpable end range is detrimental. When the symptomatic end range is avoided over a period of time, symptoms at end range are more difficult to elicit, and eventually the Postural Syndrome resolves. When static loading at the symptomatic end range is frequently pursued, it perpetuates the syndrome and may diminish the delay regarding elicitation of symptoms. Constant vigilance regarding avoidance of the symptomatic end range is required to resolve this condition, which generally is accomplished over a period of several weeks.

P.S. REASONS FOR FAILURE OF PATIENT STRATEGIES

When patients do not successfully resolve this syndrome on their own, it is because they are not avoiding the symptomatic end range for long enough periods of time. Postural correction is required, and the patient must be vigilant to avoid the postural habit that holds the spinal joint at the "offending" end range. Patients may feel too awkward or be too concerned about their appearance if this requires them to maintain an upright, neutral, sitting posture. The patient may experience a sense of fatigue in the corrected sitting position, or may experience new discomfort when performing proper sitting posture. The Postural Syndrome is a mechanical problem for which pain or antiinflammatory medication is inappropriate and ineffective. It has a specific mechanical correction—to *avoid* the symptomatic end range.

P.S. HYPOTHESIZED PATHOANATOMY

When joints are held at end range, whether they are extremity joints or spinal joints, noncontractile structures such as ligaments and joint capsules are stressed. An example is the bent finger illustration. If the index finger is hyperextended, discomfort is experienced almost immediately. If it is held just short of the point of immediate discomfort, discomfort would be experienced within 20 minutes. No pathologic condition need exist for this abnormal stress to cause discomfort in a normal joint. These principles applied to the spine are proposed as the origin of Postural Syndrome symptoms, which occur when spinal joints are held at end range for a prolonged period of time.

P.S. RELATED TERMINOLOGY

The particular Postural Syndrome is named according to the movement plane direction of which the offending sustained position represents the end range. The particular Postural Syndrome, therefore, is named in reference to the particular end range at which static loading occurs. Some examples are: sustained extension, sustained flexion, sustained right lateral shift, and/or a combination of movement plane directions.

Sustained extension of the lumbosacral spine may be experienced during poor standing posture, especially in pregnant patients or those with a "beer belly." In addition, sustained extension of the upper cervical spine is experienced commonly with the poor sitting posture of head protraction.

Sustained flexion of the lower cervical, thoracic, and lumbosacral spine commonly occurs with poor, slouched sitting postures.

A *sustained lateral shift* may be seen when all weight rests on one leg in a standing position, thereby shifting the thorax and pelvis in opposite directions within the coronal movement plane.

P.S. SUMMARY INCORPORATING HYPOTHESIZED PATHOANATOMY

When noncontractile, ligamentous, capsular, etc. structures are held at sustained end range for long periods of time, symptoms develop in what is a *mechanically unimpeded* normal spinal joint structure subjected to abnormal stresses. Release of the abnormal stress on these structures is accompanied by immediate symptomatic relief. As this abnormal stress of static loading at end range occurs with greater frequency and/or duration, discomfort is easier to elicit. The condition develops slowly, and the pain is intermittent because it is experienced only when spinal joint structures are held at sustained end range for a prolonged period.

Examination reveals no loss of motion or deviation of movement, i.e., no abnormal mechanical responses. In addition, no symptoms occur during movement or at end range on examination. To provoke symptoms, the joint must be held at end range for a prolonged period. Therefore, the traditional examination of patients with "pure" Postural Syndromes reveals no objective or subjective findings.

Nevertheless, these patients may report having had symptoms in multiple areas of the spine, which occur because of holding multiple areas at end range. These patients are not hysterical, nor are they hypermobile. The best therapeutic avenue is one of avoiding symptoms (sustained end range) for a period of time long enough for the offended tissue to extinguish the symptomatic response to sustained end-range loading.

Dysfunction Syndrome

Dy.S. MECHANICAL AND SYMPTOMATIC RESPONSES

Symptomatic and mechanical responses characterize this syndrome.

Dy.S. FREQUENCY OF RESPONSES (COMPLAINTS)

Responses are intermittent.

Dy.S. POINT OF RESPONSE ELICITATION

Responses are elicited at a mechanically impeded end range of the *restricted end range* variety.

Dy.S. RATE OF RESPONSE ELICITATION

The Dysfunction Syndrome exhibits an immediate elicitation of symptomatic and mechanical responses at the *restricted end range* when sufficient loading overpressure is present.

Dy.S. RESPONSE PERSISTENCE AFTER LOADING CESSATION

Mechanical and symptomatic responses elicited immediately when loading at the restricted end range resolve once that loading tactic is terminated. This behavior is typical of the

Dysfunction Syndrome and contributes to the intermittent nature of complaints.

Dy.S. RATE OF SYNDROME RESOLUTION

The characteristic responses of the Dysfunction Syndrome may take as long as 6 to 20 weeks to resolve. Changes in the mechanical and symptomatic responses characteristic of the syndrome cannot be accomplished during the initial evaluation.

Dy.S. RESPONSES AT MECHANICALLY IMPEDED END RANGES

Restricted end range usually occurs in only one movement plane direction. If it occurs in more than one movement plane direction, responses at the individual restricted end range have no effect on each other. Mechanical and symptomatic responses occur immediately at the restricted end range only. These responses do not persist after loading at the restricted end range ceases. Any deviation from the intended movement plane direction occurs at the restricted end range only. Restricted end range may be accompanied by the subjective perception of mechanically impeded end range. If discomfort *is not present* at the restricted end range, overpressure creates it, but this discomfort resolves when loading at the restricted end range ceases. If discomfort *is present* at the restricted end range, overpressure increases it, but again, this increased discomfort resolves when overpressure at the restricted end range ceases. The centralization response does not occur. If the peripheralization response occurs, it is experienced only during motions containing a component that achieves the restricted end range of the flexion movement plane direction. Typical of the dysfunction pattern, symptoms that peripheralize do not persist after cessation of loading at the restricted end range of flexion.

Dy.S. MOVEMENT PLANE-SPECIFIC RESPONSES

Loading in the symptomatic movement plane direction does not result in mechanical or symptomatic responses within the opposite movement plane direction or other movement planes. Conversely, loading in the opposite direction of the symptomatic movement plane direction, or in another movement plane, has *no effect* on the mechanical or symptomatic responses in the symptomatic movement plane direction.

Frequent static or dynamic loading at or to the restricted end range helps resolve the syndrome over time. Static or dynamic loading in the opposite direction of the same movement plane, or in another movement plane, serves no therapeutic benefit. The only therapeutic action is that of pursuing the symptomatic premature end range. All other movements or positionings are equally ineffective regarding resolution of the syndrome.

Dy.S. PREFERRED LOADING STRATEGY

In the Dysfunction Syndrome, pursuing the symptomatic restricted end range is of paramount importance. Avoiding the symptomatic restricted end-range perpetuates the syndrome and perhaps permits the mechanically limited end range to become more restricted in the future. Daily frequent and repetitive motion to the symptomatic end range is required to resolve this condition, which generally occurs slowly over 6 to 20 weeks.

Dy.S. REASONS FOR FAILURE OF PATIENT STRATEGIES

Patients may avoid the restricted end range because of the discomfort involved as well as the proprioceptive cue of reaching the limits of motion. In so doing, they avoid "therapeutically beneficial" restricted end-range discomfort and perpetuate the Dysfunction Syndrome.

Pain or anti-inflammatory medication cannot correct the mechanical problem underlying this syndrome, which requires restricted end-range loading for its resolution.

Dy.S. HYPOTHESIZED PATHOANATOMY

As a result of chronic postural habits that avoid bringing spinal joints to certain end ranges, or as the result of tissue damage leading to scar formation, *adaptive shortening* or *dysfunction* of tissue may occur. A loss of elasticity occurs causing *restriction* of spinal movement. If a perfectly normal elbow is cast in a flexed position for 1 month, the ability to extend it is restricted when the cast is removed, an example of the dysfunction behaviors just described.

Scar tissue, which shortens over time, may form at the site of disk derangement or spinal surgery. After significant derangement or surgical intervention, an *adherent nerve root* may develop, exhibiting the typical mechanical and symptomatic responses of the dysfunction syndrome. The adherent nerve root condition may involve the peripheralization of symptoms to an extremity without an associated "centralization response." This peripheralization response occurs at the *restricted end range* of the flexion movement plane direction only. Other special conditions must accompany this end-range flexion to elicit adherent nerve root responses; e.g., extended knee for the lumbar spine and lateral flexion of the cervical spine combined with shoulder abduction. The peripheralization response noted with the adherent nerve root does not remain after the precipitating loading actions cease. Treatment is fashioned according to the preferred loading strategy for dysfunction; i.e., evoking the discomfort at end range, which, in this case, involves peripheralization of symptoms.

Dy.S. RELATED TERMINOLOGY

The particular Dysfunction Syndrome is named according to the movement plane direction limited by *restricted end range*. Examples include the following:

- Extension dysfunction
- Flexion dysfunction (includes "adherent nerve root")
- Right rotation dysfunction
- Left rotation dysfunction
- Right lateral flexion dysfunction
- Left lateral flexion dysfunction

• Right side-gliding dysfunction
• Left side-gliding dysfunction

Typically, rotation and lateral flexion dysfunctions apply to the cervical spine, whereas the side-gliding dysfunctions apply to the lumbosacral spine.

Because of the predominance of flexion in the industrial lifestyle, extension dysfunctions develop commonly in the lower cervical spine and lumbosacral spine by middle age. Because of poor sitting posture, protraction of the head occurs, which involves extension of the upper cervical spine. Flexion dysfunction of the upper cervical spine commonly occurs as a result.

Dy.S. SUMMARY

The cause of the syndrome is shortened, nonelastic structures that restrict spinal movement. Resolution involves stretching these structures. The loss of range of motion or deviation from the intended movement plane direction results from inelasticity. Avoiding symptoms only perpetuates the syndrome and may, in fact, slowly enable it to develop further by approximating the ends of structures that are then permitted to shorten further. Frequent and repetitive elicitation of discomfort is required to improve quality of movement. Peripheralization to the extremity occurs only when the healing process subsequent to disk injury or surgery results in the tethering of neurologic structures, which limits and is challenged by the movement plane direction of flexion. Therefore, adherent nerve root is a subcategory of flexion dysfunction.

For didactic purposes, this syndrome has been described as displaying symptomatic responses at a restricted end range that cease once loading at that end range ceases. For all intents and purposes, this description is true. To differentiate this syndrome from the Derangement Syndrome, however, one must be cognizant of the possibility of a symptomatic response that will not cease should overstretching occur. Such symptomatology is considered evidence of an inflammatory response to overstretching and damaging tissue. The potential inflammatory response to overstretching shortened tissue must be kept in mind to differentiate this contingency from the constant symptomatic response attributable to mechanical factors of the Derangement Syndrome.

Derangement Syndrome

De.S. MECHANICAL AND SYMPTOMATIC RESPONSES

Symptomatic and mechanical responses characterize the Derangement Syndrome.

De.S. FREQUENCY OF RESPONSES (COMPLAINTS)

Responses may be intermittent or constant.

De.S. POINT OF RESPONSE ELICITATION

Responses are elicited at mechanically impeded end range(s) of the *obstructed end range* variety, at mechanically unim-peded end range(s), during midrange motion, or during midrange static loading.

De.S. LOADING TIME REQUIRED TO ELICIT A RESPONSE

The Derangement Syndrome may exhibit immediate elicitation or delayed onset of symptomatic and mechanical responses at the obstructed end range, at mechanically unimpeded end ranges, during motion, or with midrange static loading.

De.S. RESPONSE PERSISTENCE AFTER LOADING CESSATION

Responses or behaviors elicited as a result of loading at an obstructed end range, at a mechanically unimpeded end range, during midrange motion, or with midrange static loading may remain after the loading tactic responsible is terminated. This persistence is typical of the *Derangement Syndrome* which is the only syndrome with constant symptoms, especially those of peripheralization.

De.S. RATE OF SYNDROME RESOLUTION

The characteristic responses of the Derangement Syndrome may change rapidly and radically during the time provided for the initial evaluation. Resolution of this syndrome may be possible within a matter of days.

De.S. RESPONSES DURING MOTION

The obstructed end range may be significant enough to prevent curve reversal. An obstructed end range exists in at least one movement plane direction, and may exist in multiple movement plane directions. Deviation from the intended movement plane direction or symptoms during motion may be noted. The centralization or peripheralization responses may be noted during motion.

De.S. RESPONSES AT MECHANICALLY UNIMPEDED END RANGES

Deviation from an intended movement plane direction and/or symptoms may occur. Overpressure may change mechanical and/or symptomatic behavior. The centralization response does not occur; the peripheralization response may occur.

De.S. RESPONSES AT MECHANICALLY IMPEDED END RANGES

Obstructed end ranges may occur in a single or in multiple movement plane directions. If an obstructed end range occurs in more than one movement plane direction, responses at the individual obstructed end range may affect each other. Mechanical and symptomatic responses may be elicited immediately or exhibit delayed onset as a result of loading at the obstructed end range. Deviation from the intended movement plane direction may occur at the obstructed end range as well as at the unimpeded end range. Loading at the obstructed end range may be accompanied by the subjective perception of a mechanically impeded end range.

If discomfort *is not present* at the obstructed end range, overpressure may create it, and this discomfort may then exhibit a centralization or peripheralization response. If discomfort *is present,* overpressure may increase or decrease it, as well as precipitate a centralization or peripheralization response. The centralization or peripheralization responses may occur at obstructed end ranges. Centralization occurs only in movement plane directions (during motion or at end range) that contain the "key" obstructed end range.

De.S. MOVEMENT PLANE-SPECIFIC RESPONSES

Loading in a symptomatic or asymptomatic movement plane direction may change mechanical and/or symptomatic responses of the opposite movement plane direction or of another movement plane direction. These changes may be therapeutically beneficial or detrimental.

In the Derangement Syndrome, the therapeutically beneficial loading action to pursue involves loading at the "key" obstructed end range. In other words, if there is more than one obstructed end range, loading at one obstructed end range may be therapeutically beneficial, whereas loading at another may be therapeutically detrimental or neutral. If there is only one obstructed end range, that is the "key." Avoiding therapeutically detrimental obstructed end ranges, movement plane directions, or other loading tactics is of paramount importance in resolving this syndrome.

In general, the *centralization response* is noted as a result of loading motions toward or static loading at the "key" obstructed end range. Symptoms generally do not occur during motion within the movement plane direction that leads to the "key" obstructed end range, especially after the first few cycles of dynamic loading are accomplished. As discussed previously, a rapidly retreating obstructed end range may mimic symptoms during motion, when in fact symptoms are occurring at a rapidly resolving obstructed end range.

The *peripheralization response* is noted as a result of loading motions toward or at end ranges that do not contain the key obstructed end range. These end ranges may be mechanically unimpeded or may contain obstructions that are not reduced as a result of loading and, in fact, may become worse.

De.S. PREFERRED LOADING STRATEGY

Pursuing and avoiding certain loading tactics, as well as the order in which they are accomplished, is critical in the care of this syndrome.

In general, symptomatic responses are pursued if characterized by the centralization response and avoided if characterized by the peripheralization response. The "key" obstructed end range is the one that exhibits the centralization response when pursued. Avoided are obstructed end ranges, mechanically unimpeded end ranges, or loading within movement plane directions that evidence the peripheralization response. Avoidance of loading tactics that elicit the peripheralization response is not sufficient, as loading at the key obstructed end range may still not be accomplished.

The preferred loading strategy revolves around reducing the key obstruction. This effort may be accompanied by the rapid resolution of symptoms, or by the temporary increased symptomatology of the centralization response, after which symptoms resolve.

Phenomena related to the resolution of derangements exhibit varying degrees of complexity. The simplest case involves only one obstructed end range in the sagittal plane, which is the key obstructed end range. The centralization response may be noted at the obstructed end range. The peripheralization response is elicited typically by means of loading within the opposite movement plane direction. Peripheralization by means of loading in the movement plane direction opposite to that of the obstructed end range may be elicited immediately or by delayed onset; i.e., mechanically unimpeded flexion may peripheralize, whereas extension to the obstructed end range centralizes. The less common, but opposite simple sagittal pattern, may also be found.

More complex situations entailing multiple *obstructed end ranges,* of which only one is the key, may mandate an initial preferred loading strategy within a coronal or transverse movement plane. Consider a case involving an obstructed end range in one sagittal movement plane direction, as well as an obstructed end range in one coronal movement plane direction. In such cases, it is possible that loading in both the unimpeded and obstructed sagittal movement plane directions elicits the peripheralization response. Loading in the coronal or transverse movement plane is at first required to elicit the centralization response. Subsequently, loading in the sagittal plane becomes necessary for further resolution of the syndrome.

It is possible in cases involving multiple obstructed movement plane directions, for loading at a single (key) obstructed end range to resolve all obstructions, without requiring the sequential end range loading just described.

De.S. REASONS FOR FAILURE OF PATIENT STRATEGIES

The centralization response that occurs at the key obstructed end range may entail a significant increase or creation of central symptoms, which patients understandably avoid. Because the centralization response is associated with an increase of more central spinal symptoms, patients may choose the therapeutically detrimental strategy of pursuing loading tactics that diminish spinal discomfort, even though lesser peripheral symptomatic complaints and significant mechanical disorders are perpetuated.

De.S. HYPOTHESIZED PATHOANATOMY

The model for this syndrome is the derangement of intradiscal material or substance, whether it is solid (nuclear, annular), liquid (water, electrolytes, etc.), or gaseous (e.g., nitrogen). The behavior of symptoms and mechanics changes according to migration and/or accumulation of intradiscal substance or material in the anterior, posterior, or lateral aspects of the intervertebral disk space.

Imagine a simple case in which intradiscal material deranged in a posterior direction, causing obstructed end range to extension. Flexion would remain unobstructed but would further promote this posterior derangement, eliciting peripheralization during, or at the end range of, the derangement-promoting flexion movement plane direction. The *centralization response* would accompany extension with overpressure, as the derangement becomes reduced. The reverse case could be imagined as well.

Consider a more complex situation in which intradiscal material migrated in a posterolateral direction; flexion may further this migration. An obstructed end range could exist not only for extension, but also for side-gliding as well. If the lateral component is significant, extension may only serve to squeeze this material more to the side. In this case, both the mechanically unimpeded flexion and the obstructed extension could elicit the peripheralization response. Loading in the coronal (side-gliding) or the transverse movement plane direction (rotation) may be needed to reduce the key lateral obstruction and elicit the centralization response. After this step, the previously avoided extension component becomes the key obstruction, and loading in extension may be needed to further promote the centralization response. The lateral component has been reduced sufficiently, and the task is then to reduce the posterior component.

When disk material has migrated, both posteriorly and laterally, obstructed end ranges exist in the respective sagittal and coronal movement plane directions. If loading in the movement plane direction of extension reduces both of the obstructed end ranges, the lateral component is not considered *relevant*. If loading in the coronal movement plane direction *is required* first, the lateral component of disk migration is considered *relevant* to a loading strategy involving a nonsagittal movement plane.

RELATED TERMINOLOGY

Postural Syndrome terminology is predicated on the positioning that precipitates symptoms. Dysfunction Syndrome terminology is predicated on the movement of the person that precipitates symptoms. Derangement Syndrome terminology refers, in part, to the *anatomic* direction of intradiscal derangement. In contrast to the Postural and Dysfunction Syndromes, *two* classification systems are used to organize Derangement Syndrome phenomena.

Similar to the Postural and Dysfunction Syndromes, the first method describes derangements based strictly on the behavior of mechanics and symptoms in response to loading tactics, and names these behavior patterns by patho-anatomic inferences—*derangement behavior nomenclature*. The second method refers to the presenting symptom topography and deformities, in addition to the derangement behaviors—*derangement behavior-topography-deformity (BTD) nomenclature*.

Derangement Behavior Nomenclature. This terminology is descriptive of the anatomic direction in which the intradis-

cal derangement is thought to have occurred. Stated another way, it is descriptive of behaviors noted *as if* derangement of intradiscal material occurred in the described anatomic direction.

The Derangement Syndromes are named according to the hypothesized anatomic direction in which disk material travelled and caused an obstructed end range: anterior, posterior, and lateral derangements.

Anterior derangement describes behaviors *as if* anterior migration of intradiscal material occurred. An accumulation in the anterior compartment of the disk makes flexion mechanically difficult to perform. In extreme cases, lordosis is fixed and irreversible. Extension promotes the migration of material to the anterior compartment. Extension may be accompanied by peripheralization of symptoms during motion or at end range as a result of deranging material anteriorly. Any limitation of extension would be due to intolerance of symptoms but not to mechanically impeded end range. Peripheralization generally does not occur below the knee because the nerve radicals are not affected by distortion of the anterior aspect of the annulus. Flexion is obstructed and accompanied by symptoms at obstructed end range. Flexion to obstructed end range with overpressure is accompanied by the centralization response corresponding to a redistribution of intradiscal material to a more central location, resulting in improved biomechanics as well.

Posterior derangement describes behaviors *as if* posterior migration of intradiscal material occurred. An accumulation in the posterior compartment of the disk makes extension mechanically difficult to perform. In extreme cases, kyphosis is fixed and irreversible. Flexion promotes the migration of materials to the posterior compartment. Flexion may be accompanied by peripheralization of symptoms during motion or at end range as a result of deranging material posteriorly. Any limitation of flexion would be due to intolerance of symptoms but not to mechanically impeded end range. The peripheralization could extend below the knee, because the nerve radicals or spinal cord may be affected by distortion of the posterior aspect of the annulus. Extension is obstructed and accompanied by symptoms at obstructed end range. Extension to obstructed end range with overpressure is accompanied by the centralization phenomena, during which intradiscal material redistributes to a more central location, resulting in improved biomechanics as well.

Lateral derangement may occur alone or in combination with anterior or posterior derangement; most frequently, it occurs in combination with the latter. Unilateral symptoms, especially if they peripheralize, are assumed to have a lateral component. If dynamic and/or static loading in the sagittal plane centralizes symptoms, it is not considered a "relevant" lateral component, i.e., the "key" obstructed end range is in the sagittal plane. If the unilateral techniques of side-gliding or rotation are required to centralize symptoms, it is considered a relevant lateral component, i.e., the lateral component is the "key" obstructed end range. With a relevant lateral component, it is thought that an accumulation of intradiscal material to one side or the other of the coronal plane is sufficient to require a unilateral loading technique. When there is a "relevant" lateral component, movement in the sagittal plane not only may fail to elicit the centralization phenomena, but also may actually elicit the peripheralization response if further lateral migration of intradiscal material results. After rotation or side-gliding is performed to reduce the lateral component in these cases, the situation may require sagittal plane techniques to reduce the central anterior or posterior derangement.

An accumulation of disk material in the lateral compartment resists side-gliding to that side because of the obstructed end range. In extreme cases, a list or lateral shift is fixed and irreversible. Side-gliding in the movement plane direction of the patient's lateral shift has the potential of promoting the further migration of intradiscal material, accompanied by peripheralization of symptoms during motion or at end range as a result of deranging material more laterally. Any limitation of movement in the direction of the lateral shift relates to intolerance of symptoms and not to a mechanically impeded end range. Peripheralization may occur below the knee because the nerve radicals are easily affected by lateral distortions of the annulus when a posterior component is present as well. Side-gliding in the movement plane direction opposite to the lateral shift is obstructed and accompanied by symptoms at the obstructed end range. Side-gliding to the obstructed end range with overpressure is accompanied by the centralization response corresponding to a redistribution of intradiscal material to a more central location, resulting in improved biomechanics as well.

Derangement Behavior-Topography-Deformity (BTD) Nomenclature. This terminology uses a numeric system, labeling various derangement presentations from 1 through 7.

The first subclassification of the derangements is according to their *behavior,* as described previously. Derangements 1 through 6 are posterior derangements, Derangement 7 is an anterior derangement.

Derangements 1 through 6 are arranged in couplets, with the odd numbers describing symptom *topography,* and the subsequent even-numbered derangements describing the same symptom topography accompanying a fixed deformity (antalgia or deviation) of the spine, preventing curve reversal. Therefore, the derangement number indicates its behavior, symptom topography, and presence or lack of deformity.

This derangement nomenclature is defined as follows:

Derangement One:
- Central or symmetric symptoms about the spine
- Rarely shoulder/arm or buttocks/thigh symptoms
- No deformity

Derangement Two:
- Central or symmetric symptoms about the spine
- With or without shoulder/arm or buttocks/thigh symptoms
- With deformity of kyphosis

Derangement Three:
- Unilateral or asymmetric symptoms about the spine
- With or without shoulder/arm or buttocks/thigh symptoms
- No deformity

Derangement Four:
- Unilateral or asymmetric symptoms about the spine
- With or without shoulder/arm or buttocks/thigh symptoms
- With deformity of torticollis or lumbar scoliosis

Derangement Five:
- Unilateral or asymmetric symptoms about the spine
- With or without shoulder/arm or buttocks/thigh symptoms
- With symptoms extending below the elbow or knee
- No deformity

Derangement Six:
- Unilateral or asymmetric symptoms about the spine
- With or without shoulder/arm or buttocks/thigh symptoms
- With symptoms extending below the elbow or knee
- With deformity of acute kyphosis, torticollis, or lumbar scoliosis

Derangement Seven:
- Symmetric or asymmetric symptoms about the spine
- With or without shoulder/arm or buttocks/thigh symptoms
- Deformity of accentuated lordosis may or may not be present

The "couplet" system of symptom topography, without and with deformity, does not extend to the anterior derangements. An anterior derangement with central symptoms, unilateral symptoms, without deformity or with deformity, is classified as a derangement seven. The BTD nomenclature is reduced to behavior nomenclature only for anterior derangements, which are assigned the number 7.

PARTIAL PATTERNS OF DERANGEMENT

One distinguishing feature of the Derangement Syndrome is the exhibition of partial patterns. Because of the complex mechanical and symptomatic responses associated with the Derangement Syndrome, the absence of some of the typical derangement responses does not diminish the ability to recognize this syndrome. Examples of partial behavior patterns of derangement are as follows:

- Peripheralization response persists without the ability to elicit a centralization response
- Peripheralization response persists after sustained end range loading only; no peripheralization elicited during movement
- Centralization response persists without the ability to elicit a peripheralization response
- Peripheralization response resolves without any clear pattern of centralization response
- No peripheralization, centralization, or other symptom changes; however, mechanical responses occur
- No mechanical responses occur; however, symptomatic responses do occur

SUMMARY

The goal in the Derangement Syndrome is to reduce the derangement of intradiscal material by having it migrate back toward the center of the disk space. Obstructed end range in purely anterior or posterior derangements occurs in one movement plane direction. Obstructed end range can exist in more than one movement plane direction with either relevant or nonrelevant lateral components. If obstruction to movement in the coronal plane is eliminated by loading in the sagittal plane, the lateral (coronal) component is not considered relevant.

Intermittent symptomatic responses with a Derangement Syndrome may involve repetitive reduction and derangement of disk material in response to the patient's movements and positionings during the day. A constant symptomatic response involving the Derangement Syndrome represents a mechanical displacement of disk material not reduced by the usual movements and positionings of the patient. Prescriptive loading (a preferred loading strategy) at the key obstructed end range is often successful in reducing Derangement Syndromes in these latter cases.

Relationships Between Syndromes

In a sense, the preferred loading strategy for the Derangement Syndrome combines those of the Postural and Dysfunction syndromes, inasmuch as certain discomforts must be avoided and certain discomforts must be pursued. Typically, a mechanically unimpeded end range is avoided while a mechanically impeded end range is pursued. Therefore, the sharp distinction made between the syndromes may be, instead, diffuse lines of demarcation; certain properties of one may merge into the other.

MIXED SYNDROMES

In the previous descriptions of syndromes, each is presented as if it exists "by itself." In clinical practice, multiple syndromes may coexist, and all three may be seen in one patient.

SIMILAR SYMPTOMS, DIFFERENT RESPONSES

The importance of investigating mechanical and symptomatic responses to loading tactics cannot be overemphasized. Information concerning a single mechanical or symptomatic response to a single loading tactic is not the necessary and sufficient condition by which to diagnose a syndrome. Symptoms associated with sitting may be attributable to a postural syndrome of sustained flexion, a flexion dysfunction syndrome, the promotion of a posterior derangement, or the reduction of an anterior derangement. Symptoms associated with standing may be associated with a sustained extension postural syndrome, an extension dysfunction, the promotion of an anterior derangement, or the reduction of a posterior derangement. A thorough investigation of mechanical and symptomatic responses to loading helps to differentiate among these possible causative factors.

The *peripheralization response* may occur during the Dysfunction Syndrome or during the Derangement Syndrome. It does not occur during the Postural Syndrome. The peripheralization response with a Dysfunction Syndrome rarely persists after cessation of the loading action that precipitates it, and this loading action typically has a component of flexion to end range. In the Derangement Syndrome, peripheralization may occur at any point of a movement plane that promotes the derangement, and peripheral complaints typically persist after being elicited. The peripheralization response of derangement is typically associated with centralization responses. The peripheralization response of dysfunction is not.

APPROPRIATENESS OF MANIPULATION

Manipulation, within the McKenzie approach, is considered inappropriate in movement plane directions that do not possess mechanically impeded end ranges. Therefore, manipulation is inappropriate for the Postural Syndrome. Only postural correction is warranted.

Regarding the Dysfunction Syndrome, manipulation may be contraindicated at first, because of the danger of overstretching shortened tissue. Symptomatic responses to loading persist only when shortened tissue is stretched too fast or too far, causing tissue injury that results in chemical, nonmechanical inflammatory pain. During a manipulative thrust on a patient with a Dysfunction Syndrome, the operator may feel as if he or she has "bounced off" as a result of the resistance offered by shortened structures. In the Dysfunction Syndrome, manipulation is appropriate only after the adaptive shortening has been reduced significantly. Manipulation is inappropriate as a main form of therapy in this syndrome because of the need to stretch this tissue repetitively during the course of the day over many weeks. This effort is best accomplished by patients themselves.

The Derangement Syndrome best represents the chiropractic concept of the manipulatable lesion or subluxation. Movement of the intradiscal substance results in asymmetric relationships of joint surfaces. The supposition that the disk is responsible for this disrelationship was noted by Gonstead,[4] although the criteria on which he predicated manipulation were radiographic findings and not the mechanical and symptomatic responses to loading the spine. The mechanical and symptomatic responses to end-range loading mobilizations (taking the slack out) performed by the patient *or* the clinician predict what the responses will be to manipulation according to similar loading strategies. A lack of response or a detrimental response to patient-generated or clinician mobilizations argues against performing the manipulation, which would represent the same loading strategy, albeit with greater force. Radiographic evaluation or the palpation of "sticky joints" does not afford the clinician this same information. The McKenzie approach recommends manipulation only after self-generated movements have been explored fully and evidence partial therapeutic responses. Loading intensity is then increased by means of clinician overpressure (taking the slack out) and frequency of loading (repetitions) to "test the waters" as to the potential benefit or detriment of manipulative thrusts. It is important to note that the movement plane direction of the manipulation contemplated is determined by mechnical and symptomatic responses to loading, including patient-generated movements, patient reports concerning centralization, and both patient and clinician observations concerning mechanical observations.

Lastly, regarding the relationship to chiropractic, the McKenzie approach does not claim to be the first or only approach to include the movement plane direction of extension as a therapeutic possibility. Reinart[5] referred to extension exercise technique, therapy, and theory at least as early as 1962. The distinguishing feature of the McKenzie approach is not the advocacy of extension in selected cases, but the fact that treatment is predicated on mechanical and symptomatic responses to loading. In many cases, extension is indicated; however, in many cases, movements *other than* extension are what is required. The McKenzie approach is equated incorrectly with an exclusive predilection for extension. The approach makes no a priori, dogmatic conclusions about what every spine needs, which is perhaps the greatest virtue of its clinical reasoning.

APPROPRIATENESS OF PROGRESSIVE RESISTANCE EXERCISES

The McKenzie approach permits a thorough exploration of which movement plane directions may be pursued and which must be avoided, based on the mechanical and symptomatic responses to spinal loading. A progressive resistance exercise program is often possible much sooner than would otherwise be permitted because the clinician possesses a clear understanding of how a patients' spine reacts to movement and positioning at the outset of such a program.

THE McKENZIE APPROACH AND DEMANDS OF REHABILITATION

The McKenzie approach distinguishes itself among other rehabilitation methods as being useful to patients with either acute or chronic spine-related complaints. As such, it is often an appropriate first step before considering passive therapy or other activity therapies. When explored first, it often proves passive therapy is gratuitous and safely guides the course of subsequent activity therapies, such as strengthening routines.

"Rehabilitation," to some, equates to therapy in general, *any* kind of therapy. Used in this manner, the term loses its intended meaning and is even applied to passive methods, such as hot packs and ultrasound. Rehabilitation is not *any* means to functional ends, but signifies *functional* means to functional ends.

The key concepts defining rehabilitation relate to establishing an individual's skill to be able to "maintain a maximum level of independent functioning such as self care and employment."[6] In rehabilitation, the actions of the patient are of paramount importance. Guidance is provided by the practitioner, but the burden of treatment involves what the patient *does,* and not what is *done* to the patient.

Functional restoration,[7] work conditioning,[8] and work hardening[9] programs use this strict definition of rehabilitation. The approach stresses the physical and psychologic advantages of rehabilitation defined as activity.

The physical advantages of these programs involve reactivating the individual who may have become fearful of movement and consequently deconditioned.[10] The psychologic advantage is to reverse or prevent abnormal illness behavior,[11] helping the patient identify with societal and worker roles rather than the role of a patient as "a passive receptacle of care."[12]

Functional restoration, work conditioning, and work hardening programs are used on chronic cases. Often patients are referred to such programs after passive methods, medication, or no therapy at all (the tincture of time) fail to resolve the chronic condition. In these circumstances, passive care has not helped the individual, but may have actually "encouraged musculoskeletal morbidity."[6]

Patients presenting to "rehabilitation" centers with acute conditions often receive passive therapy initially.[13] This therapy continues until the demands of an activity program (e.g., progressive weight resistance) can be tolerated without harm. The disadvantage of such initial passive care is that it may ultimately serve a purpose contrary to that of the physical and psychologic goals of rehabilitation. Passive therapy, if introduced first, has the potential of "spoiling" the patient's chances of progressing to unassisted, active functional activities as therapy,[14] and increases the possibility of the development of abnormal illness behaviors.[15] Some authors[16] state that much low back disability is iatrogenic and results from the medical prescription of rest for simple backache that is based on the misconception that inflammation or other pathologic change plays a significant role as a causative factor.

A rehabilitation approach in the acute phase can provide the physical and psychologic benefits of functional restoration and work conditioning/hardening programs that are used to treat chronic disorders. It can, thereby, prevent the need to resolve chronic conditions by not letting them develop in the first place. The McKenzie approach satisfies these requirements. It provides self-treatment activity techniques tolerable during the acute phase that entail the physical and psychologic benefits of more expensive and lengthier rehabilitation programs. It may even prevent the need for such subsequent rehabilitation programs, as it employs many of the same physical and psychologic principles.

If functional restoration or work conditioning/hardening programs are needed subsequently, the initial use of the McKenzie protocols is likely to enhance the possibilities of their success, because these programs are a conceptually consistent continuum from the initial acute care activity therapy. Through its physical effect, the McKenzie approach addresses the mechanical nature of the patient's disorder. Through its teaching of mechanical principles of self-treatment, it is consistent with the principles of rehabilitation that prevent the development of abnormal illness behavior.

The patient learns that therapeutic movement and positioning may be accompanied by increased pain with improved function, and that certain pains are not to be avoided. Congruent with the strictest rehabilitation principles is the "hands off" first approach. If results are limited, the application of passive approaches is always possible, but the control of treatment is returned to the patient as soon as possible.

Regarding the mechanical and physiologic principles of rehabilitation, the McKenzie approach makes activity and self treatment possible during the acute phase, permitting continuous, relatively passive spinal motion to be strategically performed by the patient. These movements enhance the organization of "new" tissue along the lines of stress, with the formation of flexible scar tissue.[17] Tasks are introduced on a demand-graded basis.

If McKenzie activity therapy is dispensed during the acute phase, fear of pain and the signs of pain avoidance or illness behaviors are not encouraged,[10] and the protracted treatment intervention for patients with chronic disorders is avoided. That it is of potential benefit during the acute phase should not subtract from considering McKenzie protocols as the logical first step for the treatment of chronic conditions, for the same reasons just given. If strength training is not needed for treatment of a chronic condition, the McKenzie protocol represents a relatively quick and inexpensive alternative.

The McKenzie protocol is an excellent intervention to prevent physical and psychologic complications of injuries. It includes individuals taking an active, responsible role in rehabilitation appropriate to their level of functioning, improvement in physical functioning rather than simply concentrating on symptomatic relief, safety practices, maintaining the worker role through minimal time away from the work place, activity control of symptoms as opposed to symptomatic control of activity, and an attempt to avoid use of analgesics or passive treatment methods.

As stated elsewhere:

"By reducing the use of therapist's technique in the initial stages of treatment and maximizing patient technique, the patient will recognize that his recovery is largely the result of his own efforts. Few patients fail to assume responsibility for active participation in their treatment, providing the instruction and education process is firmly and vigorously pursued."[18]

"If there is the slightest chance that a patient can be educated in a method of treatment that enables him to reduce his own pain and disability using his own understanding and resources, he should receive that education. Every patient is entitled to this information, and every therapist should be obliged to provide it."[19]

REFERENCES

1. McKenzie RA. The lumbar spine: Mechanical Diagnosis and Therapy. Waikanae, New Zealand, Spinal Publications, 1981.
2. McKenzie RA: The Cervical and Thoracic Spine: Mechanical Diagnosis and Therapy. Waikanae, New Zealand, Spinal Publications, 1990.
3. Haldeman S: North American Spine Society: Failure of the pathology model to predict back pain. Spine 15:718, 1990.
4. Herbst RW: Gonstead chiropractic science and art. Mt. Horeb, WI, Sci-Chi Publications, 1980.
5. Barrale R, Diamond R, Filson R, et al: Manipulative management lumbar disc bulge. Chiro Tech 1:87, 1989.
6. Deutsch P, Sawer H: Guide to Rehabilitation. New York, Matthew Bender & Co., pp 39–40, Suppl & Rev 1989.
7. Mayer T, Gatchel R: Functional Restoration for Spinal Disorders: The Sports Medicine Approach to Low Back Pain. Philadelphia, Lea & Febiger, 1988.
8. Isernhagen S: Work hardening or work conditioning—what's in a name. Indust Rehabil Q II(2);7, 1989.
9. Matheson LN, Kemp BJ: Work hardening: Occupational therapy in industrial rehabilitation. Am J Occup Ther 39:314, 1985.
10. Troup J: The perception of musculoskeletal pain and incapacity for work: Prevention and early treatment. Physiotherapy 74:435, 1988.
11. Pilowsky I: Abnormal illness behaviour. Psychiatr Med 5:85, 1987.
12. Saal J: Intervertebral disk herniation in nonoperative treatment. In Physical Medicine and Rehabilitation: State of the Art Reviews. Philadelphia, Hanley & Bellfus, 1990, p 185.
13. Mitchell RI, Carmen GM: Intensive active exercise program. Spine 15:514, 1990.
14. Dereberry VJ, Tullis WH: Delayed recovery in the patient with a work compensable injury. J Occup Med 25:829, 1983.
15. Waddell G: A new clinical model for the treatment of low-back pain. Spine 12:632, 1987.
16. Allan DB, Waddell G: An historical perspective on low back pain and disability. Acta Orthop Scand 60(Suppl 234), 1989.
17. Evans P: The healing process at cellular level. Physiotherapy 66:8, 1980.
18. McKenzie RA: The Cervical and Thoracic Spine: Mechanical Diagnosis and Therapy. Waikanae, New Zealand, Spinal Publications, 1990, p 103.
19. McKenzie RA: The Cervical and Thoracic Spine: Mechanical Diagnosis and Therapy. Waikanae, New Zealand, Spinal Publications, 1990, p 113.

13 Manual Resistance Techniques and Self-Stretches for Improving Flexibility/Mobility

CRAIG LIEBENSON

The original manual resistance techniques (MRT) have their origin in the proprioceptive neuromuscular facilitation (PNF) philosophy of physical therapy and the muscle energy procedures (MEP) of the osteopathy. These techniques involve manual resistance of a patient's isometric or isotonic muscular effort. This resisted effort is typically followed by a stretch of a tight or tense muscle. The MRT are primarily used to relax overactive muscles or to stretch shortened muscles and their associated fascia. Many different methods have been developed depending on the clinical goal. To achieve these positive clinical effects, MRT take advantage of two physiologic phenomena: postcontraction inhibition and reciprocal inhibition (RI). The MRT are invaluable workhorses in the rehabilitation of the motor system.

These techniques are also used to facilitate or train an inhibited or weak muscle. Because the doctor or therapist provides the resistance, precise patient positioning and movement can be controlled to a degree not possible with machines or even free weights. Manual contacts also allow for proprioceptive stimulation to facilitate an inhibited muscle during active resistance. The value of clinician control over resistance exercise cannot be underestimated, especially when the goal of improved coordination is as important as that of strengthening.

Publications about the use of PNF to facilitate neurologically weak muscles first appeared in the late 1940s.[1] Soon, other reports followed, stating that spasticity responded to this type of therapy as well.[2] This positive response led to the development of various forms of PNF (i.e., hold-relax, contract-relax, etc.) that could be used for orthopedic as well as neurologic problems. The osteopaths primarily used muscle energy procedures (MEP) to mobilize joints. They also developed a variety of applications designed to stretch shortened muscular and connective tissues and to strengthen weak muscles.[3]

Manual medicine practitioners in Europe were not far behind in incorporating these new methods. Gaymans and Lewit[4] wrote of success in applying these techniques for joint mobilization using specific eye movements and respiratory synkinesis to enhance the physiologic effectiveness of the procedures (see Chapter 11). Later, Lewit[5] focused on a gentle muscle relaxation technique, termed post-isometric relaxation (similar to hold-relax), which was applied to the contractile portion of an overactive muscle.

NEUROMUSCULAR AND BIOMECHANICAL BASIS OF FLEXIBILITY TRAINING

Two aspects to MRT are their ability to relax an overactive muscle (increased neuromuscular tension or "spasm") and their ability to enhance stretch of a shortened muscle or its associated fascia, when connective tissue or viscoelastic changes have occurred. When using MRT, it is important to relax the neuromuscular (contractile) component before attempting any aggressive stretching maneuver. Often a "release phenomena" occurs so that a length change occurs automatically after merely relaxing excessive neuromuscular tension (see Chapter 11). In such cases, treatment serves as a diagnostic test, differentiating neuromuscular (contractile) from connective tissue (noncontractile) problems. Even if noncontractile pathologic changes have occurred, it is still wise to relax the neuromuscular apparatus before stretching. This step will inhibit the stretch reflex and allow the patient to tolerate more vigorous stretching.

Two fundamental neurophysiologic principles account for the neuromuscular inhibition that occurs during application of these techniques. The first is postcontraction inhibition, which states that after a muscle is contracted, it is automatically in a relaxed state for a brief, latent period. The second is RI (reciprocal inhibition), which states that when one muscle is contracted, its antagonist is automatically inhibited. For instance, if the quadriceps is contracted, the hamstrings are inhibited, thus allowing for easier stretching of the latter muscles. This procedure takes advantage of Sherrington's Law of reciprocal inhibition. The purpose of RI is to allow an agonist (i.e., biceps) to achieve its action (flexion) unimpeded by its antagonist (i.e., triceps). Different explanations have been proposed for how the effects of MRT are achieved. Whereas only postcontraction inhibition and RI have been validated, other suggested mechanisms include autogenic inhibition, Golgi tendon organ stimulation, reciprocal innervation, presynaptic inhibition of Ia afferents, resetting of the gamma system, and postsynaptic inhibition.

It has been demonstrated that the receptors responsible for this inhibition are intramuscular and are not in the skin or joints.[6] Measurements of the Hoffman reflex activity (representative of the excitability of the motor neuron pool) show activity is inhibited for up to 25 to 30 seconds after an agonist or antagonist contraction, whereas inhibition only lasts about 10 seconds during static stretching.[7] This effect has been found to be neurologically mediated and not a result of any mechanical effect.[8]

Muscle fibers also have certain biomechanical characteristics that affect their stiffness. Skeletal muscle fibers are known to adapt to imposed demands. For instance, during growth, muscle length increases as new sarcomeres are added (in series) and individual fibers increase their girth.[9] Prolonged immobilization of a limb joint in an extended or shortened position results in an increase or decrease in the number of sarcomeres, respectively.[9,10] When immobilized in a shortened position, muscle stiffness increases.[10] It has been observed that an increase in connective tissue occurs with immobilization in a shortened position.[11]

Connective tissue proliferation is minimized if the immobilized muscles are placed in a lengthened position or their contractile activity is maintained with electrical stimulation.[10,11] Therefore, either passive stretching or maintenance of contractile activity in immobilized muscles can prevent muscle shortening and connective tissue proliferation.

Shortened muscles that have been immobilized require about 4 weeks of treatment to return to their pre-immobilization length.[10] Muscles stiffness in response to stretch varies on the basis of intrinsic molecular properties of muscle fibers. Muscles that are kept still increase their stiffness twofold in just a few minutes.[12] Conversely, oscillations and isometric or eccentric muscles contractions all reduce muscle stiffness.[12,13] This plasticity of muscle fibers in response to passive or active movements is described as thixotrophic behavior. This thixotrophy relates to changes in viscosity and resistance to deformation of the intrinsic molecular make-up of muscle fibers that result from shaking or stirring motions. Both intrafusal and extrafusal muscle fibers have thixotrophic properties.[14]

Thixotrophic bonds are thought to occur between actin and myosin filaments.[14,15] Such bonds or cross bridges form easily in muscles. According to Hagbarth, "After stretching or passive shortening, it may take 15 minutes or more before muscle fibers spontaneously return to their initial resting length."[14] He also stated, "Strong isometric contractions and muscle stretching maneuvers are likely to dissolve preexisting actomyosin bonds and thereby reduce the inherent stiffness of the extrafusal muscle fibers."[14]

DIFFERENT METHODS

Proprioceptive neuromuscular facilitation (PNF) is the most complex system of MRT.[16] In PNF, neuromuscular reeducation is the goal. *Manual contacts, patient prepositioning, muscle contraction against resistance, irradiation, and verbal commands are all used in concert to begin the process of improving movement.* The inhibitory techniques used most commonly are hold-relax (HR), contract-relax (CR), and rhythmic

stabilization. The HR technique involves isometric resistance and is used mostly for pain relief. Used for relaxing and stretching tight muscles and related soft tissues, CR incorporates isotonic resistance and multiplanar (usually diagonal) movement. Both agonist and antagonist muscles are used to create a neurophysiologic summation of RI and postcontraction inhibition.

When osteopathic physicians used these procedures, they applied them to mobilize joints, as well as to strengthen and relax muscles, referring to them as muscle energy procedures (MEP).[3] Using a language familiar to chiropractors, they described the area where they felt movement was limited, or if resistance is perceived prematurely after moving a joint through its full available range of motion or lengthening a muscle as far as it will allow, as a "pathologic" barrier (see Fig. 11.3). The MEP were developed by osteopaths as alternatives to thrust manipulation procedures for restricted joint mobility. In these cases, the use of fairly gentle forces are required. They were also used on muscles in a way similar to PNF.

In Europe, manual medicine physicians soon began experimenting with these methods. Gaymans and Lewit[4] wrote of success when using these techniques in an extremely gentle fashion. At first, they used the rhythmic stabilization approach borrowed from PNF. Later, Lewit[5] focused on the HR approach. He found that by positioning an overactive muscle in a full stretch position and then resisting a gentle isometric contraction, excellent relaxation and an improved resting length of the muscle could be achieved regularly. Lewit termed this approach postisometric relaxation (PIR). Gaymans and Lewit[4] also incorporated specific eye movements, asking the patient to look in the direction of contraction and then in the direction of stretch. For most muscles, breathing in facilitates contraction, and exhaling aids relaxation in the overactive muscle. Lewit believed only the gentlest force was required.[5]

Janda used HR with significantly greater forces for treating true muscular and connective tissue shortening.[17] This adaptation, termed postfacilitation stretch (PFS), is for chronically shortened muscles. The patient performs a maximal contraction with the tight muscle from a midrange position. On relaxation, the doctor quickly stretches the muscle, taking out all the slack.

Today, work by Evjenth and Hamberg stands as the most authoritative manual for these muscle stretching procedures.[18] They demonstrate the exact doctor and patient positions for performing HR for each joint and muscle. Other authors have also used MRT, including Holt,[19] describing the scientific

Table 13.1. Manual Resistance Techniques

Proprioceptive neuromuscular facilitation[16]
   Hold-relax
   Contract-relax
   Rhythmic stabilization
Muscle energy procedures[3]
Postisometric relaxation[5]
Postfacilitation stretch[17]

stretching for sport (3 S stretching); Calliet[20], using modified rhythmic stabilization; and Liebenson,[21,22] using active muscle relaxation techniques. The various MRT are summarized in Table 13.1

CLASSIFICATION OF TIGHT OR TENSE MUSCLES

According to Janda, it is possible to divide muscle hypertonicity into a variety of different treatment-specific categories.[23] Muscle dysfunction is typically attributable to either neuromuscular or connective tissue factors. Different types of dysfunction include reflex spasm, interneuron facilitation from joint dysfunction, trigger points, central nervous system influences (i.e., limbic involvement), or gradual overuse (Table 13.2). For a full discussion of these different factors, see Chapter 2.

Making a precise assessment of soft tissue functional pathology helps to guide the treatment decision-making process. In the case of muscle tightness or tension (Table 13.3), specific treatments are appropriate for each different type of dysfunction.

CLINICAL APPLICATION

Manually resisted exercises are the perfect bridge to active care because they take place in the treatment room and the doctor provides appropriate resistance to specific movements that are being trained. When performing MRT, it is helpful to realize that although many different names have been used for different techniques (PNF, MEP, PIR, etc.), there are certain common elements to successful MRT application. The MRT involve isometric, concentric, or eccentric contractions. They are used to relax muscles, stretch muscles or fascia, mobilize joints, or facilitate muscles. The clinical indications for these methods are summarized in Table 13.4

Table 13.2. Classification of Tight or Tense Muscles

Neuromuscular	Connective tissue
Reflex spasm	Overuse muscle tightness
Interneuron	
Trigger point	
Limbric	

Table 13.3. Specific Treatment for Different Types of Muscle Tension/Tightness

Type	Treatment
Reflex	Cause (i.e., remove appendix)
Interneuron	Joint manipulation
Trigger point	PIR or ischemic compression*
Limbic	Yoga, meditation, counseling
Muscle tightness	PFS or eccentric MEP

*Abbreviations: PIR, postisometric relaxation; PFS, postfacilitation stretch; MEP, muscle energy procedures.

Table 13.4. Goals of Manual Resistance Techniques

Muscle inhibition/relaxation/decontraction
Muscle stretch
Fascial stretch
Muscle facilitation
Joint mobilization

Manual resistance techniques have been presented as alternatives to thrust maneuvers, but in the context of this chapter, they are seen primarily as a complement to traditional chiropractic and manual medicine methods. *In as much as overactive or shortened muscles are related to a specific joint dysfunction, applying MRT may result in indirect mobilization of a joint or at least make an adjustment more comfortable and long-lasting for the patient. Thus, their main application is in direct treatment of the muscular component so as to enhance the efficacy of joint adjustments.* For both acute situations, which involve muscular guarding (neuromuscular tension or "spasm"), and chronic cases, which involve muscle and fascial shortening (connective tissue changes), MRT serve as invaluable clinical tools.

These techniques may be used to relax tension in muscles before thrust manipulation. If, however, we desire to stretch shortened muscles or fascia, then chiropractic adjustments should precede any aggressive stretching. Following an adjustment, MRT can be used to reinforce neuromuscular reeducation.

The MRT require active patient participation and are therefore less likely than passive methods to encourage patient dependency. They are, however, more demanding of the patient. Methods involving RI or gentle PIR typically are painless, and, with a little patient education, are simple to perform.

Compared to deep tissue massage and trigger point therapy (myotherapy or receptor tonus), MRT can be a faster and less painful way of reducing increased muscle tension or trigger points, except if the patient has poor coordination or is simply unable to relax. Patients with difficulty relaxing often need moist heat, relaxation and breathing exercises, and some type of gentle, nonpainful massage (i.e., effleurage). The combination of MRT and soft tissue procedures can be used with great effect. For instance, if an area of tension is found as the tissues are being massaged, the patient can be instructed to contract with that tissue. This combination can often overcome even stubborn "knots."

For some patients who cannot tolerate deep soft tissue manipulation (i.e., Rolfing or transverse friction massage), MRT may be used to reduce the sensitivity of the area. Following MRT application, deep massage or ischemic compression techniques usually are tolerable to the patient. Any massage or passive therapy runs the risk of encouraging patient dependency. Their use should always be combined with some form of patient education, exercise, and self-treatment.

Positional release (i.e., strain/counterstrain) or osteopathic functional techniques are preferable to MRT when it is difficult to find an active movement that does not provoke the symptoms. These positional release methods (finding a painless muscle or joint position and holding there) are a painless and effective means to reduce irritability and increase motion in a patient with soft tissue pain.

The MRT and Spray and Stretch have similar goals and may be used interchangeably. Both are considered alternatives to dry needling and injection of anesthetic for relief of painful trigger points or periosteal attachment points.[24] Spray and Stretch is passive and thus may be better in the first stages of treatment when a patient has poor motor control (incoordination and difficulty relaxing). Patients who are cold intolerant may require even more passive methods, such as heat, electrotherapy, osteopathic functional technique, joint mobilization, or massage. Spray and Stretch can be used as an alternative to PFS for lengthening shortened connective tissue. Sometimes Spray and Stretch and various MRT can be combined. Trial and error often determines which approach has a greater inhibitory effect on the muscle. Because of the negative environmental profile of fluoromethanes, PIR and intermittent cold and stretch have been proposed as alternatives.[25]

An alternative to PFS for musculofascial shortening is osteopathic myofascial release method, which typically encompasses lifting the involved soft tissues and stretching it perpendicular to its muscle fiber orientation.[26] This method is often advantageous because it avoids engaging the stretch reflex. Postfacilitation stretch, myofascial release, and deep tissue massage can often complement each other.

The use of hot packs, ultrasound, electrical muscle stimulation, and other passive thermal or electrical methods is common in musculoskeletal clinical care. Their use is sometimes appropriate in acute and subacute care, but is inappropriate in rehabilitation beyond the phase of early soft tissue healing.

Manual resistance techniques have the advantage that while easily tolerated, like passive methods, they also involve the patient in an active way, thus limiting patient dependency. The thrust of modern management of chronic pain is away from passive therapy (physical agents) and toward active patient involvement in the rehabilitation process.[27,28] This focus does not eliminate the role of passive therapies, but rather directs patients toward functional restoration in activities of daily living. The MRT are ideal bridges between passive and active care.

To summarize, when we find an abnormal restriction of motion in a certain direction, we have encountered a pathologic barrier at that point of resistance. This barrier may result from joint blockage, muscle shortening, or a combination of the two. Manual resistance techniques are one approach to eliminate this barrier and to restore normal range of motion (ROM). They achieve this end by relaxing the shortened muscle and/or mobilizing the hypomobile joint. When true joint blockage exists, a chiropractic adjustment is without peer as the treatment of choice. The MRT can stand on their own, but they are better as a complement to the adjustment and a bridge to exercise.

RULES FOR APPLICATION

When using MRT, the more specifically we can facilitate contraction in the desired muscle, the better our results will be. Table 13.5 summarizes some of the keys to achieving successful facilitation. For instance, how the patient is prepositioned affects how easy or hard it is to activate the muscle. Our verbal command is also important, not only for what we say, but also the inflection we use. Trial and error with each patient will reveal which commands activate the desired movement better. In general, saying to a patient to push to the right or left is not as good as giving them an actual target. Manual contacts are facilitative, so it is normal to place a contact on the muscle you wish to activate. Massage while the patient is attempting to contract the muscle may help to awaken a particularly inhibited muscle. Irradiation is sometimes used to facilitate a muscle that is especially "dormant." This process involves using a synergistic muscle that is stronger to pull its inhibited neighbor into action.

Various guidelines help us to avoid irritating patients when stretching. We must not put related joints in a position of strain (i.e., close packed position) during stretching. For example, when stretching the iliopsoas, allowing the lumbar spine to extend puts too much strain on the low back. When stretching in the spinal column, it is also important to avoid uncoupled movements. For instance, in the cervical spine, proper coupling occurs when rotation and side bending occur in the same direction (spinous process toward the convexity). In the lumbar spine, it is the opposite, unless the spine is flexed; in the neutral or extended positions, normal lumbar coupling takes place when rotation and side bending occur in opposite directions (the spinous process moves toward the concavity). This information is important when mobilizing joints with MRT and when stretching muscles that require taking out slack in what would be an uncoupled manner for the underlying spinal joints.

An example of an uncoupled joint position is the cervical side bending away and rotation toward an upper trapezius muscle being stretched. Because this positioning would strain the cervical spine, we stretch almost completely over the upper back and shoulder area and avoid any contraction or strong stretching in the neck area. This situation illustrates a general rule in stretching—stretch over the largest, most stable, and least painful joint.[29] Additionally, how we "wind-up" the upper trapezius will reduce the potential for neck strain. We first take out full flexion and rotation, then gently side bend the neck away from the muscle, and finally firmly take out slack in the upper back and shoulder regions. The patient's contraction would be only from the shoulder in a di-

Table 13.5. Facilitation Techniques

Prepositioning
Hand contacts
Tissue stimulation
Verbal cues or commands
Irradiation

Table 13.6. Safety Rules

Stretch over largest, most stable, least painful joint
Place joints in "loose packed" position
Avoid uncoupled spinal movements
Do not stretch nerves, if irritated

rection of elevation. During relaxation and stretch, we take out the slack over the larger, more stable shoulder and avoid taking out slack in the neck, except perhaps in flexion.

Another rule is to avoid stretching related structures, such as a nerve root, if it is irritated.[29] Hopefully, every clinician knows not to stretch the hamstrings if the sciatic nerve is irritated. Another similar area is the femoral nerve and rectus femoris, or the brachial plexus, which can be stretched when attempting to stretch the scalene or subscapularis muscle. Table 13.6 summarizes these important safety tips during stretching.

How we "wind-up" the muscle, in other words the order with which we take out the slack in the different movement directions (rotation, flexion/extension, side bending), dramatically alters when the patient feels most of the stretch.[29] Playing with this variable allows for better isolation of the relevant tissue. Most people use too great of force when they first begin to use MRT. According to Larricq, the forces used during MRT should be "as little as possible for as long as necessary."[29] According to Lewit, the time of the contraction can be lengthened for up to 30 seconds if inhibition is hard to achieve.[5] Whether to adjust joints before or after MRT is a common question. If significant joint restriction is encountered during attempts to stretch, it is crucial to adjust the joint first. Otherwise, adjustment is easier and thereby requires less force if we wait until after the contractile elements have been relaxed. Different ways to improve MRT results are listed in Table 13.7.

SPECIFIC PROCEDURES

Postisometric relaxation (PIR) is one of the most useful MRT. This method is Lewit's modification of the gentle, indirect isometric MEP that osteopaths applied to joints.[5] It is also similar to hold-relax. The main indication for PIR is relaxation (decontraction) of a hypertonic (contracted) muscle. Postisometric relaxation is the preferred method if the patient has difficulty relaxing or you simply want to use a "softer" approach until you gain the patient's trust. It is ideal for trigger points, joint mobilization, and neuromuscular tension.

Postisometric relaxation (PIR) involves the following simple steps:[5]

1. Passively lengthen tense muscle to a point just short of pain or where resistance to movement (barrier) is felt. Avoid bouncing.
2. Have patient gently contract the overactive muscle away from barrier for 5 to 10 seconds. This movement should be resisted with equal counterforce, creating an isometric contraction. For most muscles, the patient should breathe in while contracting the muscle.

3. Having "let go" and relaxed fully, the muscle is slowly, passively lengthened toward a new resting length as far as relaxation will allow.
4. Without backing away from the new end point, perform two to four additional repetitions.
5. If relaxation is not achieved, try the following:
   - Be sure the patient breathes in during contraction phase and exhales during relaxation phase
   - For most trunk and extremity muscles, the patient should look in the direction of contraction and then in the direction of stretch
   - Lengthen the time of contraction up to 30 seconds
   - Try a harder contraction, although do not resist the contraction when the muscles are in their fully lengthened position
   - Starting from a midrange position, use isotonic resistance of movement by the antagonist muscle toward the restricted barrier one to three times
6. After accomplishing the preceding steps, instruct the patient to perform active ROM exercise through the new range

Success with this method depends on precise positioning of the body part to isolate the tense muscular bundles involved. It is also essential to take out all the slack in the muscle and to stay at the end point of the available ROM throughout the procedure. Indications for its use include increased neuromuscular tension (i.e., trigger points) and joint mobilization (gentle).

A second valuable MRT, particularly for patients with myofascial shortening (viscoelastic stiffness), is postfacilitation stretch (PFS).[17] This method involves the following steps:

1. Place shortened muscle in a position approximately midway between its fully approximated and stretched positions
2. Have the patient contract isometrically with maximum effort for 7 to 10 seconds, and resist this movement to create a nearly isometric contraction
3. When the patient has "let go," perform a quick stretch to the final end point (avoid bouncing) and hold for up to 20 seconds
4. Allow the patient to relax for 20 to 30 seconds
5. Repeat three to five times
6. Instruct the patient to perform an active ROM exercise through the new range

After performing PFS, warn the patient that feeling warmth, weakness, burning, or tingling in the stretched tissue is normal. An appropriate series of such stretches would include six visits over a 2-week period.

In PNF, two of the most famous MRT are *hold-relax* (HR) and *contract-relax* (CR). The former involves positioning the patient in the stretch position and pushing into the "barrier" of resistance while asking the patient to hold. This step encourages an isometric contraction. After the resisted contraction,

Table 13.7. Ways to Maximize Results of Manual Resistance Techniques

"Wind up" muscles to maximize isolation
Start gentle and add force only if necessary
Increase contraction time up to 30 seconds
Adjust restricted joints first

Table 13.8. Matching Therapeutic Goals to Manual Resistance Techniques

Techniques*	Inhibit Muscle	Stretch Muscle	Stretch Fascia	Mobilize Joint
PIR	+			+
HR	+	+		
CR	+	+		
PFS		+	+	
Eccentric MEP		+	+	

*PIR, postisometric relaxation; HR, hold-relax; CR, contract-relax; PFS, post facilitation stretch; MEP, muscle energy procedures.

stretch may be increased either actively (by the patient) or passively (by the doctor). When performed actively, the patient is activating the antagonist to move toward the restricted barrier. This effort engages RI, which inhibits the tight muscle even more. When performed passively, the doctor must not overstretch the tight muscle to avoid activating the stretch reflex, which would only increase the tension in the muscle and defeat the purpose of the entire exercise.

Contract-relax involves taking out the slack and then commanding the patient to "push against me" or "push toward. . . . (an object or target)." This step encourages a concentric contraction because pushing implies movement (whereas holding implies staying stationary). Unlike PIR, you allow a greater force and accompanying movement. At the end of the contraction, RI may be used so it is the patient who actively takes out the slack. This combination is often called *contract-relax antagonist contraction* (CRAC). This method is preferable to HR if the patient is using a stronger muscle that would be hard for you to resist isometrically.

An alternative to PFS for stretching connective tissues is the *osteopathic eccentric MEP*, which involves starting at a midrange position and having the patient push lightly against your resistance (20% effort). Although they push lightly, you lengthen the muscle. The patient must continue to contract lightly so that it is a lengthening or eccentric contraction. This maneuver is excellent for lengthening noncontractile elements.

Table 13.8 summarizes the choice of MRT depending on the specific treatment goal.

Self-stretching should be performed on a regular basis to prevent recurrence of viscoelastic stiffness or elevated neuromuscular tension. Once or twice a day, key tense or stiff muscles may be gently stretched. Simple guidelines for self-stretching are as follows:

1. If possible, perform simple warm-ups before stretching
2. Gently take out all the slack in the involved muscle until you feel a gentle pulling
3. Maintain good body posture so no strain is felt anywhere else in the body
4. Hold the stretch position for 10 to 20 seconds, taking out further slack as relaxation is achieved
5. Breath deeply and slowly to encourage relaxation
6. Repeat stretches at least twice per session and one to two times per day
7. After stretching, actively contract the muscle and move it through a full ROM a few times

SELECTED MRT PROCEDURES

Manual resistance techniques can be used for a variety of purposes. They are alternatives to adjustments or soft tissue work. They are powerful facilitation and strengthening techniques. They are most famous, however, for their ability to stretch muscles.

PIR Procedures for Muscle Relaxation and Stretch

The format for this section is designed for easy clinical application. Readers are encouraged to refer to Chapters 5, 6, 14, and 18 for more detail regarding specific tests, related strengthening exercises, or treatment protocols. The following headings are used for most of the muscles described:

> **Referred Pain:** Location of pain complaint
> **Clinical Result of Shortened Muscle:** Related clinical findings
> **Activation or Perpetuation:** What activates or perpetuates trigger point
> **Observation:** Postural analysis
> **Trigger Point:** Location
> **Periosteal Point:** Location
> **Evaluation for Overactivity:** How muscle overactivity would be seen
> **Evaluation for Muscle Shortening:** Test for muscle tightness
> **Joint Dysfunction:** Related joint dysfunction
> **Corrective Actions:** Exercise and educational approach
> **MRT Stretch:**
> 　Patient Position
> 　Doctor Position
> 　Patient's Active Effort
> 　Stretch
> **Other MRT Stretches**
> **Self-Stretches**

HAMSTRING (Fig. 13.1)

Referred Pain
- Lower buttock to upper calf

Clinical Result of Shortened Muscle
- Recurrent pulled hamstrings

Activation or Perpetuation
- Compensation for weak gluteus maximus
- Compression of posterior thigh from a chair that is too high
- Being in a shortened position from prolonged sitting

Trigger Points
- Midbelly

Periosteal Points
- Ischial tuberosity
- Fibular head (biceps femoris)

Evaluation for Overactivity
- Knee flexion during prone hip extension test

Evaluation for Shortening
- Straight leg raising test of less than 80°

Joint Dysfunction

- L5-S1
- Fibular head

Corrective Action

- Facilitate or strengthen the gluteus maximus
- Avoid prolonged sitting

MRT Stretch

Patient Position

- Supine
- Hip flexed and knee extended on involved limb

Doctor Position

- Standing on side of treating limb
- Cephalad hand proximal to patellae maintaining knee in extension
- Patient's leg supported on doctor's shoulder or in crook of elbow

Patient's Active Effort

- Attempts to push leg down toward table
- Effort is resisted by doctor to keep contraction as close to isometric as possible

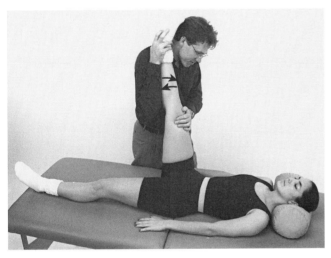

Fig. 13.1. Hamstring PIR.

Stretch

- Flexion of hip while maintaining knee in extension

Comment

Care should be taken whenever stretching the hamstrings that the sciatic nerve tension tests (Lesague's test or Straight Leg Raising test) are negative. Also, in the case of lumbar joint irritability, the opposite hip and knee may be flexed to reduce strain on the lumbar spine.

Other MRT Stretches. Additional hamstring PIR procedures are shown for the medial fibers (Fig. 13.2**a.**), lateral fibers (Fig. 13.2**b**), and the one joint hamstring—the biceps femoris (Fig. 13.3).

Self-Stretches. For hamstring self-stretches, the back must be stable. The patient should feel the stretch in the posterior thigh, but no strain in the lower back (Figs. 13.4 and 13.5). Once the final stretch position is achieved during the standing self-stretches, the patient will feel a greater stretch if instructed to perform an anterior pelvic tilt.

ADDUCTORS (Figs. 13.6 and 13.7)

Referred Pain
- Groin, inner thigh, anterior knee, and shin

Clinical Result of Shortened Muscle
- Hip or sacroiliac disorders or medial knee pain
- Difficulty with squats
- Difficulty with activation of gluteus medius

Activation or Perpetuation
- Hip arthritis, horseback riding, hill running, sudden overload (slipping)

Trigger Points
- Muscle belly

Periosteal Points
- Pubic symphysis
- Tibial tubercle (pes anserinus) (two joint adductors)

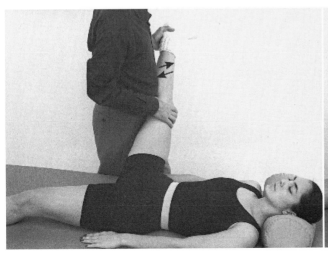
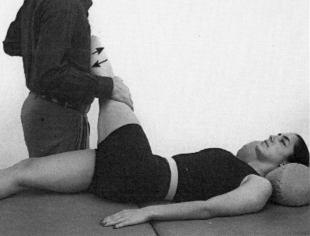

Fig. 13.2. Medial and lateral hamstring PIR.

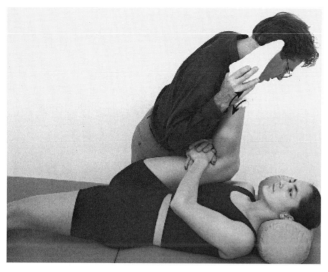

Fig. 13.3. Biceps femoris PIR.

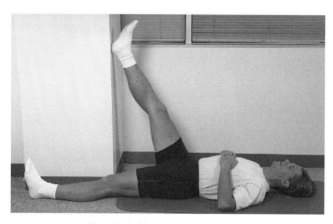

Fig. 13.4. Hamstring self-stretch.

Evaluation for Shortening
- With patient supine, abduct thigh with knee extended (normal is 40°)
- Flex knee and abduction should increase slightly

Joint Dysfunction
- Hip joint

MRT Stretch: Supine
Patient Position

- Supine
- Leg abducted (knee flexed or extended to isolate one or two joint adductors, respectively) until resistance is felt
- Opposite knee is bent

Doctor Position

- Standing with one leg between patient's abducted thigh and the table

Patient's Active Effort

- Attempts to push thigh into adduction
- Effort is resisted by doctor's leg to keep contraction as close to isometric as possible

Stretch

- Doctor then takes out slack into further abduction

MRT Stretch: Side Lying
Patient Position

- Side lying involved side up
- Nontreated leg bent at knee and hip
- Thigh abducted (knee flexed or extended to isolate one or two joint adductors, respectively) until resistance is felt

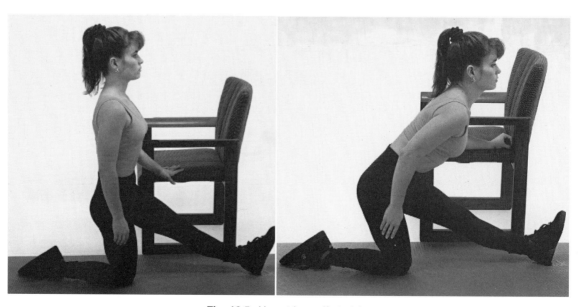

Fig. 13.5. Hamstring self-stretch.

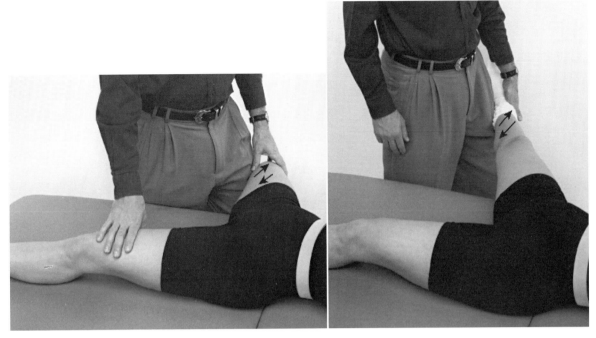

Fig. 13.6. One and two joint adductor PIR.

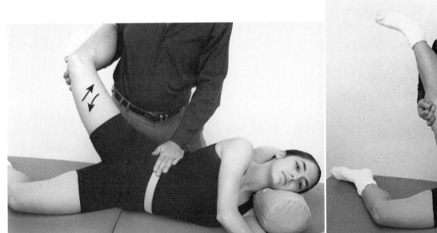
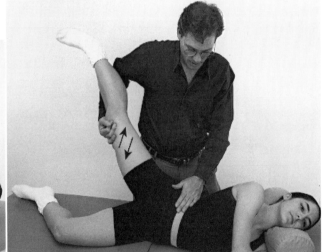

Fig. 13.7. One and two joint adductor PIR.

Doctor Position

- Standing behind patient
- Abducts patient's thigh, caudal hand hooking under patient's knee
- Cephalad hand stabilizes pelvis

Patient's Active Effort

- Attempts to push thigh into adduction toward table
- Effort is resisted by doctor's caudal arm to keep contraction as close to isometric as possible

Stretch

- Doctor then takes out slack into further abduction

Self-Stretches

- Self-stretches are shown in Figure 13.8.

ILIOPSOAS (Fig. 13.9)

Referred Pain

- Low back and sacroiliac joint, anterior thigh

Clinical Result of Muscle Shortening

- Poor hip extension
- Forward-drawn posture
- Difficulty with posterior pelvic tilt

Activation or Perpetuation

- Recent intervertebral disk syndrome

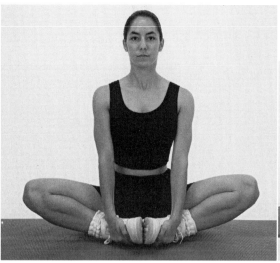
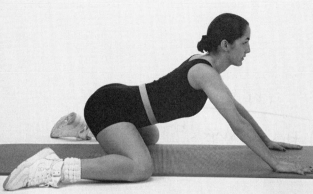

Fig. 13.8. Adductor self-stretches.

- Sway back (psoas must act as a checkrein)
- Prolonged sitting
- Compensation for weak abdominals

Trigger Points
- Anywhere in muscle belly

Evaluation for Overactivity
- Inability to keep heels on floor during knee bent sit-up

Evaluation for Shortening
- Modified Thomas test
  - Patient pulls opposite knee to chest
  - Allow tested leg to extend off table
  - Positive test if hip raises without knee extension (tight rectus femoris) or abduction (tight TFL)

Joint Dysfunction
- T10-L1

Corrective Action
- Avoid prolonged sitting
- Facilitate and stengthen abdominals
- Stretch erector spinae

MRT Stretch: Supine
Patient Position

- Supine
- Lumbar spine may be laterally flexed away from psoas
- Contralateral hip and knee held in full flexion against chest
- Involved hip freely extending off end or side of table (preferable with table height of at least 40 inches)

Doctor Position

- At same side of table as involved limb or at end of table
- One hand holds contralateral knee to chest, thereby stabilizing pelvis
- Other hand contacts proximal to knee of extended leg

Patient's Active Effort

- Raises involved thigh up toward ceiling

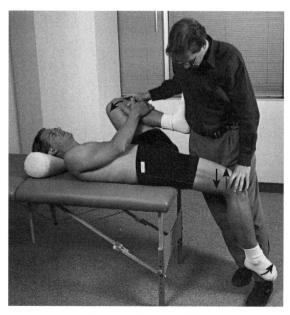

Fig. 13.9. Iliopsoas PIR.

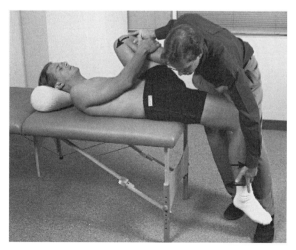

Fig. 13.10. Rectus femoris PIR.

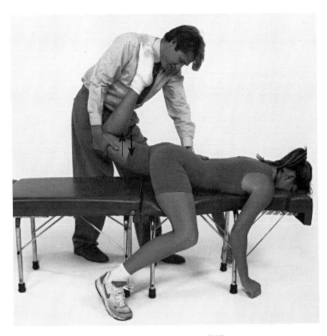

Fig. 13.11. Iliopsoas PIR.

- To enhance psoas isolation, patient told to supinate foot against resistance offered by therapist's leg
- Effort is resisted isometrically by doctor

Stretch

- Once patient has fully relaxed, doctor takes up slack by extending hip to its new end point while stabilizing opposite side

Comment

Patients often complain of discomfort in the fully flexed hip (the one not being stretched), which may be provoked by the passive overpressure required to flatten the low back. This sit-uation may require "backing off" in the attempt to take all the lordosis out of the lumbar spine. Sometimes, it is necessary to perform traction or PIR mobilization on the opposite hip, or PIR on the iliopsoas or adductors to loosen the hip sufficiently to allow for full hip flexion.

Other MRT Stretches. Other related hip flexor PIR procedures include the rectus femoris (Fig. 13.10) and prone iliopsoas (Fig. 13.11). For the prone iliopsoas, the hip should be internally rotated and the spine laterally bent away. Care is needed to avoid abducting the thigh. This procedure is perhaps the most specific iliopsoas stretch, but it is a tremendous strain on the doctor without the use of an elevation table. If an elevation table is used, start in elevation and hold the thigh up while allowing the table to lower and simultaneously stretch the muscle. A stretching belt may also be used.

Self-Stretches. When performing self-stretches for the hip flexors, the patient should feel the stretch in the anterior hip or thigh and not in the low back. For the iliopsoas, better stretch is accomplished if the patient holds a posterior pelvic tilt and internally rotates the hip while stretching (Fig. 13.12). The rectus femoris stretch requires some knee flexion (Fig. 13.13) and also benefits from a posterior pelvic tilt.

TENSOR FASCIA LATAE (TFL) (Fig. 13.14)

Referred Pain
- Lateral aspect of thigh to knee

Clinical Result of Shortened Muscle
- Knee extensor mechanism disorders
- Sacroiliac problems
- QL myofascial disorders

Activation or Perpetuation
- Repetitive strain from running
- Lateral pelvic shift
- Forefoot instability (excessive pronation)
- Prolonged sitting with hip too flexed
- Compensation to a weak gluteus medius

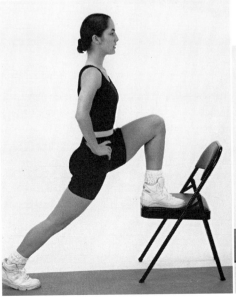
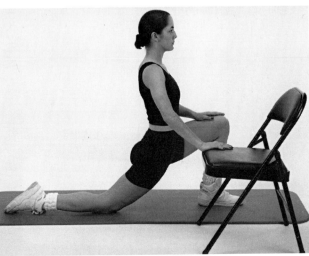

Fig. 13.12. Iliopsoas self-stretches.

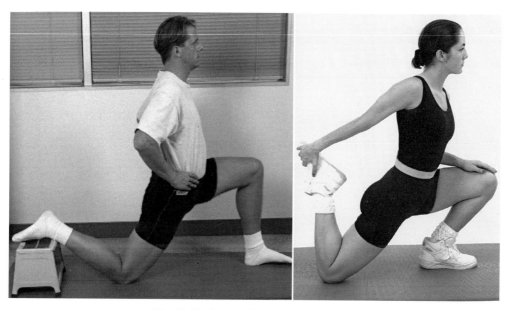

Fig. 13.13. Rectus femoris self-stretches.

Trigger Point
- Superior or mid portion of muscle

Observation
- Groove present in iliotibial band
- Lateral deviation of patellae

Evaluation for Overactivity
- Hip flexion during hip abduction (gluteus medius) test

Evaluation for Shortening
- Ober's test
- Resistance to adduction of thigh

Joint Dysfunction
- Sacroiliac joint
- Patellofemoral joint

Corrective Action
- "Short foot" exercises
- Foot orthotics
- Facilitate and strengthen gluteus medius

MRT Stretch
Patient Position

- Side lying, involved side up
- Nontreated leg bent at knee and hip
- Thigh adducted behind patient until resistance is felt

Doctor Position

- Standing behind patient
- Adducts patient's thigh with caudal hand above knee
- Cephalad hand stabilizes pelvis

Patient's Active Effort

- Attempts to push thigh into abduction toward ceiling
- Effort is resisted by doctor's caudal hand to keep contraction as close to isometric as possible

Stretch

- Doctor then takes out slack into further adduction

Other MRT Stretches. The TFL can also be stretched with the patient supine (Fig. 13.15). This stretch is felt in the quadratus lumborum (QL) if the TFL is not tight.

Self-Stretches. A self-stretch for the TFL similar to the lateral pelvic shift technique that is often used before engaging in McKenzie extension exercises.

PIRIFORMIS (Fig. 13.16)

Referred Pain
- Posterior thigh, buttock, and sacroiliac joint

Clinical Effect of Shortened Muscle
- Sacroiliac disorders
- Entrapment neuropathy (sciatic nerve)

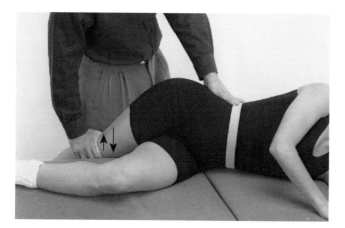

Fig. 13.14. Tensor fascia latae PIR.

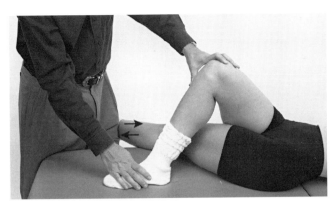

Fig. 13.15. Tensor fascia latae PIR.

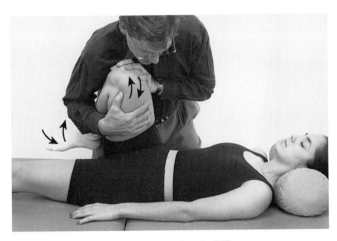

Fig. 13.16. Piriformis PIR.

Activation or Perpetuation
- Short leg
- Long drive with hip flexed and abducted
- Compensation for weak gluteus medius

Observation
- Foot turned out in standing posture

Trigger Point
- Muscle belly
- Muscular guarding elicited on light palpation over sciatic notch

Evaluation for Overactivity
- Hip external rotation or pelvic rotation during hip abduction (gluteus medius) test

Evaluation for Shortening
- Patient supine, flex hip less than 60°. Apply compressive pressure through femur to hip, and adduct fully; feel resiliency to internal rotation of hip

Joint Dysfunction
- L4-L5 and sacroiliac joint

Corrective Action
- Correct short foot
- Improve chair
- Facilitate and strengthen gluteus medius

MRT Stretch
Patient Position

- Supine
- Hip flexed about 45° (maximum of 60°)
- Knee flexed about 90°

Doctor Position

- Standing on involved side, facing patient
- Cephalad forearm on patient's thigh supported by doctor's chest
- Cephalad hand pushes through knee, down shaft of femur
- Doctor pushes patient's thigh into adduction
- Caudal hand grasps patient's calf or ankle and produces internal rotation

Patient's Active Effort

- Pushes thigh outward into doctor's chest (abduction)
- Also pushes lower leg inward in opposite direction, creating an external rotation force

Stretch

- Once patient has fully relaxed, doctor adducts and internally rotates patient's thigh to a new end point

Other MRT Stretches. PIR can also be performed on the piriformis supine in adduction (Fig. 13.17**a**), in full flexion with the hip externally rotated (Fig. 13-17**b**), or prone (Fig. 13.17**c**) with the knee flexed 90°.

Self-Stretches. Self-stretches for the piriformis are possible in a variety of positions (Fig. 13.18). Figure 13.19 shows a strong posterior hip capsule stretch that also addresses piriformis shortening.

QUADRICEPS

The quadriceps is more commonly weak than it is tight. Often, rectus femoris tightness is mistaken for quadriceps tightness. Weak quadriceps typically lead to stoop rather than squat lifting technique, which leads to lumbar overstress. Squats and lunges are the most functional exercises for training the quadriceps.

Postisometric relaxation on the quadriceps is easily performed while prone (Fig. 13.20). This procedure is like the femoral nerve stretch test in that if the associated nerve is compromised, this stretch is contraindicated. Self-stretch can be aided by the use of a belt looped around the foot (Fig. 13.21). Self-PIR can easily be accomplished with this method.

GLUTEUS MAXIMUS

Stretching this primary hip extensor is often not necessary, except for those individuals in whom this muscle is very tight. The PIR technique is also a good way to facilitate this muscle for training with posterior pelvic tilts, bridges, and other strengthening exercises. Self-stretching is performed just like the traditional Williams exercises (Figs. 13.22 and 13.23).

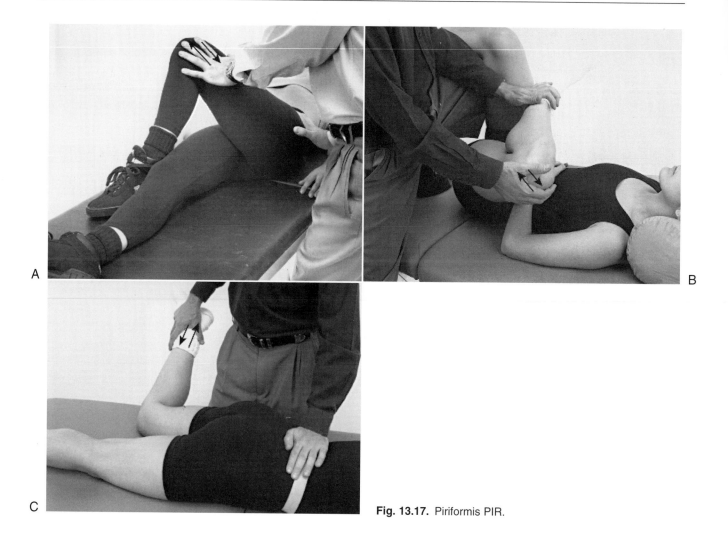

A

B

C

Fig. 13.17. Piriformis PIR.

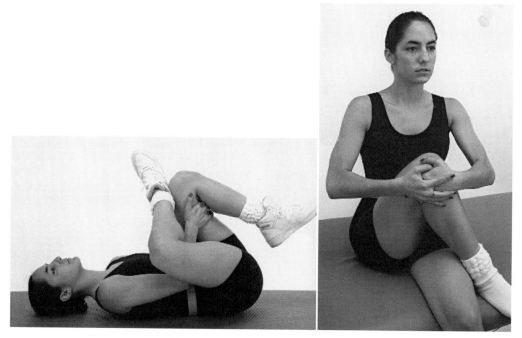

Fig. 13.18. Piriformis self-stretches.

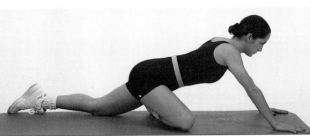

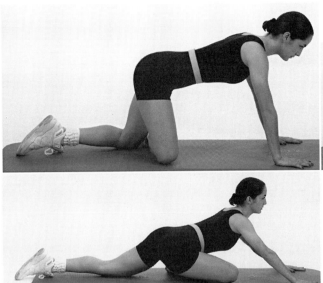

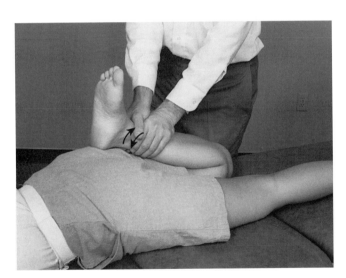

Fig. 13.19. Posterior hip capsule and piriformis self-stretch.

Fig. 13.20. Quadriceps PIR.

HIP INTERNAL ROTATORS PRONE

Postisometric relaxation for restricted hip external rotation is similar to the prone piriformis technique (Fig. 13.24). The pelvis must be firmly stabilized during this procedure.

QUADRATUS LUMBORUM (QL) (Fig. 13.25)

Referred Pain
- Lateral fibers—iliac crest and lateral hip
- Medial fibers—sacroiliac joint, deep in buttock

Clinical Result of Shortened Muscle
- Low back pain
- Perpetuation of sacroiliac disorders
- Abnormal hip hiking during gait

Activation or Perpetuation
- Lifting with trunk twisted
- Sustained overload as in gardening or working in stooped position

Trigger Points
- Beneath erector spinae muscle lateral to transverse processes
  Best to palpate with patient side lying

Periosteal Points
- Iliac crest attachment

Evaluation for Overactivity
- On hip abduction from side lying position, monitor for early pelvic elevation

Evaluation for Shortening
- Screening test: side lying patient raises trunk up with hand or forearm under shoulder. Positive result is absence of smooth convexity of lumbar spine toward down side.

Joint Dysfunction
- T10-L1

Corrective Action
- Correct short leg
- Correct unlevel pelvis when sitting
- Facilitate or strengthen gluteus medius
- Teach proper lifting technique

MRT Stretch
Patient Position

- Side lying, involved side down
- Pelvis tucked so torso is slightly rotated backward
- Hips and knees flexed 90° with ankles crossed

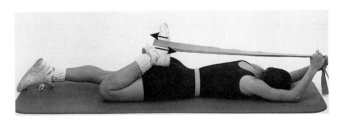

Fig. 13.21. Quadriceps self-PIR.

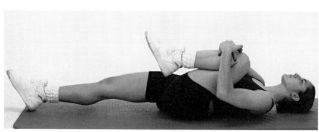
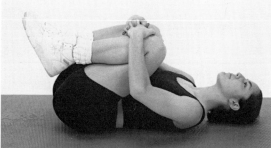

Figs. 13.22 and 13.23. Gluteus maximus self-stretch.

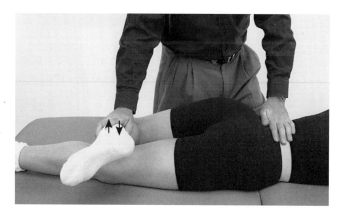

Fig. 13.24. Hip internal rotators PIR.

Doctor Position

• At side of table, facing patient
• Doctor grasps patient's ankles, raising them
• Patient's thighs rest on doctor's caudal thigh
• Cephalad hand free to palpate down side erector spinae muscles for contraction

Patient's Active Effort

• Pushes feet down toward floor
• After contracting QL for appropriate period, is encouraged to "let go" or relax

Stretch

• Pelvis in tucked position
• Hip flexion and degree of pelvic tucking may need to be modified to isolate low back muscles during both contraction and stretch

Other MRT Stretches. A tight or tense QL can be relaxed or stretched in a variety of ways. Prone (Fig. 13.26**a**) and side-lying techniques are possible (Fig. 13.26**b-d**). Sometimes, it is difficult to isolate the muscle with PIR, and intermittent cold and stretch (formerly spray and stretch) is a useful option.

Self-Stretches. A standing self-stretch is shown in Figure 13.26**e.**

ERECTOR SPINAE (Fig. 13.27)

Referred Pain
• Sacroiliac joint, diffuse area in low back, buttock

Clinical Effect of Shortened Muscle
• Low back pain
• Inhibition of abdominals

Activation or Perpetuation
• Postural overstrain (sustained slumping or stooping)
• Sudden overload when lifting with back twisted or flexed
• Compensation for weak or inhibited gluteus maximus

Observation
• Increased lordosis
• Muscle hypertrophy at lumbosacral or thoracolumbar junction

Trigger Point
• Anywhere in muscle belly

Periosteal Points
• Spinous processes of L4-S1

Evaluation for Overactivity
• During hip extension, lumbar erector spinae normally follows gluteus maximus and hamstring activity (contralateral precedes ipsilateral)

Evaluation for Shortening
• Failure of lumbar lordosis to reverse on fingertip to floor test or Sit and Reach test

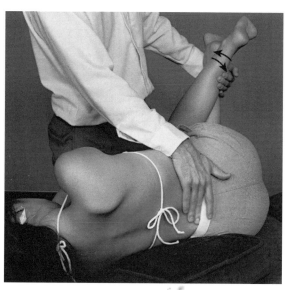

Fig. 13.25. Quadratus lumborum PIR.

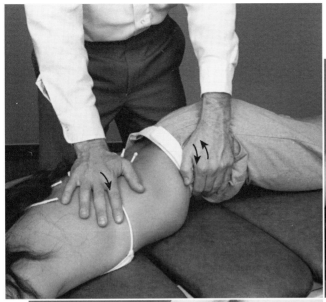

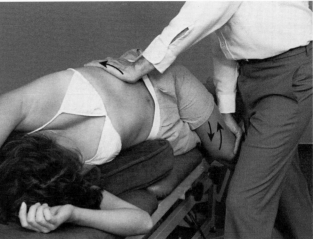

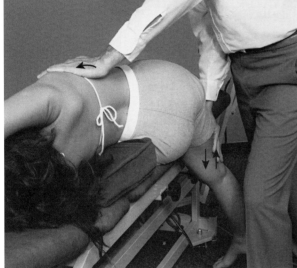

Fig. 13.26. Quadratus lumborum PIR techniques **(a-d)** and self-stretch **(e).**

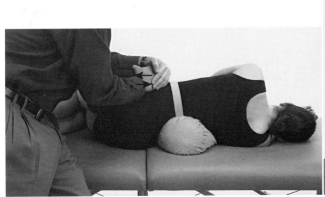

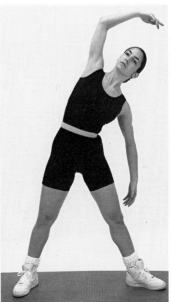

Fig. 13.26. (Continued).

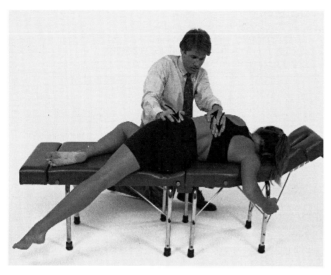

Fig. 13.27. Erector spinae PIR.

- Fingertip to floor distance not valid for lumbar flexibility because of hip motion, hamstring tension, and relative difference between arm and torso length versus leg length

Joint Dysfunction
- Segment at corresponding level, especially L4-L5 and L5-S1

Corrective Action
- Strengthen abdominals
- Facilitate or strengthen gluteus maximus
- Teach proper lifting technique
- Strengthen quadriceps
- Lumbar support for chair

MRT Stretch
Patient Position

- Side lying, involved side up
- Down side arm back and behind patient
- Upper torso rotated forward

- Up side arm hanging off table in front
- Down side leg flexed at hip and knee for stabilization
- Up side hip in slight extension so to hang leg off back of table

Doctor Position

- Standing in front or behind patient
- Fixes pelvis at anterior superior iliac spine (ASIS) with one hand
- Other hand (and forearm) takes broad contact over upside lumbar muscles
- Pulls ASIS toward himself or herself and rotates lumbar spine away (left rotation) to take up slack (i.e., engage barrier) in muscle

Patient's Active Effort

- Turns upper body backwards against resistance while breathing in (may also be instructed to look in direction of turning)

Stretch

- After contracting erector spinae, patient asked to relax and breathe out
- When doctor feels muscle has "let go," he or she takes out slack toward new barrier

Other MRT Stretches. The erector spinae may be stretched using a supine technique taught by Janda (Fig. 13.28), or in the seated position (Fig. 13.29). Care is needed to avoid uncoupled movements. If stretching in flexion, be sure to rotate and side bend to the same side. If stretching or mobilizing in a neutral or extended position, place the patient in rotation and side bending to opposite sides.

Self-Stretches. Self-stretches for the low back muscles are abundant (Fig. 13.30). A simple self-PIR technique is also an excellent way for a patient to relax their lower back (Fig. 13.31). It is pragmatic to have the patients explore which stretches seem more neutral for them.

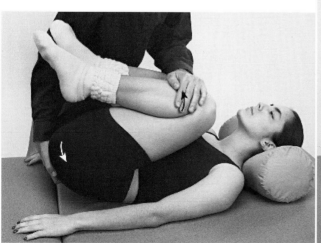
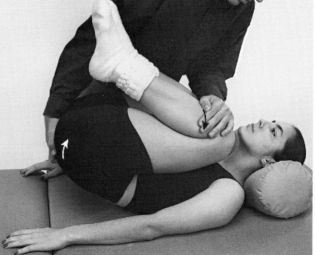

Fig. 13.28. Erector spinae PIR.

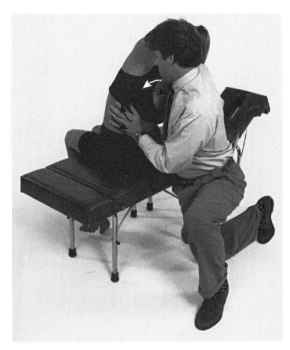

Fig. 13.29. Erector spinae PIR.

LUMBAR MULTIFIDI (Fig. 13.32)

MRT Stretch
Patient Position

- Side lying
- Torso rotated backward
- Pelvis rotated forward

Doctor Position

- At side of table on involved side
- Cephalad forearm pushed shoulder backward
- Caudal hand and wrist pull pelvis forward

Patient's Active Effort

- Rotates torso forward while moving pelvis backward
- Effort is resisted by doctor to keep contraction as close to isometric as possible

Stretch

- Once patient has relaxed fully, doctor may take slack out toward new barrier by pushing shoulder backward and pelvis forward

POSTERIOR CERVICAL MUSCLES

Referred Pain
- Up to suboccipital region
- Down to upper shoulder girdle
- Forehead

Clinical Result of Shortened Muscle
- "Short neck" or cervicocranial hyperextension
- Cervical headaches
- Dizziness of cervical origin
- Cervical zygapophyseal joint disorders

Activation or Perpetuation
- Sustained neck flexion while reading and writing
- Forward-drawn or stooped posture
- Trauma (i.e., whiplash)

Trigger Points
- Occiput, suboccipital triangle to C4-C5

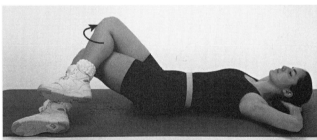

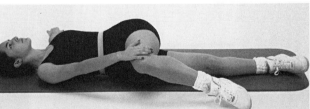

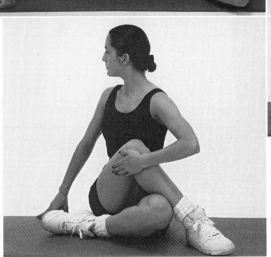

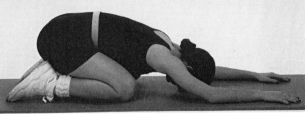

Fig. 13.30. Erector spinae self-stretches.

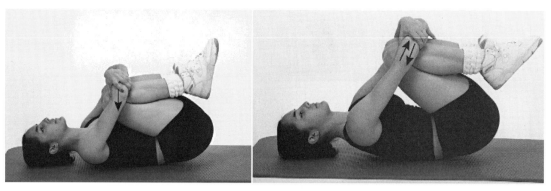

Fig. 13.31. Erector spinae self-PIR.

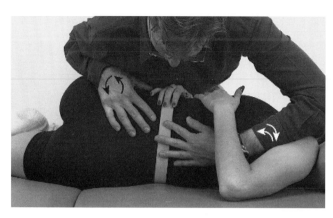

Fig. 13.32. Multifidi PIR.

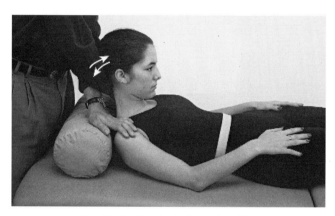

Fig. 13.33. Semispinalis capitus PIR.

Periosteal Points
- Transverse process of the atlas

Joint Dysfunction
- C0-C1 to midcervical

Corrective Action
- Train proper head on neck postural set (i.e., Alexander technique)
- Address forward weight-bearing posture (tight calves, hip flexors and pectorals)
- Facilitate and strengthen gluteus maximus and deep neck flexors

SEMISPINALIS CAPITUS (Fig. 13.33)

MRT Stretch
Patient Position

- Supine

Doctor Position

- At head of table
- Patient's head may be supported by doctor's crossed arms while doctor's hands are placed on patient's shoulders
- Bring head into forward flexion, stopping as resistance is felt or if patient perceives any stretching pain

Patient's Active Effort

- Attempts to gently push head back and breathe in while doctor offers matching resistance
- After 5 to 10 seconds, instructed to "let go"

Stretch

- When doctor perceives patient has fully relaxed, patient asked to take deep breath in and out
- As patient exhales and continues to relax, doctor takes up slack in muscle
- New resting length should be achieved that is farther into forward flexion than before stretch
- These steps can be repeated two or three more times

LEFT SPLENIUS CAPITUS/CERVICUS (Fig. 13.34)

MRT Stretch. Combine flexion with rotation and side bending to the same side (coupled motion). If the patient reports provocation of joint pain, an adjustment should be performed first. Very gentle forces should be used in this technique (intermittent cold and stretch is an option).

LEFT SEMISPINALIS CERVICUS (Fig. 13.35)

MRT Stretch. This maneuver is an uncoupled movement for the cervical spine. Therefore, if joint pain is provoked, lessen the side bending component. Very gentle forces should be used in this technique (intermittent cold and stretch is an option).

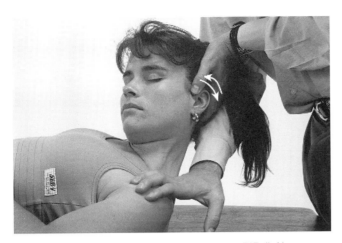

Fig. 13.34. Splenius capitus/cervicus PIR (left).

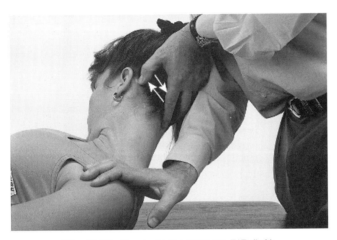

Fig. 13.35. Semispinalis cervicus PIR (left).

LEFT MULTIFIDI AND ROTATORS (Fig. 13.36)

MRT Stretch. Full rotation followed by maximal flexion of the rotated head are performed. Very gentle forces should be used in this technique (intermittent cold and stretch is an option).

UPPER TRAPEZIUS (Fig. 13.37)

Referred Pain
- To mastoid along posterior, lateral neck and occiput to forehead

Clinical Effect of Shortened Muscle
- Headaches
- Neck pain
- Altered scapulohumeral rhythm

Activation
- Occupational stress from sustained shoulder elevation
  Telephone to ear
  Chair with arm rests at wrong height or absent
  Desk, typewriter, or keyboard too high
- Compensation to weak lower fixators of scapulae
- Habitual forward position of shoulders
- Cervicothoracic kyphosis
- Inadequate support for heavy breasts

- Purse too heavy or shoulder strap too thin
- Compensation to short leg
- Shoulder elevation with respiration
- Emotional stress
  "Weight of the world on shoulders"

Observation
- Straightening of neck-shoulder line contour ("Gothic" appearance)

Trigger Points
- Midbelly, anterior, lateral

Evaluation for Overactivity
- Should not abduct with excessive upper trapezius activity or early scapular elevation

Evaluation for Shortening
- Laterally bend head away and rotate head toward side to be tested. With neck flexed, push on shoulder. Positive finding is loss of resiliency (compare bilaterally).

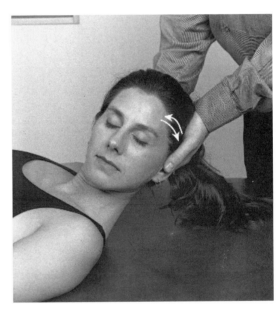

Fig. 13.36. Multifidi and rotators PIR (left).

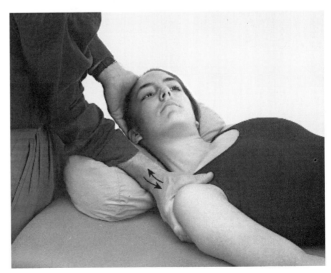

Fig. 13.37. Upper trapezius PIR.

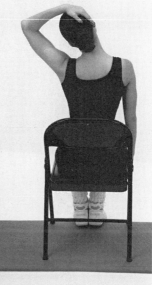

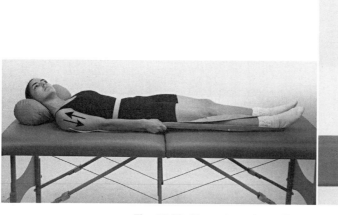

Fig. 13.38. Upper trapezius self-stretches.

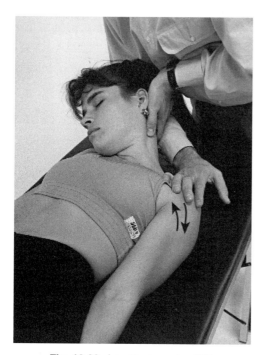

Fig. 13.39. Levator scapulae PIR.

- Tension release shoulder shrugs during "breaks"
- Proper support bra with wider strap
- Smaller purse with wider strap
- Re-educate diaphragmatic breathing
- Facilitate and strengthen lower fixators of scapulae

MRT Stretch
Patient Position

- Supine
- Head is flexed, rotated toward and laterally flexed away from side of stretch
- Arm on involved side is relaxed at patient's side

Doctor Position

- Standing at head of table on side of involvement

Joint Dysfunctional
- Atlanto-occipital, any other posterior cervical joint including the cervicothoracic junction

Corrective Actions
- Improve workstation ergonomics
  - Make sure elbows are properly supported by arm rests
  - Correct desk, typewriter, or keyboard height
  Shoulders relaxed
  Elbows bent at 90°
  Hands relaxed with wrist in "neutral position" on work surface

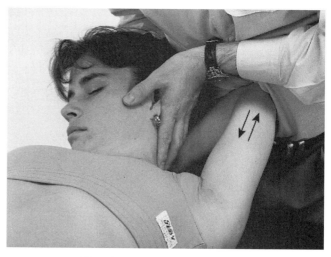

Fig. 13.40. Levator scapulae PIR.

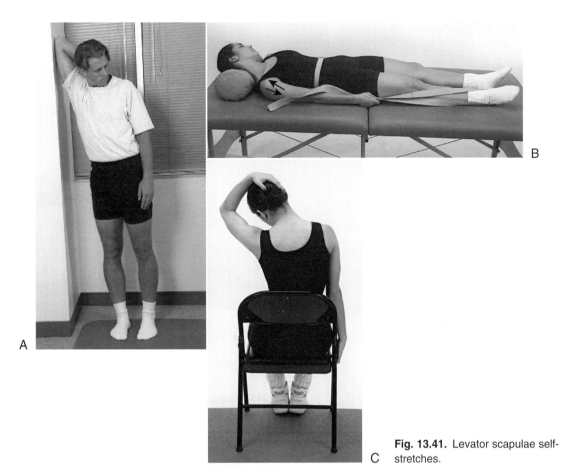

Fig. 13.41. Levator scapulae self-stretches.

- Crossed or uncrossed arm contact with one hand gently on patient's shoulder and other hand behind mastoid process
- "Wind-up" stretch by taking out slack in neck flexion and then in gently side bending away and rotation toward involved side. Finally, take out strongest slack in direction of shoulder depression.

Patient's Active Effort

- Attempts to bring shoulder into elevation toward patient's ear
- Common error is for patient to raise shoulder off table rather than elevating it toward ear
- Effort is resisted by doctor to keep contraction as close to isometric as possible

Stretch

- After contracting upper trapezius for appropriate period, patient is encouraged to "let go" or relax
- Once relaxation of muscle is felt, doctor may take up slack by depressing shoulder as far as it will allow
- Some slack may also be taken out by increasing neck flexion, but no more in uncoupled side bending away and rotation toward muscle

Self-Stretches. Excellent self-stretches are shown in Figure 13.38. Self-PIR can easily be incorporated into other self-treatment methods.

LEVATOR SCAPULAE (Fig. 13.39)

Referred Pain
- Vertebral border of scapula
- Nape of neck

Clinical Effect of Shortened Muscle
- Pain on same side as patient turns head
- Torticollis
- Altered scapulohumeral rhythm

Activation
- Postures in which patient has head turned for prolonged periods, e.g., talking to someone sitting to the side
- Excessive telephone work
- Working over a desk for prolonged periods of neck flexion

Observation
- With shortening, contour of neck line appears as a double wave where muscle inserts into scapula

Trigger Points
- Superomedial border of scapula
- Push trapezius laterally to palpate full length of muscle

Periosteal Points
- Lateral surface of spinous process of C2

Evaluation for Shortening
- Laterally bend and rotate flexed head away from tested side

- Apply gentle pressure to ipsilateral shoulder
- Positive test is lack of resiliency when pushing on shoulder

Joint Dysfunction
- C1-C2 and C2-C3, also cervicothoracic junction

Corrective Actions
- Using a headset
- Rearranging computer monitor or reading material so no need to turn head
- Facilitate or strengthen lower fixators of scapulae

MRT Stretch
Patient Position

- Same as for trapezius, except hand is turned palm up and anchored all the way under back of thigh and neck is rotated away

Doctor Position

- At head of table on side of involvement
- Arm closest to patient's head supports head while the hand contacts patient's superomedial border of shoulder blade
- Outer arm crosses in front of other arm so open hand can contact mastoid process
- Patient's head maximally flexed, laterally flexed, and rotated toward side opposite of involvement
- Take out all slack in direction of shoulder depression and minimize forces on head

Patient's Active Effort

- Tries to gently elevate shoulder blade
- Effort is resisted by doctor to keep contraction as close to isometric as possible

Stretch

- Once patient has fully relaxed, doctor takes out slack by increasing shoulder depression

Other MRT Stretches. Postisometric relaxation may also be used with resistance through the patients elbow (Fig. 13.40).

Self-Stretches. Self-stretches are shown without PIR (Fig. 13.41**a**) and with PIR (Fig. 13.41**b** and **c**).

SUBOCCIPITALS

Referred Pain
- Side of head

Clinical Effects of Shortened Muscle
- Occipital headache
- "Short neck"—cervicocranial hyperextension

Activation
- Sustained flexion
  Maladjusted eyeglass frames
  Reading or writing
- Sustained extension
  Bicycle riding
  House painting
- Forward-drawn posture
- Weak deep neck flexors

Trigger Points
- Deep to trapezius and semispinalis capitus

Evaluation for Shortening
- Supine patient draws chin to chest
- Positive finding if gap of one or more finger's breadth remains

Joint Dysfunctional
- C0-C1

Corrective Actions
- Improve forward-drawn posture
- Awareness training of "short neck" (i.e., Alexander technique)
- Book stand or writing wedge

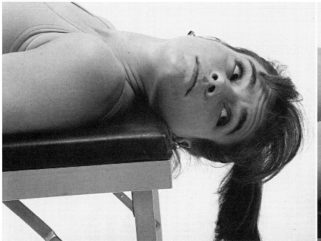
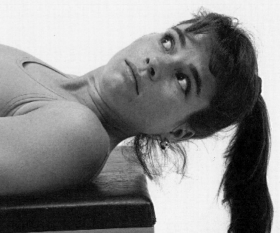

Fig. 13.42. Sternocleidomastoid PIR.

- Computer monitor at correct height (center between mouth and nose)
- Strengthen weak deep neck flexors

MRT Stretch
Patient Position

- Supine
- Chin slightly flexed

Doctor Position

- At head of table
- One hand behind neck, applying traction (slight)
- Heel of other hand on forehead with fingers pointing toward chin

Patient's Active Effort

- Attempts to tilt head backward
- Effort is resisted by doctor to keep contraction as close to isometric as possible

Stretch

- Once patient has fully relaxed, doctor increases traction force with hand supporting neck
- Doctor takes out slack with heel of hand on forehead into forward flexion
- If patient resists forward flexion, asked to actively tuck chin in and then relax; patient will have in effect taken out slack themselves and simultaneously used RI

STERNOCLEIDOMASTOID (SCM) (Fig. 13.42)

Referred Pain
- Over eye, frontal area, mastoid process

Clinical Effect of Shortened Muscle
- Headache (over eyes)
- Earache
- Decreased neck rotation

Activation
- Mechanical overload (excessive neck extension)
  Painting a ceiling
  Watching a movie from the front row
  Bicycle riding

- Sleeping on two pillows shortens SCM
- Postural stress (compensation to short leg)
- Uncorrected poor eyesight
- Forward head posture
- Weak deep neck flexors
- Shortened suboccipitals

Observation
- With shortening, visibly prominent insertion of clavicular division
- Head-forward posture

Trigger Point
- Anywhere in muscle, particularly below mastoid process

Evaluation for Overactivity
- Head flexion tested with patient supine
- Patient asked to slowly raise head into flexion in arc-like fashion
- Positive test if chin pokes during initiation of movement

Joint Dysfunction
- C0-C1 and C2-C3

Corrective Actions
- Pillow should be tucked between shoulder and chin, NOT under shoulder
- Correct head-forward posture (shortens SCM)
- Lumbar pillow may help restore both lumbar and cervical curves
- Correct nearsightedness
- Limit overhead work that overloads checkrein function of SCM
- Round-shouldered posture (tight pectoralis muscles) contributes to head-forward posture
- Strengthen weak deep neck flexors
- Stretch shortened suboccipitals

MRT Relaxation
Patient Position

- Supine
- Shoulders at edge of table, so head is supported only at base of occiput
- Head rotated away from involved side and allowed to extend slightly (Deklyne's test position)

Doctor Position

- At head of table
- Cephalad hand (hand nearest to head) cradles head
- Other hand placed on patient's forehead

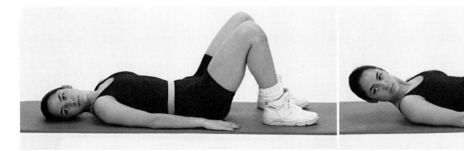

Fig. 13.43. Sternocleidmastoid PIR.

Patient's Active Effort

- Attempts to raise head slightly, without any rotation
- Effort is resisted by doctor to keep contraction as close to isometric as possible

Relaxation

- Doctor merely allows head to extend as far as it will on its own
- Gravity is only force required to take up slack
- A perfect self-treatment method as well
- Contraindicated if any signs of vertebrobasilar insufficiency noted

Other MRT Stretches and Self-Stretches. If the cervical spine is irritable, the SCM may still be treated by prepositioning in flexion, thus avoiding provocative extension positions (Figs. 13.43 and 13.44). These stretches are ideal in-office or self-treatment methods. This technique is often an excellent prethrust relaxation technique for a patient who "guards" excessively.

SCALENES (FIG. 13.45)

Referred Pain

- Pectoralis muscles, upper arm, hand, and rhomboids

Clinical Effects of Shortened Muscle

- Possible numbness or tingling in hands and/or fingers
- Differential diagnosis
  Ulnar distribution of symptoms from the brachial plexus or subclavian vein
  Radial distribution from myofascial referral

Activation

- Forward head posture
- Paradoxic breathing pattern (excessive upper chest respiration)
- Anxiety
- Tension in other fixators of shoulder girdle

Trigger Points

- Anywhere within anterior, medial, or posterior divisions of muscle
- Palpate and treat scalenes with caution because of proximity of extremely sensitive neurovascular tissue

Joint Dysfunction

- Flexion fixations of cervical spine (anterior cervicals)
- First rib blockage

Corrective Actions

- Retrain diaphragmatic breathing pattern
- Stress management

MRT Stretch
Patient Position

- Supine, head laterally bent to opposite side and slightly extended
- Anterior fibers must be stretched with head rotated toward involved side
- Medial fibers require no rotation
- Posterior fibers require head is rotated away

Doctor Position

- At head of table
- Anterior fibers isolated with one hand on medial clavicular origin and other hand just anterior to mastoid process
- Medial fibers require one hand on midclavicular origin and other hand on mastoid process
- Posterior fibers require one hand on lateral clavicular origin and other hand just posterior on mastoid process

Patient Effort

- Attempts to side bend back toward midline

Stretch

- Slack taken out into greater lateral flexion
- Anterior fiber lengthening with rotation toward involved side
- Medial fibers require no rotation
- Posterior fiber lengthening with rotation away

Concern

If the neck is hypersensitive or any vertebrobasilar symptoms are present, this technique is contraindicated. Joint manipulation may be necessary before using this method to ensure the joints are not compressing, especially with respect to the scalene anticus stretch (Fig. 13.45**a**).

Other MRT Stretches. An alternative way to address scalene dysfunction involves prepositioning the patient's neck in a stretch position and then contacting the origin of the muscle over the anterior chest. Resistance to inspiration can be suffi-

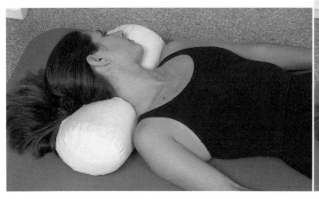
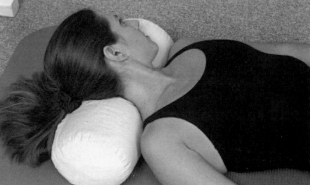

Fig. 13.44. Sternocleidomastoid PIR.

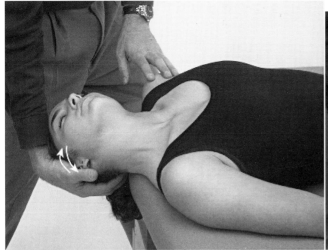

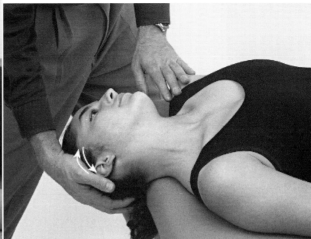

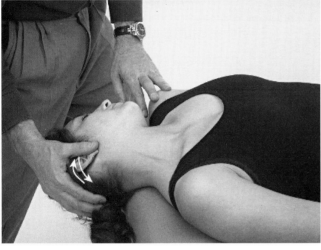

A

B

C

Fig. 13.45. Scalene PIR.

cient to achieve postcontraction inhibition. Slack can be taken out with the hand over the anterior region of the chest or clavicle to lengthen the shortened muscle.

Self-Stretches. Self-treatment is easy and safe, especially if extension is minimized (Fig. 13.46). Figure 13.47 shows a side-lying technique for performing self-PIR with gravity resistance.

PECTORALIS MAJOR (Fig. 13.48)

Referred Pain
• Anterior part of chest, breast, inner arm, and forearm

Clinical Effect of Shortened Muscle
• Pain similar to angina
• Breast hypersensitivity
• Anterior humeral position can promote shoulder impingement syndrome

Activation
• Round-shouldered, head-forward posture

Observation
• Round shoulders

• Arms internally rotated
• Scapula abducted and protracted

Trigger Points
• Anywhere in muscle belly

Periosteal Points
• Rib head attachments

Evaluation for Shortening
• Arm abducted 90° and externally rotated
• Same with 100° to 120° abduction

Joint Dysfunction
• Upper ribs

Corrective Actions
• Improve forward weight-bearing posture
• Facilitate and strengthen lower fixators of scapulae

MRT Stretch
Patient Position

• Supine
• Arm abducted 90° and externally rotated

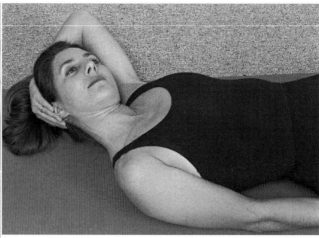

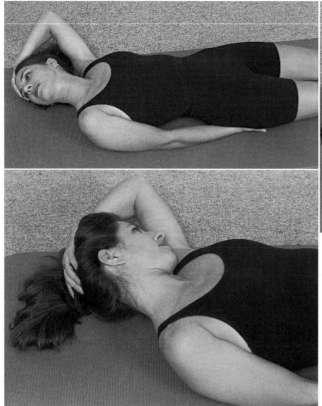

Fig. 13.46. Scalene self-stretch.

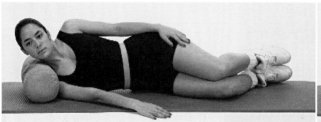
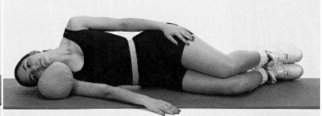

Fig. 13.47. Scalene self-PIR.

Doctor Position

- At head of table on involved side
- One hand contacts muscle belly (abdominal or sternal) or opposite clavicle
- Other hand grasps upper arm

Patient's Active Effort

- Attempts to raise arm
- Effort is resisted by doctor to keep contraction as close to isometric as possible

Stretch

- Once patient has relaxed fully, doctor may retract shoulder to new barrier
- Must firmly stabilize muscle belly over ribs while taking up slack

Concern

If brachial plexus symptoms are encountered PIR, may be performed without stretch.

Self-Stretches. Self-stretching is easy with doorway or corner stretches

PECTORALIS MINOR (Fig. 13.49)

Clinical details are similar to those for pectoralis major. Application of PIR can cause nerve entrapment related to thoracic outlet syndrome.

MRT Stretch
Patient Position

- Supine

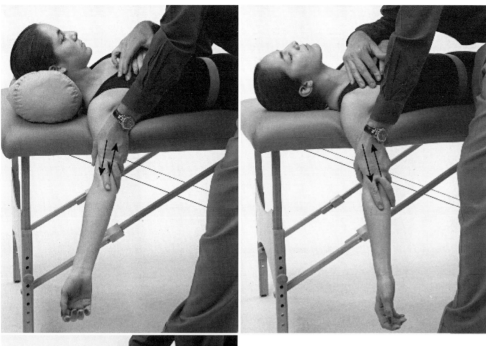

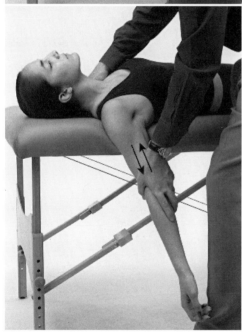

Fig. 13.48. Pectoralis major PIR.

- Arm abducted 80° and externally rotated
- Hand hanging lower than shoulder

Doctor Position

- At head of table on involved side
- Cephalad hand contacts glenohumeral joint
- Caudal hand grasps arm

Patient's Active Effort

- Attempts to raise shoulder to ceiling (keeping hand lower than shoulder
- Effort is resisted by doctor to keep contraction as close to isometric as possible

Stretch

- Once patient has relaxed fully, doctor may take slack out toward new barrier by pushing shoulder away from clavicle

Other MRT Stretches. A modified technique for prone positioning is shown in Figure 13.50.

SUPRASPINATUS

Referred Pain
- Deltoid region, lateral upper arm and elbow

Clinical Result of Shortened Muscle
- Painful abduction (painful arc)

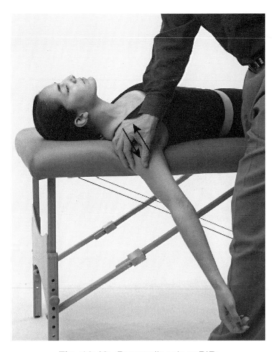

Fig. 13.49. Pectoralis minor PIR.

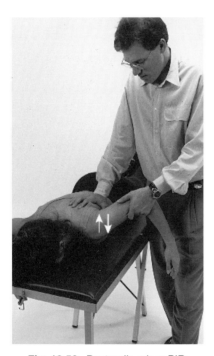

Fig. 13.50. Pectoralis minor PIR.

- Difficulty reaching above shoulder
- Rotator cuff disorders (i.e., impingement syndrome) often result from tightness of external rotators (infraspinatus, teres minor, and supraspinatus)

Activating Factors
- Overhead work (i.e., weight lifting, throwing, swimming, etc.)
- Poor scapulohumeral rhythm

Trigger Points
- Supraspinatus fossa deep to trapezius

Corrective Actions
- Avoidance of overhead work
- Cross-fiber massage
- Improve scapulohumeral rhythm

MRT Stretch
Patient Position

- Prone

Doctor Position

- Standing at same side of table as involved shoulder
- Arm extended behind patient
- With elbow flexed 90°, upper arm adducted as far as will go comfortably

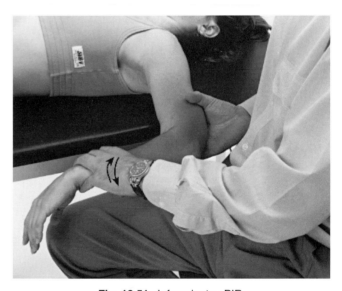

Fig. 13.51. Infraspinatus PIR.

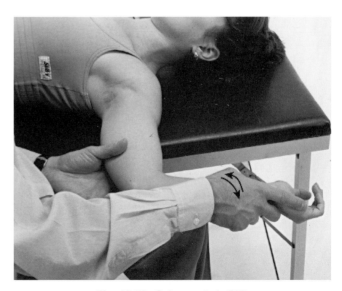

Fig. 13.52. Subscapularis PIR.

• Place one hand against upper arm and grasp patient's wrist with other hand

Patient's Active Effort

• Gently pushes upper arm out into abduction
• Effort is resisted isometrically
• Patient should follow normal breathing procedure

Stretch

• As patient relaxes, doctor takes up slack in adduction

INFRASPINATUS (Fig. 13.51)

Referred Pain
• Anterior deltoid—shoulder, down arm to hand

Clinical Effects of Shortened Muscle
• Pain when sleeping on either side
• Difficulty reaching behind back to unhook bra
• Difficulty reaching back pocket for wallet
• Rotator cuff disorders (i.e., instability syndrome) often result from tightness of external rotators (infraspinatus, teres minor, and supraspinatus)

Activation
• Neglected shoulder overuse syndrome
• Altered scapulohumeral rhythm

Trigger Points
• Infraspinatus fossa (especially superomedial)

Corrective Actions
• Sleep with involved side up and pillow under involved arm
• Improve scapulohumeral rhythm

MRT Stretch
Patient Position

• Supine
• Involved shoulder supported by table

Doctor Position

• Abduct arm and flex elbow to 90°
• Allow forearm to fall into as much internal rotation (forearm toward thigh) as gravity will force it
• Ensure shoulder does not begin to lift off table

Patient's Active Effort

• With one hand on arm above elbow and other hand on dorsal aspect of forearm, gently pushes forearm up or backward toward external rotation
• Effort isometrically resisted (again ensuring shoulder does not rise off table)

Stretch

• When patient has fully relaxed, take up slack toward new barrier in internal rotation

Concern

Although this method is simple to perform, care is needed if the shoulder joint is hypersensitive.

Other MRT Stretches. An alternative method that reduces strain on the shoulder joint is accomplished with the arm brought into full internal rotation and adduction across the front of the chest. To prevent subacromial impingement, strong traction is applied to the shoulder joint. This technique allows for the contraction and stretch to be felt at the scapular attachment rather than the shoulder attachment of the infraspinatus.

SUBSCAPULARIS (Fig. 13.52)

Referred Pain
• Posterior deltoid and posterior arm

Clinical Effects of Shortened Muscle
• Difficulty reaching back as in throwing
• Involved in "frozen shoulder"
• Promotes subacromial impingement and rotator cuff syndromes

Activation
• Shoulder overuse syndrome
• Lack of variety of motion in shoulder area
• Forward-drawn posture, especially tight pectorals

Trigger Points
• Ventral scapula

Joint Dysfunction
• Glenohumeral joint

Corrective Actions
• When lying on involved side, place pillow between arm and chest to maintain abduction
• When lying on uninvolved side, place pillow in front to prevent excessive abduction
• Improve scapulohumeral rhythm
• Stretch pectoralis major

MRT Stretch
Patient Position

• Supine
• Involved shoulder supported by table

Doctor Position

• Facing patient on same side as involved shoulder
• Abduct arm and flex elbow to 90°
• Allow forearm to fall into as much external rotation (forearm toward head) as gravity will force it
• Ensure shoulder does not begin to lift off table

Patient's Active Effort

• With one hand on arm above elbow and other hand on ventral aspect of forearm, gently pushes their forearm up or forward toward internal rotation
• Effort is isometrically resisted (shoulder should not rise significantly off table)

Stretch

• When patient has fully relaxed, take up slack toward new barrier in external rotation

Concern

This technique is contraindicated if anterior instability is present. It also will provoke extreme pain if a "frozen shoulder" is the problem. In either case, the functional range for PIR may be limited to less than 90° of shoulder abduction.

GASTROCNEMIUS (Fig. 13.53)

Referred Pain
• Calf, posterior knee, and instep

Clinical Result of Shortened Muscle
• Forward weight-bearing posture
• Achilles tendinitis

Activation
• Seat height too high
• High heels
• Too much driving (pushing on accelerator)

Trigger Points
• Medial and lateral border of muscle

Evaluation for Shortening
• Supine dorsiflex ankle without allowing knee to bend. Should have 10° dorsiflexion.

MRT Stretch
Patient Position

• Supine with legs extended

Doctor Position

• Standing at end of table; grasps heel of foot with hand
• Passively dorsiflexes patient's foot by leaning cephalad
• Patient's knee not allowed to flex

Resisted Effort

• Patient attempts to plantarflex foot (not toes)
• Effort is isometrically resisted

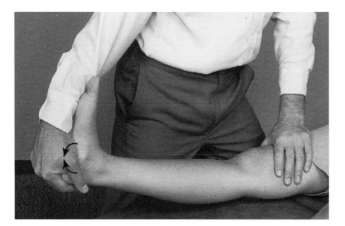

Fig. 13.53. Gastrocnemius PIR.

Stretch

• When patient has fully relaxed, take up slack toward new barrier in ankle dorsiflexion

Self-Stretches. Self-stretching the gastrocnemius is best performed with the standing wall lean and its modifications (Fig. 13.54). It is essential that the knee is extended and the heel does not rise up.

SOLEUS (Fig. 13.55)

Referred Pain
• Heel, posterior calf

Clinical Result of Shortened Muscle
• Forward weight-bearing posture
• Difficulty squatting

Activation
• High heels
• Excessive running

Trigger Points
• Superior and inferior muscle belly

Evaluation for Shortening
• Prone with knee bent 90°, dorsiflex ankle; should have 20° dorsiflexion

MRT Stretch
Patient Position

• Prone

Doctor Position

• Standing at side of table, places patient's leg in 90° knee flexion
• Passively dorsiflexes patient's foot by pulling up on heel while pushing down on metatarsals

Resisted Effort

• Attempts to plantarflex foot (not toes)
• Effort is isometrically resisted

Stretch

• When patient has fully relaxed, take up slack toward new barrier in ankle dorsiflexion

Self-Stretch. Self-stretch is accomplished as for the gastrocnemius, except that knee flexion is allowed (Fig. 13.56).

Postisometric Relaxation Joint Mobilization Procedures

HIP JOINT (Fig. 13.57)

Patient Position
• Supine
• Involved leg flexed at knee and draped over seated doctor's shoulder

Doctor Position
• Seated at same side of table as involved hip, facing patient

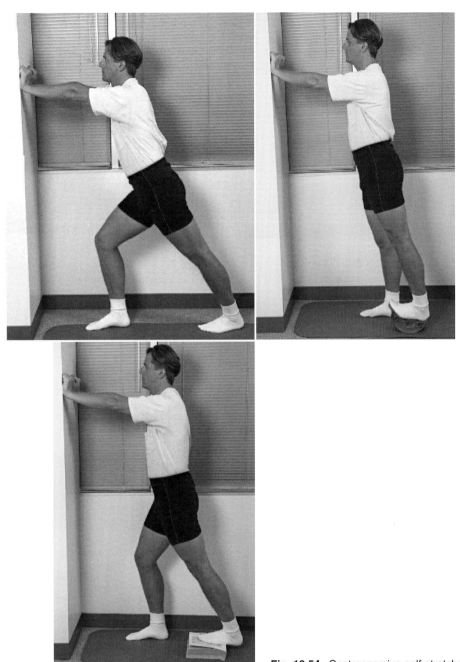

Fig. 13.54. Gastrocnemius self-stretches.

- Patient's leg draped over doctor's shoulder
- Contact made over patient's anterior hip with both hands and pulls A to P to take out all available slack in posterior glide

Resisted Effort
- Patient instructed to pull thigh toward abdomen
- Effort should be isometrically resisted by doctor
- Patient and doctor should feel contraction occurring in anterior hip region

Stretch
- Once patient has fully relaxed, doctor takes up slack by increasing posterior glide to its new end point

LUMBAR SPINE (EXTENSION MOBILIZATION) (Fig. 13.58)

Patient Position
- Side lying with hips and knees flexed

Doctor Position
- Facing toward patient
- Places fingers over spinous processes (one hand over the other)
- Patient's knees in contact with doctor's anterior thigh
- Doctor must take out all slack in lumbar extension by pushing with thigh into patient's knees while stabilizing vertebral segment above joint fixation with hand contact

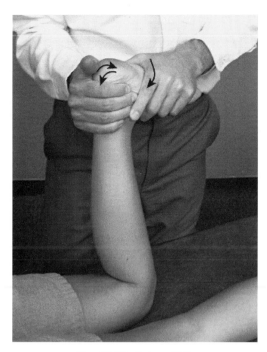

Fig. 13.55. Soleus PIR.

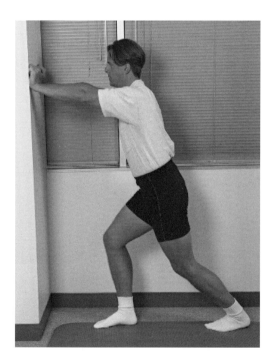

Fig. 13.56. Soleus self-stretch.

Resisted Effort
- Patient attempts to push knees into doctor's thigh
- Kyphosis of patient's spine should result

Stretch
- Once patient has fully relaxed, doctor extends patient's spine by pressing hands anterior to stabilize segment above fixation, while pushing with thigh against patient's knees in a direction toward fixed lumbar segment

Self-Treatment. Self-treatment of the lumbar spine into extension can be accomplished by performing the McKenzie prone on elbows, prone press-up, and standing extension exercises (Fig. 13.59). If these exercises are uncomfortable, the back extension stretch on the exercise ball is an effective extension mobilization self-treatment (see Figure 14.54 in Chapter 14).

THORACIC SPINE EXTENSION MOBILIZATION (Fig. 13.60)

Postisometric relaxation can be used to improve extension mobility in the thoracic spine. The seated patient pushes with their elbows downward against the practitioner's resistance. Mobilizing the thoracic spine into extension is then accomplished by raising the patient's elbows while pressing into the spine with an opposing hand.

Self-Treatment. The thoracic region can easily become kyphotic. A simple stretch to increase extension mobility is shown in Figure 13.61.

RIB MOBILIZATION

Postisometric relaxation can be used to help mobilize an upper costotransverse joint. The technique requires that the doctor contact the dysfunctional joint and reach the barrier in

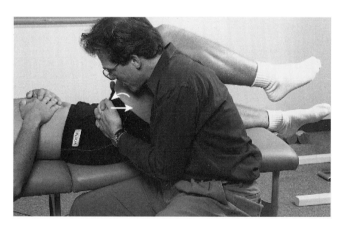

Fig. 13.57. Hip joint posterior glide PIR mobilization.

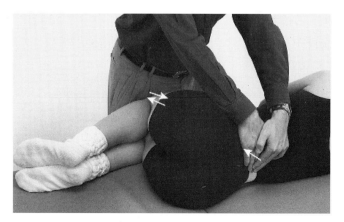

Fig. 13.58. Lumbar spine extension PIR mobilization.

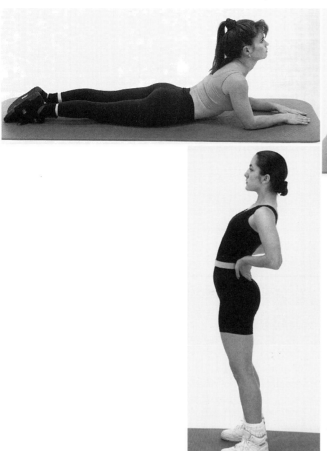

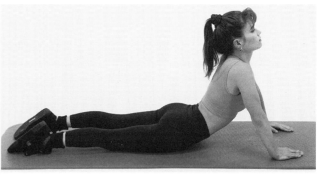

Fig. 13.59. Lumbar spine extension automobilization.

extension by raising the ipsilateral elbow. The patient is instructed to push his or her elbow downward. After resistance is applied to this movement and the patient relaxes, the joint may be mobilized (Fig. 13.62).

Facilitation Techniques

LOWER FIXATORS OF THE SCAPULAE (LOWER & MIDDLE TRAPEZIUS) (Fig. 13.63)

Patient Position
• Supine

Doctor Position
• Standing to side of patient
• Grasps patient's arm with both hands and pulls shoulder blade into protraction/abduction

Resisted Effort
• Patient pulls should back toward table and in toward spine, avoiding hiking shoulder toward their ear or use of triceps (elbow is seen to bend)
• Effort is isometrically resisted by doctor

Other Facilitation Techniques. The PNF DE2 pattern shown in Figure 13.64 is another excellent way to facilitate the lower fixators of the scapulae.

RHYTHMIC STABILIZATION OF SHOULDER JOINT

A well-known PNF technique for the shoulder involves resisting contractions by the internal and external rotators in various degrees of abduction (Figures 13.65 and 13.66).

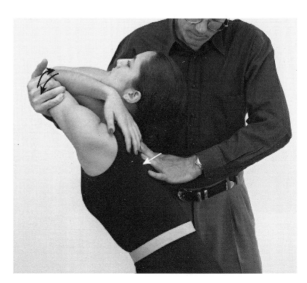

Fig. 13.60. Thoracic spine extension PIR mobilization.

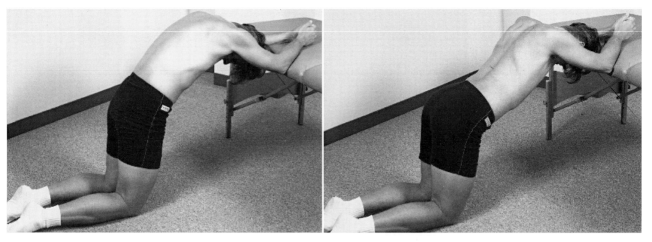

Fig. 13.61. Thoracic spine extension self-stretch.

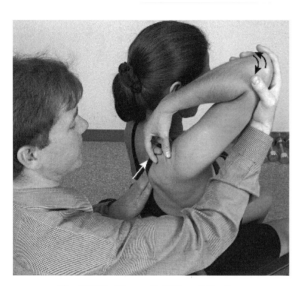

Fig. 13.62. Upper rib PIR mobilization.

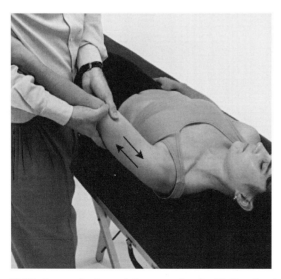

Fig. 13.63. Lower fixators of the scapulae facilitation (contract-relax).

MIDDLE TRAPEZIUS (Fig. 13.67)

Patient Position
- Prone with arms at sides

Doctor Position
- Standing at side of table

Patient's Active Effort
- Raises arms into extension with external rotation
- Attempts to pull shoulder blades together without shrugging shoulders
- Resistance may be applied to medial border of scapulae
- Hand weights added for progressive training

Greater challenge will result from performing this same movement with the arms partially abducted, abducted 90°, and fully abducted. A bench or exercise ball may be used. None of these exercises should be performed, however, unless the patient can avoid shoulder shrugging (upper trapezius activation) during the movement.

Other Facilitation Techniques. This area may also be exercised with the elbows bent by simply squeezing the shoulder blades together (Fig. 13.68). Resistance to the medial border of the scapulae will facilitate the middle trapezius (Fig. 13.69).

LOWER FIXATORS OF THE SCAPULAE (LOWER AND MIDDLE TRAPEZIUS) (Fig. 13.70)

Patient Position
- Side lying
- Involved side up
- Arm fully abducted

Doctor Position
- Sitting behind patient
- Places thumb or finger contact at inferomedial border of scapulae

Patient's Active Effort
- Pulls shoulder blade back toward spine while avoiding any tendency to shrug shoulders

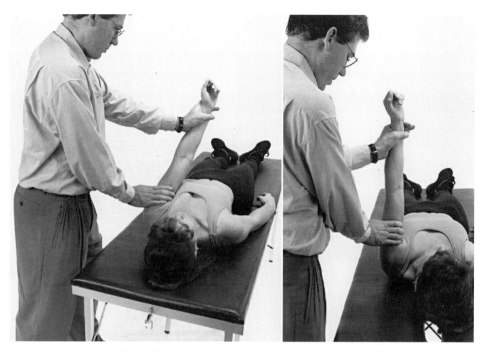

Fig. 13.64. DE2 proprioceptive neuromuscular facilitation pattern.

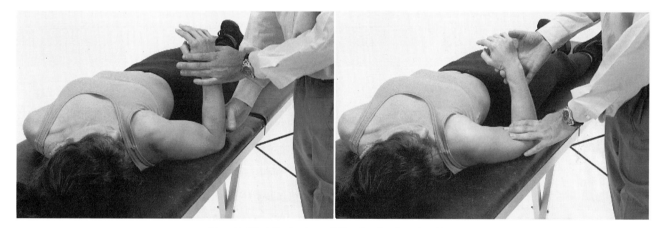

Fig. 13.65. Rhythmic stabilization for the shoulder.

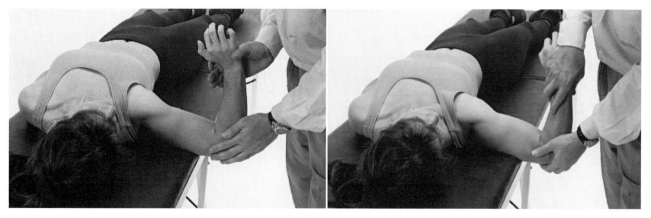

Fig. 13.66. Rhythmic stabilization for the shoulder (90° abduction).

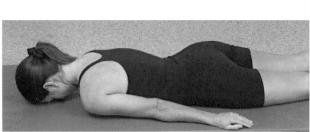

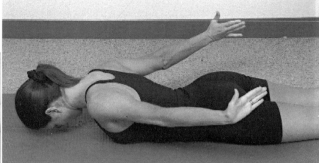

Fig. 13.67. Middle trapezius facilitation exercise.

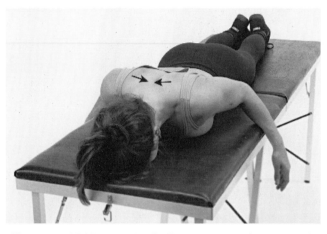

Fig. 13.68. Middle trapezius facilitation exercise (elbows bent).

- Effort should be isometrically resisted by doctor at inferomedial border of scapulae (or posterior shoulder)
- Patient may isometrically hold adducted and depressed (back and down) position of scapulae and perform:
  - Shoulder adduction/abduction
  - Shoulder flexion/extension

- Hand weight may be added
- If patient tends to hyperextend the low back, place a pillow under abdomen

GLUTEUS MEDIUS FACILITATION (Fig. 13.71)

Patient Position
- Side lying with lower hip and knee flexed

Doctor Position
- Standing behind patient
- Contacts gluteus medius insertion onto greater trochanter
- Grasps patient's leg around knee

Facilitation
- Rapid mobilization into abduction while applying "goading" stimulation to tendinous insertion
- Each mobilization should incrementally increase range into hip abduction (may be performed in fast, ratchety manner four to eight times)
- After mobilization, leg placed into abduction, internal rotation, and slight extension; patient holds leg up as doctor suddenly lets leg drop
- Muscle should be seen to quickly contract so leg does not drop

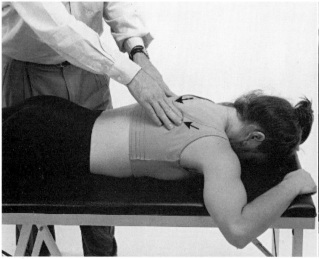

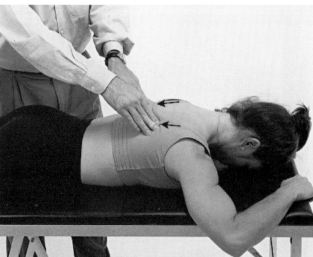

Fig. 13.69. Middle trapezius contract-relax facilitation.

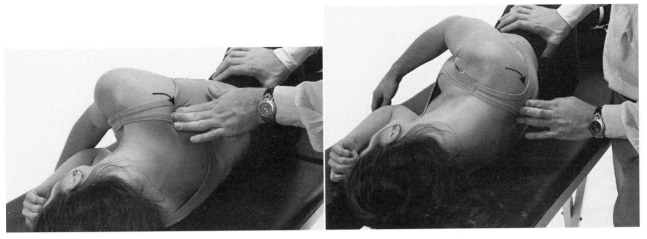

Fig. 13.70. Lower and middle trapezius contract-relax facilitation.

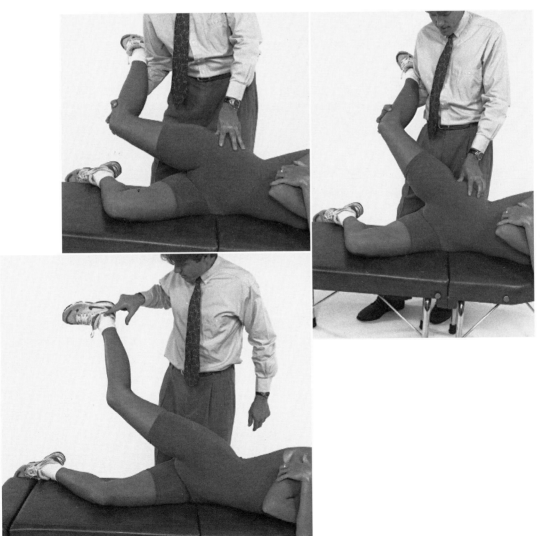

Fig. 13.71. Gluteus medius facilitation.

CONCLUSION

The MRT are invaluable tools when soft tissue lesions are considered primary or significant in the patient's functional pathology. If chiropractic adjustments are unsuccessful in relaxing contracted musculature, MRT should be applied. High velocity adjustments are still the most potent tool available, especially when a joint lesion is primary. In patients with significant guarding, however, MRT relax the patient and inhibit muscle tension, thereby making the adjustment easier to perform and longer lasting.

Generally, tense muscles should be relaxed and shortened myofascial tissue stretched before weak muscles are exercised. Therefore, MRT should be used at the beginning of any rehabilitation program before initiating a strengthening program.

Manual resistance techniques are simple and allow a patient to learn self-treatment. Their use enhances the doctor-patient relationship, encouraging the patient to become more actively involved in their own health care. Well-prepared patients are better able to manage minor aggravations of their symptoms on their own. Self-treatment does not replace chiropractic or manual medicine treatment, but it is increasingly valuable in an era of diminishing third-party reimbursement.

ACKNOWLEDGEMENTS

I thank Joanne Larricq, Jerry Hyman, Vladimir Janda, and Karel Lewit for their suggestions and contributions to this chapter.

REFERENCES

1. Kabot H: Studies on neuromuscular dysfunction. XIII: New concepts and techniques of neuromuscular reeducation for paralysis. Permanente Found Med Bull 8:121, 1950.
2. Levine MG, Kabat H, Knott M, et al: Relaxation of spasticity by physiological techniques. Arch Phys Med Rehabil 35:214, 1954.
3. Mitchell Jr F, Moran PS, Pruzzo NA: an Evaluation of Osteopathic Muscle Energy Procedures. Valley Park, Pruzzo, 1979.
4. Gaymans F, Lewit K: Mobilization techniques using pressure (pull) and muscular facilitation and inhibition. In Lewis K, Gutmann G (Eds): Functional Pathology of the Motor System. Rehabilitacia Supplementum, 10-11. Bratislava, Obzor, 1975, pp 47-52.
5. Lewit K: Postisometric relaxation in combination with other methods of muscular facilitation and inhibition. Manuelle Med 2:101, 1986.
6. Robinson KL, McComas AJ, Belanger AY: Control of soleus motoneuron excitability during muscle stretch in man. J Neurol Neurosurg Psychiatry 45:699, 1982.
7. Guissard N, Duchateau J, Hainaut K: Muscle stretching and motoneuron excitability. Eur J Appl Physiol 58:47, 1988.
8. Schieppati M, Crenna P: From activity to rest: Gating of excitatory autogenetic afferences from the relaxing muscle in man. Exp Brain Res 56:448, 1984.
9. Williams PE, Goldspink G: Longitudinal growth of striated muscle fibres. J Cell Sci 9:751, 1971.
10. Tarbary JC, Tarbary C, Tardieu C, et al: Physiological and structural changes in cat's soleus muscle due to immobilization at different lengths by plaster casts. J Physiol Paris 224:231, 1972.
11. Williams PE, Catanese T, Lucey EG, et al: The importance of stretch and contractile activity in the prevention of connective tissue accumulation in muscle. J Anat 158:109, 1988.
12. Lakei M, Robson LG: Thixotrophic changes in human muscle stiffness and the effects of fatigue. Q J Exp Physiol 73:487, 1988.
13. Habarth KE, Hagglund JV, Nordin M, et al: Thixotrophic behaviour of human finger flexor muscles with accompanying changes in spindle and reflex responses to stretch. J Physiol (Lond) 368:323, 1985.
14. Hagbarth KE: Evaluation of and methods to change muscle tone. Scand J Rehabil Med Suppl 30:19, 1994.
15. Hutton, RS: Neuromuscular basis of stretching exercises. In Comi P (ed): Strength and Power in Sport: The Encyclopedia of Sports Medicine Series. London, Blackwell Scientific, 1992.
16. Voss DE, Ionta MK, Myers BJ: Proprioceptive Neuromuscular Facilitation, Patterns and Techniques. 3rd Ed. Philadelphia, Harper & Row, 1985.
17. Janda V: Seminar notes. Los Angeles College of Chiropractic, May 1988.
18. Evjenth O, Hamberg J: Muscle Stretching in Manual Therapy, A Clinical Manual. Vol. 1. Alfta Rehab, 1984.
19. Holt LE: Scientific Stretching for Sport. Halifax, Dalhousie University Press, 1976.
20. Cailliet R: Shoulder Pain. 2nd Ed. Philadelphia, F.A. Davis, 1981.
21. Liebenson CL: Active muscle relaxation techniques. Part I: Basic principles and methods. J Manipulative Physiol Ther 12:446, 1989.
22. Liebenson CL: Active muscle relaxation techniques. Part II: Clinical application. J Manipulative Physiol Ther 13:2, 1989.
23. Janda V: Muscle spasm—a proposed procedure for differential diagnosis. J Manual Med 6:136, 1991.
24. Lewit K, Simons DG: Myofascial pain: Relief by post-isometric relaxation. Arch Phys Med Rehabil 65:452, 1984.
25. Travell J, Simons D: Myofascial Pain and Dysfunction: The Trigger Point Manual. Vol. 2. Baltimore, Williams & Wilkins, 1992.
26. Greenman PE: Principles of Manual Medicine. Baltimore, Williams & Wilkins, 1991.
27. Spitzer WO, LeBlance FE, Dupuis M, et al: Scientific approach to the assessment and management of activity-related spinal disorders: A monograph for clinicians. Report of the Quebec Task Force on Spinal Disorders. Spine 12 (Suppl 7):S1, 1987.
28. Bigos S, Bowyer O, Braen G, et al: Acute Low Back Problems in Adults. Clinical Practice Guideline. Rockville, U.S. Department of Health and Human Services, Public Health Service, Agency for Health Care Policy and Research, December 1994.
29. Larricq J: Lecture. Los Angeles College of Chiropractic, April 1994.

14 Spinal Stabilization Exercise Program

JERRY HYMAN and CRAIG LIEBENSON

Repetitive strain is the most common reason people develop pain. Improving load handling ability is instrumental in preventing chronic or recurrent pain. Ironically, by redirecting the patient's focus from chronic pain to functional integrity, the pain is more likely to "go away." The result of controlling loads in a more biomechanically effective manner is less tissue strain and, therefore, fewer painful episodes. Stabilization exercises train a patient to control posturally destabilizing forces. These exercises may start by requiring isometric postural stabilization of a key area, such as the lumbopelvic junction during trunk or extremity movements, and progressing to involve control of lumbopelvic posture during functional activities such as sitting, lifting, squatting, lunging, etc. Such exercises are *therapeutic* in that they teach the patient how to maintain postural control in activities of daily living. By focusing primarily on reducing lumbar overstress during functional exercises, the quadriceps, gluteals, and abdominals are trained without increasing back or hip pain. With this program, it is possible to achieve strength and endurance gains because the back is not stressed, thus the individual can train muscles to the point of exhaustion. Postexercise muscle soreness without symptom exacerbation is one of the essential stepping stones to returning to full participation in the activities of daily living.

Physical training addresses key functional deficits of strength, mobility, or motor control (endurance, coordination, balance). Functional stabilization (FS) exercises begin with identification of a functional range, especially of lumbopelvic movement. This is the range of movement that is both safe and appropriate for the task at hand. Pathoanatomic diagnosis is of secondary importance in these patients. Assessment of functional deficits or pathology (specific joint or muscular dysfunction and abnormal movement patterns) and identification of a safe training range (neutral spine position and functional range) are of primary importance in successful physical training of the patient with back pain.

Functional stabilization achieves muscular reconditioning without aggravating presenting symptoms by focusing on control of the lumbopelvic junction (maintaining a functional range) while exercising the "weak link" with the necessary intensity to achieve a training effect. Neuromuscular control, mobility, pain-free range, endurance, and willingness are all assessed during this process. Basic exercises such as pelvic tilts, bridges, trunk curls, lunges, and others are included. It is necessary for the practitioner to experience their own abilities through active learning during such a training regimen to elicit proper responses from the patient. Maintaining proper lumbopelvic stability requires limiting and controlling excessive or undesired lumbopelvic movement strategies; e.g., performing a lunge with too much anterior pelvic tilt and resultant lumbar hyperlordosis.

Patient education about the importance of good function for preventing pain recurrences is essential to motivate the patient to work on creating a healthier back. Explaining that fitter backs have fewer symptoms is helpful. Therefore, it is wise for patients to remediate function rather than just to seek pain relief. Learning to stabilize their back and gain self-management skills is the key to preventing recurrences. Educating our patients about the importance of this process and seeking a commitment from them is one of our most crucial functions.

STABILIZATION PROGRAM AND OVERALL PATIENT CARE

The stabilization program starts by identifying the training or "functional range" in which movement can be performed in a biomechanically correct and painless manner. Staying within this range may initially require performing isometric stabilization exercises by co-contracting the gluteal and abdominal muscles (i.e., posterior pelvic tilt). If a patient is asked to hold a posterior pelvic tilt and then move either arms or legs or both ("dead bug"), they find that holding the pelvic tilt "burns" the abdominals. Kinesthetic awareness, coordination, strength, and endurance are all trained in the process. A simple trunk curl is another example of an exercise that requires proper lumbopelvic control. During a trunk curl, the patient must control the natural tendency to recruit hip flexors that would tilt the pelvis anteriorly. Floor, pulley, machine, and gymnastic ball routines may all be used to increase the stabilizing demands. The stabilization routine can begin in non-weight-bearing positions and thus achieves intense training effects, such as postexercise muscle soreness in failed back surgery, postsurgical, subacute, and chronic pain patients without causing harm.

The main goal of this program is reconditioning key spinal stabilizers through building strength and endurance while insisting on proper neuromuscular control and coordination. The program also is of value as a mobilization approach that gently shows the path to movement exploration and re-education. In this case, the desired end result is less a conditioning effect (postexercise soreness) and more increasing patient confidence, muscle relaxation, circulation, and joint movement. In addition, while performing stabilization exercises, structural limitations are clearly identified (i.e., inability to perform a posterior tilt during a bridge as an indicator of tight anterior hip structures) that may require remediation through stretching techniques.

This exercise progression is often facilitated by the addition of manipulative therapy to improve joint or muscle function. Sometimes an exercise that is painful at first becomes painless after an adjustment or muscle inhibition technique. The combination of passive and active care is ideally suited to enhance the effects of either alone. Adjustments should last longer and pain recurrences diminish in frequency as a patient begins to gain greater lumbopelvic control and thus improved spinal stability.

This exercise program was first formulated for patients with low back pain by Vollowitz and Morgan, and is called functional stabilization or spinal stabilization.[1,2] It has been adapted for use by orthopedists and has reduced the need for surgery.[3,4] Its integration with other rehabilitation methods in a chiropractic setting has been discussed previously.[5] In a study of various treatments for chronic low back pain following unsuccessful L5 laminectomy, stabilization exercises along with McKenzie-type exercises were the most effective.[6] These low-technologic exercises were found to be superior when compared with passive methods, joint mobilization, and high-technologic exercise experimental groups. All treatments were administered three times per week for 8 weeks. Specifically, increased function as measured by lumbar range of motion (modified-modified Schober for flexion and extension), spinal muscle strength during lifting (Cybex Liftask), and self-report of disability (the Oswestry Low Back Pain Disability Questionnaire) showed greater improvement with the active approaches than with passive methods. Finally, the mean interval for pain relief was highest in the low-technologic exercise group (91.4 weeks) compared to 52.8 weeks for the high-technologic group and less than 10 weeks for the other groups.

FUNCTIONAL OR TRAINING RANGE

Many chronic pain, subacute, postsurgical, or failed back surgery patients are fearful that exercise will increase their pain. Some simple concepts can be applied that enable nearly anyone to begin to stabilize their spine. Training an area requires first that the range of motion (ROM) for the particular movement is defined. The goal is to find a range in which the patient can exercise without eliciting symptoms other than physiologic soreness (postexercise soreness). This range may be narrow, leading initially to only isometric exercise (i.e., a pelvic tilt). Some patients demonstrate a flexion or extension "bias" that must be respected. Some patients may not tolerate sagittal motions, but are fine with rotary or side-bending active movements. *When the painfree range or "bias" has been determined to be biomechanically safe or stable, it should be used in progressive exercise therapy.* This range may change depending on the position the patient assumes or the movement being tested. This training range has been labeled the

"functional range" for the particular task at hand. *Identifying the training range is important for performing therapeutic exercise in any part of the body. With respect to spinal problems, however, the lumbopelvic motion is of greatest value.* The beauty of this exercise approach is that the patient learns that it is possible to exercise without pain. As a result the patient gains confidence that some control over symptoms can be achieved with the use of specific self-treatment procedures.

RULE FOR TRAINING THE "FAILED" BACK
Find the painfree range of motion or functional range

Identifying the training range involves uncovering postural, movement, and weight-bearing sensitivities.[7] Individuals with postural sensitivities usually must sit or stand a specific way to avoid pain. For instance, an individual with a flexion bias is not able to stand for prolonged periods because of an inability to tolerate lumbar extension. They must preposition their spine in some flexion, e.g., using a foot stool.

Patients with movement sensitivities may have pain during certain activities. An individual who experiences pain when bending forward to tie shoes or put on pants may have an extension bias. The functional range of such a patient may not include flexion of the lumbar spine. A weight-bearing sensitivity or gravity intolerance may be revealed by a history of pain that occurs during sitting or standing and is relieved when resting. Compression usually aggravates these symptoms, as does coughing, sneezing, or any strong muscular contractions. This situation is common in patients with acute disk syndromes, who may have no functional range when upright, but can train effectively when recumbent. Another option for the weight-bearing sensitive patient is water exercises. Exercise performed in water should not mimic land-based exercises because motor programming may be inappropriately altered by the combined effects of water contact on the skin and reduced weight bearing.

Finding the training range is somewhat like a provocative examination used in the McKenzie system (see Chapter 12). The goal is to determine what movements and positions relieve, aggravate, or have no effect on symptoms. Those movements and positions in which symptoms are relieved or are unchanged can be used as part of a training program.

Activity within the training range is best tolerated by the patient when attempting repetitive and prolonged exercise training. The pain-free range is not always one and the same with the most stable or biomechanically correct movement. For example, a posterior pelvic tilt during trunk flexion is biomechanically efficient, because an anterior tilt can overstrain the lumbar spine and encourages substitution of the hip flexor muscles (i.e., iliopsoas) for the abdominal muscles (see Chapters 6 and 18). Many patients, however, report more pain with this positioning than with the anterior tilt of the pelvis. In cases in which the less stable or biomechanically inefficient movement is more pain-free, the joints and related soft tissues should be analyzed for dysfunction, with a focus on poor mobility or flexibility because of adaptive shortening or poor soft tissue extensibility.

Because of the individuality of each patient's functional range, how much anterior or posterior pelvic tilt is feasible will vary for everyone. Finding the painless range, along with assessing for short muscles and capsular restrictions and diagnosing structural pathology (i.e., spondylolisthesis) will lead to determining the functional or training range for each patient.

The bridge exercise provides another example of when altered mechanics because of poor mobility or flexibility can result in the exercise being less painful when performed incorrectly than when it is performed correctly. Biomechanically, the bridge is most stable and efficient when a sufficient posterior tilt is used, thus reducing lumbar stress and increasing gluteal activity. If, however, the patient has tight hip flexors, shortening of the hip joint capsule, and/or tightness of the lower lumbar erector spinae muscles, little if any posterior pelvic tilt will be tolerated by the patient. This case is one in which muscle relaxation and/or stretching and joint mobilization and/or adjustment would be required before the bridge could be used as a stabilization exercise.

PROGRESSIVE STABILIZATION EXERCISE TRAINING

Exercise therapy should be simple and painless to promote patient confidence. Initial reactivation exercises are designed specifically for a patient emerging from an acute episode or for a patient with chronic pain with fear of movement ("kinesiophobia") and symptom magnification to allow them to exercise without exacerbating their symptoms. *The patient should learn to explore basic lumbopelvic movements, such as the pelvic tilt, and perform gentle stretches and light cardiovascular exercise.* Weight bearing or gravity stress can be minimized by focusing on supine, prone, and sitting positions during exercise. The stress may be greater during upright activities of daily living.

Initial exercises wherein the patient explores movement at the lumbosacral junction in a variety of postures demonstrates the patient's neuromuscular control (or kinesthetic awareness). These exercises also reveal any structural limitation. Such a limitation may be present as a result of viscoelastic stiffness, elevated neuromuscular tone, bony abnormality, or structural pathology.

When acute pain is accompanied by inflammation, the patient will have pain with most or all movements. "Relative rest" and physical agents are necessary for this "chemical" pain. As inflammation subsides, symptoms will begin to behave "mechanically," meaning certain movements will provoke symptoms whereas other movements will relieve symptoms. As symptoms become mechanical, active exercise is indicated.

The starting point for the exercise is determined by appropriate history and examination. The answers one receives are determined by the questions one asks. Movements and positions that provoke symptoms are best avoided, and those that relieve symptoms should be included in an exercise regimen. *Post-training checks of pain-provoking movements or posi-*

tions, along with other additional outcome measures (i.e., limited range of motion, areas of tenderness), should be performed. This postcheck is a crucial step in increasing patient confidence about the positive benefits of exercise. It can allay fear and anxiety about pain and convert the patient from a pain-avoider to a pain manager. Also, showing the patient that they can move easier and with less pain after the exercises have been performed enhances patient compliance and motivation.

Evaluation of the prospective stabilization rehabilitation patient is summarized in Table 14.1.

STABILIZATION CONCEPTS

The important concepts that pertain to this therapeutic exercise philosophy are defined as follows.

Functional or training range: Painfree and stable joint range of motion (usually with respect to lumbopelvic motion) and appropriate for the task at hand

Passive prepositioning: Using body position and/or supports to passively place joints within the functional range (i.e., lumbar roll to preposition lumbar spine in extension during sitting)

Active prepositioning: Patient actively puts his or her lumbopelvic joint into the functional range and holds it isometrically during the course of an exercise (i.e., posterior pelvic tilt as a prelude to a "dead bug")

Dynamic stabilization: Gradual movement of the lumbopelvic junction into the functional range during exercise (gradually changing a pelvic tilt from squatting to standing)

Facilitation: Process of activating ("waking up") a muscle that is inhibited

Labile surfaces: Support surfaces that are unstable, such as styrofoam rolls, balance or wobble boards, and "gymnastic" balls

Functional tasks: Tasks which one would perform during the normal course of daily work, recreational, or sports activity. Performing these tasks with stability and coordination is the final goal of therapeutic exercise.

The purpose of stabilization exercises is to train proper coordination during posture, movement, and exercises of progressing levels of difficulty. The stabilization program teaches an individual to: identify correct posture, find their training range, maintain postural control while performing intensive exercises, and automatize coordinated, stable movements and postures during activities of daily living (Table 14.2).

When training a patient with back pain, improving stability involves more than just adding resistance and repetitions. Table 14.3 lists important variables to consider as patients progress through a routine.

In the office setting, stabilization exercises can be used like other conditioning programs by increasing repetitions and resistance according to standardized protocols (i.e., goal of 3 sets/15 reps). According to Morgan, it is customarily ad-

Table 14.1. Identifying the Training Range

History of static, dynamic and weight-bearing intolerance
Identification of the movements that provoke or relieve symptoms
Identification of the positions that provoke or relieve symptoms

Table 14.2. Trunk Stabilization Routine

1. Identify and explore training or functional range
2. Train lumbopelvic control during dynamic exercise using
   - Passive prepositioning
   - Active prepositioning
   - Other facilitation methods
3. Automatize coordinated posture and movement in daily skills

Table 14.3. Increasing Factors that Progress Training

Gravity load
Movement complexity
Balance requirement
Repetitions
Resistance

vantageous to perform stabilization exercises to a point of exhaustion independent of repetitions,[4] the end point being when the patient can no longer maintain the spine in the functional range during movements. Even then, the patient may be instructed to perform a similar exercise in an easier position ("peel back") so they can continue to exercise the muscles toward greater physiologic exhaustion. *Gaining kinesthetic awareness of the functional range and then exercising to fatigue is the best way to derive full benefit from this program. It is the quality and not the quantity of movement that is most significant.*

Peeling back is an important consideration as a patient progresses through a therapeutic exercise program. In this process, an exercise in the patient's training range is identified during which the individual can feel a "burn." After exhausting the muscle over a minimum of 2 minutes of training, the patient then "peels back" to another exercise in which the functional range can be maintained. The end result is a more intense conditioning effect while maintaining stability of the spine.

Achieving post-exercise muscle soreness requires a certain minimum intensity of exercise. From 30 to 40 minutes or hundreds of repetitions are needed to attain such a training effect in just a handful of lumbopelvic muscles (e.g., abdominals, gluteals, quadriceps, hamstrings). These same exercise principles, however, can be used in a less intense fashion to help promote better neuromuscular control without actually accomplishing a muscle conditioning effect. Such an application may be successful for certain patients, but it may fall short of the mark for a patient with lumbar instability or chronic pain.

CLINICAL APPLICATION

Therapeutic intervention with stabilization exercises requires a clinical problem-solving approach. *Typical problems encountered when progressing patients through a stabilization routine are poor flexibility, muscle inhibition, weight-bearing intolerance, or low motivation.* Addressing these situations as one encounters them is essential.

Stabilization exercises are often painful if extensibility is poor. When this situation is identified, it must be addressed before the patient can successfully perform stabilization exercises. For instance, difficulty in activating the gluteal muscles is often related to "lower crossed syndrome" with tight anterior hip structures. Any attempt at hip extension exercises typically results in lumbar overstress and hamstring and erector spinae overactivation. In this example, the first line of treatment would be flexibility training, followed by gluteus maximus muscle facilitation and then exercise (see Chapters 2 and 18).

Often during therapeutic exercise training, a muscle is hard to activate. The muscle may not be weak from loss of innervation or disuse atrophy, but may only be inhibited. Reflex inhibition from related joints and reciprocal inhibition from antagonist muscles are both potential therapeutic targets that should be addressed (see Chapters 2 and 18). Such reflex therapy can facilitate a "dormant" muscle. Other methods to wake up such an inhibited muscle include techniques from the proprioceptive neuromuscular facilitation philosophy, such as optimum patient positioning, verbal command, tone of voice, irradiation, and proprioceptive contacts. The value of these methods in facilitating an apparently weak muscle should not be underestimated.

When the muscle is adequately facilitated so that perception or awareness is present, volition alone can enable the patient to train the muscle therapeutically. With practice and repetitions, the muscle can be strengthened and its inclusion in everyday or even stressful activities can be automatized. Such "reprogramming" is the ultimate goal of FS exercises.

Depending on the level of deconditioning or structural pathology, patients may present with a gravity intolerance. These patients can still be trained using nonweight-bearing positions. Gradually, they can move from supine and prone loading to quadruped and kneeling and eventually to standing. Slide board or shuttle apparatuses (i.e., Total Gym) with incremental adjustments from horizontal to vertical can facilitate the transition from nonweight bearing to weight bearing.

Individuals with low motivation often are noncompliant with active care regimens. These patients can be "converted" or problems can be avoided by determining mutually acceptable functional goals and creating simple, painless exercises tailored to their individual needs. Additionally, postexercise checks of functional outcomes provide the patient with evidence demonstrating the benefits of self-treatment. If they see progress, they will be motivated to a greater extent than if asked to proceed on the doctor's word alone.

Treating failed back surgery, lumbar instability, or highly anxious patients represents the most difficult challenge to the physician. These patients have nearly invisible "functional ranges," but they may initiate training in the following manner. After identifying and exploring their functional range, they may begin by performing isometric floor stabilization exercises in the recumbent (nonweight bearing) position with traction assistance (see Figure 14.56). The patient may progress with or without traction assistance to other more demanding positions, such as quadruped, seated, or standing. If

Table 14.4. Lunge Test as a Functional Screen

- Trunk drifts forward during lunge: tight hip flexors, weak gluteal muscles
- Increased hyperlordosis during lunge: tight erector spinae, weak abdominals
- Front leg's heel lifts off floor: tight soleus
- Excessive knee shaking: weak quads, poor balance
- Front knee in front of foot: too short of a stride or torso moves too far forward

the patient has difficulty maintaining their functional range through active prepositioning, they may use passive prepositioning. For instance, supine hook lying with a cushion under the knees keeps the spine in a posterior pelvic tilt and allows easier stabilization training with either trunk (sit-up) or extremity movements (respecting any flexion or extension bias). The exact progressions chosen depend on the patient's response to training and the individual work or activity demands to which they must return safely.

Training can also progress by increasing the movement complexity. For instance, movements may begin in cardinal planes (sagittal or coronal) and advance to include torsional, coupled, and functional movements. Once a patient has learned to explore lumbopelvic motion and to identify their asymptomatic and stable functional range, they can perform various exercises while isometrically holding their spine within this range. Adding extremity movements to basic trunk exercises further challenges the patient's lumbopelvic control.

The goal of FS exercises is to perform skilled functional movements with the spine stabilized as the patient moves from one position to another. Examples include moving from sitting to standing, standing to kneeling, and quadruped to standing. At times, the functional range may change during a movement. A classic example of a transitional stabilization exercise is performing a lift from a squat position to standing with overhead reaching. In the squat position, an anterior pelvic tilt is held, and in the standing, overhead reaching position, a relative posterior tilt is maintained. This change is necessitated by the tendency of the lumbar spine to hyperlordosis when reaching overhead.

Another type of progression involves increasing the balance requirement during exercise. Progressing from floor to gymnastic ball or balance board exercises heightens the balance demands. This increase allows for a training effect that simultaneously improves strength, coordination, and balance. The freedom of movement provided by a labile surface allows subcortical training of reflexes that helps the patient to automatize better spinal stability. Improved reflex, automatic control of lumbopelvic motion during activities of daily living is the final goal of spinal stabilization training. When the patient has automatized this behavior, they can be considered re-educated.

Two types of functional testing are described. One type provides baseline information that shows overall progress. This form of testing can be used to motivate the patient and to inform third party payers of the patient's status. If this type is quantifiable, it is an ideal outcomes assessment tool. Another type of functional testing seeks to identify functional deficits that are correctable with specific prescribed interventions. For the purpose of spinal stabilization training, such prescriptive functional testing would assess the patient's ability to perform anterior and posterior pelvic tilts in a variety of positions (hook lying, quadruped, seated, standing), lunges, squats, trunk curls, sit backs, single leg balances, and bridges. Other tests could be singled out, but a few simple tests, such as those listed, can provide information about coordination, strength, and flexibility. Table 14.4 shows how the lunge can be used as a screening test.

STABILIZATION EXERCISE TRACKS

Stabilization training as described in this chapter deals with a progressive program of exercises designed to reverse the effects of deconditioning or to maximize performance potential. Exercises are organized into various "tracks," each one challenging the patient's ability to stabilize their spine in a different way. Within each track, the exercises are ordered so that they progress from simple to more complex movements. Each track is in effect a progress chart of a patient's spinal stability. The patient who can successfully perform only the first few exercises in a specific track is more deconditioned than the patient who can execute all the exercises in that track. It is best to find the exercise within each track where "breakdown" occurs, and then "peel back" to the one in which control is regained. Finding the patient's limit and peeling back is the art of spinal stabilization.

Progressing through a stabilization program does not mean mastering one track before moving on the next. When difficulty or weakness is encountered in one track, switching to another is often a catalyst to progress. Progress can be monitored by using a checklist (Appendix 14.1).

One key element to stabilization exercises is the emphasis on maintaining the spine in a functional range during training, often incorrectly termed the "neutral spine position." Most abdominal and gluteal exercises require a posterior pelvic tilt. Just how much flexion each patient needs should be determined individually. Most individuals do not have a "neutral spine posture" but rather have a functional range. Each patient, with the help of their clinician, must learn how to control excess motion to avoid exceeding the boundaries of their functional range. Some patients indeed have a "bias" toward more extension or flexion of the lumbar spine, again emphasizing the need for individualized training. Similarly, certain universal biomechanical principles dictate that when sitting, standing, or lifting, the spine should be upright (lordotic). How much lordosis will vary. Some people tend to be "slumpers," whereas others are more "swayback." Each group of individuals needs to develop reflex, automatic control of their lumbopelvic junction a little differently to avoid excessive loading. This fine tuning is what FS exercises are all about. Training may start with increasing awareness through facilitation methods, then progress to exhausting exercises and daily hypervigilance (for about 6 weeks), but it will ultimately fail unless normal movement patterns are not reprogrammed so that the individual "catches themselves doing it right."

The following specific exercises are designed as different avenues to travel with a patient. Each patient will proceed at a different rate. Sessions may vary from 10 minutes to more than 1 hour depending on the needs of the patient, and not those of the practitioner. In general, each regimen carries the potential for patient frustration because a great deal of coordination is required by the patient. Clear goals must be laid out and the practitioner must be patient and empathetic. A 6-week course of stabilization sessions is often adequate to begin the process of "reprogramming" better neuromuscular control and spinal stability.

Office sessions should occur no more than three to four times per week. At first, the patient is simply trying to feel a "burn" in the "big" muscles while feeling no strain in the spinal areas. Exercise intensity is increased until postexercise soreness is achieved without symptom exacerbation. A few sessions may be required to find the training range and achieve this result. Once this task is accomplished, the program quickly gathers momentum. As long as an exercise causes postexercise muscle soreness, it should not be repeated daily. Without the intensity of training required to achieve this effect, the motor control necessary to achieve spinal stability in daily life is not likely to result. Once a patient is discharged from the program, intensity and frequency may be decreased to a maintenance level.

1. Floor Stabilization Exercises

A. LUMBOPELVIC FUNCTIONAL RANGE EXPLORATION

Lumbopelvic range of motion is explored by performing posterior and anterior pelvic tilts.

- Hook lying (Fig. 14.1)
- Supine legs extended (ensure only minimal downward heel pressure) (Fig. 14.2)

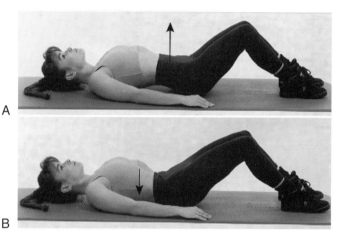

A

B

Fig. 14.1. Anterior **(a)** and posterior **(b)** pelvic tilt (hook lying).

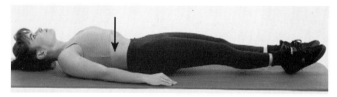

Fig. 14.2. Posterior pelvic tilt (supine).

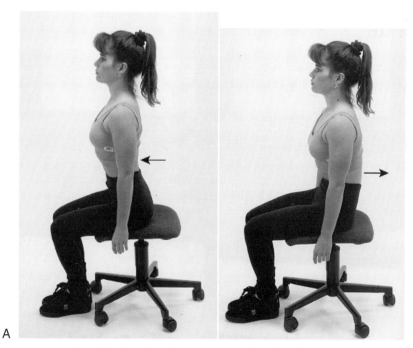

A

B

Fig. 14.3. Anterior **(a)** and posterior **(b)** pelvic tilt (seated).

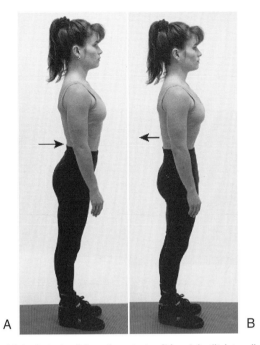

Fig. 14.4. Anterior **(a)** and posterior **(b)** pelvic tilt (standing).

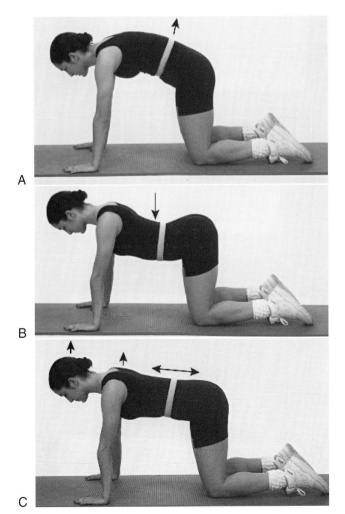

Fig. 14.5. Posterior **(a)**, anterior **(b)**, and partial **(c)** pelvic tilt (quadruped).

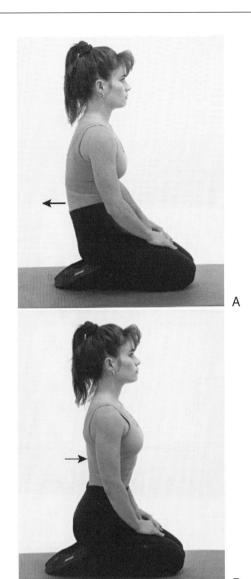

Fig. 14.6. Posterior **(a)** and anterior **(b)** pelvic tilt (kneeling with buttocks on heels).

- Seated (Fig. 14.3)
- Standing (Fig. 14.4)
- Quadruped (Fig. 14.5)
- Kneeling with buttocks on heels (Fig. 14.6)
- Kneeling with thighs vertical (Fig. 14.7)
- Sitting on floor with feet (soles) together (Fig. 14.8)
- Prone

Difficulty performing pelvic tilts often is a result of poor neuromuscular control. Appropriate verbal commands, facilitative cues, passive prepositioning, and appropriately directed resistance are all helpful aids in achieving the ability to perform these basic movements.

Adjustment or mobilization to the lumbar spine in either flexion or extension is often helpful, as is relaxation of overactive erector spinae muscles.

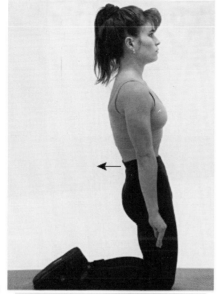

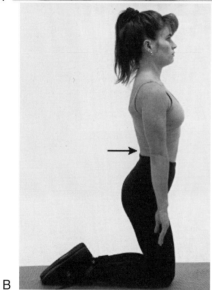

Fig. 14.7. Posterior **(a)** and anterior **(b)** pelvic tilt (kneeling with thighs vertical).

B. "DEAD BUG" TRACK (ABDOMINALS)

For each exercise in this track, ensure that the patient maintains the posterior pelvic tilt not only at the beginning of the movement, but also to the end of the exercise.

1. Hook lying, active preposition in posterior tilt, raise one arm at a time overhead
2. Hook lying, active preposition in posterior tilt, raise both arms overhead
3. Hook lying, active preposition in posterior tilt, raise one foot a few inches off the floor at a time, switching to the other foot so as to "march"
4. Hook lying, active preposition in posterior tilt, bring one knee to chest at a time.
5. Hook lying, active preposition in posterior tilt, bring one knee to chest at a time while raising opposite arm, return foot to floor (Fig. 14.9)
6. Hook lying, active preposition in posterior tilt, perform alternating kicks without letting feet touch the floor (the lower the legs, the harder the exercise) (Fig. 14.10)
7. Dead bug (Fig. 14.11)
8. Add ankle and wrist weights

When a patient has developed the neuromuscular skill to perform exercise 6 properly, then they have an exercise that, if performed repetitively, will bring about the required training effect to condition the muscles.

Difficulty with the "dead bug" track is usually associated with poor neuromuscular control or weak abdominals. Shortened psoas and/or erector spinae (hip flexors) muscles may also be a factor.

C. BRIDGE TRACK (GLUTEALS AND QUADRICEPS)

1. Supine, hook lying, with active prepositioning in posterior pelvic tilt bridge, slowly raising the pelvis and lumbar spine one segment at a time and then lowering one segment at a time (keeping kyphosis of lumbar spine throughout) (Fig. 14.12)
2. Bridge up, alternate heel lifts while holding bridge
3. Perform bridge, then "march" with only one foot on the floor (shift weight before marching) (Fig. 14.13)

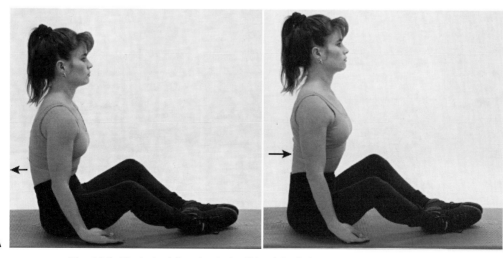

Fig. 14.8. Posterior **(a)** and anterior **(b)** pelvic tilt (sitting with soles together).

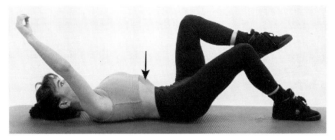

Fig. 14.9. Posterior pelvic tilt with opposite arm and leg raised.

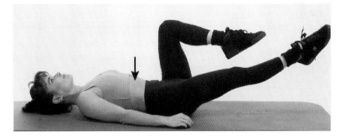

Fig. 14.10. Posterior pelvic tilt with alternating leg kicks.

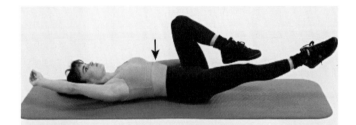

Fig. 14.11. "Dead Bug."

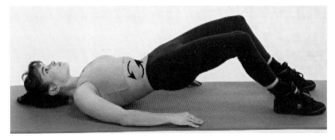

Fig. 14.12. Bridge.

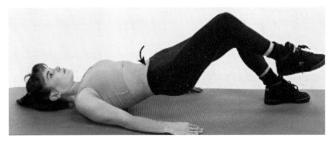

Fig. 14.13. Bridge with "marching."

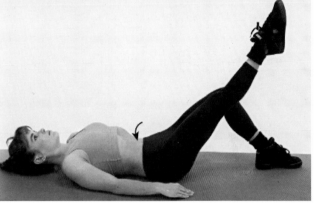

A

B

Fig. 14.14. One leg bridge ("dips").

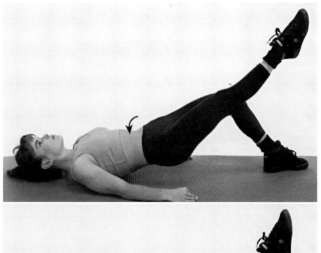

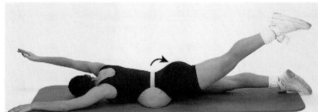

Fig. 14.15. Opposite arm and leg raise.

4. Bridge up, extend one knee, keeping both thighs parallel, perform one-leg bridges or "dips" (Fig. 14.14)
5. Holding bridge with straight leg, lower and raise leg

A training effect is possible with application of exercises from exercise 2 on. Difficulty with the bridge track is often associated with a shortened psoas muscle or overactivity in the lumbar erector spinae muscles. The one-leg bridge exercise involves use of the gluteal medius, and its difficulty may be associated with piriformis or thigh adductor tightness/overactivity. Additionally, lumbar segments may have decreased flexion motion. Sacroiliac and thoracolumbar joint dysfunction should also be considered.

D. PRONE TRACK (GLUTEAL MAXIMUS)

1. Single arm raise with pillow
2. Arm and opposite leg raise with pillow (Fig. 14.15)
3. Without pillow

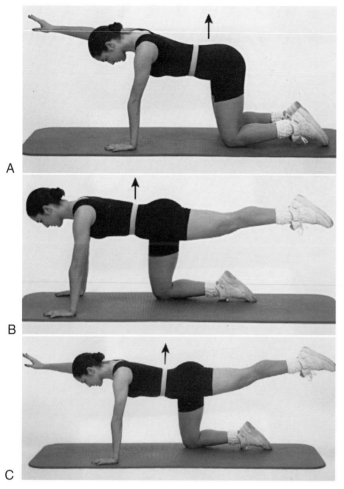

A

B

C

Fig. 14.16. Quadruped progression.

Difficulty often arises because of decreased spinal and hip extensibility. A tight psoas (hip flexor) muscle or hip capsule may be involved. Decreased lumbar spine mobility in extension (fixed kyphosis) is also a factor.

E. QUADRUPED TRACK (GLUTEUS MAXIMUS, MEDIUS)

- Preposition in neutral position and raise one arm (Fig. 14.16**a**)
- Raise one leg (Fig. 14.16**b**)
- Raise opposite arm and leg (Fig. 14.16**c**) (may add wrist and ankle weights)
- Add external resistance with doctor pushes (Fig. 14.17)
- With one arm raised, perform trunk rotation (Fig. 14.18**a**)
- Support arm on balance board, perform trunk rotation (Fig. 14.18**b**)

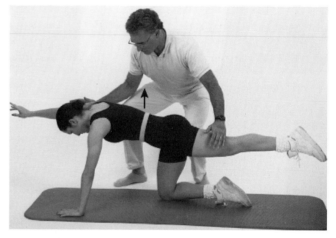

Fig. 14.17. Quadruped with external resistance.

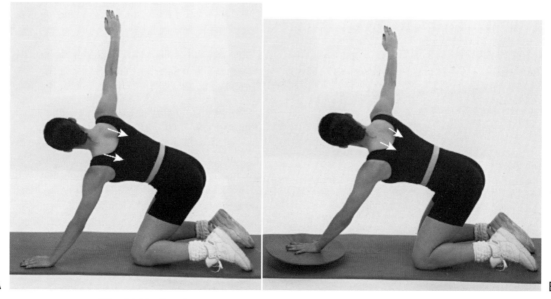

A

B

Fig. 14.18. Quadruped with trunk rotation **(a)** and on balance board **(b)**.

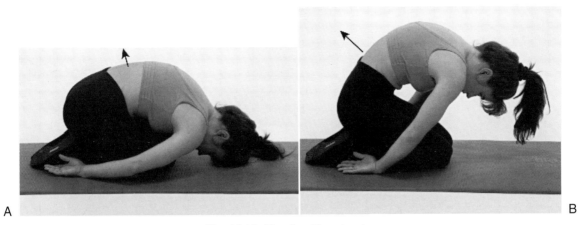

Fig. 14.19. Kneeling hip extension.

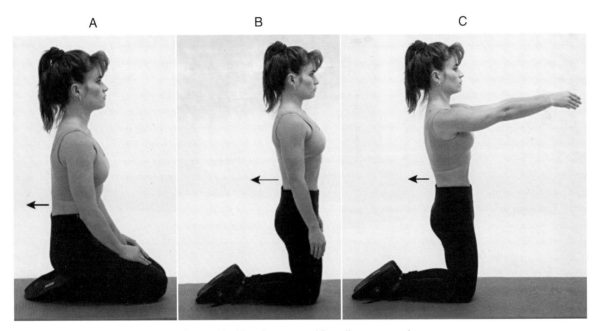

Fig. 14.20. Kneeling to semi-kneeling progression.

Difficulty with the quadruped track is encountered when the prone track is not mastered. Also, gluteus medius weakness/inhibition on the support leg side may be present because of adductor, piriformis tensor fascia lata, or quadratus lumborum hyperactivity/tightness.

F. KNEELING TRACK (QUADRICEPS, GLUTEUS MAXIMUS)

1a. Sitting on heels, trunk and hips flexed, posterior pelvic tilt, raise torso by extending hips (abdominals and gluteus maximus) (Fig. 14.19)

1b. Sitting on heels, trunk upright, posterior pelvic tilt, raise torso by extending hips (Fig. 14.20 **a** and **b**)

2. Same position as shown in Figure 14.20B with arms raised (Fig. 14.20**c**)

3. With weights (Fig. 14.21)

4. Hold raised position while flexing and extending arms (Fig. 14.21c)

Kneeling may be difficult because of knee problems or tightness in the erector spinae or rectus femoris. Erector spinae shortening or decreased lumbar flexion motion is also a factor.

G. ABDOMINALS

• Crunch with passive prepositioning (hips and knees positioned at 90° flexion as on a chair)

• Crunch with active prepositioning (Fig. 14.22)

• Trunk curl (with knees bent and partially extended) (Figs. 14.23 and 14.24)

    Posterior pelvic tilt

    Keep chin tucked, raise head then upper back until shoulder blades are off floor

    Feet should not lift up

A   B   C

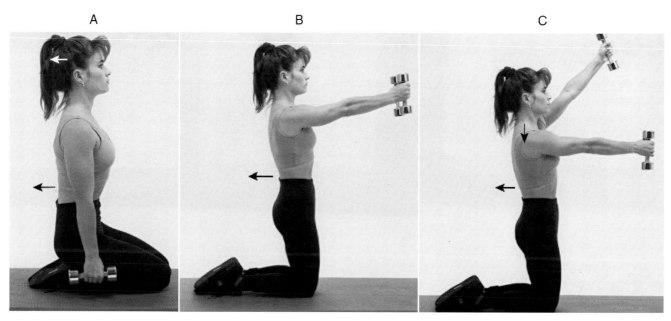

Fig. 14.21. Kneeling to semi-kneeling progression with hand weights.

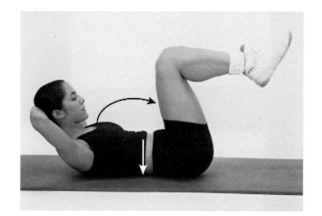

Fig. 14.22. "Crunch" abdominals (active prepositioning).

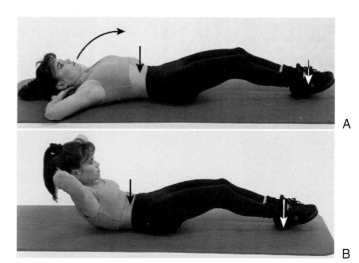

A

B

Fig. 14.24. Trunk curl with legs extended.

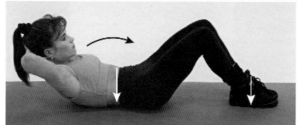

A

B

Fig. 14.23. Trunk curl with knees bent.

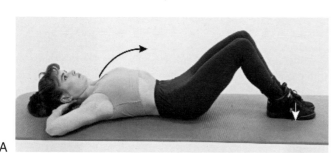

- Sit back
    Posterior pelvic tilt and lower trunk one segment at a time,
    then raise back up without lordosis (Fig. 14.25)
- Lower abdominal hip thrust with back flat and hips and knees
    flexed 90° (Fig. 14.26)
- Oblique

    Difficulty is often encountered when the erector spinae or
hip flexors are overactive/tight. Lumbar spine joint dysfunction may also be present.

H. LUNGE (QUADRICEPS) (FIG. 14.27)

- Feet should be shoulder width apart
- Maintain slight lumbar lordosis throughout lunge (front knee 90° flexion)
    Slight posterior pelvic tilt may be needed near completion of descent
    Stride should be long enough so knee is just over toes
- Lunge forward until back knee touches floor (Fig. 14.27B)
- Add hand weights, medicine ball, or weight bar
- Add resistance from behind with pulley or exercise tubing hooked onto patient's belt
- Backward lunge
- Sideways lunge

Difficulty can be encountered when hip flexors (back leg) or hamstrings (front leg) are tight. Observe balance errors, in-

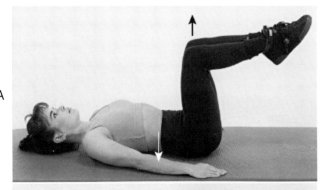

Fig. 14.25. Sit back.

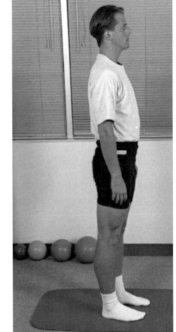

A

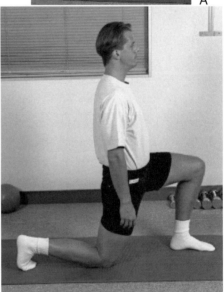

B

Fig. 14.27. Lunge.

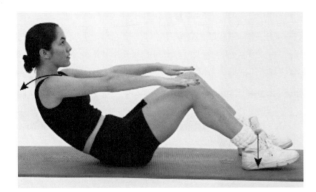

A

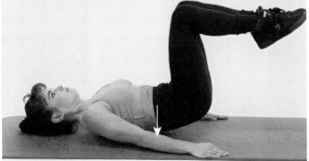

B

Fig. 14.26. Lower abdominal hip thrust.

appropriate neck/shoulder movements (i.e., chin poke, shoulder shrug), and small jerky transitional movements.

I. SQUATS

- With feet shoulder width apart, actively preposition in partial anterior pelvic tilt and perform partial squat (no more than 90° knee flexion) (Fig. 14.28)
- Progress to leaning forward to touch floor with hands without losing anterior pelvic tilt

Difficulty can be encountered if adductors are shortened. Heels will lift up if soleus is tight.

2. Styrofoam, Medicine Ball, Stick, Exercise Tubing Stabilization Exercises

A. ON STYROFOAM

- Perform posterior pelvic tilt with hands on floor (½ circle) (feet closer together is harder) (Fig. 14.29**a**)

Note: These movements are more difficult on circular-tubular foam
- Alternately lift one foot slightly off floor (Fig. 14.29**b**)
  Progress to 90° hip flexion
- Repeat above with arms overhead (Fig. 14.29**c**)
- Repeat above with both hands above chest (Fig. 14.29**d**)
- On circle wedge, hands on chest, one knee to chest

B. ISOMETRIC ABDOMINALS (WITH DOCTOR OR THERAPIST)

- Active preposition in crunch position with foam held between knees
  Patient resists movement of foam when doctor pushes or pulls foam (Fig. 14.30)
- Active preposition in crunch position (90/90 hip/knee flexion) with medicine ball or light object held between feet
  Doctor throws ball to patient overhead (Fig. 14.31)
- Active preposition in crunch position with ball held between feet and gymnastic ball on abdomen
  Patient resists movement of gymnastic ball by the doctor in different directions slowly

3. Gymnastic Ball Exercises

To increase patient confidence, gymnastic ball exercises can be done between two chairs for balance support. The ball is of the proper height if the hips and knees of the patient sitting on the ball are at 90° angles.

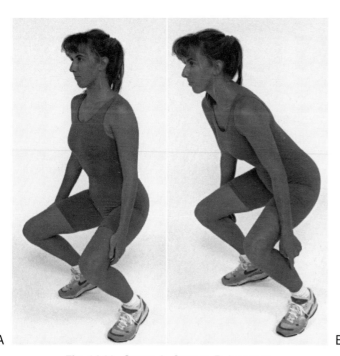

Fig. 14.28. Squat. **A.** Correct. **B.** Incorrect.

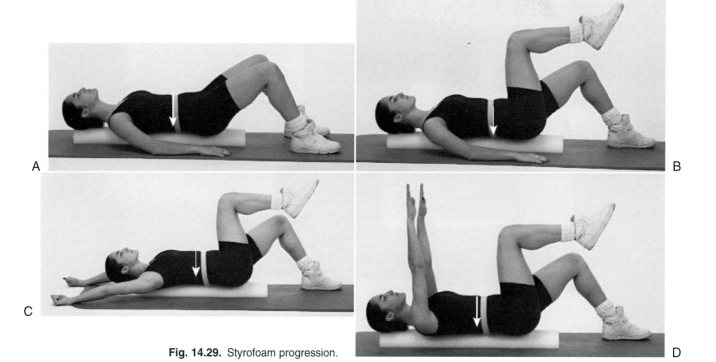

Fig. 14.29. Styrofoam progression.

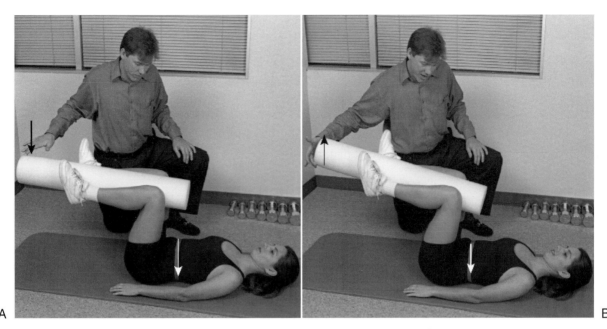

Fig. 14.30. Isometric abdominal "crunch" position with resistance.

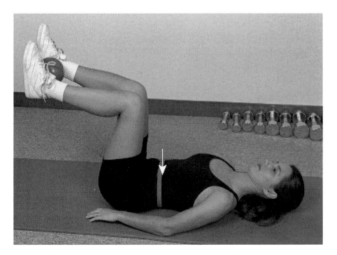

Fig. 14.31. Isometric abdominal "crunch" position with medicine ball.

A. SEATED

- Perform anterior and posterior pelvic tilt on ball (Fig. 14.32)
- Active preposition in neutral position, perform single leg raise (Fig. 14.33**a**)
- Single leg raise and roll back (maintain slight lumbar lordosis) (Fig. 14.33**b**)

B. BRIDGE (QUADRICEPS, GLUTEALS)

- Seated, perform posterior pelvic tilt and roll down ball to bridge (Fig. 14.34)
- Return to sitting position with posterior or anterior tilt (small steps do not stop)

Be careful that the head does not shift forward ($+Z$) or that the chin pokes out causing cervicocranial hyperextension
- Seated, posterior tilt, and roll down ball part way until abdominals begin "working" (Fig. 14.35)
  Hold position and slowly lift one foot at a time (gluteus medius)
- Shoulders on ball, active preposition in posterior pelvic tilt and bridge up (Fig. 14.36)
- Hold bridge and flex one leg with knee bent (Fig. 14.37)
  Keep posterior tilt and prevent opposite hip from falling and/or hiking
- Hold bridge and flex one leg with knee extended (Fig. 14.38)
- Bridge up and down with one leg on floor

C. ABDOMINALS

- Middle of back on ball, trunk curls
  Start low on ball (passively prepositioned in flexion) and progress higher on ball until exercising in extended position (Figs. 14.39 and 14.40)
- Middle of back on ball, perform partial trunk curl, catch ball thrown by doctor (Fig. 14.41)
- Progress to harder positions on ball
- Middle of back on ball, perform partial trunk curl, pull pulley or exercise tubing in rotary direction (elbows should stay extended, movement occurs from waist and not shoulders or arms)
- Progress by adding resistance
- All fours, front roll (feet off the ground) (Fig. 14.42)

D. HAMSTRINGS

- With legs extended and feet on ball, bridge up and roll ball toward buttocks by flexing knees, then roll ball away (Fig. 14.43)
- With hips and knees at 90/90 flexion, perform bridges (Fig. 14.44)

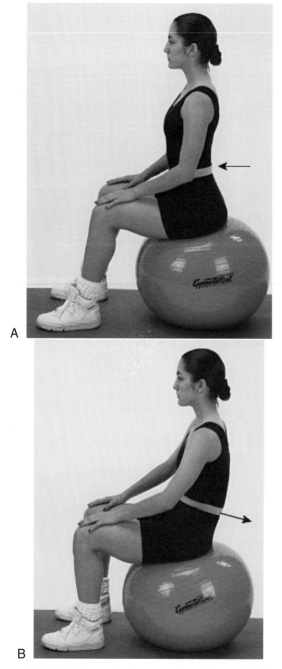

Fig. 14.32. Seated anterior and posterior pelvic tilt.

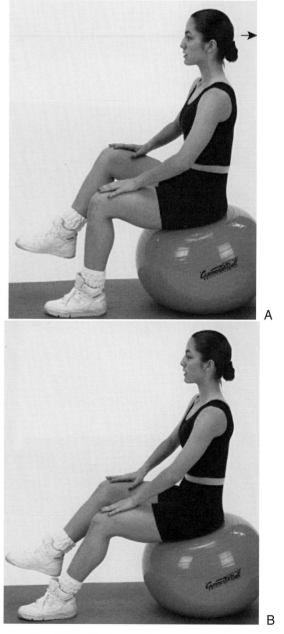

Fig. 14.33. Single leg raise and roll back.

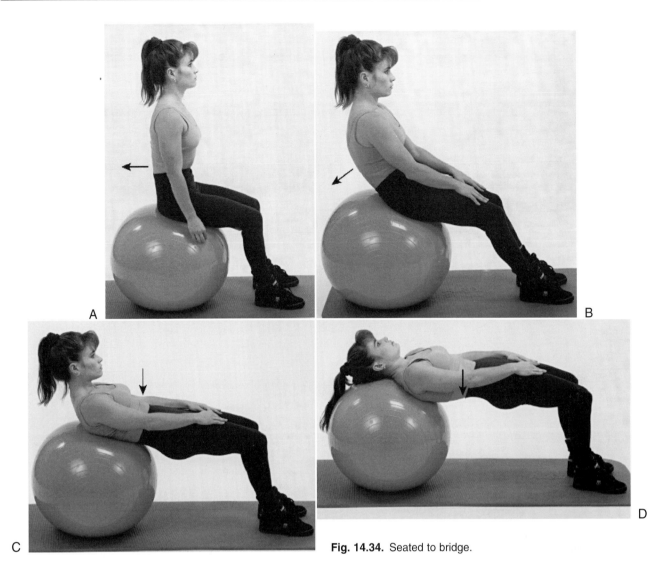

Fig. 14.34. Seated to bridge.

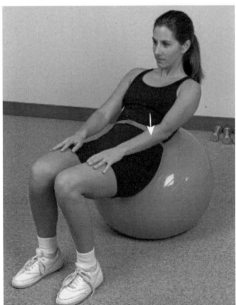

Fig. 14.35. Half sit-up with alternating leg raise (progress to partial bridge).

- Roll ball from extended position to knee flexion position with single leg (Fig. 14.45)
- 90/90 bridge with single leg (Fig. 14.46)
- Raising the arms vertically increases the stabilization demands on the trunk

E. SUPERMAN

- Prone on ball with feet against the wall, perform posterior pelvic tilt and then extend the trunk by pushing off from wall and straightening the back. Make sure to maintain some gluteal and abdominal co-contraction throughout movement (Fig. 14.47**a** and **b**)
- In extended position, swing one arm up overhead while holding posterior pelvic tilt (Fig. 14.47**c**)

If this exercise is difficult to perform, retreat to the kneeling track exercise shown in Figure 14.19.

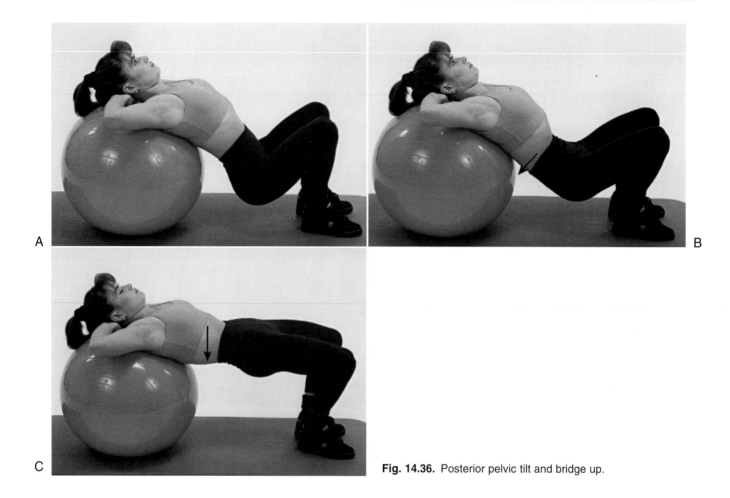

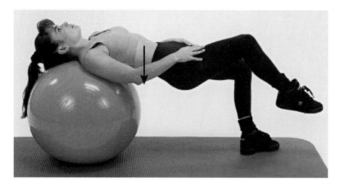

Fig. 14.36. Posterior pelvic tilt and bridge up.

Fig. 14.37. Hold bridge and flex bent leg.

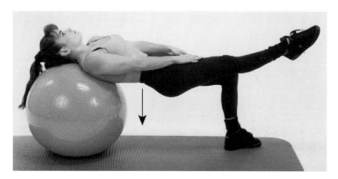

Fig. 14.38. Hold bridge and flex straight leg.

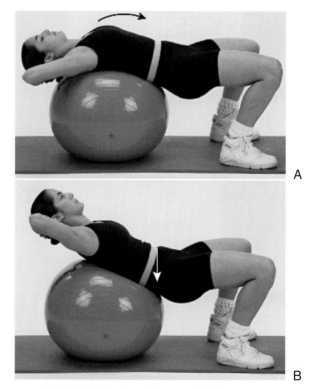

Fig. 14.39. Trunk curl lower on ball (easier).

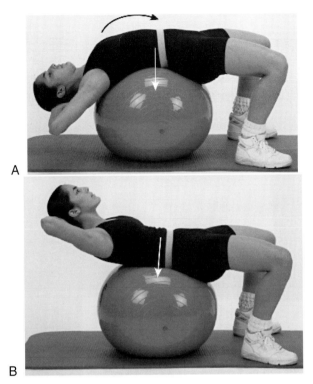

Fig. 14.40. Trunk curl higher on ball (harder).

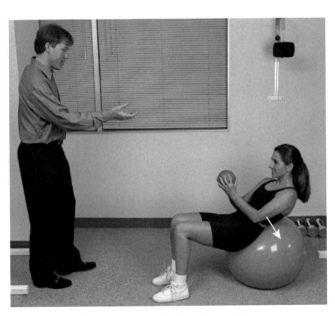

Fig. 14.41. Trunk curl and catch medicine ball.

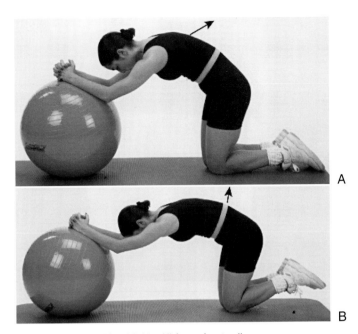

Fig. 14.42. All fours front roll.

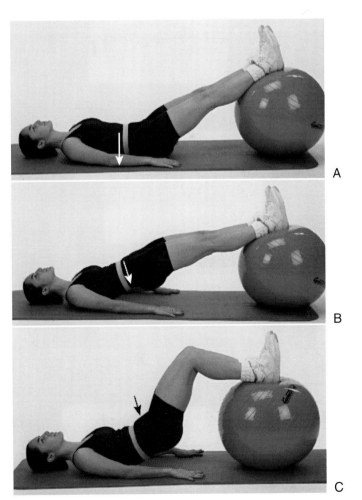

Fig. 14.43. Bridge and roll ball in and out.

F. SEE-SAW

- Anterior thighs on ball, hands on floor, active preposition in neutral position, raise and lower upper and lower body alternately (see-saw) (Fig. 14.48a and **b**)
- Raise one leg to perform the scissor (Fig. 14.48c)

Difficulty can be encountered if erector spinae or hip flexors are tight.

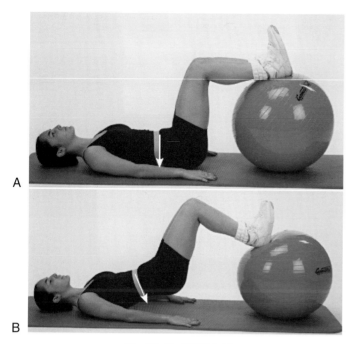

Fig. 14.44. 90/90 bridge.

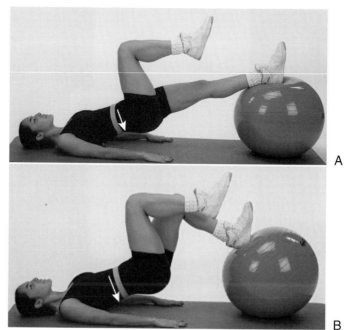

Fig. 14.45. One leg bridge with roll.

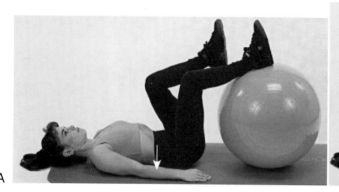

Fig. 14.46. One leg bridge 90/90.

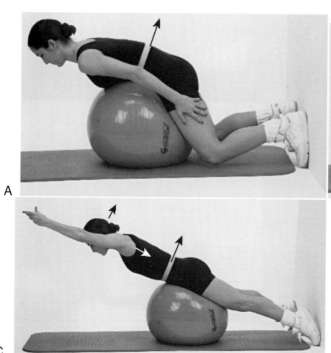

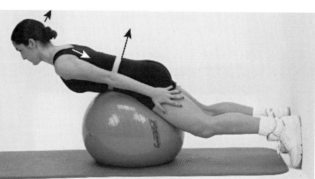

Fig. 14.47. Superman progression.

G. SQUATS

- Wall slide with lower back against wall and slight anterior pelvic tilt (Fig. 14.49)
- Perform with a weight in hands; as legs extend, gradually raise the weight overhead

  When the arms reach horizontal, transition from an anterior to a posterior pelvic tilt
- Perform a squat with one foot on floor (Fig. 14.50) (one-legged squats with the ball may not be as deep)

H. KNEE ON BALL FRONT ROLL

- Knees on ball and hands on floor, circumduct pelvis (Fig. 14.51)

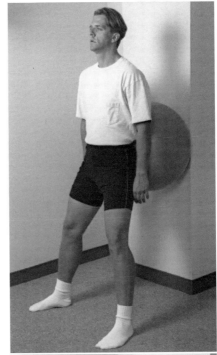

A

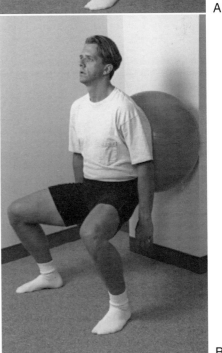

B

Fig. 14.49. Squat.

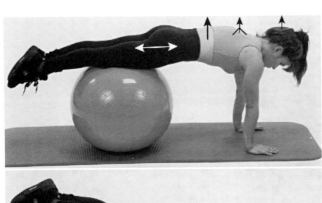

A

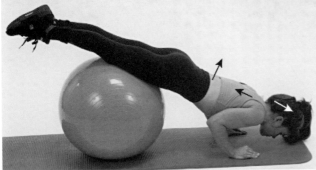

B

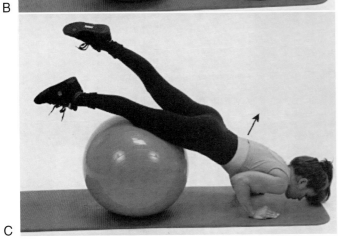

C

Fig. 14.48. See-saw progression.

I. OTHER BALL EXERCISES

- Prone on ball back extension (Fig. 14.52)
- Prone on ball upper back extension (Fig. 14.53)

  Adduct shoulder blades and then lift sternum off ball

  Keep chin tucked in
- Back stretch on ball (Fig. 14.54)

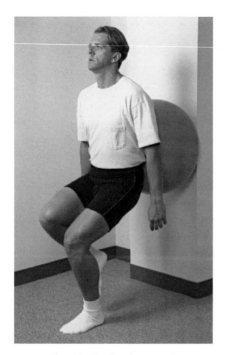

Fig. 14.50. One leg squat.

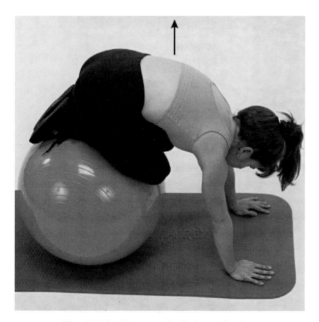

Fig. 14.51. Knees on ball circumduction.

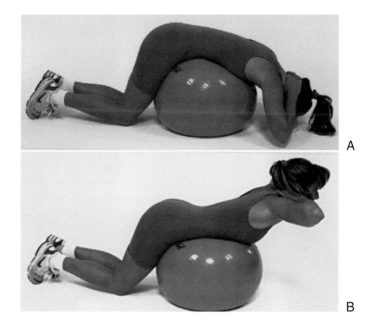

A

B

Fig. 14.52. Lumbar extension.

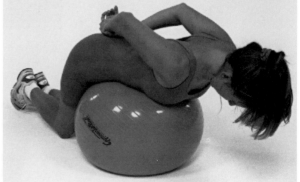

A

B

Fig. 14.53. Dorsal extension.

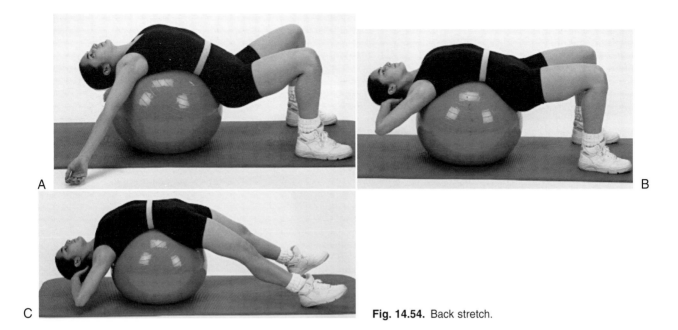

Fig. 14.54. Back stretch.

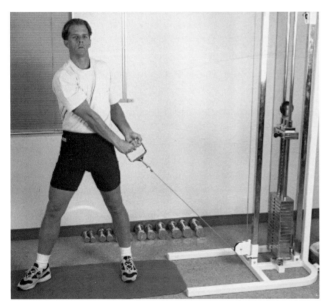

Fig. 14.55. Shoulder rotation with trunk stabilization.

4. Pulleys and Bicycle

A. TRUNK TWISTS

- Isometric stabilization with abdominal/gluteal co-contraction, perform trunk twist against resistance (hold elbows in extended position) (Fig. 14.55)

B. GRAVITY-ASSISTED PULL DOWNS

- Perform posterior pelvic tilt against resistance while bringing hands to abdomen against resistance (Fig. 14.56)

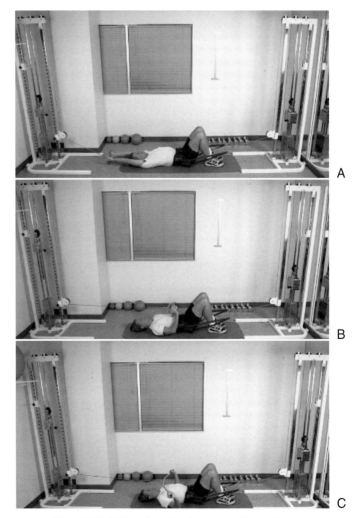

Fig. 14.56. Pelvic tilt and pull downs with traction.

C. RECUMBENT BICYCLE

- Supine on floor or lay back on large ball while riding stationary bicycle (Fig. 14.57)

REFERENCES

1. Morgan D: Concepts in functional training and postural stabilization for the low-back-injured. Top Acute Care Trauma Rehabil 2:8, 1988.
2. Morgan D: Seminar, Los Angeles College of Chiropractic, 1992.
3. Saal JA, Saal JS: Nonoperative treatment of herniated lumbar interverte-bral disc with radiculopathy. Spine 14:431, 1989.
4. Saal JA: Dynamic muscular stabilization in the nonoperative treatment of lumbar pain syndromes. Ortho Rev 19:691, 1990.
5. Liebenson CL: Rehabilitation of the chronic back pain patient: Functional restoration techniques. Cal Chir J 16:26, 1991.
6. Timm KE: A randomized-control study of active and passive treatments for chronic low back pain following laminectomy. J Orthop Sports Phys Ther 20:276, 1994.
7. Vollowitz E: Furniture prescription for the conservative management of low-back pain. Top Acute Care Trauma Rehabil 2:18, 1988.

ACKNOWLEDGMENTS

We are grateful for the example and guidance of Dennis Morgan and Joanne Larricq in the completion of this chapter.

APPENDIX 14.1 Exercise Checklist:

1. FLOOR STABILIZATION EXERCISES

a. Lumbopelvic functional range exploration
____Hook lying
____Supine legs extended
____Seated
____Standing
____Quadruped
____Kneeling with buttocks on heels
____Kneeling with thighs vertical
____Sitting on floor with feet (soles) together

b. "Dead bug" Track (abdominals)
____Raise 1 arm at a time overhead
____Raise both arms overhead
____"March"
____Bring 1 knee to chest at a time
____Bring 1 knee to chest at a time while raising opp. arm
____Alternating kicks
____Dead bug
____Ankle and wrist weights

c. Bridge Track (gluteals and quadriceps)
____Bridge
____Bridge w/ heel lifts
____Bridge w/ "march"
____1 leg bridge
____Bridge and lower and raise leg

d. Prone Track (gluteus maximus)
____Single arm raise w/ pillow
____Arm/opp. leg raise w/ pillow
____W/out pillow

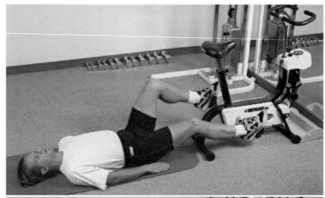

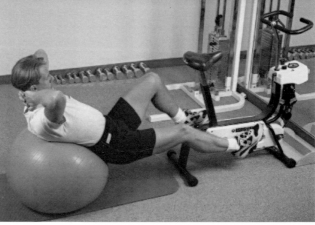

Fig. 14.57. Recumbent bicycle.

e. Quadruped Track (gluteal maximus, medius)
____Raise 1 arm
____Raise 1 leg
____Raise opposite arm and leg
____Wrist and ankle weights
____External resistance
____1 arm raised perform trunk rotation
____Balance board perform trunk rotation

f. Kneeling Track (quadriceps, gluteal maximus)
____Sitting on heels raise torso
____Sitting on heels, trunk upright raise torso
____Sitting on heels, trunk upright raise torso w/ raised arms
____W/ weights
____Flexing and extending arms

g. Abdominals
____Crunch
____Trunk curl
____Sit back
____Hip thrust
____Obliques

h. Lunge (quadriceps)
____Lunge
____W/ weight
____W/ pulley or exercise tubing
____Backward lunge
____Sideways lunge

i. Squats

_____Squat

_____W/ forward bend

2. STYROFOAM, MEDICINE BALL, STICK, EXERCISE TUBING STABILIZATION EXERCISES

a. On styrofoam

_____Posterior pelvic tilt

_____1 knee to chest

_____1 knee to chest w/arms overhead

_____On circle wedge hands on chest 1 knee to chest

b. Isometric Abdominals (w/doctor or therapist)

_____Crunch position with foam between knees doctor pushes or pulls

_____Medicine ball between feet/ doctor throws ball

_____Ball between feet and gym ball on abdomen/doctor pulls ball

_____Medicine ball held between feet/sticks

3. GYMNASTIC BALL EXERCISES

Isometric Stabilization

a. Seated

_____Anterior and posterior pelvic tilt

_____Single leg raise

_____Single leg raise and roll back

b. Bridge (quadriceps, gluteals)

_____Seated and roll down ball to bridge

_____Return to sitting position

_____$\frac{1}{2}$ sit up and "march"

_____Bridge up/down

_____Bridge and flex 1 leg w/ knee bent

_____Progress to only upper back and head on ball

_____Bridge and flex 1 leg w/ knee extended

_____Bridge up and down w/ 1 leg on floor

c. Abdominals

_____Middle of back on ball trunk curls

_____Trunk curl and catch ball thrown by doctor

_____Progress to harder positions on ball

_____Trunk curl/pulley or exercise tubing in rotation

_____All fours front roll

d. Hamstrings

_____Feet on ball bridge w/roll in

_____90/90 bridges

_____Roll ball w/ single leg

_____90/90 w/ single leg

e. Superman

_____Superman

_____W/ arm swing

f. See-saw

_____See-saw

_____Raise 1 leg scissor

g. Squats

_____Wall slide

_____W/ something in hands

_____W/ 1 foot off floor

h. Knee on ball front roll

_____Front roll

i. Other ball exercises

_____Back extension

_____Upper back extension

_____Stretch

4. PULLEYS AND BICYCLE

_____Trunk twists

_____Gravity-assisted pull downs

_____Recumbent bicycle

15 Sensory Motor Stimulation

VLADIMIR JANDA and MARIE VA´VROVA´

Therapeutic approaches have changed along with our increasing knowledge and understanding of physiology. In the original approach to therapy, we viewed the motor system as an effector only, and did not consider its role with the afferent system as one functional unit. The conclusion was drawn that motor performance is a result of isolated and separate, although coordinated, activation of individual muscles. The focus of these techniques was activation of individual muscles or muscle groups in the hope that the new motor pattern would develop automatically. Examples of such thinking are exercises prescribed according to muscle testing or the progressive resistance exercise program.

The next step in the evolution of therapeutic approaches accepted that a movement cannot be accomplished without coordination of the afferent pathways and centers. Along with this knowledge came the realization that the motor system and the afferent system were closely linked.

VARIETY OF THERAPEUTIC APPROACHES

Kabat developed and introduced into practice the concept of activation of afferent pathways as an approach to movement re-education.[1] In therapy, this concept is the basis of the Proprioceptive Neuromuscular Facilitation (PNF) technique. This approach, as well as others such as those developed by Temple Fay, the Bobaths, Vojta, and Brunnstrom, systematically stresses muscle coordination and the importance of proprioceptive information. At present, it is understood that the afferent system not only has an informative role, but also participates substantially in motor programming and motor system regulation. Therefore, proprioceptive stimulation is stressed more and more.

The term *proprioception* was used for the first time in 1907 by Sherrington to describe the sense of position, posture, and movement.[2] This term has since been defined in a broader way, and today, although not quite correctly, it is used to describe the function of the entire afferent system.

It is now understood that to split the function and/or dysfunction of the myo-osteo-articular system from central regulatory nervous mechanisms is wrong. Both parts function as one inseparable functional unit and cannot be separated. Thus, any lesion or impaired function of any part of the peripheral motor system leads to adaptive mechanisms in the central nervous system and vice versa.

Kurtz was probably the first to notice, from a clinical point of view, the relationship between the lesion (injury) of the foot joints and incoordinated muscle function of the lower leg.[3] Apart from fundamental experimental work, such as that by Wyke[4] and Skoglund,[5] it was Freeman and co-workers (1964, 1965, 1967) who, in the clinical setting, systematically considered some aspects of joint traumatology and the importance of impaired afference in the genesis of an unstable ankle joint.[6-8] Freeman and colleagues also introduced, in non-neurologic cases, a detailed evaluation of coordination, and stressed the importance of muscle inhibition as an integral part of the clinical picture. Since the publication of this initial report by Freeman and Wyke, interest in this problem has increased. One of the most extensive works on this topic is by Hervéou and Mésséan.[9]

In 1970, we started to work out our program for clinical use, based to some extent on the published reports just mentioned. To avoid problems in terminology and/or confusion with terms such as PNF, we named our technique "sensory motor stimulation" with the hope of stressing the unity between the afferent and efferent system without implicating any specific structure or function.

BASIC CONCEPTS OF MOTOR LEARNING

The principle of sensory motor stimulation is based on the concept of two stages of motor learning.[10] The first stage is characterized as an attempt to achieve new movement performance and to work out the basic motor program. The brain cortex (predominantly the frontal and parietal lobes) are strongly involved in this process. This type of motor regulation has some advantages as well as disadvantages. It enables the individual to achieve new skills, although it is rather slow as it passes several synapses, and it is tiring given the necessary conscious participation of the cortex. Therefore, the brain tries to minimize the pathways and to simplify the regulatory circuits. This mechanism has been named as the second stage of motor learning. It enables a reduction of cortical participation, and thus is less tiring and much faster. If such a motor program has become fixed once, however, it is difficult, if not impossible, to change it. Therefore, in motor re-education, the goal is to achieve a quality of movement patterns that is as close to normal as possible.

To prevent injury, and microinjury in particular, fast reflex muscle contraction is needed to protect the joints. The second stage of motor learning enables such a faster response, which may, in fact, play a decisive role in prevention. Bullock-Saxton and colleagues[11] reported it is possible to

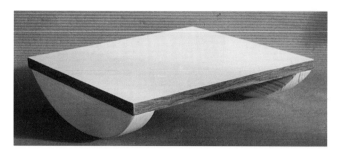

Fig. 15.1. Rocker board.

Many exercise aids of various types are used, including wobble and rocker boards, rolls from plastic material, balance shoes, various types of twisters and trampolines, and the Fitter. Wooden wobble and rocker boards are preferable to those made of plastic material, because wood stimulates the receptors to a greater extent. For the same reasons, toys made of wood more readily stimulate proprioception in children.

The average dimensions (length × width × height) for the rocker board are 35 cm × 25 cm × 15 cm.[16] The radius of the wobble board is 35 cm on average and the height is 15 cm. Exercises on the rocker board are easier than on the wobble board, and therefore it is advisable to start with its use (Figs. 15.1 and 15.2).

The size of balance shoes (Fig. 15.3) depends on the size of the foot. Sandals must have a firm, inflexible sole that is modeled and has metatarsal support; these features help to configure the small foot. There should be just one strap over the forefoot and the heel should remain free, again to help to activate the intrinsic muscles of the foot. The hemispheres are of solid rubber, 5 to 7 cm in diameter, and are placed in the center of gravity.

The twister enables activation of the trunk and buttock muscles. Exercising before a mirror helps to visualize any asymmetry in muscle strength and/or asymmetrically performed exercise. We prefer to use a flat twister that is 40 cm in diameter.

The Fitter, like the twister, is strictly speaking not a device for proprioceptive training, although it helps to improve coordination. Several devices with similar function are currently available. We use one developed by Fitter International from Canada (Fig. 15.4).

A minitrampoline (Fig. 15.5) is an excellent device for stimulating the proprioceptors of the entire body. Unfortunately, the material used for most trampolines is not sufficiently resilient. The stimulatory effect is thus reduced. Springs that are 15 to 18 cm in length provide a suitably unstable base; springs of less than 7 cm do not provide enough proprioceptive stimulation.

Other devices include balance balls that vary in size from 60 to 120 cm in diameter. They are efficient for kinesthetic stimulation and balance training. Rolls from polyester are widely used in the United States and help to activate the trunk muscles in general. Because these rolls are used mostly while the patient is supine, they do not overstress the spine and

accelerate muscle contraction approximately twofold with increased proprioceptive flow and balance exercises. In sensory motor stimulation, an attempt is made to facilitate the proprioceptive system and those circuits and pathways that play an important role in regulation of equilibrium and posture.

From the point of view of afference, receptors in the sole of the foot,[7] from the neck muscles,[12] and in the sacroiliac area[13] have the main proprioceptive influence.

Receptors from the sole can be facilitated in different ways, e.g., by stimulation of the skin receptors or, more effectively, by active contraction of the intrinsic muscles of the foot by forming the so-called "short or small foot." Clinical experience has revealed that isolated activation of the intrinsic muscles without activation of the long toe flexors is most effective. Therefore, it is difficult to agree with Ihara and Nakayama, who recommended the "foot fist" to activate proprioceptors.[14]

The deep neck muscles contain many more proprioceptors than are found in other striated muscles.[12] Abrahams has shown that these muscles should be considered for maintaining posture and equilibrium rather than for producing dynamic movement. It should be mentioned that deep tonic neck reflexes are the result of muscle activation and do not involve the neck joints, as was described originally.

In clinical practice, the sacral region is now recognized as an important area in the control of posture and equilibrium. This observation was confirmed by Hinoki and Ushio.[13] At present, however, it is not possible to differentiate whether it is the sacrum itself and its position or the sacroiliac joints that play the decisive role.

A special role has been recognized for the cerebellum and the whole spinovestibulocerebellar regulatory circuit.

SENSORY MOTOR DEVICES AND AIDS

The sensory motor approach is not a rigid program or system. It can be used in all cases and can be tailored to each patient. Various balance exercises are used. Any equipment required is simple and inexpensive. The principles are not new and were introduced by Bobath and Bobath for motor re-education of children with cerebral palsy.[15] The application of this approach to patients with chronic back pain patients, however, was introduced only recently.

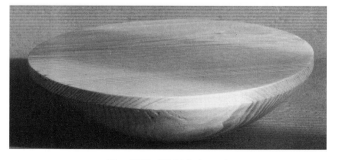

Fig. 15.2. Wobble board.

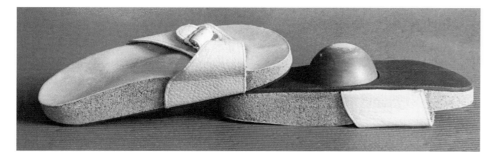

Fig. 15.3. Balance shoes.

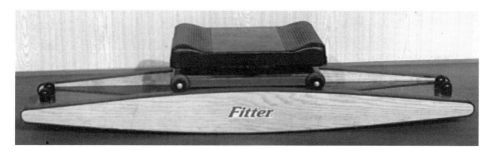

Fig. 15.4. The Fitter.

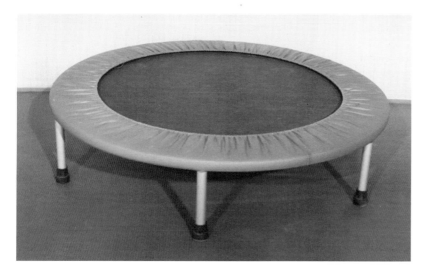

Fig. 15.5. Minitrampoline.

therefore can be used by individuals with an acute low back pain syndrome.

INDICATIONS FOR USE

Sensory motor stimulation is beneficial when used as a part of any exercise program in that it helps to improve muscle coordination and motor programming or regulation and increases the speed of activation of a muscle. Used originally to improve the unstable ankle after an injury, sensory motor stimulation can be of value to individuals with a variety of conditions (Table 15.1). Chronic back pain syndromes represent one of the most important indications. Better control of the trunk, improved activation of the gluteal muscles, and thus better stability of the pelvis are achieved. There is a broad indication for its application for sensory defects of neurologic origin. Carefully (to avoid injury), the method can help to compensate proprioceptive loss in aged subjects and

thus help in preventing falls. This technique cannot be recommended, however, for patients with acute pain syndromes.

METHODOLOGY

In this chapter, we describe only the main methodologic principles. A detailed description is available elsewhere.[17]

One of the most important advantages of this program is that it helps to improve not only muscle imbalance but, in par-

Table 15.1. Indications for Sensory Motor Stimulation

- Unstable knee
- Sprained or unstable ankle
- Idiopathic scoliosis
- Faulty posture
- Postural defects in general
- Chronic back or neck pain
- Prevention or treatment of ataxia

ticular, the most important motor activities, such as standing, i.e., posture and gait. Therefore, the most important exercises are those performed in the upright position.

Respecting the approach of motor learning and motor regulation, any dysfunction in the periphery should be normalized first, because any pathologic or unwanted proprioceptive information from the periphery results in functional adaptive processes of the entire central nervous system. Therefore, attention is first paid to the skin, joints, and their adjacent structures, followed by muscles and their fascia. The trigger points, either active or latent, should be treated, and muscle imbalance, which is always present to some degree, is improved by a reasonable stretching program.

To increase proprioceptive flow, special attention is paid to forming the small (short) foot, the locking mechanism of the knee, stabilization of the pelvis, and the position of the head and shoulder girdles.

The exercise program in the upright position follows several rules:

1. Correction begins in distal areas and gradually continues proximally. Modeling of the foot (feet) comes first, followed by correction of the position of the knee, then the pelvis, and finally the head and shoulders.
2. Exercises are performed in bare feet, which increases proprioceptive stimulation and forces the therapist to pay attention to better control. Last but not least, while using the balance aids, it helps to decrease the potential danger of injuries.
3. Exercise should by no means provoke pain and should not lead to physical (somatic) fatigue.
4. From the beginning, the awareness of posture warrants special attention.
5. Exercises should begin on stable surfaces and then progress to more labile surfaces.

Exercises can be divided into those that focus on training the transfer of weight or the center of gravity and those that focus more on balance and muscle coordination in general.

The term "small (short) foot" (Fig. 15.6) is used to describe the shortening and narrowing of the foot while the toes are relaxed as much as possible. The small foot helps to increase afferent input, mainly from the sole. It improves the position of the body segments and the stability of the body in the upright position, and helps to improve the required springing movement of the foot during walking.

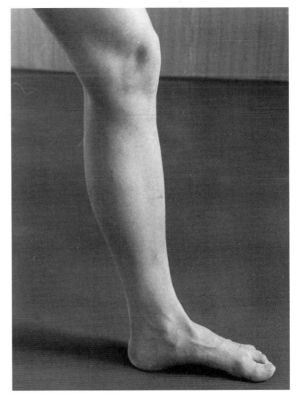

Fig. 15.6. The short foot.

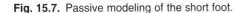

Fig. 15.7. Passive modeling of the short foot.

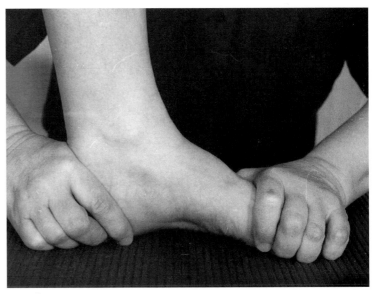

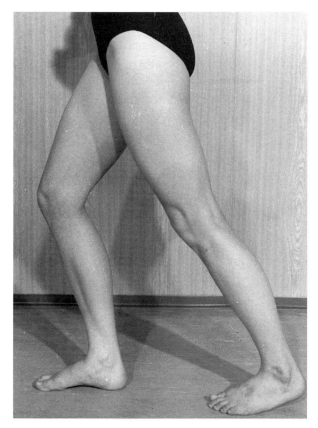

Fig. 15.8. Short feet and half step forward stance.

Initially, the formation of the small foot is difficult to perform in erect posture. Therefore, it is advisable to start the formation while sitting, usually in three steps: (1) sitting, with passive modeling by the therapist; (2) semiactive (passive modeling by the therapist in combination with active patient effort); and (3) active self-formation (Fig. 15.7). Proprioceptive stimulation can be increased by additional pressure applied toward the knee and thus via the shin to the foot.

In standing, one training exercise begins with the small feet parallel and slightly apart. Then, the body sways slowly forward and back, the heels remain fixed toward the floor, and the lower extremities and the trunk are in alignment. The range of motion must be controlled to prevent falls. The therapist controls the sways by touching the chest from the front and the buttocks from the back.

In another variation the knees are bent to 20 to 30°. The hips are slightly abducted so that the knees are slightly apart. Both positions and additional swaying movements help to increase the body awareness and the feeling of a well-balanced and controlled posture.

The next steps are body control in a *half step forward stance,* the corrected stance on both legs, and in one leg stance. To increase proprioceptive flow, slow pushes and then even strokes in different directions toward the pelvis, shoulders, and both areas are added by the therapist (Fig. 15.8).

When the patient achieves sufficient skill, similar exercises on the rocker board and later on the wobble board are added. The demands can be increased by additional variations, such as maintaining the balance in one leg stance or in a semisquat with a slight external rotation in the hip joints. This position is recommended especially for patients with an unstable knee joint. Almost specifically, the activation of the vastus medialis is increased.

Another step is the performance of *lunges* (Fig. 15.9), first on the firm floor, then on the rocker, and finally on the wobble board. Fast lunges accelerate reaction and control and are thus effective for preventing knee injuries and, in particular, falls resulting from incoordination.

The program continues with *jumps* (Fig. 15.10), again on both legs on a firm floor. Progressions include performing on one leg, on labile boards, and/or on the trampoline.

Pushes toward the pelvis, trunk, shoulder girdles in different directions, combined with perpendicular pushes toward the labile boards (Fig. 15.11), significantly increase the proprioceptive flow to the central nervous system, which facilitates the spinovestibulocerebellar circuits. This activation brings sometimes quite surprising and fast therapeutic effects. This technique has been introduced into therapeutic practice only recently. Its application for diagnostic purposes was described by the French neurologist Foix in 1903 and has since been used clinically in the diagnosis of cerebellar lesions.[15]

Balance shoes (Fig. 15.12) are exceptionally useful, and most patients like them more than most other exercises. Balance shoes increase the demands on the entire postural mechanism and automatically, without a conscious effort, help to correct posture. Because this exercise does not require special control and can be used throughout the day, it is usually easy to maintain the patient's motivation to cooperate. In general, the improved posture becomes evident within a few weeks of training. Better coordination and increased speed of muscle contraction can be noticed within 1 week of training, attributable to improved activation of the gluteal muscles.[11] In an unpublished study, we demonstrated that the abdominal recti, if hypotonic or inhibited, were better activated after using the shoes for 1 week. This improvement could be related to both the speed of muscle contraction as well as the total amount of electromyographic activity during a curl up.

When using balance shoes, several important aspects must be considered:

- The small feet must be maintained if possible during the whole gait cycle.
- The subject should try to control the posture, in particular the position of the pelvis, shoulder girdles, and head.
- The steps should be short but quick.
- The feet should be held parallel.
- Lateral and vertical shift of the pelvis should be avoided.

Gait should be trained in place first, if necessary with some support to avoid instability and falls. At the beginning of the training program, it is advisable to control the gait in balance shoes before a mirror. According to our clinical ex-

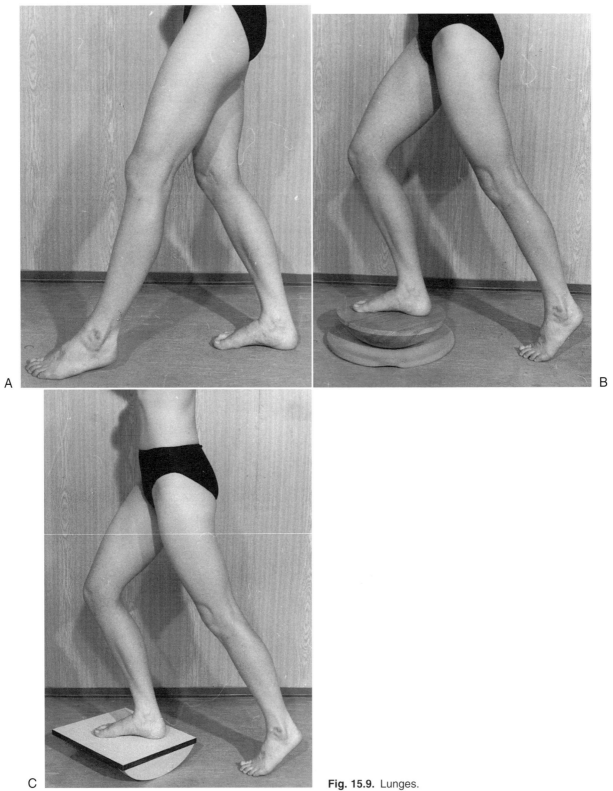

Fig. 15.9. Lunges.

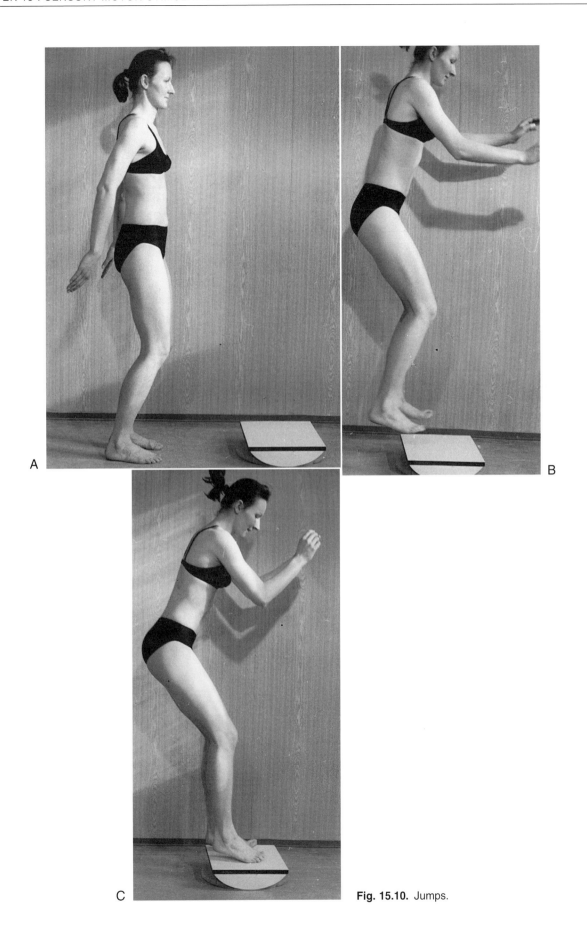

Fig. 15.10. Jumps.

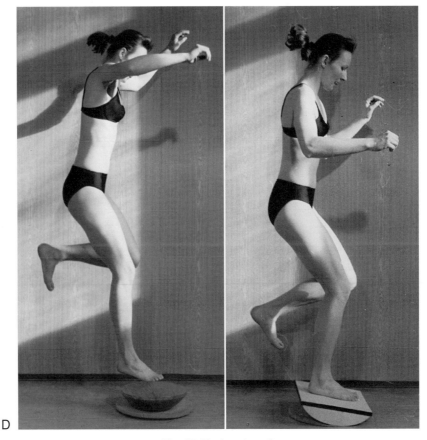

D   E

Fig. 15.10. (continued)

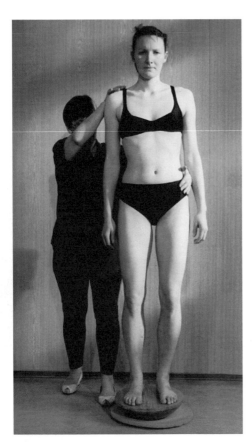

Fig. 15.11. Therapist pushes.

perience, it is more effective to walk in the balance shoes for a short time, just several steps may be sufficient (1 to 2 minutes), several times per day.

The *twister* helps to improve the activation of the trunk and buttock muscles. In addition, the twisting movements specifically activate the deep intrinsic spinal muscles. During its use, it is easy to control the symmetry of the exercise. This device is valuable because it helps correct asymmetries that develop in patients with back pain as a rule and are sometimes difficult to recognize. The twister does not specifically increase proprioception, but it improves coordination and automatizes trunk and pelvic control.

The *Fitter*™ functions in a similar way as the twister, although the estimation of body asymmetries is less recognizable. It also emphasizes the gluteus medius muscle and its lateral stabilizing functions (Fig. 15.13).

The use of *rollers and balance balls* in the treatment of back pain has gained popularity, although they were used for decades in the treatment of children with cerebral palsy. One advantage in using balls is that they are safe, minimize the danger of an injury almost to nil, and help to activate proprioception, balance, and equilibrium control. The incredible variety of possible exercises, especially with regard to the potential positions, helps to establish improved kinesthetic awareness, spinal stability, and new movement patterns.

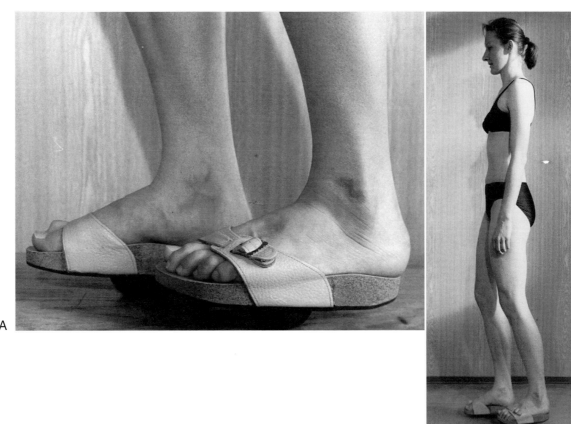

Fig. 15.12. Standing on balance shoes.

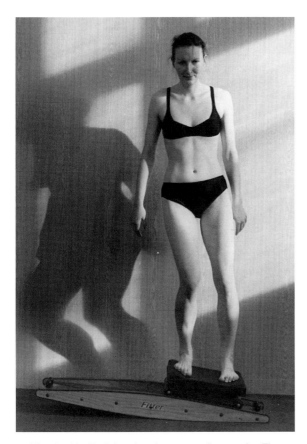

Fig. 15.13. Training the gluteus medius on the Fitter.

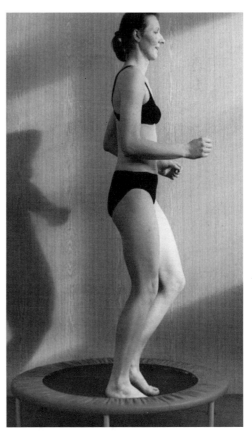

Fig. 15.14. Walking on a minitrampoline.

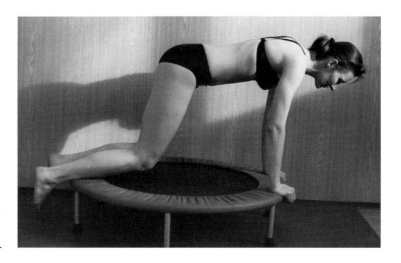

Fig. 15.15. Four point kneeling on the minitrampoline.

The *minitrampoline* is a particularly useful device. Jogging or jumping activates proprioceptors more effectively than a similar exercise performed on a firm floor. In addition, it protects the joints because it functions as a shock absorber. Exercises on a trampoline do not need to be performed in an upright position only. Exercises performed while sitting are particularly effective in strengthening the abdominal muscles, and four point kneeling is recommended for elderly women with kyphosis related to osteoporosis (Figs. 15.14 and 15.15).

CONCLUSION

The sensory motor stimulation approach represents an essential part of the therapeutic program for patients with chronic back pain as well as for individuals with postural defects, such as idiopathic scoliosis or faulty posture, and for all situations in which defects in afference are presumed. Such a program can also be used effectively to improve the ability of the "healthy" motor system to respond more quickly. Given that the speed of muscle contraction is one of the most important means to protect the joints, it seems proprioceptive facilitation can contribute substantially to the prevention of recurrences of acute pain. The sensory motor stimulation program is not a fixed or rigid program; rather, it must be adapted to the individual problems of the individual patient. The need to stimulate proprioceptors is even greater than a few decades ago; our lifestyle has changed substantially and is associated with a general decrease in sensory (proprioceptive) stimulation.

REFERENCES

1. Kabat H: Central mechanisms for recovery of neuromuscular function. Science 112:23, 1950.
2. Sherrington CS: On reciprocal innervation of antagonistic muscles. Proc R Soc Lond [Biol] 79B:337, 1907.
3. Kurtz AD: Chronic sprained ankle. Am J Surg 44:158, 1939.
4. Wyke BD: The neurology of joints. Ann R Coll Surg Engl 41:25, 1967.
5. Skogland S: Anatomical and physiological studies of knee joint innervation in the cat. Acta Physiol Scand 36 (Suppl 124):1, 1956.
6. Freeman MAR, Dean MRE, Hanham IWF: The etiology and prevention of functional instability of the foot. J Bone Joint Surg [Br] 47:678, 1965.
7. Freeman MAR, Wyke BD: Articular contributions to limb muscle reflexes. J Physiol (Lond) 171:20P, 1964.
8. Freeman MAR, Wyke BD: Articular reflexes at the ankle joint. An electromyographic study of normal and abnormal influences of ankle joint mechanoreceptors upon reflex activity in leg muscles. Br J Surg 54:990, 1967.
9. Hervéou C, Mésséan L: Technique de reeducation et d education proprioceptive. Paris, Maloin, 1976.
10. Guyton AC: Basic Neuroscience. Philadelphia, WB Saunders, 1987.
11. Bullock-Saxton JE, Janda V, Bullock MI: Reflex activation of gluteal muscles in walking. Spine 18:704, 1993.
12. Abrahams VC: The physiology of neck muscles. Their role in head movement and maintenance of posture. Can J Physiol Pharmacol 55:332, 1977.
13. Hinoki M, Ushio N: Lumbosacral proprioceptive reflexes in body equilibrium. Acta Otolaryngol 330(Suppl):197, 1975.
14. Ihara H, Nakayama A: Dynamic joint control training for knee ligament injuries. Am J Sports Med 14:309, 1986.
15. Bobath K, Bobath B: The facilitation of normal postural reactions and movement in treatment of cerebral palsy. Physiotherapy 50:246, 1964.
16. Burton AK: Trunk muscle activity induced by three sizes of wobble (balance) boards. J Orthop Sports Phys Ther 8:70, 1986.
17. Janda V, Vavrova M: Sensory Motor Stimulation: A Video. Presented by JE Bullock-Saxton. Brisbane, Australia, Body Control Systems, 1990.

16 Postural Disorders of the Body Axis

PIERRE-MARIE GAGEY and RENE GENTAZ

POWER OF THE POSTUROLOGIST

When posturologists undertook the study of postural control, they did not suspect how much power would fall into their hands.[1] Slowly, year after year, they discovered their ability to manipulate muscle tone by manipulating the input into the postural system. Preceding generations of neurologists had conducted studies of muscle tone and that ended in failure. In 1948, Thomas and de Ajuriaguerra wrote, "Le tonus varie à tout moment, il est continuellement en jeu . . . Toutes les excitations périphériques, de quelque nature qu'elles soient, sont capables de provoquer des réactions toniques" (The tone varies at every turn, it is continuously at work. Any peripheral excitation of whatever kind can bring about tonic reactions).[2] At present, posturologists are finding that they do know how to manipulate tone, and this knowledge empowers them. This power is indeed extraordinary in its novelty, but not always in its reliability; posturologists are reminded from time to time that they do not yet know everything about manipulating muscle tone. The basis of this new knowledge is worth explaining.

BASIS OF POSTUROLOGY

Ever since Bell[3] asked how a person maintains an upright or inclined posture when facing into the wind, physiologists have asked the same difficult question. Over many years, the contributions of various types of sensory input to the control of upright posture were discovered one by one: vision[4] and signals from the legs and feet,[5] the vestibular apparatus,[5] paraspinal muscles,[6] and oculomotor system.[7] Not until the concept of the system appeared was it possible to understand how all these different senses work together to control posture. Researchers could not observe and record the subtle phenomenon of upright posture[8–15] adequately until the resources of electronics[16] and computers were available to allow them to make recordings that do not modify the phenomenon and can be interpreted by signal analysis.

Today, after many years of study, Bell's question can be answered in terms of a simple and consistent model of the mechanisms participating in the control of orthostatic posture: the model of the fine postural system. The term *system* is used here in accordance with control system theory, i.e., we do not need a detailed understanding of the nervous centers and pathways participating in this control in order to study the input and the output of this black box and to analyze its transfer function.

Input into the Fine Postural System

EXTEROCEPTIVE INPUT

To remain upright and steady in their surroundings, people use all the information about their position provided by their sensory organs in relation with the surroundings, including the electromagnetic field,[4,17–19] the gravitational field,[20–22] and the pressure field underfoot.[23–27] Three outwardly directed sensors, or exteroceptors—vision, vestibular apparatus, and baroreceptors from plantar soles—provide information; we do not know of any others apart from these three captors (Fig. 16.1).

PROPRIOCEPTIVE INPUTS

The eye moves about in the socket, while the vestibular apparatus is enclosed in a bony mass. The system cannot integrate positional information from these two sensors unless it knows their relative positions, which are given by the oculomotor system.[28–30] Thus arises the idea of another kind of sensor, inwardly directed, a proprioceptor, which has no direct relation to the surroundings but is nevertheless indispensable to a steady posture within them. Likewise, the feet can move by many degrees in relation to the head, but postural information from the feet and the head cannot be used together unless the system knows the relative positions of the head and the soles. This type of information is assessed by proprioception of the whole body axis.[31–36]

Central Integration

NECESSARY BUT PRECARIOUS INTEGRATION

Retinal, otolithic, and plantar exteroceptive information, combined with proprioceptive information from the 12 oculomotor muscles, all the paraspinal muscles, and the muscles of the legs and feet, unite to give the relative positions of skeletal elements from the occiput–atlas to Lisfranc's joint. This combination generates a considerable amount of information that the system must integrate, in real time, if the posture is not to waver. Therefore, problems with the control of orthostatic posture do not necessarily indicate that a sensor has failed. Rather, it may involve faulty integration,[37] which may occur for many reasons.

DISORDERS OF INTEGRATION OF VISUAL INPUT

Faulty integration of visual input is easier to analyze than that relating to other types of input, because it is easy to record a steadiness of stance with and without the help of vision, and to reckon the contribution of the visual input using the so–called "Romberg's quotient."[4] Postural sway is often measured on a statokinesigram, a record of the successive positions of the subject's center of gravity projected onto the surface beneath the feet, and the Romberg's quotient is the ratio of the "area" of the statokinesigram with the eyes closed to the area with the eyes open, multiplied by 100. With this simple test, some patients are found to be just as steady with their eyes closed as with them open. They might as well be blind as far as their standing posture is concerned. Such "postural blindness" is a frequent finding, occurring in association with many disorders, including vestibular neuritis (Fig. 16.2),[38] strabismus,[39] and low back pain.[40]

Deficiencies of integration of visual input are so frequent in clinical practice that visual input, despite its powerful effect (usually postural steadiness is 250% better when the eyes are open[41]), seems also to be easily disrupted. Its integration is thought to depend on the normal functioning of the other sensors. By itself, the signal of retinal slip is ambiguous; it may be related to movement of the body, of the surroundings, or of the eyes. Its postural significance must be determined by comparison with signals from other sensors: oculomotor input (is it the result of movement of the eyes?) or vestibular or plantar input, in the latter case combined with proprioceptive input concerning the body axis (is it the result of body movement?). One might predict that integration of visual input is poor when other input into the fine postural system is malfunctioning, and that situation is precisely what is observed clinically.

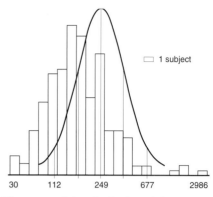

Fig. 16.2. Histogram of the distribution of Romberg's quotient in 182 patients with vestibular neuritis. The gaussian curve shows the theoretic normal distribution of Romberg's quotient in a normal population. Logarithmic scale. 253, mean for normal subjects; 152, mean for patients with vestibular neuritis; CL 95% confidence limits; p < 0.001, Student's t-test.

Output of the Fine Postural System: Muscle Tone

Few would argue that maintaining an upright position is achieved by means other than muscle–postural tone. At the beginning of the last century, Bell noted that it is only by the use of muscles that the limbs stiffen and the body is firmly balanced and kept upright.[3] What is new is the knowledge that postural tone is controlled by a postural system. Therefore, by manipulating the input into the postural system, one can manipulate postural tone almost at will.

Observations Relating to the Fine Postural System

The most striking feature of the control of orthostatic posture is its fineness; every normal person keeps his or her gravitational axis inside a cylinder less than 1 cm^2 in cross section.[41–44] We know that the fine stretching of the neuromuscular spindles is accurately controlled[45]; that the stretching of oculomotor muscles acts on postural tone only if it is fine[28]; and that the fineness of postural sway is below the theoretic threshold of the semicircular canals.[46] Clinically, we observe that, standing upright with their eyes closed, patients with vestibular neuritis are as steady as normal subjects (Fig. 16.3).[38] Only when postural sway becomes abnormally great (area of the statokinesigram is more than 2000 mm^2) do the semicircular canals perceive it. A clear break exists between the neurophysiologic control of fine movements and the control of wider movements. Theoretically, in posturology, this break would be at a statokinesigram area of about 2000 mm^2, and clinical findings confirm the theory: a group of 800 dizzy patients comprised two subpopulations, divided at precisely that breaking point (Fig. 16.4).[37]

It is important to avoid confusing behaviors controlled by different neurophysiologic mechanisms; such confusion leads to difficulty in interpreting data.[47] It is to prevent such confusion that the set of mechanisms controlling orthostatic posture is called the fine postural system.

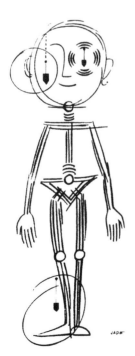

Fig. 16.1. The postural man.

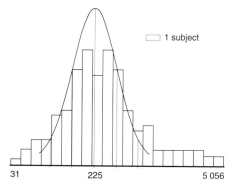

Fig. 16.3. Histogram of the distribution of statokinesigram areas in 182 patients with vestibular neuritis (eyes closed). The gaussian curve shows the theoretic normal distribution of the parameter of statokinesigram area in a normal population (eyes closed). Logarithmic scale. CL, 95% confidence limits; 225, mean for normal subjects; 282, mean for patients with vestibular neuritis. (From Gagey PM, Toupet M: Orthostatic postural control in vestibular neuritis. A stabilometric analysis. Ann Otol Rhinol Laryngol 100:971, 1991.)

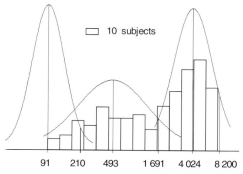

Fig. 16.4. Histogram of the distribution of statokinesigram areas for 800 unstable patients (eyes open). The gaussian curve (left, heavy line) shows the theoretic distribution of this parameter in a normal population. The fine curves have been superimposed merely to emphasize the bimodal aspect of the distribution. Logarithmic scale. 91, mean for normal subjects; 210, upper 95% confidence limit.

Limits of Posturology

To consider the central nervous system as a "black box" is certainly an avowal of weakness. Until neuroanatomy can explain where and how the multimodal information that helps people stand upright is integrated,[48] however, we have no other choice. We cannot pretend to know enough about the nervous centers and pathways controlling posture to be able to propose a neuroanatomic model useful in clinical practice. The scientific way forward is to establish what links we can observe between the input of the fine postural system and its output.

POSTURAL DISORDERS OF THE SPINE

The subject that particularly interests the therapist is how posturology can help the person for whom standing upright is difficult or painful.

The Postural Patient

The person whose spine hurts for a postural reason is said to have a functional disorder. Radiographic and laboratory tests have eliminated rheumatic disease, orthopedic illness, and obvious nucleus pulposus herniation, but pain continues for unknown reasons. Often, the patient feels better after manual therapy, but the pain keeps coming back. Such recurrences likely have a cause that the manual therapy has not addressed. In fact, one can observe in these patients abnormal asymmetry of postural tone. Is this the mysterious cause of the recurrences?[49]

Identifying Postural Tonic Asymmetry

PHYSIOLOGIC ASYMMETRY

A human being does not have the perfect symmetry of a Greek statue; rather, the statistical norm is postural asymmetry. Not only have we seen asymmetry of orthostatic posture in tens of thousands of "normal" subjects, but also we have established that such asymmetry is not random (p < 0.001 on the χ^2 test).[50] Therefore, it is reasonable to think that such asymmetry is characterized by laws. The practitioner must not conclude that every type of postural asymmetry is abnormal.

PATHOLOGIC ASYMMETRY

To distinguish pathologic from physiologic asymmetry, the gains of neck reflexes are measured during a stepping test.
Fukuda–Unterberger Stepping Test. A normal subject stepping in place blindfolded rotates up to, but not more than, 20°/30° after 50 steps.[51,52] This finding is easy to verify, but several technical points must be considered. Testing conditions should include no sound or light source that could indicate a direction. The thighs should be raised neither too far nor too little at each step (about 45° is right). The pace should be neither too slow nor too fast (1.4 Hz is good).[53] When putting on the blindfold, the eyes should be in the "primary position" (looking straight ahead).[54] The head should be neither rotated nor tilted,[55] and the arms should be stretched forward, horizontal and parallel.[51,52]

Although this simple test, with the head in a neutral position, provides useful information, we prefer a more rigorous test that makes use of the postural neck reflex.
Measuring the Gain of Neck Reflexes. When a normal subject keeps his or her head turned to the right, the tone of the extensor muscles of the right leg increases, and vice versa for the left side.[56,57] When a normal subject performs the Fukuda–Unterberger stepping test with the head turned to the right, he or she rotates farther leftward than if the test is performed with the head facing forward (Fig. 16.5). The difference between these two angles of rotation is a measure of the gain of the right neck reflex. The same applies, mutatis mutandis, if the head is turned left.[55]

The test must be carried out methodically to avoid confusion. The results are tabulated, following clearly defined conventions. Angles of rotation are denoted ("+" if rightward

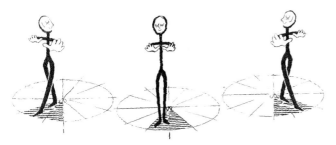

Fig. 16.5. Fukuda-Unterberger's stepping test with head rotation. When the subject performs the test with the head rotated to the right rather than straight ahead, he or she rotates farther leftward and vice versa.

and "−" if leftward; +10° means the patient had turned 10° to the right at the end of the test and −30° means the patient turned 30° to the left). Calculating the absolute value of the gain of the neck reflex requires paying attention to the signs: +10° and −30° make 40° of difference, not 20°! It is important to adopt new conventions for the gain of the neck reflex; for instance, a gain in the "normal" (predicted) direction as just described is denoted "+," otherwise "−."

An example of how to calculate the predominance of neck reflexes is provided in Table 16.1. The following explanation relates to this sample.

HL, +50°: Head turned left; the patient rotated 50° rightward
HA, −10°: Head straight; the patient rotated 10° leftward
HR, +20°: Head turned right; the patient rotated 20° rightward
LG, +60°: Absolute value of the gain of the left neck reflex is 60°, noted with a "+" because it is in the normal direction
RG, −30°: Absolute value of the gain of the right neck reflex is 30°, noted "−," because it is not in the normal direction
Left predominance 90°: The best gain is the gain of the left neck reflex because it is in the normal direction; the difference between the two gains is 90°. (If both gains are in the normal direction, the larger is considered best. If neither gain is in the normal direction, the smaller is considered best.)

This method allows testing of the muscle tone as it varies in accordance with a postural tonic reflex. Although it is accepted that a predominance of more than 50° is surely pathologic, the risk of error in accepting this limit is not yet known.

Table 16.1. How to Calculate the Predominance of Neck Reflexes

HL	HA	HR	LG	RG	Predominance
+50°	−10°	+20°	+60°	−30°	Left 90°

HL, +50°: Head turned left; the patient rotated 50° rightward. HA, −10°: Head straight; the patient rotated 10° leftward. HR, +20°: Head turned right; the patient rotated 20° rightward. LG, +60°: The absolute value of the gain of the left neck reflex is 60°, noted with a + sign, because it is in the normal direction. RG, −30°: The absolute value of the gain of the right neck reflex is 30°, noted −, because it is not in the normal direction.

Left predominance 90°: The best gain is the gain of the left neck reflex because it is in the normal direction; and the difference between the two gains is 90°. (If both gains are in the normal direction, the larger is considered best, if neither gain is in the normal direction, the smaller is considered best).

How to Manipulate Input into the Fine Postural System

If the patient shows abnormal asymmetry of postural tone, the posturologist must try to restore symmetry by modifying the input into the system that controls orthostatic posture. The system is delicate, however, and must be manipulated carefully, with gentle stimulations; otherwise, it does not respond.[28]

Three types of input are accessible to the clinician: spinal, oculomotor, and plantar.

SPINAL INPUT

Manual therapy of the spine is well known, and for the patients considered in this chapter, it is assumed that clinical success is only temporary. That assumption does not always apply to other postural patients, such as those labeled unstable and the squinter. The practitioner should consider the possibility of acting on the fine postural system through this sensory route.

OCULOMOTOR INPUT

Oculomotor (and possibly visual) input can be manipulated by putting a weak prism, of 1 to 4 prism diopters, in front of the patient's eye.[58] An optical prism deviates light rays toward its base. For pedagogic purposes, think of a weak prism put in front of a normal eye as moving the eyeball by eliciting the fusion reflex opposing diplopia. This movement stretches various oculomotor muscles in accordance with the various positions of the base of the prism. (In fact, this cannot be the true explanation of the action of such prisms because they act even in the absence of binocular vision.)

Conventions of Notation. Imagine an optical prism, base down in front of a subject's eye and with one of its dioptric faces perpendicular to the subject's visual axis. If the prism is rotated around this axis, its base describes successive tangents on a trigonometric circle centered on the subject's visual axis. By convention, degrees on this circle are counted counterclockwise from the observer's viewpoint. Regarding the subject's left eye, 0° is toward the subject's temple, 90° at the zenith, and 180° toward the nose, whereas for the subject's right eye, 0° is toward the nose, 90° at the zenith, and so on (Fig. 16.6).

Strabismologists consider that each of the six oculomotor muscles has a main direction of action (at 0°, 55°, 125°, 180°, 235°, or 305°).[59] Because a prism deviates light rays toward its base, the main oculomotor muscle it forces to work is the one with the main direction of action that is opposite the base of the prism (see Fig. 16.6). Table 16.2 illustrates the correlations between prism positioning and activation of oculomotor muscles. The formula RLR 3 refers to a prism of 3 diopters, in front of the right eye, base tangent at 0°, activating the right lateral rectus.

Law of the Semicircular Canals. Even when considering only the main direction of action of each oculomotor muscle, there are 12 directions and 12 possible positions of the prism.

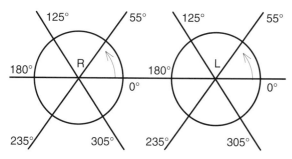

Fig. 16.6. Main directions of action of the oculomotor muscles and positions of prism bases.

Table 16.2. Relations Between the Positions of the Base of Prism and Oculomotor Muscles

Base of Prism At	Stretched Muscle	
	Right Eye	Left Eye
0°	RLR	LMR
55°	RIR	LOS
125°	ROS	LIR
180°	RMR	LLR
235°	ROI	LSR
305°	RSR	LOI

LR: lateral rectus; MR: medial rectus; IR: inferior rectus; SR: superior rectus; SO: superior obliquus; IO: inferior obliquus.

Six oculomotor muscles increase the gain of the left neck reflex, and the other six increase that of the right neck reflex. It is better to decide in advance which oculomotor muscles may bring about better balance of the muscle tone than to proceed solely by trial and error. The law of the semicircular canals can help in the decision.

According to the law of the semicircular canals (Table 16.3), deviation of light rays away from the main direction of action of an oculomotor muscle acts on the tone of the extensor muscles of the legs in the same way as deviation of the endolymph stimulating the cupula of the semicircular canal governing the reflex activity of this oculomotor muscle.[60–64] If you know on which side you wish to increase the gain of the neck reflex, six oculomotor muscles can be eliminated immediately by referring to law summarized in Table 16.3.

PLANTAR INPUT

Plantar input can be modified with microwedges under the soles. The mechanoreceptors of the soles are accurate to within 1 g, and the wedges used to stimulate them must be correspondingly thin (about 1 mm in thickness). Thick wedges do not alter postural tone.

Microwedges act on plantar baroreceptors. They may also stimulate deeper proprioceptive sensors, such as capsular or ligamentous Pacini's and Ruffini's corpuscles, Golgi tendon organs, and neuromuscular spindles. Microwedges placed under certain regions of the sole modify the sensory input into the fine postural system.

Because the technology of conventional orthopedic shoes does not correspond to that for postural stimulation, we pro-

pose new terminology to describe these new plantar orthoses. Any construction crossing the foot transversally is called a *bar*, and any more circumscribed construction is called a *spot*. The front–to–back position of bars can be designated as follows:

- Infracapital, under the metatarsal heads
- Anterior, behind the metatarsal heads
- Median, at the level of the scaphoid and cuboid bones
- Posterior, under the distal part of the calcaneus
- Infratuberous, under the calcaneal tuberosity

For spots, side–to–side positioning is also specified:

- Medial infracapital and lateral infracapital, under the heads of, respectively, the first and second and the fourth and fifth metatarsals
- Anteromedial and anterolateral, behind the heads of the corresponding metatarsals; and so forth (mediomedial, mediolateral; posteromedial, posterolateral; and medial and lateral infratuberous)

Any construction must be positioned in accordance with the podographic footprint, with due attention to dysmorphisms of the feet. The footprint can be achieved by using a light layer of ink under the foot and then having the subject place that foot onto white paper.

Foot Pain. The effectiveness of these exteroceptive stimulations may be limited by any pain in the foot of which the patient may not even be aware. Therefore, we recommend both questioning the patient and pressing with the thumb on various regions of the soles to discover any painful area that the patient had not noticed. In such cases, antalgic elements should be provided in addition to the element for postural stimulation.

Proprioceptive Disorders of the Legs and Feet. When free movement of the joints of the legs and feet is impaired to the extent that proprioception is affected greatly, plantar postural stimulations are less effective. Such disorders must be corrected before stimulatory wedges are used.

Identifying the Right Input

In principle, the therapist can modify any input discussed in this chapter. In practice, however, there may be only one that

Table 16.3. Law of the Semicircular Canals

		Increases the gain of the neck reflex	
		Right	Left
Oculator muscle	Right eye	RMR	RLR
		RSR	RIO
		RIR	RSO
	Left eye	LLR	LMR
		LIO	LSR
		LSO	LIR

LR: lateral rectus; MR: medial rectus; IR: inferior rectus; SR: superior rectus; SO: superior obliquus; IO: inferior obliquus.

will effectively alter the patient's postural tone, and the practitioner must look for it. Then, the quickest and most adaptable clinical test is the rotators test.

ROTATORS TEST

Our team has used this clinical test of the tone of the hip rotator muscles since the work of Constantinesco and Autet.[65] This test has the great advantage that the patient is lying down and does not get tired, and that the effectiveness of each manipulation is known within seconds. Seen for the first time, it looks like a conjuring trick, so before explaining how to do it, we explain the underlying ideas.

Clinical Investigation of Muscle Tone. Clinical investigation of muscle tone is a delicate subject indeed. Despite the longstanding agreement, going back to Galen, to define "tone" as muscular activity that does not bring about any movement, most authorities agree that the term is ambiguous. The idea of "light tension that any muscle at rest is usually subject to," or some such usual definition confuses the effects of the viscoelastic properties of muscle tissue with the effects of contractile processes originating in the nervous system.[66] Therefore, tone is a trap, representing one of those words the meaning of which may unconsciously be distorted, to the great detriment of clarity of discussion.

Because the concept of tone is so elusive, criteria for its clinical investigation must be all the more rigorous. This need is particularly great when we manipulate tone to test it, for what is observed then is not "tone," but rather certain tonic reactions to certain changes imposed by the clinician. In the unavoidable "action–reaction" pair, the reaction will have epistemologic value only insofar as the action is known. We must know what we are doing before we can understand what we are observing.

Sherrington led the way in the rigorous study of muscle tone by quantifying the tone of a muscle by its resistance to passive stretching in terms of the physical quantities length, time, and force applied. It is reasonable to continue stretching muscles to test their resistance to stretching, and thus their "tone," but each maneuver must be defined in physical terms. Regarding stretching movement, the amplitude, speed, acceleration, time elapsed since the previous movement, and applied force must be specified. Each parameter matters: amplitude for the properties of elasticity and for secondary spindle endings; speed for the properties of viscosity; speed and acceleration for primary spindle endings; and time elapsed between two successive stretchings for muscular thixotropy.[67]

We cannot adequately stress the limitations of the clinical examination of tone. In such a moving world, the posturologist must be wary and accept only those excitation–reaction sequences that are repeatable and uncontaminated.

Performing the Test. The subject is supine, in a strictly controlled posture: arms lying loosely beside the body, head facing straight up, eyes in the primary position, jaw relaxed (the teeth should not touch). Stand at the end of the table, facing the patient's feet, and take the heels in your palms, with your hypothenar eminences and little fingers resting at the edge of the soles without touching them, and the medial edge of your thenar eminences pressing on the anterior edge of the patient's external malleoli (Fig. 16.7).

Lift the subject's feet just 2 or 3 cm from the table; your arms should be extended and your body should be straight and leaning slightly back, so that you are pulling gently on the patient's legs. With the subject relaxed with feet slightly apart, perform five or six successive medial rotations of both feet at once to test the passive resistance of the external thigh rotators to these movements. Nine out of ten times, the external rotators of the right thigh offer the stronger resistance. We say they are hypertonic relative to the symmetric muscles.

This test is not as easy to carry out as it may seem. Your pronation movements to rotate the feet should be supple, relaxed, and fairly fast—at a frequency of about 2 Hz, which is the resonant frequency of the hip joint in such axial rotation movements (Walsh EG, personal communication). Thus, this rapid test mainly investigates the viscous component of mechanical properties and the primary spindle endings; it eliminates the effects of muscle thixotropy. (We recommend practicing with volunteers; after about 100 exercises, you will start doing it easily.)

Preparing to Perform the Test. The amplitude of tonic responses to manipulations of the postural system varies among subjects. Therefore, it is important to take some time at first to become acquainted with the amplitude of each patient's own reactions, to feel how the rotators respond when the head, eyes, or arms are turned.

Usually, the tone drops in the rotators on the side to which the head is turned (or increases in the other side—the test fundamentally is a comparison). The same holds true when the eyes are turned, but for unknown reasons the eyes must be closed. Medial rotation of the arm (as when the right hand is placed on the left shoulder) brings about a decrease of the tone of the ipsilateral rotators, and lateral rotation of the arm (as when the left hand is placed under the neck) brings about a decrease of the tone of the contralateral rotators.

Once the practitioner can accurately detect the patient's responses, the next step is to eliminate any interference related to malocclusion.

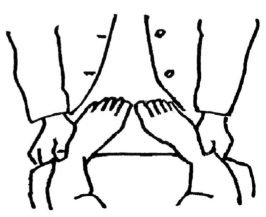

Fig. 16.7. Rotators test.

MANDIBULAR INTERFERENCE

Why or how mandibular disorders can change the rules of the game of postural tone is unknown. This still mysterious phenomenon must be borne in mind from the outset when examining any postural patient, for experience has taught us that it is a waste of time to put prisms in front of the eyes or microwedges under the feet of a patient whose postural tone is altered by a mandibular disorder. Only after mandibular disorders have been cured, so that they no longer interfere with postural tone, is it reasonable to use prisms or microwedges, if the patient still needs them.

The back teeth—molars and premolars—have protrusions or cusps that engage the cusps of the opposite teeth during closing movements or occlusion of the jaw, for instance, during swallowing. The positioning of cusps makes great demands on precision, with which occlusodontists are familiar. The posturologist need know only how to be sure that some modification of this "intercuspidation" is not altering postural tone.

Testing Procedure. The principle of the test for interference by malocclusion is simple: the tone of the rotators must not alter when the intercuspidation is modified.

To begin, test the rotators with the subject's teeth in the usual intercuspidation position. Ask the patient to swallow spittle and keep the teeth in contact—the usual intercuspidation position; now, test the rotators.

Next, put a small piece of Bristolboard, cut to size, between the back teeth and have the patient walk around and swallow spittle several times before testing the rotators again, with the modified intercuspidation.

If the results of the two tests are not the same, modification of the intercuspidation has altered the tone. To verify this finding, use other tests (such as the Fukuda–Unterberger stepping test or the thumbs test) and refer the patient to an occlusodontist.

The bite planes can be more sophisticated and more effective than the piece of Bristolboard recommended here, but how to make them and fit them is beyond the scope of this chapter. Even if better options are not available, this crude method is useful.

After establishing that mandibular input is not playing havoc with the patient's postural tone, the practitioner then considers which of two types of input into the fine postural system to modify to effect treatment.

LOOKING FOR AN EFFECTIVE PRISM

Measuring the gains of the neck reflex reveals which side has the stronger tone, left or right; the law of the semicircular canals identifies which of six oculomotor muscles have the best chance of modifying postural tone in the desired direction. The next step is to test those six muscles, one after the other, using the rotators test. The patient puts on trial spectacles with a 4 diopter prism. With the base of the prism positioned successively at each of the six orientations associated with these muscles, the rotators are tested for altered tone. (Before testing the tone of the rotators, the patient should

adapt to the new visual surroundings by turning his or her eyes to look around in all directions.) If one or two muscles bring about tonic reactions, this information is noted for a possible prescription. If none of them produces a response, we recommend testing the other six muscles anyway before going on to the next step; the practitioner need not be a slave of the law of the canals.

LOOKING FOR AN EFFECTIVE PLANTAR AREA

Manipulating plantar input is easy: test the rotators in the standard conditions, stimulate the sole at a particular spot, and immediately test rotators again. The stimulation is done simply by applying light pressure with a finger, just enough to stimulate the baroreceptors in the soles—200 g at most. If the results of these two tests differ, the plantar spot stimulated may be able to modify postural tone, and is worth keeping in mind for a possible prescription.

The entire area of both soles, one after the other and spot by spot, may be tested, but spots under the scaphoid at the top of the arch and under the cuboid at the lateral edge of the foot should be tested first, followed by spots in bars under and just behind the heads of the metatarsal bones and then spots in bars under the anterior part of calcaneum.

Prescribing

Tonicity is such an elusive phenomenon that measuring the gains of neck reflexes and testing rotators is not sufficient to ensure that the correct manipulation has been identified. Faced with this uncertainty, the practitioner has various choices, depending on the circumstances.

If the patient can be re–examined promptly, e.g., within a fortnight, it is acceptable to try the simplest and most efficient modification (a press–on prism affixed to the patient's glasses or wedges made quickly). A therapeutic trial is one way of making clear determinations.

If, however, the patient cannot be re–examined soon, the prescription must be based on the convergence of several tests. From the battery of possible tests—posturologic, chiropractic, osteopathic, kinesiologic—each practitioner chooses the ones with which he or she is most comfortable. Normally, we use the stepping test and the test of Barré's vertical (see subsequent discussion), which we consider fairly reliable, and

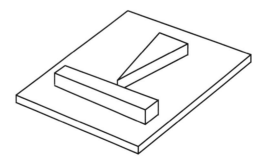

Fig. 16.8. Device for Barré's test. Heels are 2 cm apart and blocked behind. Feet are fanned out at 30°.

the thumbs' test (see following section), which is sensitive. None of these tests, however, is absolutely necessary. What is necessary is to base the prescription on more than one test.

BARRÉ'S TEST

For this test, Barré observed his patients in relation to a vertical plane, the intermalleolar median sagittal plane. Each adjective matters. The unclothed patient is positioned between two motionless plumb lines that are aligned with the main medial axis of his or her support base. Positioning the feet is accomplished most easily by using a simple arrangement such as a block behind the heels and a block with a 30° angle between the feet, with the heels 2 cm apart for the sake of steadiness (Fig. 16.8). The subject must stand still, relaxed, looking forward at eye level, with the arms hanging beside the body. The observer, behind the patient, aligns his or her eye with the two plumb lines and notes the mean positions, at the midpoint of postural oscillations, of the gluteal cleft, the spinal processes of L3 and C7, and the vertex relative to the plumb lines.

The observation is repeated with and without the corrective device—the prism or plantar insert—that is being evaluated (Fig. 16.9)[68]. Often, the result of this test is not immediately altered by a manipulation that later proves to be effective. Therefore, we consider the test to be fairly reliable.

THUMBS TEST

The patient stands upright, with feet apart by the width of the pelvis. The practitioner, from behind, puts his or her thumbs gently on the patient's skin, without pressing (a pressure of about 10 g is appropriate), making sure they are positioned symmetrically relative to the patient's body axis, starting at the level of the posterior superior iliac spine. The patient is then asked to roll downward slowly, i.e., to start by dropping

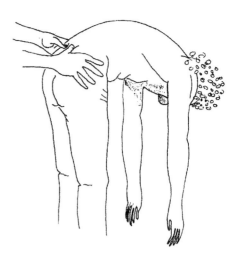

Fig. 16.10. Thumbs test.

the head completely, then letting the shoulders fall, and finally the trunk, as if attempting to touch the feet with the hands, without bending the knees (Fig 16.10).[69]

The practitioner, meanwhile, notes whether his or her thumbs are dragged symmetrically, or if one is dragged higher than the other. The test is repeated with the thumbs at various levels of the spine, for instance L3, D12, D7, D4, C7, and the occiput. The results obtained with and without manipulating an input into the system are written in a table for comparison.

Using a test the mechanism of which is not fully understood has its dangers, but with this reservation, we can say that the thumbs test is sensitive, revealing slight differences that other tests miss—the results of the thumbs test are altered by a change of only one diopter of the prism. This sensitivity is the reason we include it in our battery of tests.

Just which tests are used—Barré's vertical, the thumbs test, or some other test—matters less than the need to prescribe on the basis of a group of converging arguments, so that on each test, the prescribed corrective device alters the result in the desired direction.

Treatment Follow-up

Within 1 or 2 months after the start of treatment, the patient must be seen again. Within this time, a prism can induce an iatrogenic postural hypertonicity contralateral to the original hypertonicity. The patient then merely stops wearing the prism.

After 2 weeks, an area of plantar stimulation may have lost its effectiveness. If the patient's pain has not been fully relieved, another plantar area may be better—the change in postural tone having changed the distribution of pressures under the feet. For this reason, we prefer treating by prism insofar as possible, because postural tone does not change continuously, as it tends to do in response to plantar stimulations. Prisms must be used with caution, however. Small prisms are powerful; they can modify an antalgic posture, and one can imagine the effect on the patient's suffering.

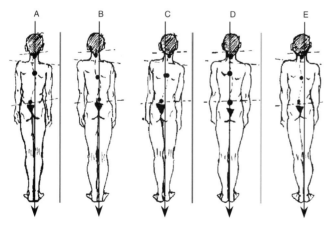

Fig. 16.9. Barré's test. **A,** Try the plantar input first. **B,** Try the oculomotor input first. **C,** Try both of them. **D,** Be careful, do not try either oculomotor input or plantar input without looking at the spine, the mandible, and joints of the feet. **E,** A whiplash injury is a possibility. (From Guillaume P: L'Examen clinique postural. Agressologie 29:687, 1988.)

Contribution of Stabilometry

Although we have mentioned only clinical examination, a noteworthy means to record the functioning of the fine postural system is the standardized computerized platform for clinical stabilometry.[70] The reason for not mentioning this apparatus previously is simple: in effect, the platform reduces the subject to a single point, the center of gravity, and analyzes the stability of this point relative to the surroundings. It is difficult for a clinician to accept such a reduction of patients. Nevertheless, stabilometry remains a basic tool, because it provides much needed certainty regarding the elusive phenomenon of muscle tone. It provides documentary evidence useful for treatment follow–up and also for compiling statistics on groups of patients, making it possible to see beyond the random variability encountered in everyday clinical practice. In addition, stabilometry is indispensable to the clinician, because disorders of the regulation of orthostatic posture often are not clinically apparent and are manifested only in patients' complaints and abnormal stabilometric parameters. Without its stabilometric underpinnings, posturology would not have the certainties it has at present.

ROMBERG'S QUOTIENT AND LOW BACK PAIN

The first objective indication that low back pain is improving is a stabilometric criterion: a shift of Romberg's quotient toward a normal value. From 600 patients with low back pain who had been followed using stabilometry, Guillamon and co–workers[40] selected 125 for statistical analysis because they showed no other impairment, they had received the same treatment, and they had not received any other treatment that could have modified their postural tone. Seventy–one subjects of this group benefited from the treatment, and of these, 63

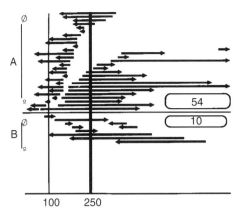

Fig. 16.12. Changes in Romberg's quotients of patients whose condition did not improve. Each arrow represents changes in Romberg's quotient of one patient, from the start to the end of follow-up. 250, normal value; 100, limit for postural blindness. **A,** 54 patients whose condition did not improve and whose Romberg's quotients move away from normal. **B,** 10 patients whose condition did not improve and whose Romberg's quotients shifted toward normal.[40]

showed a shift of the Romberg's quotient toward normal (Fig. 16.11).

The condition of 54 subjects, however, was not improved by treatment; of these, only 10 showed a shift of the Romberg's quotient toward normal values (Fig. 16.12), and all 10 showed obvious stabilometric signs of "overcontrol" of their orthostatic posture (sinusoidal intercorrelation function) suggesting malingering or "oversimulation."[71]

Although stabilometry potentially is widely applicable, it can be carried out only by a specialist, the posturologist. It is in the interest of all therapists to know about stabilometry, however, for all can benefit from its contribution.

Contribution of Postural Orthoptics

Because oculomotricity plays a major role in the fine postural system, knowing how well patients' eyes are functioning is as important as knowing how well their vestibular apparatus is functioning. Posturologists cannot work effectively without collaboration with neuro–ophthalmologists as well as neuro–otologists. Neuro–ophthalmologists working with posturologists have developed orthoptic examinations useful in posturology, e.g., tests of oculomotor balance in various postures (standing, sitting, head straight ahead or rotated, eyes in the primary position or in different versions) or tests of oculomotor balance under the effect of postural prisms.[72] Case management is greatly facilitated if the results of such tests and of the clinical postural examination are consistent and in agreement. Although it is beyond the scope of this chapter to describe these orthoptic techniques in more detail, the contribution of postural orthoptics deserves mention. We never put a prism in front of an eye unless the patient has had an orthoptic evaluation. In this collaboration, we are fortunate, and we wish every therapist the same good fortune.

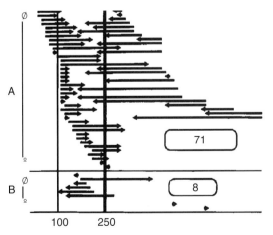

Fig. 16.11. Changes in Romberg's quotients of patients whose condition improved. Each arrow represents changes in Romberg's quotient for one patient, from the beginning to the end of follow-up. 250, normal Romberg's quotient; 100, limit for postural blindness. **A,** 71 patients whose condition and Romberg's quotients both improved. **B,** 8 patients whose condition improved but whose Romberg's quotient moved away from the normal mean.[40]

Postural Training Platform

Postural rehabilitation can be accelerated by the use of a wobbly platform, similar to that described by Freeman et al[73] but adapted to the fine postural system. The dome on which the platform rests has a large radius of curvature and the platform construction limits its mean range of movement to 4 or 5° (the normal range of body sway in orthostatic posture that is controlled by the fine postural system). Therefore, a subject standing on the platform commonly remains within these limits of the fine postural system (Fig. 16.13).

The subject is asked to stand upright on the platform, keeping it as horizontal and as steady as possible for about 1 minute. The exercise is repeated several times a day. Admittedly, this platform cuts down the plantar input into the fine postural system, because information perceived by plantar baroreceptors is not the same as when the subject is standing on firm ground. This condition probably increases the contribution of visual input to the control of orthostatic posture.

For whatever reason, we have observed that postural blindness responds to this form of treatment within 3 months.[74] As wearing a prism can result in iatrogenic postural blindness, it is advisable to prescribe exercises on a postural training platform every time a prism is prescribed, especially in the absence of a stabilometric platform that could be used to detect the appearance of postural blindness. These exercises also seem useful in treating mild low back pain.

Psychologic Aspect

How reductive it would be if the posturologist considered a standing person as merely an assemblage of exteroceptors and proprioceptors, the information from which is integrated to produce the reactions needed for stabilization in his or her surroundings. To stand upright means much more. To stand on one's feet means to have the hands free to act and the joy of control over one's body. Phylogenetically speaking, humankind is the outcome of this impulse toward more freedom, more control, more power. To reduce the standing person to posturologic terms is to condemn ourselves to misunderstand the "mis-standing" person.

No longer being able to stand upright is shaming, the opposite of being upright and proud of it; to lose this ability is to be powerless and dependent. With a postural patient, therefore, we must assess the psychologic aspect of this disorder on his or her behalf, for the patient will not be aware of the extent of this break. We are then faced with a difficult situation, because the significance of psychologic disorders that accompany postural disorders is double-sided: the individual may have experienced a profound wound to the bodily ego that is expressed as depression and anguish, or the patient may feel depression or anguish that is being expressed in bodily language. Some postural disorders can be ameliorated with purely psychiatric treatment. All practitioners must remember that a purely posturologic point of view does not reflect the entire person.

CONCLUSION

Everything said about the control of orthostatic posture seems obvious, but we must not forget that an "obvious fact" may assume its true weight only after gradually emerging through many experimental confrontations. Thanks to the pioneers of posturology, and in particular of stabilometry, a few facts are now known about the person standing upright, but there is still a long way to go before this knowledge comes into its own.

ACKNOWLEDGMENTS

We thank Susan Miller for her help with the English translation and Sylvie Villeneuve-Parpay for her help with illustrations.

REFERENCES

1. Gagey PM, Baron JB, Ushio N: Introduction à la posturologie clinique. Agressologie 20E:119, 1980.
2. Thomas A, de Ajuriaguerra J: L'axe Corporel. Musculature et Innervation. Paris, Masson, 1948, pp 37–38.
3. Bell C: The Hand. Its Mechanism and Vital Environment. 4th Ed. London, V. Pickering, 1837, pp 234-235.
4. Van Parys JAP, Njiokiktjien C: Romberg's sign expressed in a quotient. Agressologie 17B:95, 1976.
5. Flourens P: CR Acad Sci [III], 1829.
6. Longet FA: Sur les troubles qui surviennent dans l'équilibration, la station et la locomotion des animaux après la section des parties molles de la nuque. Gazette Médicale de Paris 13:565, 1845.
7. Cyon E de: L'oreille Organe d'Orientation dans le Temps et dans l'Espace. Paris, Alcan, 1911.
8. Vierordt K: Grundzüge der Physiologie des Menschen. Berlin, Springer, 1864.
9. Mitchell SW, Lewis MJ: The tendon jerk and muscle-jerk in disease and especially in posterior sclerosis. Am J Med Sci 92:363, 1886.
10. Bullard WN, Brackett EG: Observations on the steadiness of the hand and on static equilibrium. Boston Med Surg J 109:595, 1888.
11. Hancock JA: A preliminary study of motor ability. Pediatr Semin 3:9, 1894.

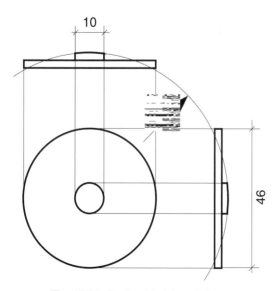

Fig. 16.13. Postural training platform.

12. Bolton JW: The relation of motor power to intelligence. J Physiol (Lond) 14:619, 1903.

13. Miles WR: Static equilibrium as a useful test of motor control. J Ind Hyg 3:316, 1922.

14. Fearing FS: The factors influencing static equilibrium. J Comp Physiol Psychol 4:90, 1924.

15. Hellebrandt FA: Standing as a geotropic reflex. Am J Physiol 121:471, 1938.

16. Ranquet J: Essai d'Objectivation de l'Equilibre Normal et Pathologique. Paris, Thèse Médecine, 1953.

17. Lee DN, Lishmann JR: Vision - The most efficient source of proprioceptive information for balance control. Agressologie 18A:83, 1976.

18. Bles W, Brandt T, Kapteyn RS, et al: Le vertige de hauteur un vertige de distance par déstabilisaton visuelle? Agressologie 19B:63, 1978.

19. Paulus WM, Straube A, Brandt T: Visual stabilization of posture: Physiological stimulus characteristics and clinical aspects. Brain 107:1143, 1984.

20. Nashner LM: A model describing vestibular detection of body sway. Acta Otolaryngol (Stockh) 72:429, 1971.

21. Walsh EG: Standing man, slow rhythmic tilting, importance of vision. Agressologie 14C:79, 1973.

22. Bizzo G: Tentative de détermination de la fonction de transfert du système de régulation posturale chez l'homme en orthostatisme à la suite de stimulation électriques labyrinthiques. Paris, Thèse de Sciences (Paris V), 1974.

23. Okubo J, Watanabe I, Baron JB: Study on influences of the plantar mechanoreceptors on body sway. Agressologie 21B:61, 1980.

24. Gagey PM, Bizzo G, Debruille O, et al: The one hertz phenomenon. In Igarashi M, Black FO (eds): Vestibular and Visual Control on Posture and Locomotor Equilibrium. Basel, Karger, 1985, pp 89-92.

25. André-Deshaye C, Revel M: Rôle sensoriel de la plante du pied dans la perception du mouvement et le contrôle postural. Méd Chir Pied 4:217, 1988.

26. Asai H, Fujiwara K, Toyama H, et al: The influence of foot soles cooling on standing postural control. In Brandt T, Paulus W, Bles W (eds): Disorders of Posture and Gait. Stuttgart, Georg Thieme, 1990, pp 198-201.

27. Magnusson M, Enbom H, Johansson R, et al: The importance of somatosensory information from the feet in postural control in man. In Brandt T, Paulus W, Bles W (eds): Disorders of Posture and Gait. Stuttgart, Georg Thieme, 1990, pp 190–193.

28. Baron JB: Muscles Moteurs Oculaires, Attitude et Comportement Locomoteur des Vertébrés. Paris, Thèse de Sciences, 1955.

29. Tokumasu K, Tashiro N: Relationship between eye movement and body sway during standing. In Ushio N, Kitamura H, Matsunaga T (eds): Postural Reflex and Body Equilibrium. Nara Tenri, 1980, pp 35–49.

30. Roll JP, Roll R: Perceptual and motor effects induced by extraocular muscle vibration in man. 3rd European Conference on Eye Movements. Dourdan, September 1985. Excerpta 13:3, 1985.

31. Aggashyan RV: On spectral and correlation characteristics of human stabilograms. Agressologie 13D:63, 1972.

32. Nashner LM: Vestibular and reflex control in normal standing. In Stein RB, Pearson KG, Smith RS, et al (eds): Control of Posture and Locomotion. New York, Plenum Press, 1973, pp 291–308.

33. Mauritz KH, Dietz V: Characteristics of postural instability induced by ischemic blocking of leg afferents. Exp Brain Res 38:117, 1980.

34. Lund S, Broberg C: Effects of different head positions on postural sway in man induced by a reproducible vestibular error signal. Acta Physiol Scand 117:307, 1983.

35. Hlavaka F, Njiokiktjien C: Postural responses evoked by sinusoidal galvanic stimulation of the labyrinth. Acta Otolaryngol (Stockh) 99:1, 107, 1985.

36. Roll JP, Vedel JP, Ribot E: Exp Brain Res 76:213, 1989.

37. Gagey PM: Non-vestibular dizziness and static posturography. Acta Otorhinolaryngol Belg 45:335, 1991.

38. Gagey PM, Toupet M: Orthostatic postural control in vestibular neuritis. A stabilometric analysis. Ann Otol Rhinol Laryngol 100:971, 1991.

39. Marucchi C, Weber B, Gagey PM, et al: Maturation and evolution of Romberg's quotient: Influence of abnormal oculomotor equilibrium. In Amblard B, Berthoz A, Clarac F (eds): Posture and Gait: Development, Adaptation and Evolution. Amsterdam, Elsevier, 1989, pp 85–92.

40. Guillamon JL, Gentaz R, Baudry J: The Postural Disturbances Induced by Low Back Pain. 10th International Symposium on Disorders of Posture and Gait. Münich, September 1990.

41. Normes 85, Published by the Association Française de Posturologie, 4, avenue de Corbéra, 75012 Paris, 1985.

42. Hirasawa Y: Study on human standing ability. Agressologie 14C:37, 1973.

43. Guidetti G: Stabilometria clinica. Istituto di clinica Otorinolaringoiatrica dell' universita di Modena, 1989.

44. Sugano H, Takeya T, Kodaira N: A new approach to the analysis of body movement. Agressologie 13B:15, 1970.

45. Matthews PBC, Stein RB: The sensitivity of muscle spindle afferents to small sinusoidal changes in length. J Physiol (Lond) 200:723, 1969.

46. Gagey PM, Toupet M: What Happens at Around 2000 mm^2? 9th Symposium of the International Society for Postural and Gait Research. Marseille, May-June, 1988.

47. Toupet M, Heuschen S, Gagey PM: Postural dyscontrol in the elderly and vestibular pathology. In Woollacott M, Horak F (eds): Posture and Gait: Control Mechanisms. Portland, University of Oregon Books, 1992, pp 307-310.

48. Gagey PM: A critique of posturology: Towards an alternative neuroanatomy? Surg Radiol Anat 13:255, 1992.

49. Gagey PM: Les asymétries du tonus de posture peuvent être toxiques, vérifiez-les. Kinesither Sci 294:4, 1990.

50. Gagey PM, Asselain B, Ushio N, et al: Les asymétries de la posture orthostatique sont-elles aléatoires? Agressologie 18:277, 1977.

51. Fukuda T: The stepping test. Two phases of the labyrinthine reflex. Acta Otolaryngol (Stockh) 50:95, 1959.

52. Weber B, Gagey PM, Noto R: La répétition de l'épreuve modifie-t'elle l'exécution du test de Fukuda? Agressologie 25:1311, 1984.

53. Tsutsumiuchi K, Okubo J, Kotaka S, et al: Stepping movement control and response. Two dimensional analysis of dynamic control mechanisms. Agressologie 24:115, 1983.

54. Gagey PM, Baron JB: Influence des mouvements oculaires volontaires sur le test de piétinement. Agressologie 24:117, 1983.

55. Ushio N, Hinoki M, Baron JB, et al: The stepping test with neck torsion: Proposal of a new equilibrium test for cervical vertigo. Practica Otologica Kyoto 69(Suppl 3):1369, 1976 (Japanese).

56. Magnus R: Körperstellung. Berlin, Springer, 1924.

57. Fukuda T: Studies on human dynamic postures from the viewpoint of postural reflexes. Acta Otolaryngol (Stockh) Suppl 161, 1961.

58. Utermöhlen GP: De prismatherapie getoest aan 160 lijders aan het syndroom van Ménière. Ned Tijdschr Geneeskd 91:124, 1947.

59. Krewson W: Action of the extraocular muscles. Trans Am Ophthalmol Soc 48:443, 1950.

60. Lorente de Nò R: The regulation of eye positions and movements induced by labyrinth. Laryngoscope 42:233, 1932.

61. Szentagothaì J: The elementary vestibulo-ocular reflex arc. J Neurophysiol 13:395, 1950.

62. Ito M, Nisimaru N, Yamamoto M: Pathways for the vestibulo-ocular reflex excitation arising from semicircular canals of rabbits. Exp Brain Res 24:257, 1976.

63. Cohen B, Suzuki J, Shanzer S, et al: Semi-circular control of eye movements. In Bender MB: The Oculomotor System. New York, Harper & Row, 1964, pp 163-172.

64. Gagey PM, Dujols A, Fouché B, et al: The law of the canals: Systematic variations of the spin movement during Fukuda's stepping test depends on the position of the prism base. In Taguchi K, Igarashi M, Mori S (eds): Vestibular and Neural Front. Amsterdam, Elsevier, 1995, pp 537–540.

65. Autet BM: Examen Ostéopathique Prenant En Compte L'activité Tonique Posturale. Montpellier, Mémoire de la Sereto, 1985.

66. Paillard J: Tonus, posture et mouvements. In Kayser C (ed): Physiologie. Vol. 2. Paris, Flammarion, 1976, pp 521–728.

67. Walsh EG, Wright GW: Postural thixotropy at the human hip. Q J Exp Physiol 73:369, 1988.

68. Guillalume P: L'examen clinique postural. Agressologie 29:687, 1988.

69. Bassani B: Les sciatiques et la vertébrothérapie. Proceedings of the 5th Symposium "Journées d'Acupuncture et de Vertébrothérapie." Vichy 1965. de Bussac Clermond-Ferrand, de Bussac, 1966, pp 57–61.

70. Bizzo G, Guillet N, Patat A, et al: Specifications for building a vertical force platform designed for clinical stabilometry. Med Biol Eng Comput 23:474, 1984.

71. Ferrey G, Gagey PM: Le syndrome subjectif et les troubles psychiques des traumatisés du crâne. Encycl Méd Chir (Paris), Psychiatrie, 37520 A10, 1988.

72. Marucchi C, Fouché B: Amblyopie profonde et prismes posturaux. Agressologie 32:169, 1991.

73. Freeman MAR, Dean MRE, Hanham IWF: The etiology and prevention of functional instability of the foot. J Bone Joint Surg [Br] 47:678, 1965.

74. Gagey PM: La plate-forme de rééducation posturale. Ann Kinésithér, 20:331, 1992.

17 Lumbar Spine Injury in the Athlete

ROBERT G. WATKINS

Low back pain has been a significant factor in many different types of athletic activity. The severity and extent of back pain often determines the actual ability to compete and is a worry to the athlete, the family, coaches, trainers, and those persons responsible for paying the bills. Treatment of the athlete with a lumbar spine injury involves an understanding of basic anatomy and biomechanical function of the spine, the diagnosis of conditions affecting the lumbar spine, proper use of diagnostic studies, and a systematized, all-inclusive history and physical examination. We must also recognize some factors that predispose the athlete to lumbar spine problems, as well as training and therapeutic techniques to prevent lumbar spine problems in athletes.

Obtaining a proper diagnosis in the athlete presenting with low back pain is crucial. It is the key to initiating an appropriately aggressive diagnostic and therapeutic plan.[1,2] A variety of pathologic conditions can be diagnosed on the basis of plain film radiography and their relationship to the athlete and his or her sport can be addressed more specifically.[3] Especially in the adolescent and younger athlete, a high index of suspicion must be maintained to accurately diagnose conditions such as stress fractures and spondolytic defects.[4] The bone scan is a vital diagnostic tool for the physician caring for athletes with lumbar spine problems. An adolescent athlete with significant back pain that persists for longer than 3 weeks should be evaluated radiographically and a bone scan should be obtained. Unusual conditions ranging from osteoid osteoma, infections, and stress fractures of the sacroiliac joint, to the more routine spondolytic defects can be found. *Approximately 30 to 38% of young athletes presenting with significant lumbar pain have positive bone scan.*[4,5] Predisposing factors to back pain in athletes include increased trunk length and stiff lower extremities.[6] There is an increased prevalence of occulta spina bifida in patients who develop lower lumbar spondolytic defects.[7]

The study of exercise and back pain in athletics and in the average population demonstrated no higher incidence of back pain in athletes participating in organized sports relative to regular students. Fairbank et al found that back pain was more common in students who avoided sports than in those who participated. Fisk et al[8] found that prolonged sitting was the important factor in the pathogenesis of Scheurmann's disease as opposed to athletes lifting weights, undergoing compressive stresses, or doing heavy lifting and part-time work. This study involving 500 17- and 18-year-old students showed that 56% of young men and 30% of young women had some radiographic evidence of changes similar to Scheurmann's disease.[8]

Keene et al[9] found that 80% of back injuries occurred during practice, 6% during competition, and 14% during preseason conditioning. Of those who sustained injury, 8% were men and 6% women, which was of no statistical significance. The nature of injury usually was acute (59%); 12% were related to overuse and 29% involved aggravation of a pre-existing condition.

ANATOMY

The vertebral column is a series of linked intervertebral joints. The joint consists of the intervertebral disk, its two facet joints, concomitant ligaments, vessels, and nerves, referred to as a neuromotion segment. A neuromotion segment is considered as one of the basic units of spine anatomy and function. The lumbar spine has a lordotic curve and plays an important role in the biomechanics of the lumbar spine.

The spine comprises two basic columns; an anterior column consisting of the disk and vertebral bodies and the accompanying longitudinal ligaments, the anterior longitudinal ligament and the posterior longitudinal ligament. The posterior column consists of the facet joints, lamina, spinous process, ligamentum flavun, and pars inarticularis. The disk itself may be described as a circular, multilaminated ligament that connects the two vertebrae. The nucleus pulposus is the central, more gelatinous portion of the disk. The annulus is the multilayered woven basket with fibers at precise angles to resist torsional and compression forces. This structure is firmly anchored to the end-plate of the vertebrae. The annulus, nucleus, and the accompanying end-plates resist compressive forces well and torsional forces less efficiently.

The orientation of the facet joint is different at every level of the spine. In the lumbar spine, the facet joints are oriented in a transitional phase from parasagittal in the upper lumbar spine to a more coronal orientation in the lower lumbar spine. This parasagittal orientation allows good motion in flexion and extension, and less motion in lateral flexion. The parasagittal orientation of the facet joints would naturally resist rotation; high torsional forces can overcome the strength of the joint, tearing the annulus and injuring the facet joints.

When considering the anatomy of the spine, one must consider the important role of the entire cylinder of the trunk and its supporting muscles. The static ligamentous structures provide considerable resistance to injury, but this resistance in itself would be insufficient to produce proper spine strength without the additional support provided through the trunk musculature and lumbodorsal fascia. Muscle control of the lumbodorsal fascia allows greater resistance to bending and loading stresses. The role of lumbosacral fascia may be compared to the anchoring devices of a circus tent, which pull on the side of the tent to stabilize the pole in the middle. The fascia stabilizes the spine and allows it to right mechanically. The lumbodorsal fascia and the muscles attaching to it are of equal importance to the more specialized function of the intervertebral disk and facet joints.

DIAGNOSIS

In determining the exact etiology of lumbar spine pain in athletes, age is an important factor. Younger athletes are more likely to have stress fractures and congenital predispositions to stress fractures. Diseases that affect growing cartilage are more common in young athletes, such as Scheurmann's disease. In the mature athlete, radiologic assessment often involves distinguishing between age-related, asymptomatic changes and symptomatic recent trauma. Is the L5-S1 disk degeneration at the symptomatic level in a 30-year-old athlete or is it an asymptomatic finding? The diagnostic plan must be organized to allow diagnosis of the most common conditions as well as such rare conditions as herniation of the inferior lumbar space[10] or osteoid osteoma.

Important diagnoses to make in the athlete with back and leg pain are peripheral nerve injury and peripheral nerve entrapment. The variety of peripheral nerve problems ranges from a generalized peripheral neuropathy to carpal tunnel syndrome, pyriformis syndrome, peroneal nerve injury, femoral neuropathy, and interdigital neuroma. The chief reason for electromyographic and nerve conduction studies of the lower extremities is to identify a peripheral nerve problem. The nerve conduction study, combined with a careful physical examination, can at least raise the distinct possibility of a peripheral nerve problem and heighten the diagnostician's skepticism concerning small, potentially asymptomatic spinal lesions in the role of the patient's extremity nerve pain.

Spondylolysis and Spondylolisthesis

Age is important in the natural history of these conditions. An incidence of 4.4% at age 6 years increases to 6% by adulthood. It is unusual for children to present with spondylolysis before the age of 5 years or with severe spondylolisthesis, grade III or IV. Most symptoms appear in adolescence. Fortunately, however, but the risk of progression after adolescence is low (about 15%). Symptoms cannot be correlated with the degree of slip. Rapid progression to spondyloptosis is more common in 9 to 11 year olds and in children with occult spina bifida and doming of S1. Children with high degree slips may present with deformity and minimal pain. Many times, it is the pain of an injury that leads to the identification of a significant spondylolisthesis.

Isthmic spondylolisthesis most commonly develops as a stress fracture. A hereditary predisposition to developing the stress fracture is likely, and there is certainly the predisposition in conditions in which the bone of the pars inarticularis is not sufficient to withstand normal stresses. Also, certain mechanical activities that expose the patient to repeated biomechanical challenge, increasing stress concentration on the pars interarticularis, have a higher incidence of spondylolisthesis. The concept of repeated microtrauma with concentration of these stresses in the pars has become increasingly recognized in adolescent athletes who participate in sports such as gymnastics and weight lifting.

The most common site for spondylolysis and spondylolisthesis is L5-S1. The slippage in the latter disorder results from the lack of support of the posterior elements produced by the stress fracture of the pars. The spectrum of neurologic involvement runs from rare to more common with higher degree slips. The majority of neurologic deficits are an L5 radiculopathy with an L5-S1 spondylolisthesis. Cauda equina symptoms are more likely in grade III or IV slips. Cauda equina neurologic loss is rare.

The diagnostic and therapeutic plan for spondylolisthesis begins with a high degree of diagnostic suspicion in the adolescent athlete with low back pain. As many as one third of adolescent athletes presenting with low back pain have evidence of a stress fracture on bone scans. Bone scanning is warranted for patients with low back pain that has not resolved within 3 weeks. If the results of the bone scan are positive, CT scanning is performed to determine if there is a demonstrable stress fracture or if the bone is "hot" because of an impending fracture. If the results of the bone scan are negative and the patient persists with lumbosacral pain, magnetic resonance imaging (MRI) is indicated. Using a combination of MRI, bone scanning, and CT, it is possible to diagnose most significant pathologies in the lumbar spine.

The treatment plan for spondylolisthesis is rest or restriction of enough activity to relieve the symptoms. This plan may vary from simply removing the athlete from participating in the sport until the pain has significantly improved to immobilization in a lumbosacral corset, Boston brace, or TLSO, or bed rest and casting.

The goal is to stop the pain through whatever amount of inactivity is required. For an athlete with a "hot" bone scan, we routinely prescribe a brace and restrict activity for 3 months. At the end of this period, if the bone scan is repeated and the results are negative, sufficient healing has occurred to allow the patient to begin a rehabilitation program. If the findings of the bone scan are still positive, and the athlete is asymptomatic, it may be difficult to decide whether to begin the rehabilitation program or to continue further restriction. We usually initiate the rehabilitation program and observe carefully for any return of symptoms. If the patient is asymptomatic in a full, rigorous, trunk stabilization program (level II Back Class) and aerobic conditioning program, we allow their return to their sport and continue the rehabilitation program.

Patients with unilateral "hot" bone scans, with or without demonstrated fracture, have a reasonably high incidence of healing, and adolescent athletes in general should be treated with the idea of healing the defect. Bilateral stress fractures are less likely to heal despite comprehensive nonoperative therapy.

If the bone scan findings are negative in a patient with a spondylitic defect, the treatment plan should be like that for any patient with mechanical low back pain. This plan usually involves a progressively vigorous trunk stability rehabilitation program. We put no permanent restrictions on athletes with spondylolysis or spondylolisthesis. Clearly, patients with grade III to IV spondylolisthesis are less likely to be able to participate in vigorous sports activities without pain and discomfort. They should probably avoid the heavy strength sports, such as football, weight lifting, etc.

The incidence of spondylolysis and grade I spondylolisthesis in sports participants is high. In the long term, this condition is not considered to be a significant factor in an athlete's ability to play.

BIOMECHANICS

The understanding of the basic biomechanics of the lumbar spine begins with an understanding of the forces and stresses applied to the spine as related to its normal curvatures. Because of the lordotic shape of the spine, the results of vectoral force on the spine usually consist of a vertical axial loading compressive force perpendicular to the surface of the disk and one horizontal to the disk, producing a shear strain. The combination of these two forces produces both tensile stress in the annulus fibrosis and a shear force on the neural arch.

The center of gravity of body weight is anterior to the spine. This weight times the distance back to the spine produces a lever arm effect of the weight of the body. This effect is resisted by the erector spinae muscles, the lumbodorsal fascia, and the gluteus maximus. Abnormal stresses applied to this equation may result in annular tears of the intervertebral disks or stress fractures on the neural arch related to this excessive resistive force. The most common place for stress fractures is the pars interarticularis.

The basic mechanisms of injury produce a combined vector of force that may be difficult to analyze in a force diagram. Three common mechanisms of injury to consider are: (1) compression or weight loading to the spine; (2) torque or rotation, which may result in various shear forces in a more horizontal plane; and (3) tensile stress produced through excessive motion on the spine.

The compressive type of stress is more common in sports that require high body weight and massive strengthening, such as football and weight lifting. Torsional stresses occur in throwing athletes, e.g., the javelin, baseball players, golfers, etc. Motion sports that put tremendous tensile stresses on the spine include gymnastics, ballet, dance, pole vaulting, high jump, etc.[11]

Some injuries result from direct blows. Certainly, sports such as football are associated with muscle contusions, muscle stretches, and tears of fascia, ligaments, and, occasionally, muscle.

Lumbar fractures can occur as a result of direct blows to the back with fracture of the spinous process or twisting injuries that avulse the transverse process. Vertebral body endplate fracture from axial compression load on the disk is a relatively common source of compressive disk injury. The annulus is more likely injured in rotation. The end-plate is more vulnerable to compression than the annulus. Axial loading compression injuries can result from jarring injuries in motor sports or boating. Flexion rotation fracture dislocations of the cervical and lumbar spine are certainly possible. In any sport in which one athlete falls on another, the mechanism is similar to that of the coal face injury with the rock falling on the coal miner while on all fours. An athlete can suffer an asymmetric loading, rotational injury to the thoracolumbar spine.

The intervertebral disk is injured predominantly through rotation and shear, which produce circumferential and radial tears. Initially, the layers may actually separate or the inner layers break. As the inner layers weaken and are torn, added stress is placed on the outer layers. This increase can produce a radial tear of the intervertebral disk. With the outer layers torn, the inner layers of annulus break off and, with portions of the nucleus, are forced with axial loading to the place of least resistance, the weak area in the annulus. The outer areas of annulus are richly innervated, producing tremendous pain and reflex spasm when the annulus tears. The nuclear material can produce a chemical neuritis and inflammation. The spasm and pain is mediated through the sinuvertebral nerve with anastomosis through the spinal nerve and the posterior primary ramus. As the herniated material extrudes and it produces pain from the transversing or exiting nerve root itself, the patient may develop sciatica or radiculopathy. Intradiscal infiltration of the granulation tissue adds increased potential for painful sensation in the annulus. The annulus, with time, can heal, although the healing annulus will not retain the same biomechanical function capability as the original intervertebral disk.

Biomechanical functioning of the spinal column and its relationship to the biomechanics of nerve tissue involves several basic concepts:

1. Flexion of the lumbar spine increases the size of the intervertebral canal and the intervertebral foramina.[12]
2. Extension decreases the size of the intervertebral canal and the intervertebral foramina.[12]
3. Flexion increases dural sac and nerve root tension.[13]
4. Extension decreases dural sac and nerve root tension.[13]
5. Front flexion, axial loading, flexion, and upright posture increase intradiscal pressure.
6. With flexion, the annulus bulges anteriorly.[14]
7. With extension, the annulus bulges posteriorly.[14]
8. Nuclear shift in an injured disk is poorly documented, but probably corresponds with annular bulge.[12]
9. Rotation and torsion produces annular tears and disk herniations.[15]

Conclusion of these facts indicate that motion does have an effect on the nerves and the neuromotion segments of an injured area. For example, in the presence of a spinal obstructive problem, such as spinal stenosis, extension exercises can further compress the neurologic structures and make them worse. In the presence of a nerve root tension problem, such as disk herniation, flexion can produce increased tension in an already tense nerve and increase symptoms.

HISTORY AND PHYSICAL EXAMINATION

The key to a proper history and physical examination is to have a standardized format that accomplishes the needed specific objectives.

1. Quantitate the morbidity. Use a scale value of pain, function, and occupation to understand how sick the patient is. Converse with the patient to hear the inflections and manner of pain description. Detail the time of disability and the time of origin of the pain.
2. Delineate the psychosocial factors. Know what psychologic effect the pain has had on the patient. Know the social, economic, and legal results of the patient's disability. Understand what can be gained by his or her being sick or well. Derive an understanding of what role these factors are playing in the patient's complaints.
3. Eliminate the possibility of tumors, infections, and neurologic crisis. These diseases have a certain urgency that requires immediate attention and a diagnostic therapeutic regimen that is different from that for disk disease.
4. Diagnose the clinical syndrome:
   - Nonmechanical back and/or leg pain. Inflammatory, constant pain, minimally affected by activity, usually worse at night or early morning.
   - Mechanical back and/or leg pain. Made worse by activity, relieved by rest.
   - Sciatica. Predominantly radicular pain, positive stretch signs, with or without neurologic deficit.
   - Neurogenic claudication. Radiating leg pain or calf pain, worse with ambulation, negative stretch signs, worse with spine extension, relief with flexion.

Pinpoint the pathophysiology causing the syndrome. Important determinations are: (1) What level? Which neuromotion segment? (2) What nerve? (3) What pathology? What is the exact structure or disease process in that neuromotion segment that is causing the pain?

The history and physical examination represent the first step in determining the clinical syndrome. Some key factors are:

1. The time of day during which the pain is worse
2. A comparison of pain levels during walking, sitting, and standing
3. The effects on pain of valsalva, coughing, and sneezing
4. The type of injury and duration of the problem
5. A percentage of back versus leg pain. We insist on getting an accurate estimate of the relative amount of discomfort in the back versus the legs. There must be two numbers that add up to 100%.

The physical examination should address:

1. The presence of sciatic stretch signs
2. The neurologic deficit
3. Back and lower extremity stiffness and loss of range of motion
4. The exact location of tenderness and radiation of pain or paresthesias
5. Maneuvers during the examination that reproduce the pain

The history determines whether it is an axial (back pain) or extremity (leg pain) problem. What is the exact percentage of back versus leg pain? Is the pain made worse by the mechanical activity or is it a constant resting pain? Does the pain worsen with maneuvers that increase intradiskal or intraspinal pressure? Is there significant night pain? Do maneuvers that decrease spinal diameter increase the pain? Do maneuvers that increase nerve root tension increase the pain?

Classic radiculopathy is radicular pain radiating into a specific dermatomal pattern, with paresis, muscle weakness, loss of sensation, and reflex loss. The radicular pattern of the pain and neurologic examination determines the nerve involved.

The classic history for radiculopathy resulting from a disk herniation is back pain that progresses to predominantly leg pain. It is made worse by increases in intraspinal pressure such as coughing, sneezing, and sitting. Physical examination shows positive nerve stretch signs. A dermatomal distribution of leg pain is made worse by straight leg raising, sitting or supine; leg–straight foot dorsal flexion; neck flexion; jugular compression; and direct palpation of the politeal nerve or sciatic notch is characteristic of radiculopathy. A source of radicular pain not found in this description is that caused by spinal stenosis. Spinal stenosis usually lacks positive nerve stretch signs, but has the characteristic history of neurogenic claudication (i.e., leg and calf pain produced by ambulation). Pain that does not go away immediately on stopping is made worse with spinal extension and is relieved by flexion. The pain progresses from proximal to distal.

The pain drawing, completed by each patient, is a major help in accomplishing the objectives of the physical examination. The pain drawing distinguishes organic from psychologic pain fairly well. It also helps in localizing the symptoms for future reference with pain reproduction studies, such as with diskography and postoperative evaluations.

The initial history and physical evaluation determine the aggressiveness of the diagnostic and therapeutic regimen. The morbidity rating and the duration of the problem are important facts that help to determine the aggressiveness and invasiveness of the diagnostic plan. The leg pain versus back pain ratio is an important factor in determining which diagnostic tests are indicated. Leg pain leads to tests for nerve function and obstructive pathology in EMG/NC, myelograms, contrast CT scans, and MR images. Back pain evaluation includes bone scans, MR images, and diskograms. The clinical syndrome should be divided into predominantly mechanical pain, axial pain, and leg pain. An appropriate treatment program can begin, based on the initial evaluation.

Most athletic injuries to the lumbar spine fall under the category of mechanical, axial, back or leg pain. Included within this grouping are several different syndromes. First is an annular tear of the intervertebral disk, usually a loaded compressive rotatory injury to the lumbar spine producing severe, disabling back spasm and pain. The pain is usually worse in flexion with coughing, sneezing, straining, upright posture, sitting, and any other situations that increase intradiscal pressure. Other clinical evidence includes referred leg pain, low back pain with straight leg raising, and anterior spinal tenderness. Annular tears can be produced with as little as three degrees of high torque rotation.[16] Facet joint alignment that protects the disk from rotatory forces may lead to facet joint injuries as the annulus fails in rotation.

Second is the facet joint syndrome, more typically occurring in extension with rotation, reproduced with extension rotation during the examination. Patients may present with pain on rising from flexion, with a lateral shift in the extension motion. Point tenderness in the paraspinous area over the facet joint is reported and may be associated with referred leg pain.

Third are tears of the lumbodorsal fascia and muscle injuries and contusions present with muscle spasm, stiffness, and many of the characteristics of facet joint syndrome in annular tears.

Finally, athletic injury may result in sacroiliac joint pain and pain in the posterior superior iliac spine, the most common area for referred pain from the annulus in the intervertebral disk and the neuromotion segment of the spine. Sciatic pain can hurt in the sciatic joint area as well as in the sciatic notch and buttocks. Although injuries to the sacroiliac joint can occur, most sacroiliac joint pain is thought to be the result of referred pain from a neuromotion segment in the spine.

The most important goal in the physical examination of the athlete is demonstrating what types of motions reproduce the patient's pain. Where exactly is the area of tenderness? What deformity is present in the spine? If there is a lateral shift, in which direction? The chief advantage for physical therapists in the treatment of the athlete with lumbar spine pain is the hands-on approach directed specifically to motions and activities that produce and relieve the pain. Local techniques can be directed specifically to localized areas of inflammation and pain. Treatment of referred pain areas through localized treatment in the area from which the pain is referred plays a major role in the relief of symptoms and return to performance. Therefore, techniques of treatment of referred pain should be understood and used, including injections of local anesthetic, cortisone injections, TENS units, ultrasound, and ice.

Another important diagnostic goal of the physical examination is to identify areas of contracture and weakness. The physician and therapist can make the diagnosis by carefully examining the patient for areas of muscle atrophy and loss of range of motion. Sophisticated testing techniques and dynamic EMG function analysis have identified localized areas of weakness in the shoulders as well as in the abdominal musculature of baseball pitchers.[18] Recognizing these deficiencies during the physical examination and designing a rehabilitation program to correct them requires a great deal of skill on the part of the physician.

NONOPERATIVE CARE

The nonoperative treatment plan consists of several basic rules.

1. Stop the inflammation
2. Restore strength
3. Restore flexibility
4. Restore aerobic conditioning
5. Restore balance and coordination
6. Adapt the rehabilitation program to sports–specific training and exercises
7. Start slowly back into the sport
8. Return to full function

Rest and/or immobilization are often required to stop inflammation of the spine in an injured athlete. We try to keep the period of rest and immobilization to a minimum. Bed rest produces stiffness and weakness, which cause the pain to persist. Stiffness and weakness are the antithesis of the body functions necessary for athletic performance. Every day of rest and immobilization may produce weeks of rehabilitation before the athlete is able to return to performance. As in motion treatment of lower extremity injuries, i.e., fracture bracing and postoperative continuous motion machines, rapid rehabilitation of lumbar injuries in athletes requires effective means of mobilizing the patient. Bed rest for longer than 3 to 5 days is not of any benefit in the natural history of the disease.

Rapid mobilization requires the use of strong anti-inflammatory medications, ranging from epidural steroids, oral Medrol Dose pak, and Indocin SR to other nonsteroidal anti-inflammatory agents and aspirin; ice; a TENS unit; and mobilization with casts, corsets, and braces. Corsets and braces are used for only limited periods of time. Strengthening techniques begin when the brace is applied so braces can be removed as soon as possible. Braces in themselves can cause a significant amount of stiffness and weakness.

Exact timetables are difficult, but determinations should be based on information obtained during the history and physical examination. As a general rule, our patients with acute disk herniation are treated with 3 to 5 days of bed rest; see the physical therapist within 7 days; use a corset for no longer than 10 to 14 days; receive Indocin, occasionally Medrol, and less commonly, epidural injections. The therapist begins the neutral position, isometric trunk strengthening program that, depending on the response of the patient, evolves into resistive strengthening, motion, and aerobic conditioning as tolerated.

Part of the key to being able to initiate early therapy is understanding, based on the physical examination, what makes the patient symptomatic. Nonoperative care should be the basis of any therapeutic approach to athletes with lumbar spine injuries. With the exception of cauda equina injuries, this type of care should also apply for the athlete with neurologic deficit. The key to effective nonoperative care is well thought out, balanced biomechanical approach. Common questions are whether to do extension, flexion, or twisting exercises, what type of aerobic exercising should be done, when can someone lift weights, what role does Nautilus beautification exercises have in rehabilitation of the athlete, and what type of nonoperative rehabilitation is best for the individual athlete's sport?

A common concern is the risk of producing or increasing a neurologic deficit through nonoperative care. So often, nonoperative care, in the face of a neurologic deficit, has consisted of no care. A short period of bed rest is the usual, initial stage of treatment of the athlete with a disk herniation and neurologic deficit. Bed rest is thought to protect the patient from increasing injury to the spine and therefore increasing neurologic deficit.

Unfortunately, bed rest also produces profound weakness and loss of biomechanical function, which actually increases the risk of injury. If the purpose of bed rest is to decrease inflammation, the logical substitute is aggressive anti-inflammatory medication. If the objective of bed rest is to prevent motion, braces and casts can be substituted. If the objective of bed rest is to prevent abnormal motion that could injure the spine, it is with the understanding that certain mechanical functions have to take place. Patients get on and off of bed pans, they get up to go to the bathroom. They roll over in bed. They cough, they sneeze, and eventually have to walk. It seems logical that if we could design an exercise system that would prevent abnormal motion while restoring strength and flexibility in a biomechanically sound fashion, we could protect the spine from the abnormal motion that produces injury, and possibly enhance healing. This enhancement takes place through normal biomechanical motion in the injured part through increasing strength and flexibility in the adjacent portions of the body that can absorb the stress potentially directed to the injured part and in preventing the atrophy, weakness, and stiffness caused by inactivity.

Lumbar spine injuries in athletes demand prevention of atrophy and stiffness and restoration to maximum function as early as possible. It follows that if this restoration can be achieved in athletes, it can function just as effectively in steelworkers, secretaries, weekend athletes, and housewives. The key to the program, obviously, lies in safety and effectiveness. If you could summarize an overall basis to our preferred rehabilitation program, it would lie in the concept of neutral position isometric strengthening for the spine. *This program is derived from work by Jeff Saal, M.D., Arthur White, M.D., and others including Celeste Randolph, Ann Robinson, Clive Brewster and others at the Kerlan Jobe Orthopedic Clinic.*

Trunk Stretching and Strengthening Program

This exercise program concentrates on trunk strength and trunk mobility, balance, coordination, and aerobic conditioning. A practical application of the use of trunk strengthening in back treatment, injury prevention, and improved performance in athletes.

It appears that the place to begin the rehabilitation program in an injured lumbar spine, with or without neurologic deficit, neutral position isometric strengthening. The basis of the trunk stability program is to have the patient find a neutral, painfree position while supine with the knees flexed and feet on the ground. Not only is this beginning to rehabilitation as nontraumatic as possible, but also it forms the basis of an important concept in terms of both athletic function and activities of daily living for everyone. We retrain muscles to work to support the spine while the patient is using his or her arms and legs. It is not only theoretically ideal, but also practically possible. Teaching muscle control with tight, rigid contraction of the muscles, controlling the spine through the lumbodorsal fascia, with the gluteus maximus, oblique abdominals, latissimus dorsi, not only produces protection of the lumbar spine, but also can improve athletic performance. The power and strength of any throwing athlete comes from the trunk. Lifting weight requires functioning of the lumbodorsal fascia.

Trunk strength is an important treatment method for back pain, and it also can prevent back injuries. Although treatment plans for symptomatic back pain patients may include similar exercises, each plan should be designed to match the examination and the symptoms. Any trunk strengthening plan puts strain on the spine and can produce back pain related to overload. Therefore, it should be conducted in a controlled, progressive manner.

The key to safe strengthening is the ability to maintain the spine in a safe, neutral position during the strengthening exercises. For upper body strengthening, the spine must be well aligned with the chest-out posture. Doing isometric trunk exercises and upper body exercises emphasizing this chest-out posture strengthens the support for the cervical spine, strengthens the postural muscles necessary for maintaining proper body alignment, and prevents neck pain caused by bad postural alignment.

For the lower body, trunk control plays a vital role in the ability to rotate and transfer torque safely. Trunk strengthening exercises such as sit-ups and spine extensions produce strength. Flexibility produces a protective range of motion, but often the key is providing trunk strength and control at the proper moment during the athletic activity. For example, a baseball hitter goes from flexion through rotation to extension. If the trunk musculature does not maintain rigid control, despite these changes in the axis of alignment, the player may lose power or sustain a back injury. An athlete can have strong muscles, but if they do not fire in sequence at the proper time, they offer no protection from injury and certainly will not enhance performance. A key to producing a safe range of motion is to begin trunk control in the safe, neutral position, establish muscle control in that position, and maintain control through the necessary range of motion to perform the athletic activity.

We begin our identification of the neutral spine position with the dead–bug exercises (Fig. 17.1). To perform these exercises, the individual is supine with the knees flexed and feet on the floor. With the assistance of the trainer or therapist, the

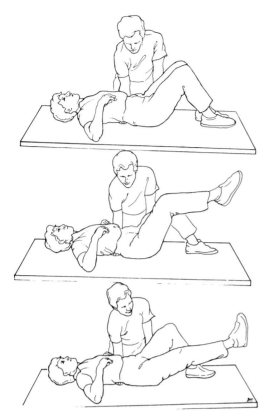

Fig. 17.1. Begin identification of the neutral position with dead–bug exercises. The patient is supine with the knees flexed and feet on the floor. With assistance from the trainer or therapist, the patient pushes the lumbar spine toward the mat until a moderate amount of painless force is exerted on the examiner's hand. The patient then maintains this same amount of force through abdominal contraction while: 1. Raising one foot; 2. Raising the other foot; 3. Raising one arm; 4. Raising the other arm; 5. Raising one leg; 6. Raising the other leg; 7. Doing a leg flexion and extension with one foot; 8. Doing a leg flexion and extension with the other foot. These same exercises can be performed with weights on arms or legs.

player pushes the lumbar spine toward the mat until a moderate amount of painless force, not exaggerated, back flattening, extreme force, is exerted on the examiner's hand. The player then learns to maintain this same amount of force through abdominal and trunk muscle contraction while:

1. Raising one foot.
2. Raising the other foot.
3. Raising one arm.
4. Raising the other arm.
5. Raising one leg.
6. Raising the other leg.
7. Doing a leg flexion and extension with one foot.
8. Doing a leg flexion and extension with the other foot.

These same exercises can be performed with weights on arms or legs.

The next stage for torque transfer athletes is resistance to rotation, first supine, then sitting, then standing, in which the player maintains the neutral spine control position while resisting rotation of the upper body on the lower body. The player resists the rotational activity exerted by the therapist or trainer.

In the next stage, the player maintains trunk control while actively rotating through a short range of motion against the trainer's resistance. This maneuver is done in numerous positions to teach trunk control regardless of the positions assumed by the patient (Fig. 17.2).

Beach ball exercises can also be of benefit. A ball that is 4 feet in diameter can be used to do partial sit-ups while maintaining control of the ball. With the trunk in neutral position, the sit-ups and resistive sit-ups are done on the ball (Figs. 17.3 and 17.4).

Lower extremity, trunk, and upper extremity strengthening must be done with concentration on maintaining the neutral trunk control position. It must be taught away from the sport, without a bat or ball, on the training table or floor. A routine is established for the player: think trunk control—neutral position—tense contractions. Trunk control is incorporated into throwing or batting. This control will ultimately produce a more efficient transfer of torque from the lower to the upper extremities, i.e., better bat control for a hitter and better endurance and ball control for a pitcher. An additional valuable benefit can be prevention of spine injuries and spinal pain associated with the athletic activity.

After establishing neutral position isometric control of the spine, extremity strengthening can begin. Probably the most important muscles needed to protect the spine itself are the quadraceps. The ability to return to work after a back injury is directly related to quadraceps strength. Yet, quadracep strengthening should not be done in the standard, sitting, full knee extension position in a patient with severe lower back pain. The goal is to accomplish quadracep strengthening without irritating the lumbar spine mechanical pain. Also, the ability to move a weight from 90° to zero may not relate as specifically to lumbar spine function as quadraceps strength obtained through functional strengthening. Functional strengthening initially involves wall slides—sliding down the wall, holding the position for 10 seconds and back up at varying depths of slide. We begin this exercise immediately after surgery for our patients. Throwing the medicine ball in a flexed knee position. Exercise that involves the use of such devices as a Versiclimber or stationary cycle as well as other techniques are used to teach quadraceps function while maintaining trunk control and during sports-related activity.

Gluteal and hip extensor strengthening is important, but must be done without inadvertently hyperextending the lumbar spine. Exercise bands that provide resistance to hip extension without much spine extension are optimal, as are other techniques that de-emphasize spine motion while producing isometric extensor strength.

Weight machines, with a safe, protected range of motion, can be of value in extremity strengthening. The key to the

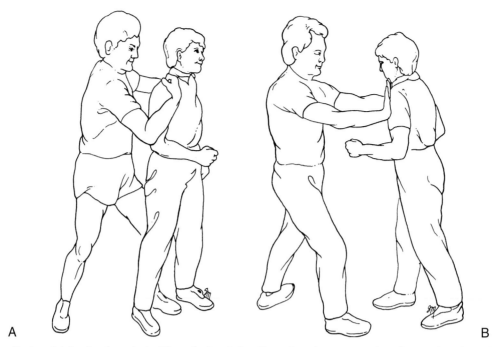

A   B

Fig. 17.2. The patient maintains trunk control while actively rotating through a short range of motion against the trainer's resistance. This maneuver is performed in numerous positions to teach trunk control regardless of the position of the patient.

successful use of these machines is good isometric trunk control in a painfree neutral position. By first establishing trunk control, it is possible to determine a safe, protected range of motion and a good position for the spine. Therefore, military presses as well as lats, arm, and lower extremity leg strengthening with machines can be of benefit while protecting the spine. Spine strength testing machines have been shown to be of benefit in predicting return to work. The ability to perform flexion extension exercises or resistance rotational exercises on a machine, however, may not translate to functional spine activity during athletics. We have not recommended a specific back machine for treatment of lumbar injuries; we greatly prefer the trunk stabilization program.

Stretching exercises are an important part of any rehabilitation program. The more flexible the legs, arms, and upper body, the more likely the proportional decrease of motion stress on the injured lumbar spine. If trunk muscle control is established first through the strengthening program, then the spine can be held in a stable position while stretching of the extremities takes place. It is important to note that hamstring stretching too often is taken to the extent that produces abnormal lumbar spine motion. Stretching the leg past the point of pelvic motion only strains the spine and does not increase hamstring looseness. Too often, lumbar spine conditions are irritated because of excessive lumbar motion during hamstring stretching. The spine should be held in a neutral, stable position during hamstring stretching exercises. Lumbar spine motion is important also, but it is not the initial stage of the rehabilitation program. Lumbar spine motion begins with good muscle control of the spine during the motion exercises. The most common initial stage

of motion is the CAT/COW position on all fours, for example, a position in which muscle control can be easily maintained.

The stretch exercises are a critical component of the program. Stretching increases the functional range of motion of the trunk and legs, which in turn decreases the likelihood of lumbar spine injury during the strengthening program during play.

Most low back injuries occur when the player exceeds the strength of the spine and its range of motion. The stretching program provides a greater area of painfree and injury-free function. For example, if a player who is stiff, having 10° of spine extension and 20° of spine rotation, suddenly reaches for a ball producing 25° of extension and 40° of rotation, injury to the back can occur through tearing stiff tissue. If mobility exercises produce a functional range of motion of 40° of extension and 50° of rotation, injury is less likely to occur. This is a protective range of motion.

The chief findings in our ball players with back pain are weak abdominal musculature, loss of spine extension, loss of rotation (usually more in one direction), and poor mechanics in rotation. Once the back pain starts, the weakness and contractions increase. This program is designed for performance enhancement and injury prevention, as well as treatment of back pain.

Aerobic Conditioning

Numerous methods are available for aerobic conditioning. Often we see athletes who prefer a specific technique, such as running, but have developed pain and problems directly related to its performance.

Cross-training is critically important in recovering from aerobic exercise-induced injury. Not only does the runner with an injured back have to do the stretching and strengthening rehabilitation program, but also they must learn cross-training for aerobic exercise. Water running, swimming, cycling, crosscountry skiing machines, Versiclimber, and rowing machines can produce the needed aerobic conditioning outside of the injurious sport. The benefit of swimming and water running program[19] should be obvious. The total unweighting of the spine in water removes many of the compressive loads and allows good physical activity without the tremendous pounding and straining of running. The cross-country skiing machine builds tremendous conditioning with strong use of the arms and increasing cardiac output without the pounding of running.

The Versiclimber and cycling have several things in common. First, it is possible to assume a beneficial position for back protection while still getting good aerobic conditioning. The cycling position is slightly bent forward, which helps the stenotic spine. The Versiclimber position is erect, which removes as much nerve root tension as possible. Both devices are associated with the same potential hazard: lateral tilt of the pelvis. For the Versiclimber, taking short steps should prevent a lot of pelvic tilting, and in cycling, the legs should not become fully extended when reaching for the peddles. The goal is to keep the pelvis and spine in a firm, neutral position with good isometric control during the aerobic conditioning.

Running stairs or stair-walking machines produce good leg strength and good hip extensor strength. Rowing machines can result in injury to the back, but if they are used properly, with muscle control of the spine in a limited range of motion, the benefit of upper extremity and lower extremity function and quadricep strengthening can produce good aerobic conditioning without spine stress. The better the aerobic condition of the athlete, the less likely he or she will sustain

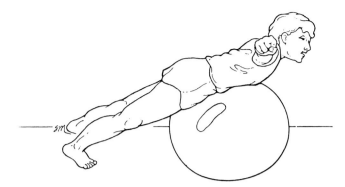

Fig. 17.4. Extension exercises on the exercise ball while maintaining control of the ball and the trunk in the neutral position.

injury, including lumbar spine injury. Therefore, aerobic conditioning is an important part of every spine rehabilitation program.

Restore Balance and Coordination

Restoration of balance and coordination is vital to an effective return to full activity and sports. Incorporation of balancing techniques into the strength program as is done in the Spine Stabilization Rehabilitation Program, begins the process of retraining muscles to fire at the right time with the proper strength. Balance and coordination are the key to friction-free performance; it is safer and more effective. Coordination is the key to swinging the golf club, throwing a baseball, or even lifting weights. Using the Swiss exercise ball, balance beam, standing positions for resistive exercises, exercises bands, and techniques such as one leg squats while resisting an exercise band pulling on the waist uses balance with strengthening exercises. Therefore, it is important to incorporate balance and coordination into all strengthening, stretching, and aerobic conditioning aspects of a rehabilitation program.

Sport-Specific Exercise

After relief of inflammation and pain; restoration of strength, flexibility, conditioning, and coordination; and establishing the rehabilitation exercises, the physical therapist, trainer, physician, and coach come together in the rehabilitation program to incorporate these techniques into the sport. Much will be lost and injury will likely reoccur if this application does not take place properly. New exercises are added that more closely simulate the sport. Proprioceptive neuromuscular facilitation-type techniques of resistive rotation and others blend in with techniques used by the athlete normally to prepare for the sport. The coach may be able to change certain techniques such as slight external rotation of the lead foot in golf, or a different foot plant in baseball.

All athletes should *start slowly back into the sport*. The return is comparable to spring training all over again. They must take the time to test out the new techniques and the new awareness of trunk muscle function and body alignment. Too fast a return is too fast back into the same old rut that often

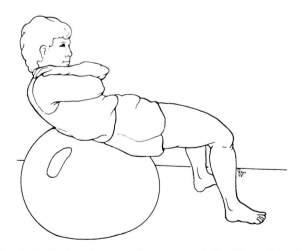

Fig. 17.3. Partial sit-ups on the exercise ball while maintaining control of the ball and the trunk in the neutral position can be of benefit.

led to the injury. It is important to build up to the maximum performance.

The summary of an effective nonoperative treatment program for lumbar spine injuries is as follows:

1. Stop the inflammation. We prefer anti-inflammatory medications; Indocin SR is our standard medication. Patients should be advised of potential complications of any anti-inflammatory medications. Medrol dose pack may be used in increasingly difficult clinical situations, as well as epidural cortisone injections.
2. Restricted activity. This limitation may vary from 24 to 72 hours of bedrest to immediate immobilization in a lumbosacral corset and restriction of painful activities.
3. Spine stability rehabilitation program. This program begins as soon as practically possible. It may vary from in bed in the hospital at 24 hours to the first available outpatient appointment in physical therapy.
4. Follow with extremity stretching, lumbar motion, extremity strengthening, aerobic conditioning, sport–specific exercises and return to full function.

Responses to some questions asked previously follow.

1. *Do you start flexion or extension exercises?* You start neither. You start neutral isometric control exercises.
2. *Do you do twisting exercises?* Twisting exercises can be the most injurious exercises in any rehabilitation program, yet torsional rotation is an important part of many sports. The answer lies in producing tight, rigid trunk control that controls the spine during rotational activities with the motion occurring predominantly in shoulders, hips, and legs. The athlete is then able to produce a parallelism between the shoulders and pelvis during rotation, especially during the contact portion of the rotational sport. A twisting exercise that allows loss of muscle control of the spine during exercise can be injurious, and may not be of benefit.

   Rotational strengthening can be important, but it must be initiated with close observation and control. We twist many times in an average day and twisting is a part of many sports. Having a painfree rotational range of motion is important; therefore, proper, slow-active stretching in rotation is important. The recommendation is: do not twist—learn to rotate the entire body.
3. *What type of aerobic conditioning should be done?* The type that holds the spine in its most advantageous position and best unweights the spine from injurious compressive loads. Cross-train using a variety of aerobic conditioning techniques.
4. *When can someone lift weights?* They can lift weights when they can do it safely, i.e., they have tight, rigid trunk control. They can protect their spine while strengthening their extremities. They can lift weights when they can understand the role of balance, speed, and proper mechanical advantage in weight lifting. The key to functional weight lifting for the athlete is not to lift the weight at the greatest mechanical disadvantage, but to simulate positioning used in their sport. Isometric trunk control and position protection first, then resistive weight lifting.
5. *What role do weight machine exercises have?* Weight machines can be a distinctly advantageous control situation for resistive weight lifting. All machines that strengthen the extremities require proper spine control first. We have not used trunk strengthening machines, such as the flexion, extension, or rotation machine, in patients with back problems. Questions still linger as to their benefit. The key probably lies in proper use of the equipment and combining the equipment with a functional isometric control-

type system such as the trunk stability rehabilitation program. A disadvantage of machines is that the individual must move the weight in an arc motion established by the machine. Free weights allow the use of the arc that is to the best advantage of the individual. This difference between the machine and free weights can be important for an athlete with an injured shoulder.
6. *What type of nonoperative rehabilitation is best for the individual athlete's sport?* It depends much on the sport and the demands as to rotational activity, compressive load, and tensile extremes of range of motion.

Individual Sports

The lumbar spine is a highly vulnerable area for injury for participants in a number of different sports. The incidence varies from 27%[20] to 7%[9] to 13%.[2] Although the incidence is significant and the amount of time lost may be significant, probably the most important problems lie in fear of spinal injuries and the necessity of a therapeutic plan. Lumbar pain is a big part of many sports, but an organized diagnostic and therapeutic plan can prevent permanent injury and allow full function and maximum performance.

GYMNASTICS

With reference to lumbar spine injuries, gymnastics is probably the sport mentioned most commonly. The motions and activities of gymnastics produce tremendous strains on the lumbar spine. The hyperlordotic position used with certain maneuvers such as the back walkovers exerts tremendous forces on the posterior elements and requires a great deal of flexibility. The amount of lumbar flexion/extension used during flips and vaulting dismounts requires a great deal of strength to support the spine during these extremes of flexibility.[21]

Jackson[7] reported that female gymnasts have an incidence of spondylolysis of 11%. Spondylolysis is a fatigue fracture of the neural arch that, in gymnastics, is thought to result from vigorous lumbar motion in hyperextension. Jackson also found spina bifida occulta in 9 of 11 gymnasts with pars interarticularis defects. It is known that there is a hereditary predisposition to the stress fracture of spondylolysis, and the findings of occult spina bifida may point out a weakness of the dorsal arch in some of these gymnasts. Certainly, however, the sport itself plays a tremendous role in a higher incidence of spondylolysis and a higher incidence of back pain in general. Garrick and Requa[22] observed a high incidence of low back pain in female gymnasts and recommended the vigorous trunk strengthening exercises that are used today to properly prepare gymnasts for their sport.

BALLET

Many motions used in ballet are similar to those in gymnastics. The classic maneuver that produces back pain problems is the arabesque position, which requires extension and rotation of the lumbar spine. Performing this maneuver properly is the key to preventing lumbar strain. Several points have been emphasized: keep the pelvis stable, keep the extension of the spine symmetric over all levels of the spine, and obtain good extension through the hip joints.[23]

Ballet involves the lifting of dancers, especially lifting in awkward positions. The outstretched hand produces tremendous level-arm stresses across the spine of the lifting partner. Off-balance bending and lifting is a hallmark of back problems in industrial workers, and yet ballet, although a sport of balance, often involves some of the most difficult lifts. Male dancers follow the body weight of their female partners very closely.

Spondylolysis and spondylolisthesis play a critical role in dancers and may often produce severe mechanical back dysfunction.

WATER SPORTS

In addition to injuries to the wrist and cervical spine, diving is associated with added strain to the lumbar spine that results from rapid flexion/extension changes and severe back arching after entering the water. Although swimming and water exercises are a major part of any back rehabilitation program, certain kicks, such as the butterfly, produce vigorous flexion/extension of the lumbar spine, especially in young swimmers. The swimmer must learn good abdominal tone and strength in order to protect his or her back during a vigorous kicking motion. Thoracic pain and round back deformities in young female breast-strokers can be a problem because of the repeated round shoulder-type stroke motion.

POLE VAULTING

Pole vaulting is another sport that involves maximum flexion/extension and muscle contraction. The range of motion of the lumbar spine has been documented with high speed photography from 40° of extension to 130° of flexion in 0.65 seconds. One can imagine the tremendous forces generated across the spine with these functional demands.[24]

WEIGHT LIFTING

Moving from the motion sports—those sports that require tremendous flexibility and strength and involve large degrees of changes in range of motion, we go to the "heavier"—those that require strength, lifting, and high body weight. The most common such sport is weight lifting.

The incidence of lower back pain and problems in weightlifters is estimated to be 40%.[25] The tremendous forces exerted on the lumbar spine by lifting weights over the head produces tremendous lever arm effects and compressive injury to the spine. Weight lifting begins with the spine in tight rigid position of flexion, and the lifter lifts with the legs. Tremendous extension force is exerted at the hips and knees with the spine in a rigidly stable position. Success in this portion of the lift requires the body to generate tremendous rigid immobilization of the spine in the power position of slight flexion.

To perform a forward bent motion with the spine out of proper position can be dangerous. Lifting weights with the spine flexed at 90°, whether they are lighter arm weights or weights across the upper back, generate tremendous lever arm effect forces. The weight times the distance back to the spine results in tremendous shear forces across the lumbar spine, especially if weight is to be moved in this position. One cannot imagine muscles that must be strengthened in this dangerous and mechanically disadvantageous position.

A dangerous time for weight lifters is the shift from spinal flexion to extension that occurs with lifting the weight over the head as in the clean jerk maneuver or the "snatch." Making this transition must be done with rigid, tight muscle control. Inexperienced lifters, especially, have no muscle control as the spine shifts from flexion to extension. A trained lifter, again, controls that shift with rigid muscle control of the lumbodorsal fascia.

Holding weight over the head invariably draws increased lumbar lordosis. These tremendous extension forces of the lumbar spine naturally lead to discussion of spondylolysis and spondylolisthesis. The incidence of spondylolysis in weight lifters has been estimated at 30%, and the incidence of spondylolisthesis is 37%.[26] Many newer training techniques in weight lifting emphasize the role of general body conditioning, flexibility, aerobic conditioning, speed, and cross-training, in addition to the ability to lift weight.

FOOTBALL

Football players lift weights. It is part of the sport. For most athletes involved in the sport, football requires tremendous upper body forces and leg strength. Some football players rely on great agility and jumping ability, throwing ability, and eye–hand contact, but strength is the backbone of football.

Every year, professional teams need heavier, stronger athletes, especially for the offensive line. Players go through their period of mechanical back pain as training camp begins, it is difficult to prepare an athlete in the off-season for the tremendous, rapid back extension against weight necessary for blocking in the offensive line. Extension jamming of the spine produces facet joint pain, spondylolysis, and spondylolisthesis. The effect is similar to the weight-lifting position of weight over the head, except that it must be generated with forward leg motion, off-balance resistance to the weight while trying to carry out specific maneuvers such as blocking a man in a specific direction. Lumbar spine problems in these athletes requires specific training in back strengthening exercises to prevent injuries.[27,28]

Safety in weight lifting is an important part of football. Having a promising football player injured in the weightroom is a relatively common occurrence. It has been estimated that more injuries occur in training than competition.[29] This situation can be avoided by using proper weight-lifting techniques.

In addition to extension lifting-type forces, football involves sudden off-balance rotation, which may produce transverse process fractures, torsional disk injuries, and tears in the lumbodorsal fascia. Sudden off-balance twisting is part of the game and may be caused by tremendous loads or a loose, unloaded position. Football has the added dimension of receiving unexpected, severe blows to the lumbar spine that may produce contusion or fracture: impact from a helmet to the ribs produces rib fractures, and similar impact in the flank can produce renal contusion, retroperitoneal hemorrhage, and fracture of the transverse and spinous processes. Many aerobatic receivers and runners suffer spondolytic defects for the same reasons as gymnasts and ballet dancers, but the most common cause of problems is the weight lifting. The role of the strength coach in teaching proper lifting techniques and designing training schedules that prepare the lumbar spine for what is expected with football is important to prevent lumbar spine injuries in football players.

RUNNING

Another sport that produces stiffness is running. Distance runners must cross-train with flexibility to prevent injury. Running involves maintenance of a specific posture with tremendous muscle exertion over a long period of time. Low back pain as well as interscapular and shoulder and neck pain are commonly reported by runners. The majority of runners with mechanical low back pain are "cured" with stretching exercises. Runners also have a natural tendency to develop isolated abdominal weakness. Running does not naturally involve constriction of abdominal and spine-stabilizing musculature. A significant inbalance is often noted between flexor and extensor muscles, not only in the legs but also in the trunk. Intrascapular and back pain also results from abnormal posture during running. As stated previously, the key to posture is good isometric trunk strength that holds the body in an upright chest out position.

Treatment for runners with low back pain should include the following:

1. Vigorous stretching program that stretches trunk as well as lower extremities
2. Cross–training and muscle strengthening techniques that also strengthen the antagonist muscles, such as hip extensors and knee extensors.
3. Abdominal strengthening, using isometric trunk stability exercises to enhance abdominal control
4. Chest–out strengthening exercises, beginning with abdominal strengthening and adding upper body shoulder shrugs, arms behind the back–type exercises to emphasize chest–out posturing and tight abdominal control. The basis of back pain prevention in runners is stretching exercises.
5. Proper footwear for cushioning and enhancement of foot function.

ROTATIONAL AND TORSIONAL SPORTS

Rotational and torsional sports have certain characteristics in common despite the exact sport itself. Baseball, golf, and the javelin all require rotation and have distinctly different demands on the spine.

Javelin Throw. The javelin throw requires an athlete to generate a tremendous amount of force to go from a hyperextended position to a full flexion forward through position. Athletes do not throw a javelin 200 feet with their arm. Although shoulder and arm injuries are common in javelin throwers, the key is rigid abdominal strength that produces the torque necessary to throw the javelin. Attempting to throw with the arm only results in arm injury and in no way can generate any type of distance. Every arm injury in a javelin thrower must be treated with trunk exercises and trunk strengthening. A rotatory lumbar spine injury in a javelin thrower is a completely debilitating injury that requires tremendous care and correction before returning to the sport.

Golf. Golfers notoriously have the highest incidence of back injury of any professional athlete. In one review by Callaway and Jobe of injuries on the 1985–1986 PGA tour, 230 of 300 professional golfers were injured (an incidence of 77%). Of the total injuries, 43.8% were related to the spine; 42.4% were lumbosacral. Lumbar spine pain in golfers results in torsional stress on the lumbar spine, and the key to pain prevention is to minimize the torsion stress by absorbing the rotation in the hips, knees, and shoulders and spreading the rotational stresses on the spine over the entire spine. Maintaining rigid, tight control through the power portion of the swing is critical. Proper technique in golf begins when addressing the ball. The knee flexion of the address position tenses the abdominal musculature. This tension is initiation of the trunk control necessary for a properly placed swing. The emphasis is on maintenance of parallel shoulders and pelvis through the majority of the swing, which requires rigid abdominal control and rotation between shoulders and hips. Loss of this rigid parallelization of the shoulders and pelvis can generate rotational strain on the lumbar spine. Rotation occurs between the hips and shoulders in the back swing, and the amount of back swing is not as important to the power of the swing as the ability of the golfer to regain tight muscle control as he or she proceeds from maximum back swing down through the power portion of the swing. It is the ability to obtain and maintain tight control and parallelism that produces the power and protection for the lumbar spine.

Advice for any recreational golfer with back pain is as follows. First, cut down the back swing and the follow through. Concentrate on the power portion of the swing. Concentrate on tight abdominal control during the power portion and minimize the excesses of rotation with back swing and follow through. Keep the golf swing symmetric. The same amount of extension on back swing and follow through is important. Avoid lateral bending, especially in the follow through. There is a tendency to bend to the left side; an off-balance lateral bending position and asymmetric loading of the spine produces injury. Golf is usually self–restricted according to the player's symptoms.

There is no condition of the lumbar spine for which we specifically restrict golf. Many people with spondylolisthesis, through superb conditioning and care, can play relatively painfree. Premature, symptomatic degenerative disk disease is common among golfers who play a great deal, especially among professionals who not only play, but also practice long hours. People can return to golf after decompressive lumbar spine operations or spinal fusions. The effect of a spinal fusion on an adult, professional golfer raises significant questions. The effect on adjacent segments and on overall spine function may not allow any better function. Under these circumstances, a fusion should be a last resort.

Baseball. Torsional problems develop in both pitchers and hitters. Throwers require a rigid cylinder of strength to transfer torque from their legs to their throwing arm. Trunk and leg strength generate the velocity of the throw and the arm provides the fine control strength. Fatigue reduces the control of the pitching motion and ball location. A major factor in ball control is a loss of tone and strength in the trunk caused by trunk muscle fatigue. A loss of the rigid trunk cylinder produces a loss of synchrony between the legs and arms, which in turn causes abnormalities in pitching mechanics. Our initial attempts at scientific study of the role of trunk musculature in throwing athletes started with throwers and progressed to professional pitchers. We used electromyographic evaluation of muscle activity.

As abdominal musculature weakens because of fatigue, lumbar lordosis increases and the back arches. The subtle change of a few degrees puts the arm behind in the pitching motion, promoting earlier ball release, and the pitch comes up. Arm strain increases as the trunk musculature fatigues. Attempts to compensate for loss of trunk strength and a "slow arm" increase the use of the arm musculature and predispose the shoulder to injury. Developing power in torsion depends on trunk strength, i.e., strengthening abdominal, back, buttock, and thigh muscles. Trunk strengthening exercises are designed not only to enhance the performance, but also to prevent arm injury. Trunk strength is superceded only by balance and coordination. The firing sequence of trunk muscles in a professional baseball player follows a consistent median pattern. Any alteration produces an inconsistent, uncoordinated pattern that leads to arm strain and back injury.[8]

Hitters are required to initiate a violent lumbar rotation based on instantaneous occular information, and so the role of the lumbar spine in a baseball hitter begins with visualization of the ball. If a hitter does not see the ball properly, the mechanics of the swing are disturbed. The most common situation is the delayed recognition of the ball producing a rotation with the hips in front of the shoulders, a loss of parallelism of shoulders and hips, and increased torsional strain of the lumbar spine. The successful player sees the ball properly and initiates a symmetric swing. The trunk should move quickly as a solid unit, through the baseball swing.

TENNIS

When reporting on racquet sport injuries, Chard and Lachmann[30] separated incidence data according to squash (59%), tennis (21%), and badmitton (20%). It has been reported that 38% of professional tennis players have missed tournaments because of back pain. Trunk strengthening should be a major part of the tennis player's regimen.[31]

Tennis involves speed, rotation, and extremes of flexion, lateral bending, and extension, as well as the power aspects of the overhead serve—the effect of trunk strength on shoulder function—many of the aspects brought out in other sports. The most consistent and important factor in protecting the spine in tennis is bending the knees. Leg strength, quadricep strength, and the ability to play in a bent-knee, hip-flexed position while protecting the back is the key to prevention of back pain. In the serve, trunk strength in proceeding from the back extended to the follow-through position requires strong abdominal control. Gluteal latissimus dorsi, abdominal obliques, and rectus abdominus strength control the lumbodorsal fascia and deliver the power necessary through the legs up into the arm.

SUMMARY

The keys to proper management of lumbar spine problems for athletes:

1. Make a comprehensive diagnosis.
2. Provide aggressive, effective nonoperative care.
3. Pinpoint operations that do as little damage as possible to normal tissue but correct the pathologic lesion.

REFERENCES

1. Keene JS: Low back pain in the athlete from spondylogenic injury during recreation or competition. Postgrad Med 74:209, 1983.
2. Spencer CW, Jackson DW: Back injuries in the athlete. Clin Sports Med 2:191, 1983.
3. Cacayorin, ED, Hochhauser, L, Petro, GR: Lumbar thoracic spine pain in the athlete: Radiographic evaluation. Clin Sports Med 6:767, 1987.
4. Micheli LJ: Back injuries in gymnastics. Clin Sports Med 4:85, 1985.
5. Papanicolaou N, Wilkinson RH, Emans JB, et al: Bone scintigraphy and radiography in young athletes with low back pain. AJR Am J Roentgenol 145:1039, 1985.
6. Fairbank JC, Pynsent PB, Van Poortvliet JA, et al: Influence of anthropometric factors and joint laxity in the incidence of adolescent back pain. Spine 9:461, 1984.
7. Jackson DW: Low back pain in young athletes: Evaluation of stress reaction and discogenic problems. Am J Sports Med 7:364, 1979.
8. Fisk JW, Baigent ML, Hill PD: Scheuerman's disease: Clinical and radiological survey of 17 and 18 year olds. Am J Sports Med 63:18, 1984.
9. Keene JS, Albert MJ, Springer SL, et al: Back injuries in college athletes. J Spinal Dis 2:190, 1986.
10. Light HG: Hernia of the inferior lumbar space. A cause of back pain. Arch Surg 118:1077, 1983.
11. Keene JS, Drummond DS: Mechanical back in the athlete. Compr Ther 11:7, 1985.
12. Schnebel BE, Simmons JW, Chowning J, et al: A digitizing technique for the study of movement of intradiskal dye in response to flexion and extension of the lumbar spine. Spine 12:309, 1988.
13. Schnebel BE, Watkins RG, Willin WH: The role of spinal flexion and extension in changing nerve root compression in disc herniations. Spine 14:835, 1989.
14. White AA, Panjabi MM: Clinical Biomechanics of the Spine. Philadelphia, Lippincott, 1978.
15. Farfan HF: Mechanical Disorders of the Low Back. Philadelphia, Lea & Febiger, 1973.

16. Farfan HF: Muscular mechanism of the lumbar spine and the position of power and efficiency. Orthop Clin North Am 6:135, 1975.

17. Farfan HF: The biomechanical advantage of lordosis and hip extension for upright activity. Spine 3:336, 1978.

18. Watkins RG, Dennis S, Dillin WH, et al: Dynamic EMG analysis of torque transfer in professional baseball pitchers. Spine 14:404, 1989.

19. Watkins RG, Buhler B, Loverock P: The Water Workout Recovery Program. Chicago, Contemporary Books, 1988.

20. Sieman RL, Spangler D: The significance of lumbar spondylolysis in college football players. Spine 6:174, 1981.

21. Schnook GA: Injuries in women's gymnastics: A five year study. Am J Sports Med 7:242, 1979.

22. Garrick JG, Requa RK: Epidemiology of women's gymnastics injuries. Am J Sports Med 8:261, 1980.

23. Howse AJG: Orthopedist's aid ballet. CORR 89:52, 1972.

24. Gainor BJ, Hagen RJ, Allen WC: Biomechanics of the spine in the pole-vaulter as related to spondylolisthesis. Am J Sports Med 11:53, 1983.

25. Aggrawal, ND, Kaur, R, Kumar, S, et al: A study of changes in weight lifters and other athletes. Br J Sports Med 13:58, 1979.

26. Kotani PT, Ichikawa MD, Wakabayashi MD, et al: Studies of spondylolisthesis found among weight lifters. Br J Sports Med 9:4, 1981.

27. Cantu RC: Lumbar spine injuries. In Cantu RC (ed): The Exercising Adult. Lexington, Collamore Press, 1980.

28. Ferguson RJ, McMaster JH, Staniski CL: Low back pain in college football linemen. J Sports Med 2:63, 1974.

29. Davies JE: The spine in sports injuries, prevention and treatment. Br J Sports Med 14:18, 1980.

30. Chard MD, Lachmann SM: Racquet sports – patterns of injury presenting to a sports injury clinic. Br J Sports Med 21:150, 1987.

31. Marks MR, Haas SS, Weisel SW: Low back pain in the competitive tennis player. Clin Sports Med 7:277, 1988.

18 Active Rehabilitation Protocols

CRAIG LIEBENSON

Symptomatic treatments for pain relief are important, but they should be used to promote active rehabilitation rather than as an end in themselves.[1,2] Rehabilitation is of value for the patient with a chronic problem, but its early use can also prevent deconditioning and disability.[2] Rehabilitation focuses on functional restoration and reducing illness behavior, not the promotion of soft tissue healing. The goal of rehabilitation is to control rather than cure symptoms. This changes the doctor's role from one of healer to helper. Functional restoration takes place within a biopsychosocial context, in contrast to the pathoanatomic model, which emphasizes treatment of injured tissues. Most spinal pain syndromes are nonspecific conditions that may become disabling because of physical and psychologic deconditioning. The aim of rehabilitation is to address the pain, impairment, and disability of the suffering individual. Accomplishing this task requires a new paradigm and new protocols.

Rehabilitation involves more than just exercise. It is a comprehensive management approach incorporating patient education, physical training, and identification of complicating factors (i.e., psychosocial issues). Passive interventions such as chiropractic adjustments are useful as catalysts for functional improvement. Rehabilitation permits the use of passive interventions if they are used with the goal of promoting functional restoration. Within the biopsychosocial model, it is possible to direct treatment at both functional restoration and providing pain relief. What is important is to make functional restoration the primary aim and therefore active care the primary method. Rehabilitation is the highest quality approach because it addresses disability prevention by promoting patient reactivation and functional restoration.

FUNDAMENTALS OF REHABILITATING THE MOTOR SYSTEM

Identifying Appropriate Candidates for Rehabilitation

Patient selection is crucial to successful functional restoration. Those patients with serious pathology (spinal or nonspinal) should be referred to the appropriate specialist. Individuals with traumatic injuries should be stabilized before functional restoration is attempted. Patients with nerve root conditions also require aggressive conservative care to reduce their nerve tension signs before rehabilitation can be pursued. In general, once the status of a patient is subacute, restoring function can and should become the primary goal of care.

Not every patient is a candidate for functional restoration. Some patients with pain have conditions that require emergency medical attention or urgent referral, which are called *red flags* (see Table 18.1).[1,2]

Patients presenting with low back pain initially should be classified into one of three categories[1,2] (Table 18.2) (see Patient Classification, p. 361). As stated previously, those with red flags identified by a medical history and physical examination should be referred to the appropriate specialist (emergency room, oncologist, rheumatologist, etc.). Simple backache accounts for the majority of patients who seek care. Their prognosis for recovery is good; 80 to 90% of these individuals recover spontaneously within 4 to 6 weeks. Spinal manipulation is advocated because it hastens this process. Other pain-relieving approaches, such as activity modification, over-the-counter pain medication, light aerobic exercise, and reassurance are recommended for use within the acute stage. Unfortunately, the recurrence rate is high. Therefore, active rehabilitation principles are important to improve the quality of care.[2]

Persons with signs of nerve root compromise also have a high rate of resolution (80%).[1,2] For these individuals, however, bed rest as many as 7 days and stronger pain medication may be required until the severe pain or impairment abates. Management strategies similar to that for nonspecific back pain are recommended, but progress is usually slower. High-velocity thrust manipulation is used with caution in these patients.

Patients whose recovery progresses rapidly (within 2 to 4 weeks) do not need a sophisticated rehabilitation approach. Patients with chronic or recurrent pain, those considered of subacute status but with significant symptomatology after 2 to 4 weeks, and postsurgical patients, however, are ideal candidates for aggressive, active rehabilitation. Rehabilitation involves a functional and biopsychosocial approach. Functional testing to identify valid return-to-work or activity outcomes is important. Other functional tests that can direct the choice of therapeutic intervention, such as identification of specific mechanical sensitivities or functional pathologies, are also necessary. A biobehavioral approach is stressed, because the longer the patient suffers, the greater the likelihood that illness behavior will become entrenched. This approach involves patient reassurance, education, and promotion of self-reliance.

Table 18.1. Red Flags[1,2]

Fracture
Trauma
Strain in osteoporotic individual
Medical pathology
Infection
Tumor
Inflammatory
Cauda equina syndrome

Table 18.2. Low Back Classifications[1,2]

Simple backache
Nerve root pain (<5%)
Serious spinal pathology (<1%)

Functional Testing

Functional testing is the first step down a rehabilitation pathway. Functional testing seeks to uncover various functional pathologies and mechanical sensitivities (Table 18.3).

Functional testing performs two basic functions. First, it provides a baseline level of functional capacity. Second, it identifies targets for functional restoration. The baseline functional deficits are objective, quantifiable, and measurable. Thus, they are ideal outcome assessment tools. The most valid tests relate specifically to relevant job traits. They do not, however, usually tell us what dysfunction in the motor system is causally related to the patient's symptoms or "pain generators." Such information is obtained through a rigorous analysis of biomechanical and neuromuscular links in the arthrokinematic chains of the body. These all-important functional chains are concerned with our most important activities (see Chapter 11). Examples, include gait, sitting posture, standing posture, prehension, respiration, mastication, and lifting or bending.[3]

Depending on the patient's work requirements or lifestyle activities, other skills may also be targets for analysis, such as overhead reaching, pushing, pulling, kneeling, crouching, and the like. *The thrust of such an analysis of functional chains in the body is to link a specific dysfunction or series of dysfunctions to the patient's area of complaint. Successful treatment hinges on finding the key functional pathologies that are biomechanically or kinesiologically related to the symptomatic area.* Unfortunately, the results of these tests are often "soft" and only qualifiable. Because many outcomes related to return to work are valid, they often are mistakenly considered an aid to the clinician in decision making. This information does provide a quality check for the clinician, but the practitioner "in the trenches" with the patient must have the freedom to use tests of a "softer" variety if they can change the course of treatment.

The utility of a functional test is based on an overview of its safety, validity, and reliability. Rissanen found that "nondynametric tests correlated better with disability than did dynametric tests."[4] If reliability overshadows validity as a criterion for a good functional test, then we may falsely conclude

that nothing is wrong with many of our patients (false negative result). Grabiner addressed this point when he found abnormal asymmetric muscle activity during bilateral electromyographic (EMG) assessment of trunk extension on patients who passed Cybex dynametric extension evaluations.[5] The Cybex test proved to have poor sensitivity (high false-negative rate). Limiting ourselves to only quantitative examinations may result in mismanagement and an overdiagnosis of psychogenic disorders as a result of the low sensitivity of these tests to truly identifying meaningful functional pathology.

Complicating Factors of Recovery

Complicating factors may interfere with patient recovery. Our history and examination should uncover these factors to allow us to form an accurate prognosis. No one has a crystal ball for seeing when a patient will recover, but various clues can help to identify who might take longer to do so. Such factors are helpful in making projections, which are increasingly important in the utilization review process associated with managed care. Table 18.4 summarizes the Mercy, Agency for

Table 18.3. Functional Testing Evaluates

Joint mobility
Muscle flexibility
Muscle strength/endurance
Movement coordination
Static and dynamic balance
Posture and gait
Lift capacity
Weight-bearing sensitivity
Movement sensitivity (i.e., flexion or extension bias)
Postural sensitivity (i.e., sitting intolerance)

Table 18.4. Complicating Factors

History/consultation
Previous history of low back pain[2]
More than 4 episodes[6]
Total work loss in past 12 months[2]
Heavy smoking[2]
Personal problems: alcohol, marital, financial[2]
Adversarial medicolegal problems[2]
Longer than 1 week of symptoms before presenting to doctor[6]
Low education attainment[2*]
Heavy physical occupation[2*]
Questionnaires/pain drawings or scales
Radiating leg pain (pain diagram)[1,2,6]
Severe pain intensity[6]
Low job satisfaction[2,6]
Psychologic distress and depressive symptoms[1,2,6]
Examination
Pre-existing structural pathology or skeletal anomaly (i.e., spondylolisthesis) directly related to new injury or condition[6]
Reduced straight leg raising[1,2]
Signs of nerve root involvement[1,2]
Reduced trunk strength and endurance[2]
Poor physical fitness (aerobic capacity)[2]
Disproportionate illness behavior (Waddell's signs)[1,2,6]

*Only slightly increase the risk of chronicity, but significantly increase the difficulty of rehabilitation.

Health Care Policy and Research (AHCPR), and British Guidelines conclusions with respect to this vital issue in case management.

Finding the Key Link

Regardless of the structural diagnosis or "pain generator" (facet, myofascial, disk, etc.), rehabilitation involves the entire locomotor system. Uncovering key functional pathologies that are linked to the patient's symptoms is the goal of functional assessment. *Rehabilitation of the patient with spinal stenosis, a recovering sciatica, or a facet syndrome involves identifying the "clusters" of functional pathology of the locomotor system that are related biomechanically or neurophysiologically to the hypothesized pain generator.* When a key functional pathology is found, its successful improvement has far-reaching effects.

Biomechanically, the body consists of a series of functional chains. The lower extremity functions in human beings as a closed kinetic chain. Any dysfunction in the foot, such as poor ankle dorsiflexion, inevitably involves the knee, hip, and lumbar spine. A stiff hip joint may develop as a result of hip flexor tightness, in turn leading to compensatory lumbar hypermobility and paraspinal trigger points. The result may be low back or buttock pain or, even worse, a lumbosacral nerve root syndrome. In regard to back or buttock pain, local treatments involving manipulative (joint or soft tissue) therapy may improve the situation. To prevent recurrences or to treat chronic pain, however, a more comprehensive approach is required. Treatment aimed at relaxing a tight psoas and strengthening a weak gluteus maximus may be the primary treatment for lumbosacral facet pain or paraspinal myofascial pain. Although theoretical, this model incorporates biomechanical and neurophysiologic rationale into the transition from manipulative therapy to active rehabilitation. *While clinicians should adhere to newly established guidelines, they should not become prisoners to them.* In fact, future research questions emerge as a result of the creativity of clinicians.

HISTORY

Functional improvement is difficult if not impossible to achieve unless inappropriately handled external demands are identified. For example, any activity, sport, or work demand that is unusually repetitive involves great external load, or requires a biomechanically improper movement (i.e., bending and twisting) must be flushed out. Such factors can be uncovered during the *history* by asking the patient in what activities they are involved, when they typically get their symptoms, and what aggravates the pain. Examples of key information gained are provided in Table 18.5.

External demand and internal functional capacity are equally important in the prevention of recurrences (see Fig. 2.4). The individual involved in many high risk activities will require greater functional capacity. In contrast, the sedentary individual may only require a slight increase in functional capacity and some basic advice.

Table 18.5. Prognostic Factors

High risk activities
Prolonged sitting
Driving
Heavy lifting
Repetitious bending and lifting
Torsional sports (tennis, hockey, baseball)

Pain-provoking activities
After prolonged sitting
After prolonged standing
After prolonged walking
With bending
In the morning
When changing positions
With weight bearing

PHYSICAL EXAMINATION

Once a functional evaluation has been performed, it is essential to attempt to differentiate the key functional pathologies from those that are secondary. Lewit said we must not mistake the pain for the problem, but instead identify and then treat the dysfunction responsible for the pain.[7] First, we must tap the patient's history for all relevant information. Pain location and what aggravates it often helps make the diagnosis before any testing is performed at all. Therefore, this information is the crucial starting point. The next step includes various tests to localize the source of the pain (palpatory and mechanical). It is validating for the patient to have their examiner find their pain either through palpation or specific provocative testing. To be able to provoke the patient's pain experience is to hit "pay dirt." This information gives the doctor and patient a baseline or ideal outcome assessment tool that can serve as a "barometer" of the success of our interventions. It also helps the examiner "zero in" on what tissues are involved. Although trigger point palpation or McKenzie or Cyriax provocative testing is not as reliable as an anesthesiologist's needle, such an assessment can be useful in day-to-day practice.

Provocative tests, whether static (e.g., prolonged sitting), dynamic (e.g., lumbar flexion), or palpatory (e.g., trigger point identification), are invaluable as signs of irritability or dysfunction.[8,9] These results, however, should not be mistaken for the dysfunction itself or its cause. *Once a pain generator is found, the all-important job of identifying why that tissue is irritated ("the perpetuating factors") begins.*[9,10]

For instance, if a patient has buttock pain and a trigger point is found in the quadratus lumborum that refers to the region of the primary complaint, we may have found the "irritable focus" of pain, but we have not necessarily found the "problem" or source. To find the *key link,* we must discover what could be responsible for the quadratus lumborum becoming an "irritable focus." Evaluating gait and movement patterns may help to identify this patient as a "hip hiker" with a muscular imbalance involving gluteus medius weakness and overactivity of the piriformis and quadratus lumborum. Recurrent sacroiliac dysfunction may also be explained by this kinesiopathology. The entire kinetic chain from the foot up should be evaluated with the goal of finding the joint or muscle dysfunction that is "upstream" of the "irritable focus." This assessment is the only way in which we can separate the adaptive compensations of the locomotor system from the true source of functional pathology.

To rule out the chances of a short-term effect, treatment may be repeated over a period of 2 to 6 weeks to change neuromuscular patterning. If long-lasting results prove difficult to achieve, it is best to perform functional re-evaluation for other key links and to reinvestigate complicating factors (i.e., psychosocial or high external demand).

CASE MANAGEMENT

General Principles

According to recent American and British back pain guidelines, patient reassurance, pain-relief methods, and exercise should be included in case management.[1,2] Patient reassurance is required to allay fears of back pain resulting from a serious disease. It also helps to inform patients about a favorable prognosis if back pain is managed properly. Pain-relieving methods such as time-limited passive care (i.e., manipulation), pain medication, avoidance of biomechanically deleterious activities, and reactivation with light exercises are appropriate. Exercise or active rehabilitation gains in importance as the acute pain phase subsides. Exercises should be aimed at restoration of function and prevention of deconditioning. In particular, trunk strength, endurance, flexibility and cardiovascular fitness should all be addressed.

Treatment aimed at pain relief should not be the only goal of care. Even if a primary pain generator is identified, it is important to restore function in the locomotor system to reduce the likelihood of painful recurrences. Rehabilitation has two primary goals: (1) through education, ergonomics, or training in load handling, to decrease extrinsic mechanical stress (i.e., sudden or repetitive overload) on the painful area; and (2) by functional restoration to improve the intrinsic functional capacity of the spine or its stability.

Patient education helps to decrease mechanical stress placed on a painful region. The combination of manipulation and exercise restores function in the locomotor system, thus improving the ability of a painful region to adapt to increased mechanical stress. Essential ingredients in achieving a successful outcome are finding the key sources of tissue overload and identifying the key functional pathologies to address.

Key Link

It is easy to become overwhelmed when attempting to separate important from trivial functional pathologies or deficits. *So many structural and functional pathologies are present in asymptomatic individuals that they may not be clinically significant when seen in symptomatic patients.* Lewit and Janda outlined a biomechanical and kinesiologic approach that "culls out the wheat from the chaff."[7,11] The primary goal of assessment is finding the key functional pathologies of the

motor system, the associated dysfunction of which can lead to mechanical overload at a distance throughout a kinetic chain of a particular posture or movement. We must carefully analyze historical data and observe the motor system of our patients in action to identify the key functional pathology. This approach enables us to find a relevant dysfunction that can significantly alter the treatment program.

Pathokinesiology that results in tissue overload and thus pain can be identified by evaluating posture, gait, and key stereotypic movement patterns.[7,11] The implications of this analysis for chiropractors and those involved in manual medicine is that specific muscle imbalances (tight and weak muscles) that are functionally related to the painful area can be identified. Thus, we can form a prescription of which muscle needs to be stretched or relaxed, those that need to be strengthened or facilitated, and the joints that need to be adjusted. *By finding the specific pathokinesiology related to a painful area, an exercise prescription can be rationally linked to the manipulable lesion.*

Pathokinesiology in a kinetic chain can be flushed out through postural and movement analysis.[11,12] Posture, gait, skills analysis, and key movement patterns all play a part in evaluation of the motor system. Low back pain may have arisen after an overstrain. On examination, a paraspinal trigger point may be discovered. Treating the local functional pathologies may be all that is necessary. If the condition persists, however, further evaluation of the locomotor system will be required. The problem may be found in a dysfunctional chain of events involving a biomechanical foot fault, shortened iliopsoas, gluteal inhibition, and lumbosacral joint dysfunction with accompanying trigger points. Finding the chain reaction is crucial to removing key perpetuating factors for motor system disorders. A further and more difficult situation arises when longstanding abnormal posture and movement patterns have been learned by the cerebellum. This situation requires treatment of not only peripheral tissues but also the central nervous system (e.g., propriosensory retraining).[13]

Each stereotypical movement pattern is important for its relationship to basic skills performed many times each day.[3] These skills include *gait, sitting posture, standing posture, prehension, respiration, mastication, and lifting or bending* (Table 18.6). For instance, hip extension (psoas, hamstring/gluteus maximus muscle imbalance) relates to gait (toe off and forward propulsion), standing posture, and lifting. Hip abduction (tensor fascia latae [TFL], adductors, quadratus lumborum [QL], piriformis/gluteus medius muscle imbalance) relates to foot strike and stance phase of gait (pelvic stability). Trunk flexion (erector spinae, hip flexor/rectus abdominus muscle imbalance) relates to lifting and trunk stability in general (during carrying, reaching, pushing, and pulling). Shoulder abduction (upper and lower fixators of the scapulae muscle imbalance) relates to prehension, reaching, grasping, and holding activities. Trunk lowering from a push-up (pectorals/serratus anterior muscle imbalance) relates to pushing and pulling activities. Head/neck flexion (sternocleidomastoid [SCM], suboccipital/deep neck flexors muscle im-

Table 18.6. Chain Reactions in the Locomotor System

Skill	Movement Pattern	Tight or Overactive Muscle	Weak or Inhibited Muscles	Stiff Joints	Hypermobile Joints
Gait/toe off, lifting, and standing posture	Hip extension	Psoas, hamstring, erector spinae	Gluteus maximus	Hip joint	Lumbar
Gait/stance	Hip abduction	TFL, QL, adductors, piriformis*	Gluteus medius	Hip joint	SI joint and LS joint
Lifting and trunk stability	Trunk flexion	Psoas, erector spinae	Rectus abdominus	Lumbar flexion	Lumbar extension
Prehension, reaching, grasping	Shoulder abduction	Upper trapezius, levator scapulae	Lower and middle trapezius	C/T junction, S/C joint	C5-C6, G/H joint
Pushing/pulling	Trunk lowering from a push-up	Pectoralis major/minor, subscapularis	Serratus anterior	C/T junction, mid-upper thoracics	G/H joint
Mastication and sitting posture	Head/neck flexion	SCM, suboccipitals	Deep neck flexors	C/T junction in flexion, TMJ	C5-C6
Respiration	Respiration	Scalenes	Diaphragm	Rib cage, lower cervical-spine	

*TFL, tensor fascia latae; QL, quadratus lumborum; SI, sacroiliac; LS, lumbosacral; G/H, gleno-humeral; C/T, cervicothoracic; SCM, sternocleidomastoid; TMJ, temporomandibular joint, S/C sternoclavicular.

balance) relates to sitting and mastication. Respiration (scalenes/diaphragm) relates to breathing. Other important activities performed include squatting, stooping, crouching, overhead reaching, and the like, depending on the particular work or sport activity in which a person is engaged. Weaknesses of specific muscles, such as quadriceps and erector spinae, that occur with deconditioning are also key links to evaluate as areas of high risk during activities like lifting or squatting.

Once the mechanical relationship between certain postures, activities, muscles, joints, or kinetic chains and the patient's symptoms has been revealed, a treatment program can be outlined. Intervention involves three levels of care. Advice (patient education about biomechanics and ergonomics), manipulation (manual or reflex therapy), and exercise (Table 18.7). In general, advice is the easiest intervention followed by manipulation and then exercise. Chiropractors have thrived on the power of manipulation, and physical therapists on advice and exercise. The use of all three elements in combination with a complete evaluation constitutes the highest quality of care available to the public.

A good guideline to follow for improving the entire kinetic chain linking key muscle or joint pathologies is listed in Table 18.8. Table 18.9 outlines principles of case management for nonspecific back pain, which includes assessment (red flags, diagnostic triage, complicating factors, outcomes, functional pathology) and treatment (advise, manipulation, exercise).

Complicating Factors Encountered With Exercise Training

Such factors include low motivation, poor flexibility, incoordination, or a mechanical sensitivity (postural, movement, or weight-bearing). Motivational problems are addressed through appropriate goal setting, gradual conversion of the patient from a pain avoider to a pain manager, explaining the

Table 18.7. Treatment of Key Functional Pathologies

Advice (patient education)
  Head set for neck pain in receptionist
  Ice and 90/90 rest position for acute pain from lumbar strain
  Lifting advice for recurrent low back pain sufferer
  Ergonomic workstation modification for carpal tunnel syndrome patient
Manipulation
  Trigger point therapy to upper trapezius muscle for neck pain
  Adjustment to lumbar spine for back pain
  Manual resistance techniques directed at scalenes or pectoralis minor for thoracic outlet syndrome
  Adjustment of foot for low back pain
Exercise
  Strengthening abdominals for low back pain
  Improving muscle imbalance between hip flexors/extensors and paraspinal muscles for back pain
  Propriosensory retraining for chronic back pain
  Trunk stabilization program for chronic back pain
  Improving scapulohumeral rhythm for rotator cuff syndrome
  Improving lateral pelvic stability by restoring muscle balance to gluteus medius, tensor fascia latae, and quadratus lumborum

Table 18.8. Addressing Functional Pathology in the Kinetic Chain

Relax/stretch overactive/tight muscles
Mobilize/adjust stiff joints
Facilitate/strengthen weak muscles
Re-educate movement patterns on reflex, subcortical basis

difference between hurt and harm, and, if necessary, referral to a pain psychologist. Flexibility deficits are addressed by chiropractic adjustments, joint mobilization, muscle relaxation, and stretching. Incoordination, if present, will lead to poor training results. Simple exercises should be prescribed that can be carried out with proper motor control. It is helpful to limit the training range to reinforce the proper quality of movement and kinesthetic awareness (see Chapter 14). Focusing on the quality or form of the exercise and not on the quantity of repetitions or resistance is essential. Restoring

Table 18.9 Case Management for Nonspecific Back Pain and Sciatica[1,2] (see Fig. 2.24 a–b)

Conservative Care	Rehabilitation (Active Care)	Biopsychosocial Assessment
Diagnostic triage • Simple backache • Nerve root pain • Serious spinal pathology Rule out red flags • Trauma (fracture, instability) • Medical pathology (tumor, infection, etc.) > **urgent referral (<3 weeks)** • Rheumatologic/inflammatory > **urgent referral (<3 weeks)** • Major neurologic compromise (cauda equina syndrome) > **emergency referral** Diagnose nerve root compromise • Motor, sensory, reflex testing • Nerve tension tests (i.e., SLR) Evaluate for complicating factors • Abnormal illness behavior (distress, depression) • Job dissatisfaction • Past history of more than 4 episodes • Preconsultation duration of symptoms >1 week • Severe pain intensity • New condition/injury related to pre-existing structural pathology or skeletal anomaly Aggressive, conservative care (symptom control) (6 weeks)* • Rest (<2 days, unless sciatica <7 days) • **Manipulation** (joint dysfunction, soft tissue dysfunction, and/or trigger points) (Maximum of two different 2-week trials if no progress documented) • **Advice** (reassurance, early activation, activity modification) • **Exercise** (light aerobic activity, McKenzie, gentle stretches) (increase over time) • Physical agents and methods (decrease over time) • Medication (NSAIDs, acetaminophen) (more important if nerve root pain) *If unresponsive, a more active approach may start within the first 2 weeks, but no later than 4 weeks.*	Functional assessment • Quantifiable, outcomes • Functional pathology Exercise (temporary increase in pain acceptable) • Stretching • Strengthening (not within the first 2 weeks) • Propriosensory *After 6 weeks* • Active care > Passive Care • Consider alternative symptomatic measures *If unresponsive after 6 weeks, a biopsychosocial assessment is indicated.*	Special studies (biologic) • Radiography • CBC, ESR • Bone scan • MRI or CT if tests indicate specific nerve root compromise Psychologic assessment • Fear avoidance beliefs • Distress, depression • Illness behavior Social assessment • Family attitudes or reinforcement • Job satisfaction • Physical demands of job • Other factors relating to missed work *If unresponsive after 12 to 16 weeks* Disability management • Job modification • Work hardening • Vocational re-education • Pain management • Multidisciplinary approach

*If nerve root compromise progress is slower and treatment less aggressive. Thrust manipulation is avoided with severe or progressive neurologic deficit.

muscle balance, correcting articular dysfunctions, and facilitating enhanced perception of the "weak link" will contribute to improved coordination.

A mechanical sensitivity, like gravity or weight bearing intolerance, is no bar to exercise therapy. Non-weight-bearing exercises can be performed on the floor. All major muscle groups can be challenged before gradual reintroduction of gravity forces is attempted. A person with a postural sensitivity, such as to sitting, can exercise while upright or recumbent. Another common sensitivity is to movement in a certain direction. A patient with pain on flexion that is relieved with extension (extension "bias") is a classic McKenzie patient (see Chapter 12). Other patients who have pain with trunk extension, but relief in the slump posture can be trained to identify their "neutral range" and to learn to stabilize their back from potential harm. They also may have a common altered movement pattern—hip extension, in which they extend their thigh at the lumbosacral joint rather than at the hip (because of hip hypomobility and/or iliopsoas tightness). Improving coordination simultaneously eliminates this movement sensitivity and expands the functional range.

Releasing Patients to a Private Health Club

Much has been said about chiropractors working with private health club facilities. Although this practice is certainly good, a few points are worth mentioning.

- Proper spinal posture must be taught
- Nautilus-type machines are open kinetic chain and thus do not train reflex control
- Nautilus-type machines and other health club exercises often encourage "trick" movements. Be on the lookout for the following:
  —Hip flexors substituting for the abdominals
  —Lumbar hyperextension during hamstring curls, seated leg extensions, and stairclimber
  —Slumping during bent-over rows, lunges, stairclimber, incline treadmill, or bicycle
  —Chin poking during pull downs, bench press, abdominal exercise, bicycle, or squats
  —Shoulder shrugging during overhead lifting, arm exercises, or rowing
- Free weights are preferable but require specific instructions
  —Lunges should be performed with proper lumbosacral stabilization ("neutral position")

—Avoid shoulder shrugging with biceps curls

—Avoid excessive shoulder external rotation during bench press

• Aerobic exercise is excellent, but with certain exceptions

—Stairclimbing is deleterious if patient has weakness of gluteus maximus or gluteus medius or overactivity of erector spinae, quadratus lumborum, or tensor fascia latae

—Stationary bicycle may not be advisable after day of desk and auto sitting

—Floor must be properly padded

—Introductory classes must be available to prevent knee injuries in the novice

• Typical postural faults and clinical consequences that result from improper exercise programs (as described in Table 18.10)

FUNCTIONAL RESTORATION OF THE LOCOMOTOR SYSTEM

Patient Classification

Different classification schemes for back pain patients have been proposed. Those dealing with pathoanatomic diagnosis were rejected for lack of proof. The Quebec Task Force proposed the following classification scheme for spinal disorders (Table 18.11).[14] This classification has been simplified by recent British and American guidelines (see Table 18.2).[1,2]

Most patients (70 to 90%) fall into the back pain category.[1,2] This nonspecific label replaces pathophysiologic hypothesis such as facet syndrome, sacroiliac (SI) syndrome, myofascial syndrome, or radiographic diagnosis such as disk or joint degeneration. Use of this label does not mean that most low back pain has no cause, just that the cause is not yet known. Recent evidence suggests that some of these causes are becoming clearer. Using a double anesthetic injection technique (one is a control block), it is possible to identify the primary pain generator in more than 50% of both chronic neck and back pain patients.[15,16-19] Sacroiliac joints are pain generators in 13%, zygapophyseal joints in 15%, and disks in 39% of patients presenting to specialized spine centers.[15,18,19] Unfortunately, no physical signs have

Table 18.10. Typical Postural Faults and Clinical Consequences that Result from Improper Exercise Programs

Postural Faults	Clinical Result
Overactive sternocleidomastoid in women performing sit-ups incorrectly	Cervicocranial syndrome and headaches
Rounded shoulders in men doing too much pectoralis work without working their upper back	Thoracic outlet syndrome, shoulder impingement syndrome, cervicocranial syndrome
Shrugged shoulders from too much upper trapezius work and not enough lower trapezius strength	Headaches and shoulder impingement syndrome
Military posture (anterior pelvic tilt with chest sticking out) from abdominal and gluteal work without lumbosacral stabilization (posterior pelvic tilt)	Low back pain

Table 18.11. Quebec Task Force Classification of Spinal Disorders

Pain without radiation
Pain + radiation to extremity, proximally
Pain + radiation to extremity, distally
Pain + radiation to extremity + neurologic signs
Confirmed nerve root compression (advanced imaging or electrodiagnosis)
Spinal stenosis
Postsurgical status <6 months
Postsurgical status >6 months
Chronic pain syndrome
Other diagnosis (tumor, infection, fracture, rheumatologic disease, etc.)

been correlated with anesthetic relief of pain.[15,16,18,19] Hopefully, anesthetic block techniques will be used as a gold standard to adjudicate less expensive physical examination procedures as diagnostic tests for specific spinal syndromes.

Moffroid and colleagues subdivided groups of patients with nonspecific back pain into discrete functional categories.[20] These authors are studying the effects of stretching versus strengthening exercises on both flexible and inflexible patients.[21]

The Quebec Task Force also classified patients according to the duration of symptoms. Acute was defined as less than 7 days; subacute as 7 days to 7 weeks; and chronic as greater than 7 weeks. They also recommended classification by working status—working or idle. An important development in the classification of spinal syndromes was revealed by Delitto and Erhard,[22,23] who found that nonspecific back pain could be subclassified into a few categories that resulted in improved treatment outcome. An extension and an SI category were identified by specific provocative movement and functional testing, respectively. Categorization and customized treatment resulted in improved results over generic treatment for all patients with nonspecific low back pain. Using reliable tests, they showed that they could subclassify cases of nonspecific back with prescriptive validity.

The Quebec Task Force recently published a promising classification scheme for whiplash-related disorders.[24] Neck complaints were divided into four categories as follows: category I: neck complaint without musculoskeletal signs (i.e., mobility tenderness); category II: with musculoskeletal signs; category III: involves neurologic signs; category IV: involves a fracture or dislocation.

Spinal Stability, Pathokinesiology, and the Importance of Muscular Imbalances

Spinal stability depends on three intact elements of the locomotor system.[25] First is the central nervous system, in particular the cerebellum, which controls posture and movement. Second is the articular and ligamentous structures, which are the major passive structures involved in the locomotor system. And third is the muscular system, which represents the active part of the motor system. This system is under the direct control of our will during conscious activities, but it is also responsible for reflex, subconscious adaptations to irritations or injuries.

Any internal structural pathology or excessive external biomechanical load causes perturbations in the motor system. An intact motor system can adapt via central nervous system control and muscle system activity. Over time, however, repetitive overload leads to perturbations to which we cannot adapt, and instability results. The adaptations of the motor system are represented by muscle imbalances that can be assessed simply. These adaptations signify that "old" trauma or repetitive strain has perturbed the spinal stability and caused an adaptation by the motor system to adapt and prevent further instability. Unfortunately, these adaptations are less than ideal and lead to new pathokinesiology. The joints, being the passive structures, are along for the ride. They are not only bony shields to the spinal cord and vital organs, but also mobile levers that allow the muscles to perform a variety of actions. They also serve the critical function of providing afferent feedback to the motor control centers of the central nervous system to maintain efferent muscle function at an appropriate level.

Pathokinesiology of the locomotor system develops as an attempt to adapt to injuries, improper alignment or posture, or perturbations such as from repetitive strains. An injury or inflammation may lead to reflex muscle inhibition or muscular splinting. Poor foot posture, such as hyperpronation, may alter the arthrokinematics of the entire lower extremity and result in pathokinesiology. For instance, hypermobility in the foot may result in compensatory hypomobility at the knee and hip joints and then hypermobility and instability in the lumbar spine. Typical pathokinesiology associated with this chain reaction would be a muscle imbalance involving tight/overactive hip flexors, hamstrings, and erector spinae and weak/inhibited gluteus maximus. These muscle imbalances, the result of adaptations to dysfunction, pathology, or overload themselves, perpetuate a downward spiral affecting spinal stability.

Both clinical and scientific studies have generated much evidence supporting the importance of muscle imbalances as key functional pathologies. Watson and Trott demonstrated that muscle imbalances in the neck can distinguish chronic headache and nonheadache sufferers.[26] Treleaven and Jull have shown that the same muscle imbalances occur in postconcussional headache patients, but not in normal individuals.[27] According to Janda, muscle imbalances occur in a predictable manner (see Chapters 2 and 6).

Certain muscles tend to become inhibited, whereas other muscles tend to become overactive. Postural or antigravity muscles are those that tend to become overactive or shortened. Phasic muscles have a predisposition to becoming inhibited or weak. This muscle imbalance seems to be reinforced by reciprocal inhibition of antagonist muscles, as well as by habitual patterns of sterotypical use. Scientific and clin-

ical evidence substantiates this model for prescribing exercises (Tables 18.12 and 18.13).

The grouping of muscle imbalances described by Janda are not isolated clinical phenomena. *Patients typically have many functional pathologies and solving the mystery of each patient's individual functional pathology requires finding a chain reaction in the motor system.* Understanding the muscle imbalances and the relationship between muscle and joint dysfunction enables the practitioner to quickly "crack the code" of the patient's dysfunction.

Chain Reactions in the Locomotor System

LOWER CROSSED SYNDROME

One of the most clinically relevant patterns of muscle dysfunction is the lower crossed syndrome, which is typified by the following pairs of tight and weak muscles (Table 18.14). Awareness of this pattern is important for low back and pelvic conditions related to abnormal sitting, standing posture, gait, bending, or twisting activities. Table 18.15 shows the signs related to various dysfunctions associated with the lower crossed syndrome.

The combined result of this posture is that the lumbosacral, thoracolumbar, SI, hip, and knees joints are all overstressed. Joint dysfunction and trigger points naturally result from these muscle imbalances, accompanied by low back pain, buttock pain, pseudo-sciatica, and knee disorders.[7,11,41,42] Each of the three muscle imbalances that contribute to the lower crossed syndrome are discussed in the context of the

Table 18.12. Clinical Evidence for Muscle Imbalances

Forward head posture and decreased isometric strength and endurance of neck flexors correlated with headache patients[26]
Upper cervical joint dysfunction, weak neck flexors, and tight suboccipitals correlated with postconcussional headache patients[27]
Cerebral lesions result in poor descending control of tonic postural reflexes[28]
Most reflexes involve reciprocal inhibition[28]
Hypertonia with antagonist paresis is the norm[28]

Table 18.13. Scientific Evidence for Muscle Imbalance

Increased tension or tightness
    Relative type I muscle fiber hypertrophy on symptomatic side in chronic low back pain (LBP)[29,30]
    Prolonged nociceptive bombardment can lead to flexion reflex from excessive contraction of skeletal muscles in the vicinity of the nociceptors[31,32]
    Fibroblastic proliferation occurs in injured tissues if inflammatory stage is prolonged[33]
Muscle inhibition, weakness, or atrophy:
    Reflex inhibition of vastus medialis oblique after knee inflammation/injury[34–36]
    Unilateral, segmental type II muscle fiber atrophy after acute onset of LBP[37]
    Bilateral, type II muscle fiber atrophy in chronic LBP[29,30]
    Atrophy of type II muscle fibers in multifidus patients with herniated disks[38–40]

Table 18.14. Lower Crossed Syndrome (See Fig. 2.22)

Imbalance in the following pairs of muscles:
  Weak gluteus maximus and short hip flexors
  Weak abdominals and short lumbar erector spinae
  Weak gluteus medius and short TFL and QL*
Seen commonly with gait, lifting, sitting, kneeling, crouching, pushing, pulling, etc.

*TFL, tensor fascia latae; QL, quadratus lumborum.

Table 18.15. Postural Signs of Lower Crossed Syndrome

Postural Finding	Dysfunction
Lumbar hyperlordosis	Shortened erector spinae
Anterior pelvic tilt	Weak gluteus maximus
Protruding abdomen	Weak abdominals
Foot turned out	Shortened piriformis
Hypertrophy of thoracolumbar junction	Hypermobile lumbosacral junction
Groove in iliotibial band	Shortened tensor fascia latae

key movement pattern that is affected—hip extension, hip abduction, and trunk flexion.

Altered Hip Extension (Table 18.16)[7,11,13]

Hip extension is important for its relationship to the propulsive phase of gait, lifting, and the standing posture.

Weak agonist: gluteus maximus
Overactive antagonist: psoas, rectus femoris
Overactive stabilizer: erector spinae
Overactive synergist: hamstrings

Symptoms

- Low back or buttock pain (facet or myofascial syndrome) (see Figs. 18.1 and 18.2)
- Coccyalgia
- Recurrent hamstring pulls
- Recurrent or chronic neck pain

Postural Analysis

- Forward-drawn posture (see Fig. 18.3)
- Anterior pelvic tilt
- Hypertrophic erector spinae (see Fig. 18.4)
- Hypotonic gluteus maximus

Gait Analysis

- Decreased hip hyperextension
- Compensatory increased lumbar lordosis

Muscle Length Tests

- Shortened hip flexors (see Fig. 18.5)
- Shortened hamstrings (see Fig. 18.6)
- Shortened erector spinae (see Fig. 18.7)
- Contralateral upper trapezius and/or levator scapulae

Evaluation of Key Movement Patterns

- Altered activation sequence during hip hyperextension (see Fig. 18.9)

Trigger Points

- Gluteus maximus
- Coccyx
- Iliopsoas
- Erector spinae
- Contralateral upper trapezius and/or levator scapulae

Mobility (Joint Dysfunction)

- Hip joint
- Lumbosacral (L/S) junction
- Thoracolumbar (T/L) junction
- Contralateral cervical spine

Altered Hip Abduction (Table 18.17)[7,11,13]

Hip abduction is important for its relationship to the stance phase of gait and any balancing activity.
Weak agonist: gluteus medius
Overactive antagonist: adductors
Overactive synergist: tensor fascia latae (TFL)
Overactive stabilizer: quadratus lumborum (QL)
Overactive neutralizer: piriformis

Symptoms (see Figs. 10.10, 10.11, and 10.13)

- Low back or buttock pain (SI or myofascial syndrome)
- Pseudo-sciatica (myofascial syndrome)
- Lateral knee pain (knee extensor disorder)

Postural Analysis

- Prominence of the iliotibial tract
- Lateral prominence of patella
- Turned out foot (see Fig. 6.11**a**)

Gait Analysis

- Hip hiking gait
- Asymmetric pelvic rotation (blocked SI joint)

Muscle Length Tests

- Shortened hip flexors (see Fig. 18.5)
- Shortened QL (see Fig. 6.12)
- Shortened adductors (see Figs. 6.10**a** and **b**)
- Shortened TFL (see Fig. 6.7)

Table 18.16. Treatment Approach for Altered Hip Extension

Relax/stretch ipsilateral hip flexors
Relax/stretch overactive erector spinae
Relax/stretch overactive hamstrings
Adjust/mobilize low back and hip
Facilitate/strengthen gluteus maximus (bridges, squats, leg raises)
Abdominal/gluteal stabilization exercises and biomechanical/
  ergonomic advice to correct lumbopelvic posture

Table 18.17. Treatment Approach for Altered Hip Abduction

Relax/stretch thigh adductors
Relax/stretch tensor fascia latae and quadratus lumborum
Relax/stretch piriformis
Relax/stretch hip flexors
Adjust/mobilize sacroiliac joint, low back, and hip
Facilitate/strengthen gluteus medius (1 leg bridge, P-S retraining)

Evaluation of Key Movement Patterns

• Altered coordination during hip abduction (see Fig. 6.17)

Trigger Points

• Gluteus medius
• Gluteus minimus
• Piriformis
• QL
• TFL

Mobility (Joint Dysfunction)

• SI
• Hip internal rotation
• T/L and L2/L3

Altered Trunk Flexion (Table 18.18)[7,11,43]

Trunk flexion is important for its relationship to lifting, trunk stability, standing posture, and spinal statics.

Weak agonist: rectus abdominus
Overactive antagonist: erector spinae
Overactive synergist: iliopsoas

Symptoms

• Low back or buttock pain (facet syndrome, instability) (see Fig. 18.1)
• Neck pain

Postural Analysis

• Increased lumbar lordosis
• Protruding abdomen

Gait Analysis:

• Increased lordosis

Muscle Length Tests

• Shortened lumbar erector spinae (see Fig. 18.7)
• Shortened hip flexors (see Fig. 18.5)

Evaluation of Key Movement Patterns

• Altered coordination during trunk flexion (see Fig. 6.18)

Trigger Points

• Erector spinae (see Fig. 18.2)

Mobility (Joint Dysfunction)

• Lumbar-spine

Table 18.18. Treatment Approach for Altered Trunk Flexion

Relax/stretch erector spinae
Relax/stretch iliopsoas
Adjust/mobilize low back
Facilitate/strengthen abdominals (dead bugs, trunk curls, sit backs)

It is important to mention the psoas paradox. According to Janda and Schmidt, the iliopsoas normally flexes the lumbar spine.[43] If, however, the erector spinae are shortened, the psoas will instead support the resultant hyperlordosis. The hyperlordotic spine can be lifted up by the psoas without the effort of the abdominals (i.e., polio). The tighter the erector spinae, the more the psoas paradox is in effect. Thus, if the erectors are tight, it is necessary to stretch them as well as perform a posterior pelvic tilt before attempting trunk curl exercises for the abdominals. Abdominal exercises that are performed with an anterior pelvic tilt or with the feet held down encourage activation of the hip flexors.[44] Such exercises maximize lumbar compressive and shear forces.[44]

UPPER CROSSED SYNDROME

Muscle imbalances affect the neck and upper extremity just as deleteriously as they do the low back and lower extremity.[26,27,45] Janda identified an upper crossed syndrome with typical pairs of tight and weak muscles[12] (Table 18.19).

Knowledge of this pattern is important for neck, shoulder, or upper back conditions related to abnormal sitting, respiration, mastication, and prehension activities. Table 18.20 provides the signs related to various dysfunctions associated with the upper crossed syndrome.

The combined result of this posture is that the cervicocranial, cervicothoracic, glenohumeral, and temporomandibular joints (TMJ) are all overstressed.[3,7,12] Joint dysfunction and trigger points naturally result from these muscle imbalances, associated with headache, neck pain, shoulder blade pain, and TMJ and shoulder disorders.[12,26,27,45,46] Each of the three muscle imbalances that contribute to the upper crossed syndrome are discussed in the context of the key movement pattern that is affected: scapulohumeral rhythm, neck flexion, and trunk lowering from a push-up. Respiration, which is also affected, is discussed as well.

Table 18.19. Upper Crossed Syndrome

Imbalance in the following pairs of muscles:
    Weak lower and middle trapezius and short upper trapezius and levator scapulae
    Weak deep neck flexors and short suboccipitals and sternocleidomastoid
    Weak serratus anterior and short pectoralis major

Table 18.20. Postural Signs of Upper Crossed Syndrome

Postural Finding	Dysfunction
Round shoulders	Shortened pectorals
Forward-drawn head	Kyphotic upper thoracic spine
C0-C1 hyperextension	Shortened suboccipitals
Elevation of shoulders	Shortened upper trapezius and levator scapulae and weak lower and middle trapezius
Winging of scapulae	Weak serratus anterior

Altered Scapulothoracic and Scapulohumeral Rhythm (Table 18.21)[3,7,12,46]

The scapoluhumeral rhythm is important for its relationship to prehension, reaching, grasping, and carrying activities.

Weak agonist: lower and middle trapezius
Overactive synergist: upper trapezius, levator scapulae, and rhomboids

Symptoms (see Figs. 10.6, 10.7, and 10.14)

- Neck pain
- Headaches
- Rotator cuff syndromes (i.e., impingement syndrome)
- Shoulder blade pain

Postural Analysis

- Gothic shoulders (see Fig. 6.25)
- Upward rotation of the scapulae

Gait Analysis:

- Altered arm swing
- Shoulder elevation with arm flexion

Muscle Length Tests

- Shortened upper trapezius and levator scapulae (see Figs. 6.1 and 6.2)

Evaluation of Key Movement Patterns

- Altered scapulohumeral rhythm (scapular fixation) (see Fig. 5.20**c**)
- Paradoxical respiration

Trigger Points

- Upper, middle, and lower trapezius
- Levator scapulae
- Subscapularis
- Mastoid process, C2 and C3 attachment points

Mobility (Joint Dysfunction)

- Upper cervical spine
- Cervicothoracic (C/T) junction

Altered Head/Neck Flexion (Table 18.22)[3,7,12,26,27,45]

Head/neck flexion is important for its relationship to standing or sitting posture and mastication.

Weak agonist: deep neck flexors
Overactive antagonist: suboccipitals
Overactive synergist: sternocleidomastoid (SCM)

Symptoms (see Figs. 18.29 and 18.31)

- Headache
- Neck and shoulder blade pain
- TMJ

Postural Analysis

- Head-forward posture (see Fig. 18.32)
- Prominence of SCM (see Fig. 6.4)

Muscle Length Tests

- Shortened SCM (see Fig. 18.33)
- Shortened suboccipitals

Table 18.21. Treatment Approach for Altered Scapulohumeral Rhythm

Facilitate/strengthen lower and middle trapezius
Relax/stretch upper trapezius and levator scapulae
Relax/stretch subscapularis
Adjust/mobilize cervicothoracic junction and sternoclavicular joint
Breathing correction and ergonomic advice

Table 18.22. Treatment Approach for Altered Neck Flexion

Relax/stretch sternocleidomastoid
Relax/stretch suboccipitals
Adjust/mobilize C0-C1 and cervicothoracic junction
Facilitate/strengthen deep neck flexors
Correct poor sitting posture
Lumbopelvic stabilization exercises

Evaluation of Key Movement Patterns

- Altered coordination during neck flexion (see Fig. 18.34)

Trigger Points

- SCM
- Suboccipitals
- Middle trapezius
- Masticatory muscles
- Mastoid process

Mobility (Joint Dysfunction)

- C0-C1 and C/T junction
- Lower cervical spine
- TMJ

Altered Scapular Fixation during Trunk Lowering from a Push-up (Table 18.23)[3,7,12,45]

Scapular fixation is important for carrying, pushing, and pulling activities.

Weak agonist: serratus anterior
Overactive antagonist: rhomboids
Overactive synergist: upper trapezius, levator scapulae, and pectoralis major, minor

Symptoms

- Neck and shoulder blade pain
- Rotator cuff syndromes
- Cervicobrachial syndrome

Postural Analysis

- Round shoulders (see Fig. 10.20)
- Winged scapulae (see Fig. 6.24)

Table 18.23. Treatment Approach for Altered Trunk Lowering from a Push-Up

Facilitate/strengthen serratus anterior
Relax/stretch pectoralis major and minor
Relax/stretch upper trapezius
Adjust/mobilize upper thoracic spine
Postural re-education

Gait Analysis

- Winged scapulae with arm movement

Muscle Length Tests

- Shortened pectoralis major (see Fig. 6.3)
- Shortened upper trapezius and levator scapulae (see Figs. 6.1 and 6.2)

Evaluation of Key Movement Patterns

- Altered scapular fixation during trunk lowering from a push-up (see Fig. 6.19)

Trigger Points

- Pectoralis major
- Upper trapezius
- Levator scapulae
- Pectoralis minor

Mobility (Joint Dysfunction)

- Decreased upper thoracic spine extension

Respiration (Abnormal or Paradoxical Respiration) (Table 18.24)

Agonist: diaphragm
Overactive synergist: scalenes, intercostals, upper trapezius

Symptoms (see Figs. 10.6 and 10.8)

- Neck pain and headaches
- Chest wall pain
- Thoracic outlet syndrome

Postural Analysis

- Round shoulders
- Forward-drawn head
- Thoracic kyphosis

Evaluation of Key Movement Patterns

- Paradoxical breathing (chest breathing predominates over abdominal breathing)

Trigger Points

- Scalenes

Mobility (Joint Dysfunction)

- Decreased lateral bending and extension of lower cervical spine
- Decreased lateral excursion of the rib cage

Table 18.24. Treatment Approach for Altered Respiration

Relax/stretch scalenes
Relax/stretch upper trapezius
Facilitate/train diaphragmatic breathing
Adjust/mobilize lower cervicals and thoracic spine
Postural re-education

CLINICAL APPLICATION OF REHABILITATION PROCEDURES

Differential Diagnosis of Myofascial Trigger Points and Joint Dysfunction

It is clear that muscle and joint dysfunction are intertwined. If you take the view that muscles are responsible for reflex compensations to joint or disk stress, then everything possible should be done to reduce joint stress before addressing trigger points. In general, trigger points require little direct treatment (needling, ischemic compression) if joints are treated first. Often, however the muscle imbalances must be addressed to prevent joint stress. The proof of the success of the therapeutic intervention is disappearance of the jump sign on post-treatment checks.

It is still important to be able to differentially diagnose myofascial from articular sources of palpable tenderness. Bogduk and Simons discussed this issue.[47] *Trigger points satisfy the following criteria:* (1) a palpable band with a local twitch response (+ jump sign); (2) reproduction of pain on palpation of the trigger point; and (3) relief with trigger point therapy. *If a joint is considered the source of pain, the following criteria apply:* (1) abnormal passive movement, especially of end-feel; (2) reproduction of pain when moving the joint; and (3) relief with joint anesthesia or manipulation. It is not possible to differentiate between joint and muscle sources on the basis of the location of the pain. Both muscles and joints can cause local or referred pain.

Myofascial Pain Syndromes

If an active trigger point (TP) is found (taut band, twitch response, + jump sign, referred pain to target area), the approach is as follows[6,48]:

1. Assess for muscular imbalance
2. Assess for joint dysfunction
3. Identify work or lifestyle factors
4. Aim treatment at restoring muscle balance and remediating joint dysfunction
5. If treatment fails to eliminate TP use
   - Ischemic compression (5 to 10 seconds of sufficient pressure to recreate referred pain)
   - Postisometric relaxation
   - Nutritional or metabolic factors may also undermine success
   - Rule out fibromyalgia and corticalization of pain (see Chapter 2)

Facet and Sacroiliac Syndromes

Many of low back disorders of the 80% presently labeled nonspecific are undoubtedly related to problems of the facet or SI joints. The SI syndrome is present in 10 to 30% of patients with chronic low back pain.[15] Unfortunately, anesthetic blocking technique is the only known way to make the diagnosis, and it has not been correlated with any physical tests. Similarly, zygapophyseal joints have been proven to be responsible for low back pain in at least 15% of patients, al-

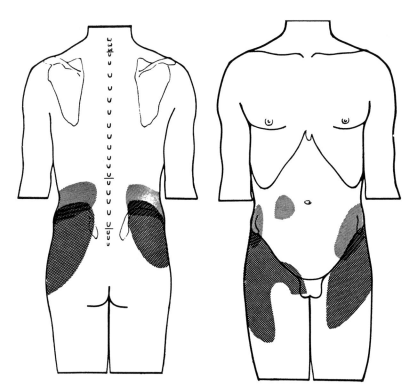

Fig. 18.1. Facet pain. (From McCall IW, Park WM, O'Brien JP: Induced pain referral from posterior lumbar elements in normal subjects. Spine 4:441, 1979.)

though no physical signs have been correlated with anesthetic relief of pain.[17,18]

Two goals when constructing an appropriate rehabilitation program for a patient with pain are as follows: (1) to reduce stress at that tissue site, and (2) to improve the ability of that tissue to handle stress. Facet syndromes are likely to correlate with pathokinesiology involving altered hip extension and trunk flexion. Improper loading in the sagittal plane, especially in a hyperlordotic individual, would be the probable pathomechanics of a facet syndrome. Predictable functional pathologies affect the hamstrings, hip flexors, and erector spinae (tightness), erector spinae (poor endurance), gluteus maximus, rectus abdominus (weakness), hip joints (hypomobile), and lumbar spine (hypermobile). Pain provocation of the hypermobile joints and trigger points (in both the tight and weak muscles) will be present. Typical findings include a forward-drawn posture (weak glutei and tight hip flexors) and increased lumbar lordosis (tight erector spinae and hip flexors with weak abdominals and glutei).

Altered hip extension synergy leads to overstress of the lumbar facets because of load transference from the stiff hip joint to the hypermobile lumbar spine. Extension of the thigh occurs through a fulcrum involving the lumbar spine rather than the hip joint. Thus, the lumbar extensor muscles, in particular the superficial erector spinae group, become overactive during hip extension motions, such as gait, standing from a chair, climbing, and jumping.

Pain referral can be expected from lumbar facet and erector spinae trigger point sources (Figs. 18.1 and 18.2). A forward drawn posture (see Fig. 18.3) and erector spinae hypertrophy (Fig. 18.4), as well as tightness of the hip flexors,

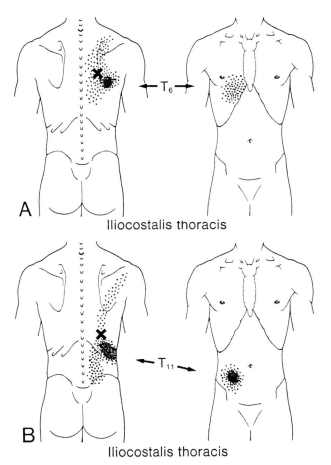

Fig. 18.2. Erector spinae trigger points. (From Travell JG, Simons DG: Myofascial Pain and Dysfunction: The Trigger Point Manual. Vol. 1. Baltimore, Williams & Wilkins, 1983.)

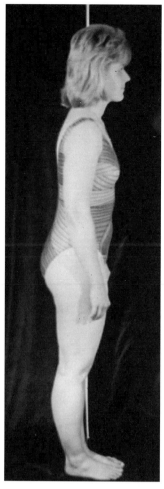

Fig. 18.3. Forward-drawn posture.

hamstrings, and erector spinae may be present (Figs. 18.5 to 18.7). Trunk extension should be tested for lack of endurance (Fig. 18.8). The hip extension movement pattern may be altered with overactivity of the erector spinae and hamstrings coupled with inhibition of the gluteus maximus (Fig. 18.9).

Rehabilitation management includes advice, manipulation, and exercise (see Table 18.7). For a typical facet syndrome, simple advice includes the following:

- Instruction about overhead activities and carrying (avoid lumbar hyperextension by performing a posterior pelvic tilt (Fig. 18.10)
- Instruction about the use of a foot stool during typical activities of daily living (Fig. 18.11)
- Avoidance of the tendency to hyperextend the back during many common health club exercises, such as the stairclimber, sit-ups, standing hip machine, lateral pull-down, step aerobics, hamstring curls, and others (Fig. 18.12)

Manipulation (i.e., adjustments, mobilization, manual resistance techniques) may address any of the following functional pathologies if present:

- CMT lumbar spine
- Mobilize hip (Fig. 18.13)
- Mobilize fibular head (Fig. 18.14)
- Relax/stretch involved hip flexors (Figs. 18.15 and 18.16)

- Relax/stretch involved erector spinae (Fig. 18.17)
- Relax/stretch involved hamstrings (Fig. 18.18)

The key is to find a specific manipulable lesion which reduces pain provocation (tender point or movement) and/or facilitates the "weak link" (gluteus maximus).

Exercises for improving strength, endurance, and flexibility should also be considered:

- Self-stretch for tight iliopsoas (Fig. 18.19)
- Self-stretch for tight erector spinae (Fig. 18.20)
- Self-stretch for tight hamstrings (Fig. 18.21)
- Strengthen gluteus maximus (Figs. 18.22 to 18.25)
- Squats and lunges (Figs. 18.26 and 18.27)
- Endurance exercise for trunk extension (Fig. 18.28)

Pathokinesiology involving altered trunk flexion also overstresses the L5/S1 joints because of poor lumbopelvic stabilization. Trunk stabilization through improved co-contraction of abdominals and gluteals is essential to prevent further lumbar overstrain.

The SI syndromes are intertwined with altered hip abduction. Weakness/inhibition of the gluteus medius will result in increased lateral shear forces across the pelvis. Often, overactivity or shortening of the adductors adds torsion to the pelvis through the pubic bones, which aggravates an SI joint problem. The gluteus medius insufficiency is also often combined with piriformis overactivity, which also causes rotation of the pelvis and adds to the SI woes. The QL may substitute for gluteus medius weakness with excessive hip hiking, and, along with concomitant lumbar problems, will refer pain into the SI joint from its trigger points.

It is always best to look for dysfunction in the feet when the gluteus medius is weak or inhibited. Hyperpronation is the most common problem and with it come many manipulable

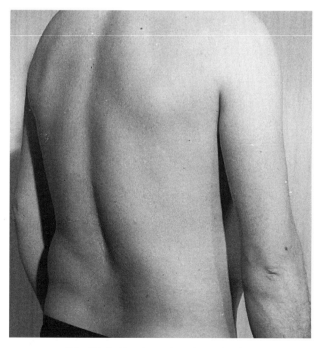

Fig. 18.4. Erector spinae hypertrophy.

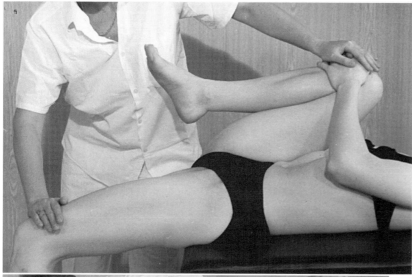

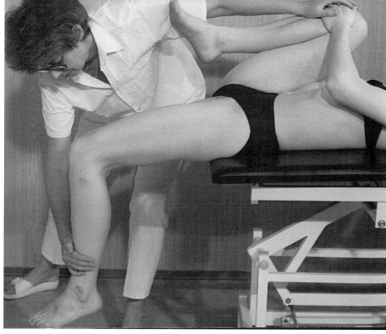

Fig. 18.5. Test for shortened hip flexors.

lesions in the talocalcaneonavicular region. Evaluation of the lower extremity kinetic chain is essential to solving the riddle of many SI and facet syndromes.

Disk Syndromes

Regardless of the cause of a clinically significant disk syndrome, the start of rehabilitation must wait until conservative care has succeeded in reducing the irritability or compression of the nerve root. As soon as nerve tension signs decrease, exercise is highly beneficial (Table 18.25).

Advice to avoid positions of increased intradiscal pressure, such as sitting, are important in the early stages (Fig. 10.18). Patients should also learn to avoid any bending or twisting movements to which the disk is particularly vulnerable (Fig. 10.5). Manipulation to improve joint

function and reduce pathokinesiology acts as a catalyst for reducing nerve root compression. Care should be taken to emphasize extension motion of the three-joint complex. McKenzie techniques have been shown to quickly

Table 18.25. Disk Protocol

Conservative care until nerve tension signs disappear
Nonweight-bearing exercise
   Aerobic exercise
   Spinal extension mobility
   Quadriceps strength/endurance
Traction assistance nonweight-bearing exercise
   Isometric trunk stabilization
Quadruped, kneeling, ball, standing stabilization exercises
Address muscular imbalances
   Seated exercises

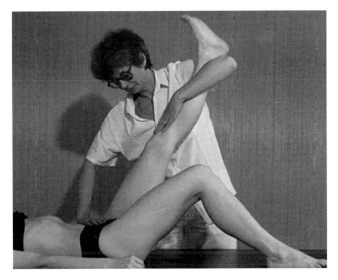

Fig. 18.6. Test for shortened hamstrings.

centralize symptoms related to nerve root compression (see Chapter 12).

Headache

The variety of types of headache includes cervical, myofascial, nutritional, vascular (migraine), other (cluster). The cervical and myofascial headaches are amenable to chiropractic and rehabilitation. Most headache sufferers have chronic or recurrent symptoms and thus rehabilitation should be included in the chiropractic care of any headache patient, regardless of the degree of cervical or myofascial involvement. As mentioned previously, Watson and Trott demonstrated that muscle imbalances in the neck can distinguish between chronic headache and non-headache sufferers.[26] Treleaven and Jull showed that the same muscle imbalances occur sig-

nificantly more often in postconcussional headache patients than in normal individuals.[27]

Patients who experience more severe headaches (usually women), occasional migraine sufferers, and those with forehead and eye pain often have weakness of their deep neck flexors and loss of lower cervical extension. Such findings certainly help us give affected patients a realistic goal. Results are often not immediate, but as head and neck flexion coordination and lower cervical extension mobility improve, the headaches will likely decrease. Any patient can clearly see the connection between not being able to hold their head up against gravity with their head flexing too far forward and the development of intractable headaches. This information is better received than the suggestion that adjustments alone will do the job, or worse, as stated by many neurologists (after brain scans and the like), that there is nothing wrong except stress (the pat diagnosis of a psychogenic disorder to explain typical symptoms of functional pathology of the motor system!).

From a rehabilitation perspective, headache syndromes are likely to correlate with pathokinesiology involving altered neck flexion and scapulohumeral rhythm. Predictable functional pathologies affect the SCM, suboccipitals, upper trapezius, levator scapulae, and pectorals (tightness), deep neck flexors, lower and middle trapezius, and serratus anterior (weakness), cervicothoracic junction (hypomobile), and C4-C5 joint (hypermobile). Pain provocation of the hypermobile joints and trigger points (in both the tight and weak muscles) is present. Typical findings include a slumped, head-forward posture (weak lower fixators of the scapulae and tight pectorals) and increased cervicocranial hyperextension (tight suboccipitals and SCM with weak deep neck flexors).

Altered neck flexion synergy leads to overstress of the cervicocranial junction because of the anterior carriage of the head. Also, the middle to lower cervical region (C4-5 and

Fig. 18.7. Test for shortened erector spinae.

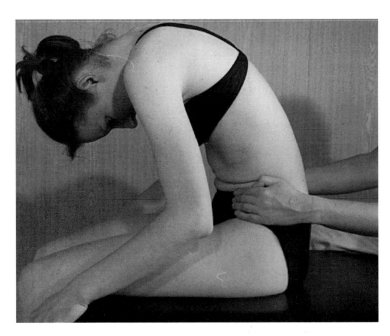

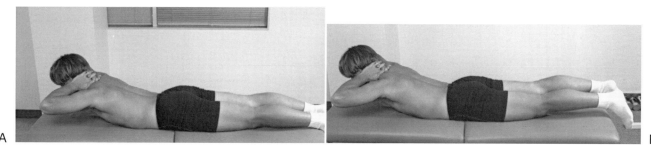

Fig. 18.8. Test for trunk extensor endurance.

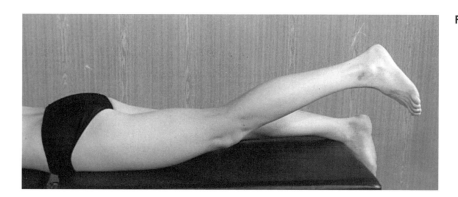

Fig. 18.9. Hip hyperextension test.

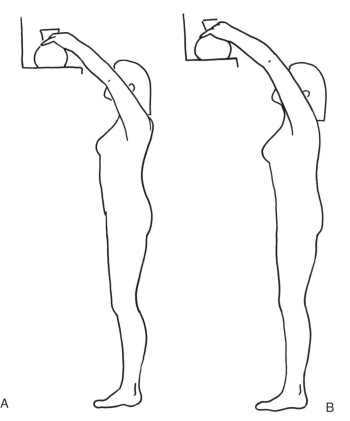

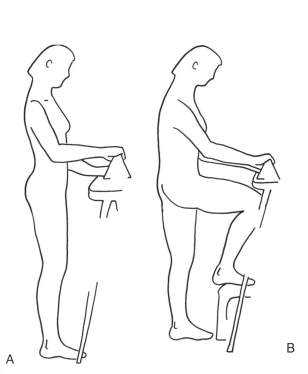

Fig. 18.10. a, Incorrect overhead reaching with back hyperextended. **b,** Correct overhead reaching with posterior pelvic tilt.

Fig. 18.11. a, Typical ironing position. **b,** Use of a foot stool to reduce lumbar lordosis.

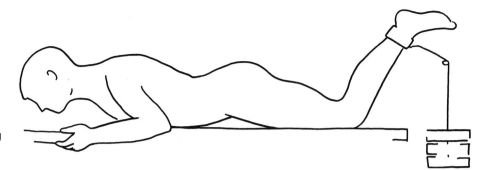

Fig. 18.12. Harmful hamstring exercise.

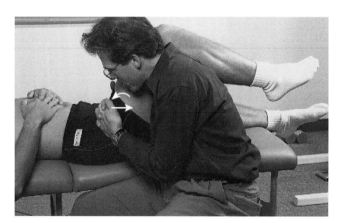

Fig. 18.13. Post-isometric mobilization of hip joint.

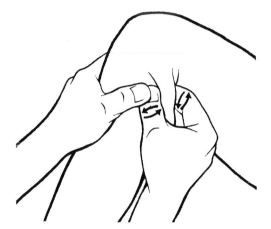

Fig. 18.14. Mobilize fibular head.

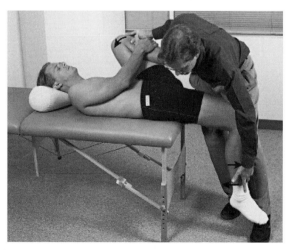

Fig. 18.15. Post-isometric relaxation rectus femoris.

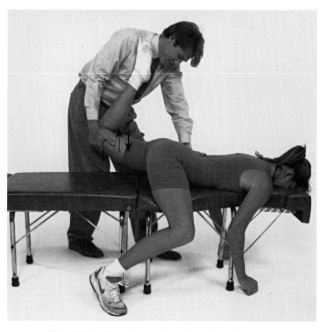

Fig. 18.16. Post-isometric relaxation iliopsoas.

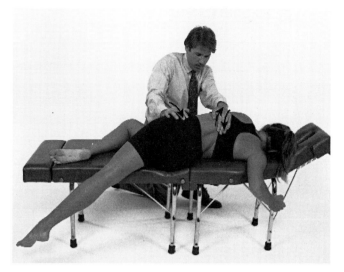

Fig. 18.17. Post-isometric relaxation erector spinae.

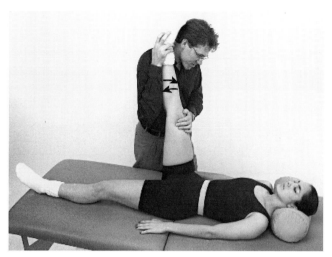

Fig. 18.18. Post-isometric relaxation hamstrings.

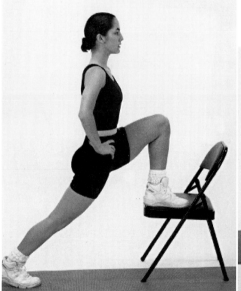

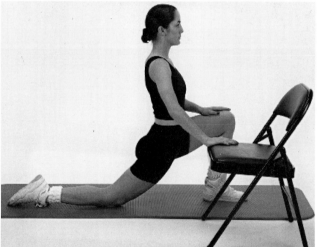

Fig. 18.19. Self-stretch for tight iliopsoas.

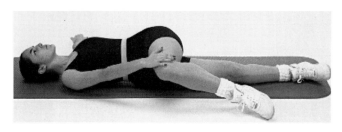

Fig. 18.20. Self-stretch for tight erector spinae.

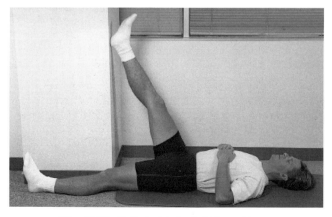

Fig. 18.21. Self-stretch for tight hamstrings.

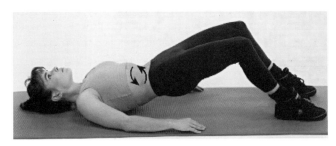

Fig. 18.22. Basic bridge.

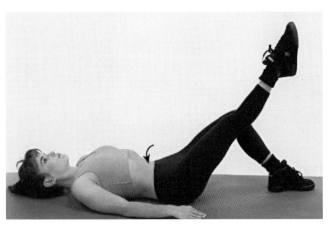

Fig. 18.23. One-leg bridge ("dips").

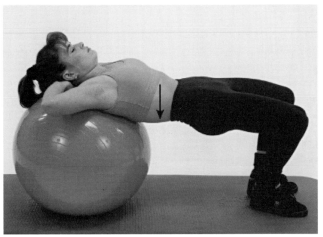

Fig. 18.24. Bridge on the ball.

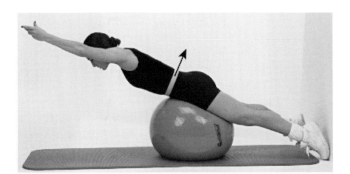

Fig. 18.25. Superman.

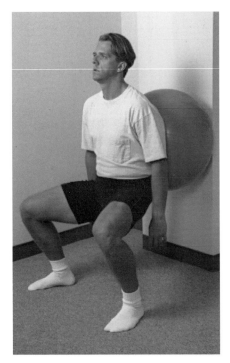

Fig. 18.26. Squat.

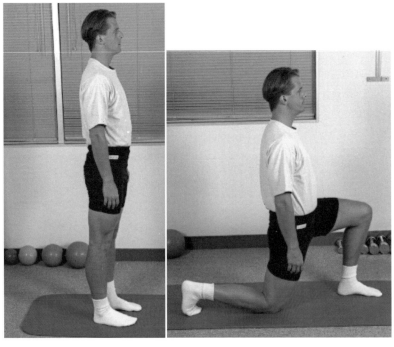

Fig. 18.27. Lunge.

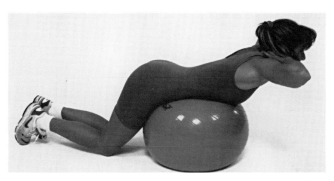

Fig. 18.28. Back extensor exercise.

C5-6) is affected by the flattening of the lower cervical curve and resultant biomechanical change in the spinal stability of the cervical spine. Patients experience typical pain referral from trigger points in the SCM and suboccipitals (Figs. 18.29 and 18.30). Joint sources of referred pain may also overlap with common referred pain patterns from muscles (Fig. 18.31).[47] Some patients may have a head-forward posture and prominence of the SCM (Figs. 18.32 and 18.33), as well as tightness of the suboccipitals, pectorals, upper trapezius, and levator scapulae (see Chapter 6). The neck flexion movement pattern may be altered (Fig. 18.34).

Rehabilitation management includes advice, manipulation, and exercise (see Table 18.7). For a typical headache syndrome, the patient is advised to: use a headset if on the telephone for prolonged periods, make available an ergonomic computer workstation (see Table 10.2), and correct poor sitting posture (Fig. 18.35).

Manipulation (adjustments, mobilization, manual resistance techniques) involve the following potential functional pathologies:

- CMT cervicocranial and cervicothoracic junctions
- Relax/stretch SCM (Fig. 18.36)
- Relax/stretch suboccipitals (Fig. 18.37)
- Manual traction cervical spine (Fig. 18.38)

- Facilitate/strengthen lower and middle trapezius (Figs. 18.39 to 18.42)

Remember, it is time saving to find the "key link" which if manipulated can affect improvement in provocative tests of the inhibited muscle (deep neck flexors).

The following exercises are recommended to improve posture and promote strength, endurance, and flexibility:

- Postural exercise for the deep neck flexors (Fig. 18.43)
- Strength/endurance exercise for deep neck flexors and lower scapulae stabilizers (Fig. 18.44)
- Strengthen lower and middle trapezius (Fig. 18.45)
- Lumbopelvic stabilization exercises (Figs. 18.46 to 18.48)
- Upper back cat (Fig. 18.49)
- Upper thoracic spine extension stretch (Fig. 18.50)

When the scapulohumeral rhythm (SHR) is abnormal, any reaching or grasping movement can trigger a headache. Prolonged static overstrain from keyboard or writing work is also a common culprit. Muscular imbalance involving overactivity of the upper trapezius and levator scapulae and inhibited lower and middle trapezius are usually responsible. Upper cervical and cranial attachments for the upper trapezius and levator scapulae can become hypersensitive and their joints become hypermobile. These headache patients sense most of their pain in the back of the head, but occasionally they describe pain over the eyes.

Advice about an ergonomic workstation helps immeasurably to improve SHR. One intervention involves the use of arm rests, which allow the arm to rest in a relaxed position. Secondly, the writing surface, typewriter, or keyboard should be at a height at which the wrists function in their neutral range, the elbow is flexed 90°, and the shoulder girdle is relaxed (see Table 10.2). Manipulation should focus on relaxing the upper trapezius and levator scapulae. Specific joints in the cervicocranial or cervicothoracic areas may need adjustment. Exercises to strengthen the lower fixators of the scapulae are necessary to avoid further overactivity in the elevators of the shoulder girdle.

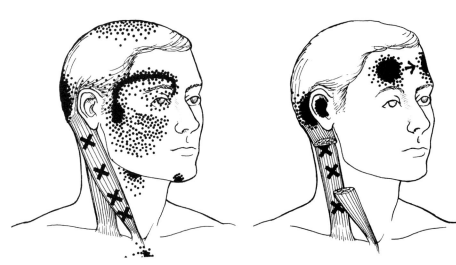

Fig. 18.29. Sternocleidomastoid trigger points. (From Travell JG, Simons DG: Myofascial Pain and Dysfunction: The Trigger Point Manual. Vol. 1. Baltimore, Williams & Wilkins, 1983.)

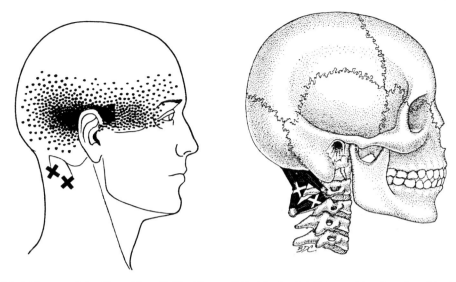

Fig. 18.30. Suboccipital trigger points. (From Travell JG, Simons DG: Myofascial Pain and Dysfunction: The Trigger Point Manual. Vol. 1. Baltimore, Williams & Wilkins, 1983.)

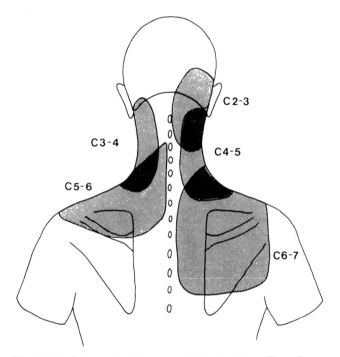

Fig. 18.31. Referred pain from cervical spine joints. (From Dwyer A, April C, Boyduk N: Cervical zygapophyseal joint pain patterns: A study in normal volunteers. Spine 15:453, 1990.)

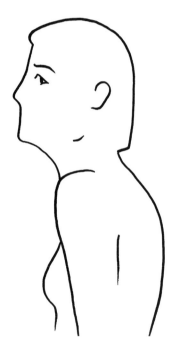

Fig. 18.32. Head forward posture.

Abnormal respiration should also be evaluated in all headache patients. Those patients with weakness of the deep neck flexors and upper thoracic kyphosis may have an aggravation of their pain if we adjust their necks too aggressively or too frequently. As the upper thoracic spine extends more (and the lumbopelvic junction stabilizes), neck adjustments will be more successful.

Thoracic Outlet and Cervicobrachial Syndromes

Shoulder blade pain, chest pain, cervicobrachial syndromes, and headaches can all come from a forward-drawn head and

downward shift of the cervicothoracic junction.[49,50] According to Janda, the cervicothoracic junction can move as low as T3/T4. This positioning is not biomechanically sound, and certainly is unattractive.

Unfortunately, such posture certainly can lead to the thoracic outlet syndrome (TOS) from scalene anticus or pectoralis minor entrapment, easily verified by the AER (abduction, external rotation) test of Roos.[51,52] Many "authorities" say TOS is an example of a psychogenic disorder, yet the dysthesia is so predictably on the pinky and not the thumb side, and is reliably reproduced by the AER test. Indeed, its origin is neurogenic and not vascular or psychogenic.

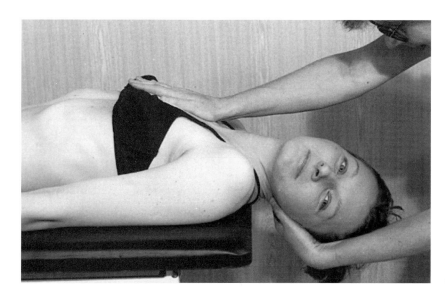

Fig. 18.33. Screening test for sterno-cleidomastoid.

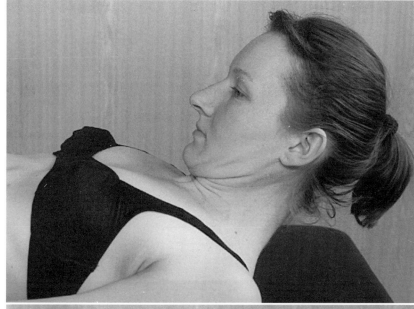

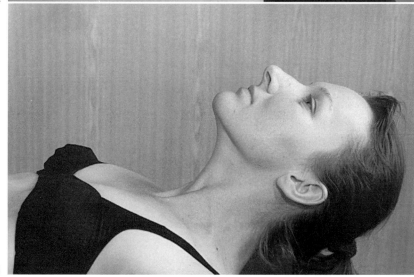

Fig. 18.34. Altered coordination during neck flexion.

A

B

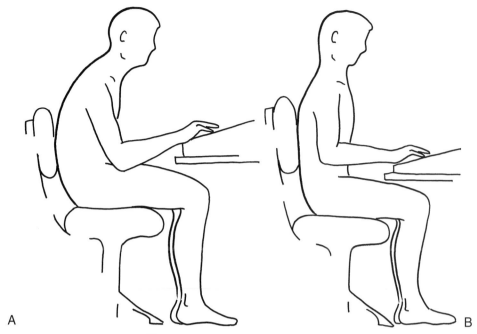

Fig. 18.35. Correct poor sitting posture.

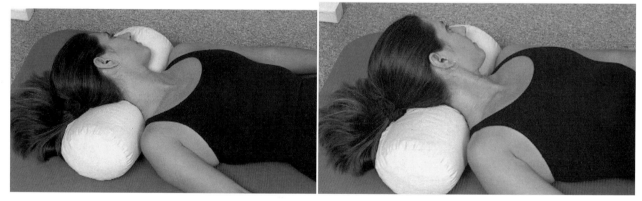

Fig. 18.36. Post-isometric relaxation sternocleidomastoid.

Advice would include avoiding slumping, especially when sitting. Manipulative treatment may start with the pectoralis minor and scalenes, but progresses often to include middle and lower trapezius facilitation. Exercises to improve posture, strengthen the lower fixators of the scapulae, stretch the pectorals and hip flexors, and stabilize the lumbopelvic region may be necessary. Improved respiration, head/neck flexion coordination, and lower cervical extension mobility are also essential. Overly eager neck adjusting may aggravate the complaint, especially if the patient has a cervical rib or weak deep neck flexors. The soundest principle to follow in TOS involves stabilizing the base of the spine and improving the mobility of the upper thoracic spine.

Cervical Acceleration-Deceleration Syndrome

Patients who have suffered motor vehicle accidents automatically must be considered differently from those with other neck or back complaints. Trauma involves inflammation, and as such, treatment follows a slower course.[6] Rehabilitation cannot begin until the "chemical" signs of inflammation decline and the pain becomes more "mechanical" (see Tables 2.15 and 2.16). The use of physical agents (ultrasound, electrical muscle stimulation, heat, ice, etc.) may be required until completion of the inflammatory phase of soft tissue healing.

Both muscles and joints have been identified as sources of chronic pain after whiplash injury or concussion.[16,27] From 50 to 70% of patients with chronic neck pain have been shown to have posterior zygapophyseal joint syndrome.[16] Typical muscle imbalances involving weakness of deep neck flexors and tightness of the suboccipitals have been identified in postconcussional headache patients.[27]

In patients who are victims of trauma, it is important to be alert to psychosocial problems that could interfere with a full recovery.[53] A biobehavioral approach is a must.

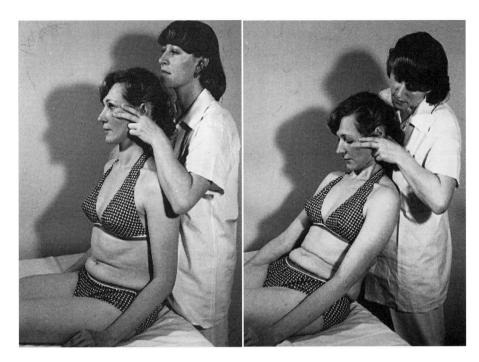

Fig. 18.37. Post-isometric relaxation suboccipitals.

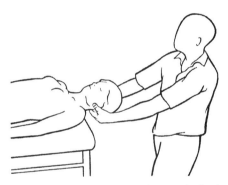

Fig. 18.38. Post-isometric traction cervical spine.

Overemphasis of the use of passive means (physical agents) to treat pain and promote soft tissue healing promote illness behavior, especially patient dependency. A rehabilitation approach should begin as soon as mechanical symptoms predominate over chemical signs of inflammation (radicular complaint subsides and relief positions other than rest are present). The goal of patient education and advice is to reassure the patient about their overall positive prognosis and the benefits and safety of early mobilization and activity.

When the inflammatory phase is subsiding, within 1 week in cases of mild to moderate trauma (see Tables 18.26 and 2.20), active rehabilitation may proceed. Manipulation may start with gentle muscle relaxation and joint traction or mobilization procedures. Typical functional pathologies targeted include overactivity of scalenes, SCM, upper trapezius, levator scapulae, suboccipitals, and the pectorals. Early rehabilitation efforts should be directed toward preventing the "programming" of any of these typical muscle imbalances. Gentle PIR (no stretching) to the overactive muscles helps in this regard. Gentle mobilization, adhering to McKenzie princi-

ples of pain centralization, aids in restoring the cervical lordosis.

Early exercises may address the gluteal/abdominal muscles to help maintain the integrity of lumbopelvic junction. Stability in this region is crucial because poor trunk stability or a forward weight-bearing position inevitably leads to cervical overstress. Calf stretching and dorsal extension flexibility exercises (cats, doorway, ball stretches) and strengthening exercises (back extension on the ball, supermans) also are tolerated well in the subacute stage, and should reduce cervical overstress.

For patients in whom excessive muscular guarding is maintained for more than 2 to 3 weeks, regaining lower cervical extension becomes a key to improving overall function. Adjustments, joint mobilization, and gentle stretching techniques are important in such cases.

The question of resistance exercises to the neck is an important one. Physical therapists have advocated that the patient apply isometric resistance to the neck. Recently, chiropractors have begun to incorporate resistance exercises to the neck (i.e., MedX or Neck Sys programs). Because of the inherent instability of the neck, such exercises should not be undertaken unless the patient is clearly out of the acute, inflammatory phase; has no peripheralization of symptoms; is performing movements that minimize joint compression (avoid uncoupled movements like side bending with contralateral rotation); and has no aggravation of local pain. Movement patterns described by Janda should be assessed before the start of any resistance training, and post-treatment checks should confirm that incoordinated movement patterns have not worsened as a result of overaggressive neck exercises. Pre- and post-treatment checks of trigger points should also adjudicate the merits of these exercises by clearly showing that soft tissue tenderness is decreasing as a result of the training.

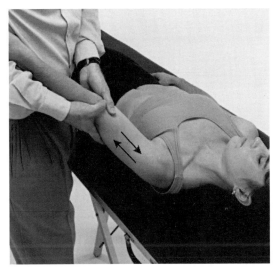

Fig. 18.39. Facilitation of the lower fixators of the scapulae.

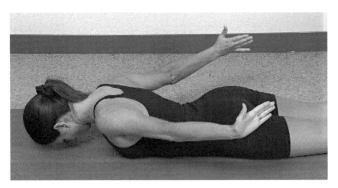

Fig. 18.40. Facilitation of the middle trapezius.

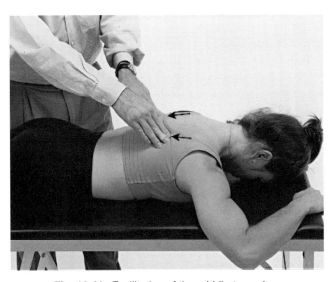

Fig. 18.41. Facilitation of the middle trapezius.

Fig. 18.42. Facilitation of the lower and middle trapezius.

Rotator Cuff (Impingement) Syndrome

Impingement syndromes in the shoulder represent one of the more intriguing rehabilitation problems. The shoulder girdle functions as part of a kinetic chain linking the neck to the hand. Many muscles in this region attach to the cervical spine and thorax; thus, addressing the shoulder is crucial to many spinal disorders. The shoulder is an inherently unstable joint—a large ball and a small socket—in contrast to the hip, which has many related joints and muscles that act in concert to allow a wide variety of movements. When we speak about the shoulder we should begin by discussing the scapulo-humeral rhythm (SHR). Especially in cases of impingement, in contrast to instability, the SHR is the most important functional phenomena related to clinical problems in the shoulder.[46] It relates to the movements of flexion, abduction, and "scaption" (scapular plane abduction).

The SHR is the pattern of joint and muscular activity occurring during shoulder abduction and flexion. Its purpose is to keep the glenoid fossa in a biomechanically optimal position to receive the humeral head. If the arm in internally rotated (impingement test), abduction will be limited by the greater tubercle striking the acromion process and cora-coacromial ligament. Total abduction is 180°. The gleno-humeral contribution is 120° and the scapulothoracic contribution is 60°. Thus, there are two degrees of glenohumeral motion for every one degree of scapulothoracic motion. In the first 30° to 60°—the setting phase—virtually all movement is glenohumeral. After that phase, abduction occurs roughly equally between the two functional joints. Two other joints also participate in this symphony of motion, namely, the sternoclavicular and acromioclavicular joints.

As the arm moves into abduction, the scapula rotates upwardly (inferior/medial border moves laterally) to position

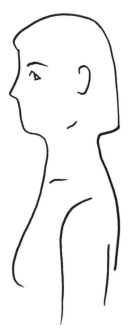

Fig. 18.43. Proper postural set of head and neck.

the glenoid fossa at the proper angle to receive the humeral head. The serratus anterior, upper trapezius, and lower trapezius help to achieve this movement. Downward rotation is promoted by the rhomboid major and levator scapulae. For the prime abductors of the shoulder—the deltoid and supraspinatus—to operate near capacity, the trapezius and serratus anterior must act synergistically. The upward rotation of the scapulae allows the deltoid and supraspinatus to keep a proper length-tension relationship, so they do not lose their strength.

Excessive elevation of the shoulder girdle caused by too much upper trapezius, levator scapulae, and rhomboid activity, along with too little lower trapezius and latissimus dorsi activity, causes impingement.

The rehabilitation of shoulder disorders is complex but rewarding because of the variety of muscles and joints interacting in a far from straightforward manner. Much more is involved than just strengthening the rotator cuff muscles in the manner laid out by orthopedists and their physical therapists (in fact, the famous "empty can" internal rotation scaption exercise is contraindicated). The key to success is focusing on the SHR, as well as joint mobilization and muscle relaxation and training. Muscle stretching aimed at improving shoulder external rotation (infraspinatus, pectoralis major and minor) often facilitates the rehabilitation. The role of a tight subscapularis (internal rotator) is still important, but typically this problem is of greater concern when assessing the stubborn "frozen shoulder."

Two new developments in shoulder rehabilitation are worth noting. The first is the inclusion of propriosensory exercises for this non-weight-bearing joint.[46,54] Wall pushes may be lead to exercises on all fours. The practitioner should watch for proper scapular fixation. Patients may then progress to tripod positioning and, eventually, the hand may be placed on a balance board or other labile surface.

The second development is the use of medicine balls and a rebounder to plyometrically train the shoulder girdle.[54] Throwing and catching is a simple, fun activity that can be varied to reintegrate the muscles into a coordinated, stable functioning. The main advantage is that eccentric and concentric actions are combined in this powerful approach.

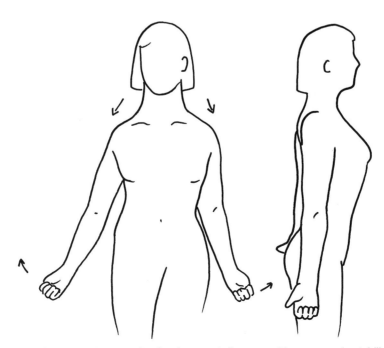

Fig. 18.44. Strengthening exercise for deep neck flexors and lower scapula stabilizers.

Hand weights and cables are mainstays for shoulder training. Exercise tubing, available in a variety of resistances, is also an inexpensive, simple training tool for home use.

Extensor Mechanism Disorders of the Knee

Knee disorders such as quadriceps (runner's knee) or patellar (jumper's knee) tendinitis are common and eventually wind up in the surgeon's parlor. Most tracking disorders are commonly thought to result from an imbalance between the quadriceps and the hamstrings. Most likely, they also may be attributed to lateral tracking of the patella caused by an overactive TFL substituting for a weak gluteus medius. Common muscular problems associated with knee problems include

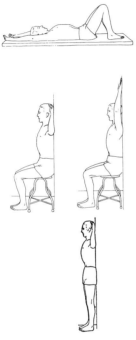

Fig. 18.45. Home exercise for middle and lower trapezius.

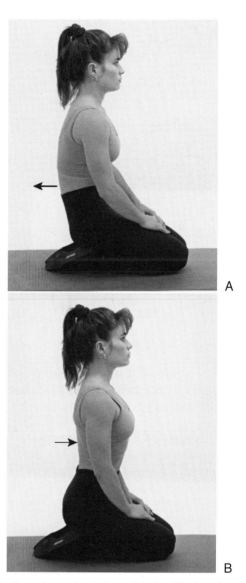

Fig. 18.46. Posterior and anterior pelvic tilt while kneeling (buttocks on heels).

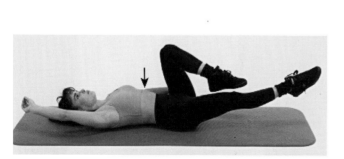

Fig. 18.47. "Dead bug."

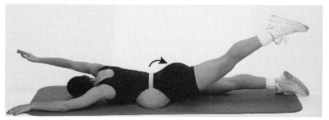

Fig. 18.48. Quadraped opposite arm and leg raise.

tightness of the TFL, hip flexors, gastrosoleus, hamstrings, adductors, and piriformis,[55] and weakness of the hamstrings and gluteus medius. Propriosensory and other biomechanical faults from the feet are also problematic. Lumbar spine, as well as SI, talocrural, and hip joint dysfunctions must also be addressed.

If the gluteus medius is weak, the TFL will only become tighter. Before an iliotibial band friction syndrome develops, knee pain can occur. Rest, ice, and the use of nonsteroidal anti-inflammatory agents are not the solution. Along with looking to the feet, assessing the gluteus medius for lower limb control during one-leg weight bearing is essential (the

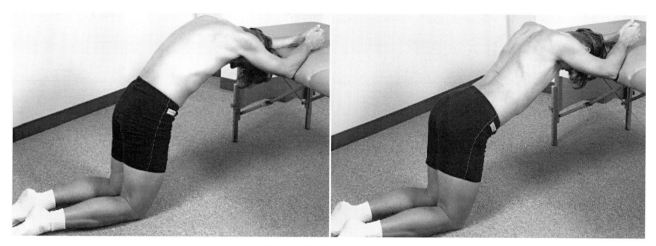

Fig. 18.49. Upper back cat.

hip abduction test is an easy screen). The key is not to wait until cartilage or meniscus damage occurs or for the surgeon to practice their lateral release procedure.

Limited range squats and lunges can be attempted. If the tracking does not allow this movement to occur painlessly, several steps are recommended that obviate retreating to open chain exercises.[56] Stretch out the tight muscles, start propriosensory balance training, and facilitate the gluteus medius. Then, return to squats and lunges and gradually increase the depth of knee flexion. The training or functional range should quickly expand.

Dizziness and Balance Disorders

The motor system depends on appropriate input from somatosensory, vestibular, and visual peripheral afferent systems.[57,58] Without one of these systems, such as in blindness, balance and equilibrium are not sacrificed. In the event of a conflict between two of the systems, however, a problem will ensue. Classic examples are the nausea that develops on a boat when the vestibule notes the motion but the feet and eyes do not, or when lying on the grass on a breezy day with big, puffy clouds floating by. The skin and vestibule register no movement while the eyes do. Dizziness or nausea may result from such a sensory conflict. Neck pain or even low back pain can result if such a sensory conflict is maintained.[59] The so-

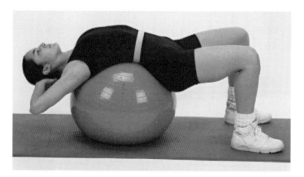

Fig. 18.50. Upper thoracic spine extension stretch.

matosensory afferent system depends on the soles of the feet, the neck, and the lumbar spine for input.

Lewit studied the relationship between cervicocranial joint dysfunction and equilibrium problems.[60] Hautant's test is an essential screening tool for finding the cervical dysfunction and then treating the related muscles or joints. Postwhiplash injury dizziness is most likely cervical in origin as well.[61,62] Gagey developed a systematic way of studying the connection between the postural system and the balance system.[59] Differentiating between primary feet, lumbar, and cervical disorders is crucial.

Vestibular dysfunction is known to be related to poor motor development in children. Children with vestibular deficits cannot stand in a darkened room (you need two of three afferent systems to maintain motor function). Longstanding vestibular exercises for the treatment of dizziness include the use of hammocks and gym balls to help train the labyrinth and tracking exercises for the eyes while the head is moving.

The visual system can be an interesting area involved in dizziness or neck pain. Optokinetic reflexes can be trained (e.g., fighter pilots and figure skaters). Gagey found that a mapping error of visual fields often results in increased tension in the upper trapezius.[59] Following correction with special prismatic lenses, the trigger points dissolve spontaneously.

Brandt found that elderly individuals with ataxia can be treated successfully with balance training.[63] Brandt reported that 2 weeks of training led to significant improvement 9 months later without any home maintenance program. Thick foam is used on the floor to deprive the feet of sensory feedback and the eyes are closed, thus forcing the vestibule and somatosensory systems to train hard. Similarly, it is possible to train the eyes and feet by leaving the eyes open, but tipping the head back (taking the otoliths out of their functioning range).

In different ways, both Lewit and Gagey reported on the relationship between the feet, balance, and vestibular problems.[59,60,64] Lewit also found that correction of a pathologic problem involving the cervical spine plays a role in improving standing postural dysfunctions.[60] Correction involved PIR to the SCM or masticatory muscles or the C0-C1 joint.

ETHICAL OFFICE PROCEDURES

Soap Notes

At the initial examination, be sure to record the presence of any red flags. Then, perform the necessary tests to identify nerve root or inflammatory conditions. Finally, review all potential complicating factors (see Table 18.4). The history, physical examination, and short form questionnaires are all that is needed to identify these complicating factors. The use of expensive pathophysiologic diagnostic testing equipment or seeking special psychologic expertise are unnecessary.

Our SOAP notes for each patient should reflect that our management strategy is rehabilitative rather than traditional. To accomplish this task, the patient's *subjective* complaints are objectified by recording a visual analog scale and a pain diagram every 2 weeks. *Objective* findings are quantified by using functional capacity measurements, which are quantifiable yet inexpensive (see Chapter 5). Even tenderness can be quantified without needing to purchase an algometer. Functional changes and results of provocative tests are noted so that treatment has some basis and progress is noted.

Assessment should indicate the presence of a functional disorder as opposed to a pathoanatomic problem. The treatment *plan* should address functional changes noted in the objective section. Active care procedures should be clearly described so they are not mistaken for passive procedures.

Report Writing

Billing procedures should also reflect the use of active approaches. Therapeutic exercise (97110) and therapeutic activities (97530) are excellent examples. Medicolegal reports should clearly state the positive results of orthopedic or neurologic tests along with findings of functional assessment. It is improper to assume that long-term care is necessary or appropriate for the majority of our "whiplash" patients.[53] Under our care, mild trauma should resolve within the same time frame as would be expected without any treatment (6 weeks). Unless we can demonstrate that a moderate or severe injury is present, it is hard to justify treatment beyond the time of spontaneous symptom resolution.

This statement does not ignore the fact that some patients take longer to get well, nor does it imply that symptomatic relief is the only goal; restoring function is an extremely important goal in rehabilitation. According to the Rand report on spinal manipulation, if a patient is progressing with manipulative intervention, then treatment should not be cut off.[65] This conclusion is in fact an albatross to insurance adjusters. If, however, a patient is not making objective improvement, then manipulative treatment can be cut off after 2 to 4 weeks.[65,66]

Be prepared to document the patient's progress and to defend the assessment with respect to injury severity. The greatest error in the treatment of patients suffering motor vehicle accidents is the assumption of a moderate to severe injury when in fact the injury is only mild to moderate.[53] It is difficult to differentiate between a mild and a moderate injury.[67] Without proper documentation, a mild or mild to moderate injury must be assumed and, with it, the appropriate type and duration of care (Table 18.26).

If an insurance adjuster or attorney questions your service codes, SOAP notes, or necessity for active care, several points can be raised to legally defend your treatments. Standards of care or guidelines have emerged in neuromusculoskeletal medicine, and this political hot potato has not been a welcome sight to many practitioners. Guidelines, however, are an accurate representation of the state of science if not the state of the art. As such, they are not meant to be applied without exceptions, but to serve as guidelines. These guidelines for care have been established as a result of review of scientific evidence and, where evidence is lacking, expert consensus opinion. Many practitioners are surprised to realize just how helpful guidelines can be. In the past, reviewers could stop payment on an insurance claim without good reason. Now, you can defend your practice and quote the guidelines. There are no longer any secrets, which can only work to the advantage of the honest, ethical doctor. Quality assurance is a goal of managed care. Thus, providers practicing to the highest standards will be sought.

The Mercy Center Conference was an example in which such a guideline process occurred.[6] Active care was distinguished from passive care in several ways. First, they addressed stages of treatment and their goals (p. 120):

Passive Care
   1. Acute intervention

Active Care
   1. Remobilization
   2. Rehabilitation
   a. Restoring strength and endurance
   b. Increasing physical work capacity
   3. Lifestyle adaptations

Second, they clearly stated that active care was essential (p 110), "It is beneficial to proceed to rehabilitation phase as rapidly as possible, and to minimize dependency upon passive forms of treatment/care." Again (p 125), "All episodes of symptoms that remain unchanged for 2-3 weeks should be evaluated for risk factors of pending chronicity. Patients at risk for becoming chronic should have treatment plans altered to de-emphasize passive care and refocus on active care approaches."

Table 18.26. Grading Injury Severity[67]

Mild =	Pain on stress of tissue, local tenderness, mild swelling, no gross instability
Moderate =	Pain on stress of tissue, generalized and marked tenderness and swelling, mild laxity, no gross instability
Severe =	Gross instability, generalized swelling, disruption of tissue, sometimes minimal pain

The British Standards Advisory Group for Back Pain similarly stated that active care was a distinct and important type of case management.[2] On page 38, "At present, the main emphasis of physical therapy for back pain is on symptomatic relief of pain, despite evidence that many of the modalities used are ineffective. Symptomatic measures to control pain are required but this should be used to embark on active rehabilitation rather than be seen as an end in itself." They went on to state (p 46) "We recommend. . . . There should be a change of emphasis and redirection of resources from symptomatic treatment, to the provision of active rehabilitation and patient education."

The American guidelines from AHCPR were emphatic in their criticism of physical agents: "Physical modalities such as massage, diathermy, ultrasound, biofeedback, and transcutaneous electrical nerve stimulation (TENS) also have no proven efficacy in the treatment of acute low back symptoms."

Convincing scientific evidence is beginning to emerge about the use of active care before the chronic stage. Refer to Chapter 1 for a full review, including the topic of chronic care. Linton demonstrated that early aggressive treatment (patient education, exercise instruction, physical therapy) was superior to traditional treatment approaches (rest and analgesics without physical therapy for 3 months), "Properly administered Early Active Intervention may therefore decrease sick leave and prevent chronic problems, thus saving considerable resources."[68] This study is particularly powerful in that the risk of developing chronic pain was eight times lower in the early active intervention group than in the traditional group.

In a comparative study of passive physical therapy versus rehabilitation, Mitchell found, "Active exercises to provide mobility, muscle strengthening, and work conditioning has shown superior results . . . substantial savings have been realized in the number of days absent from work and savings in the dollars expended for compensation benefits. There was an initial increase in health care costs resulting from the intensity of the treatment, but these costs were more than offset by savings in wage loss cost."[69]

Lindstrom et al compared a group of patients treated with exercises and education to a more traditionally treated control group and documented earlier return to work and decreased re-injury in the rehabilitation group.[70] The notion that active exercise can be harmful to an individual experiencing pain is incorrect. Guided exercise by a properly trained rehabilitation specialist is the optimal treatment program for the subacute population. A key is exercising to a pre-established quota rather than to a pain limit.[2,71] Waddell stated, "There is no evidence that activity is harmful and, contrary to common belief, it does not necessarily even aggravate the pain."[72]

Saal and Saal treated a group of patients who had back and leg pain and were referred for surgery. They concluded "All patients had undergone an aggressive physical rehabilitation program consisting of back school and stabilization exercise training . . . 92% return to work rate."[73] Active rehabil-

itation is essential for all patients, including those considered candidates for surgery. Saal and Saal said, "Failure of passive nonoperative treatment is not sufficient for the decision to operate." In a randomized, controlled trial looking at exercise and passive care in failed back surgery patients, Timm found that low-technologic exercises (stabilization and McKenzie) were of greater benefit than were high-technologic exercises (Cybex), physical methods, or joint mobilization.[74]

CONCLUSION

Rehabilitation is an exciting new way to practice. This paradigm allows us to evaluate regional conditions in light of dysfunction in the entire locomotor system. It is also a highly ethical way to practice because it reduces patient dependency on passive, pain-relieving approaches while teaching patients the self-treatment techniques needed to develop control over their symptoms. By focusing on functional restoration (instead of promotion of tissue healing), we can achieve quicker and more lasting results with spinal adjustments, because we are addressing the underlying cause of most pain syndromes. Future neuromusculoskeletal specialists will not only be experts in manipulation, but also know how to transition from passive to active care, and evaluate the biobehavioral component of musculoskeletal illness. Improved results in our practices and accompanying cost savings in the health care system will be realized by the improved management afforded by the new rehabilitation paradigm.

REFERENCES

1. Bigos S, Bowyer O, Braen G, et al: Acute Low Back Problems in Adults. Clinical Practice Guideline. Rockville, MD, U.S. Department of Health and Human Services, Public Health Service, Agency for Health Care Policy and Research, 1994.
2. Clinical Standards Advisory Group: Back Pain. London 1994, HMSO.
3. Lewit K: Chain reactions in disturbed function of the motor system. Manuelle Med 3:27, 1987.
4. Rissanen A, Alaranta H, Sainio P, et al: Isokinetic and non-dynamometric tests in low back pain patients related to pain and disability index.
5. Grabiner MD, Koh TJ, Ghazawi AE: Decoupling of bilateral paraspinal excitation in subjects with low back pain. Spine 17:1219, 1992.
6. Haldeman S, Chapman-Smith D, Petersen DM: Frequency and duration of care. In Guidelines for Chiropractic Quality Assurance and Practice Parameters. Proceeding of the Mercy Center Consensus Conference. Gaithersburg, Aspen, 1993.
7. Lewit K: Manipulative Therapy in Rehabilitation of the Motor System. 2nd Ed. London, Butterworths, 1991.
8. McKenzie RA: The Lumbar Spine: Mechanical Diagnosis and Therapy. Waikanae, New Zealand, Spinal Publications Ltd., 1981.
9. Travell JG, Simons DG: Myofascial Pain and Dysfunction: The Trigger Point Manual. Vol 2. Baltimore, Williams & Wilkins, 1992.
10. Lewit K: The functional approach. J Orthop Med 16:73, 1994.
11. Jull G, Janda V: Muscles and Motor Control in Low Back Pain. In Twomney LT, Taylor JR (eds): Physical Therapy for the Low Back, Clinics in Physical Therapy. New York, Churchill Livingstone, 1987.
12. Janda V: Muscles and cervicogenic pain syndromes. In Grant R (ed): Physical Therapy of the Cervical and Thoracic Spine. New York, Churchill Livingstone, 1988.
13. Bullock-Saxton JE, Janda V. Bullock MI: Reflex activation of gluteal muscles in walking. Spine 18:704, 1993.
14. Spitzer WO, LeBlanc FE, Dupuis M: Quebec Task Force on Spinal Disorders: Scientific approach to the assessment and management of ac-

tivity-related spinal disorders: A monograph for clinicians. Spine 12(Suppl 7):S1, 1987.

15. Schwarzer AC, April CN, Bogduk N: The sacroiliac joint in chronic low back pain. Spine 20:31, 1995.

16. Barnsley L, Lord SM, Wallis BJ, et al: The prevalence of chronic cervical zygaphophyseal joint pain after whiplash. Spine 20:20, 1995.

17. Jackson RP: The facet syndrome—Myth or reality? Clin Orthop Rel Res 279:110, 1992.

18. Schwarzer AC, April CN, Derby R, et al: Clinical features of patients with pain stemming from the lumbar zygaphophyseal joints. Spine 19:1132, 1994.

19. Schwarzer AC, April CN, Derby R, et al: The relative contributions of the disc and zygapophyseal joint in chronic low back pain. Spine 29:801, 1994.

20. Moffroid MT, Haugh LD, Henry SM, et al: Distinguishable groups of musculoskeletal low back pain patients and asymptomatic control subjects based on physical measures of the NIOSH low back atlas. Spine 12:1350, 1994.

21. Moffroid MT, Haugh LD: Prospective randomized exercise trial in two patient groups with LBP. Vermont Rehabilitation Engineering and Research Center, 1994-1998.

22. Delitto A, Cibulka MT, Erhard RE, et al: Evidence for use of an extension-mobilization category in acute low back syndrome: A prescriptive validation pilot study. Phys Ther 73:216, 1993.

23. Erhard RE, Delitto A: Relative effectiveness of an extension program and a combined program of manipulation and flexion and extension exercises in patients with acute low back syndrome. Phys Ther 74:1093, 1994.

24. Spitzer WO, Skovrom ML, Salmi LR, et al: Scientific monograph of the Quebec Task Force on whiplash-related disorders: Redefining "whiplash" and its management. Spine 20:8S, 1995.

25. Panjabi MM: The stabilizing system of the spine. Part I: Function, dysfunction, adaptation, and enhancement. J Spinal Disord 5:383, 1992.

26. Watson DH, Trott PH: Cervical headache: An investigation of natural head posture and upper cervical flexor muscle performance. Cephalgia 13:272, 1993.

27. Treleaven J, Jull G, Atkinson L: Cervical musculoskeletal dysfunction in post-concussional headache. Cephalgia 14:273, 1994.

28. Hagbarth KE: Evaluation of and methods to change muscle tone. Scand J Rehab Med Suppl 30:19, 1994.

29. Stokes MJ, Cooper RG, Jayson MIV: Selective changes in multifidus dimensions in patients with chronic low back pain. Eur Spine J 1:38, 1992.

30. Fitzmaurice R, Cooper RG, Freemont AJ: A histomorphometric comparison of muscle biopsies from normal subjects and patients with ankylosing spondylitis and severe mechanical low back pain. J Pathol 163:182, 1992.

31. Dahl JB, Erichsen CJ, Fuglsang-Frederiksen A, et al: Pain sensation and nociceptive reflex excitability in surgical patients and human volunteers. Br J Anaesth 69:117, 1992.

32. Woolf CJ: Long term alterations in the excitability of the flexion reflex produced by peripheral tissue injury in the chronic decerebrate rat. Pain 18:325, 1984.

33. Lehto M, Jarvinen M, Nelimarkka O: Scar formation after skeletal muscle injury. Arch Orthop Trauma Surg 104:366, 1986.

34. DeAndrade JR, Grant C, Dixon ASJ: Joint distension and reflex muscle inhibition in the knee. J Bone Joint Surg [Am] 47:313, 1965.

35. Brucini M, Duranti R, Galleti R, et al: Pain thresholds and electromyographic features of periarticular muscles in patients with osteoarthritis of the knee. Pain 10:57, 1981.

36. Spencer JD, Hayes KC, Alexander IJ: Knee joint effusion and quadriceps reflex inhibition in man. Arch Phys Med Rehabil 65:171, 1984.

37. Hides JA, Stokes MJ, Saide M, et al: Evidence of lumbar multifidus muscles wasting ipsilateral to symptoms in patients with acute/subacute low back pain. Spine 19:165, 1994.

38. Matilla H, Hurme M, Alaranta H, et al: Spine 11:732, 1986.

39. Lehto M, Hurme M, Alaranta H, et al: Connective tissue changes of the multifidus muscle in patients with lumbar disc herniation: An immunologic study of collagen types I and III and fibronectin. Spine 14:302, 1989.

40. Zhu XZ, Parniapour M, Nordin M, et al: Histochemistry and morphology of erector spinae muscle in lumbar disc herniation. Spine 14:391, 1989.

41. Janda V: Muscle strength in relation to muscle length, pain and muscle imbalance. In Harms-Rindahl K (ed): Muscle Strength. New York, Churchill Livingstone, 1993.

42. Sahrman SA: Posture and muscle imbalance. Faulty lumbar pelvic alignments. Phys Ther 67:184, 1987.

43. Janda V, Schmidt HJA: Muscles as a pathogenic factor in back pain. International Federation of Manipulative Physical Therapists Proceedings, Christchurch, New Zealand, 1982.

44. Johnson C, Reid JG: Lumbar compressive and shear forces during various trunk curl-up exercises. Clin Biomech 6:97, 1991.

45. Janda V: Some aspects of extracranial causes of facial pain. J Prosthet Dent 56:484, 1986.

46. Kamkar A, Irrgang JJ, Whitney SL: Nonoperative management of secondary shoulder impingement syndrome. J Orthop Sports Phys Ther 17:212, 1993.

47. Bogduk N, Simons DG: Neck pain: Joint pain or trigger points? In Voeroy H, Merskey H (eds): Progress in Fibromyalgia and Myofascial Pain. New York, Elsevier, 1993, pp 267–273.

48. Travell JG, Simons DG: Myofascial Pain and Dysfunction: The Trigger Point Manual. Baltimore, Williams & Wilkins, 1983.

49. Liebenson CS: Thoracic outlet syndrome. J Manipulative Phys Ther 11:6, 1988.

50. Matthews M: The T4 syndrome. Aust J Physiother 32:123, 1986.

51. Ribbe EB, Lindgren SHS: Clinical diagnosis of TOS. Manuelle Med 2:82, 1986.

52. Roos DB: New concepts of TOS that explain etiology, symptoms, diagnosis, and treatment. Vasc Surg 13:313, 1979.

53. Tarola G: Whiplash: Contemporary considerations in assessment, management, treatment and prognosis. JNMS 4:156, 1993.

54. Wilk KE, Arrigo C: An integrated approach to upper extremity exercises. Orthop Phys Ther Clin North Am 1:337, 1992.

55. Sommer HM: Patellar chondropathy and apicitis, and muscle imbalances of the lower extremities in competitive sports. Sports Med 5:386, 1988.

56. Tippet SR: Closed chain exercise. Orthop Phys Ther Clin North Am 1:253, 1992.

57. Schiable HG, Grubb BD: Afferent and spinal mechanisms of joint pain. Pain 55:5, 1993.

58. Proske U, Schiable HG, Schmidt RF: Joint receptors and kinaesthesia. Exp Brain Res 72:219, 1988.

59. Gagey PM: Postural disorders among workers on building sites. In Bles W, Brandt T (eds): Disorders of Posture and Gait. New York, Elsevier Science, 1986.

60. Lewit K: Disturbed balance due to lesions of the craniocervical junction. J Orthop Med 3:58, 1988.

61. Odkvist I, Odkvist LM: Physiotherapy in vertigo. Acta Otolaryngol Suppl (Stockh) 455:74, 1988.

62. Boguet J, Moore N, Boismare F, et al: Vertigo in post-concussional and migraine patients: Implication of the autonomic nervous system. Aggressologie 24:235, 1983.

63. Brandt T, Krafczyk S, Malsbendend I: Postural imbalance with head extension: Improvement by training as a model for ataxia therapy. Ann NY Acad Sci :636, 1981.

64. Gagey PM: Non-vestibular dizziness and static posturography. Acta Otorhinolarynol Belg 45:335, 1991.

65. Shekelle PG, Adams AH, Chassin MR, et al: Spinal manipulation for low-back pain. Ann Intern Med 117:590, 1992.

66. Shekelle PG: Spine update: Spinal manipulation. Spine 19:858, 1994.

67. Cox JS: Injury nomenclature. Am J Sports Med 7:211, 1979.

68. Linton SJ, Hellsing AL, Andersson D: A controlled study of the effects of an early intervention on acute musculoskeletal pain problems. Pain 54:353, 1993.

69. Mitchell RI, Carmen GM: Results of a multicenter trial using an intensive active exercise program for the treatment of acute soft tissue and back injuries. Spine 15:514, 1990.

70. Lindstrom A, Ohlund C, Eek C, et al: Activation of subacute low back patients. Phys Ther :293, 1992.

71. Fordyce WE, Fowler RS, Lehmann JF, et al: Operant conditioning in the treatment of chronic pain. Arch Phys Med Rehabil 54:399, 1973.

72. Waddell G: A new clinical model for the treatment of low-back pain. Spine 12:634, 1987.

73. Saal JA, Saal JS: Nonoperative treatment of herniated lumbar intervertebral disc with radiculopathy. Spine 14:431, 1989.

74. Timm KE: A randomized-control study of active and passive treatments for chronic low back pain following L5.

V

PSYCHOSOCIAL AND SOCIOPOLITICAL ASPECTS OF REHABILITATION

19 Psychosocial Factors in Chronic Pain

GEORGE E. BECKER

Psychological and physical factors are inextricably involved and interrelated in virtually every case of chronic back pain.[1] The art of healing begins with recognition of the several determinants of chronic back pain, and understanding that a good many of them are totally unrecognized and outside of the conscious awareness of the patient. The goals of this chapter are as follows:

- to define some of the terms helpful in describing and understanding the patient with a chronic back pain syndrome
- to describe those characteristics that will alert the clinician and enable early recognition of the problematic patient
- to review a comprehensive history format encompassing psychosocial as well as biological issues
- to describe the adjunctive diagnostic use of selected psychological tests
- to review treatment strategies for helping this extremely challenging and often frustrating group of patients

The notion of a mutual interaction between mind and body in health as well as in illness is not new. It is likely that some of the miraculous cures ascribed to the man Jesus in the New Testament attest to his charisma and the empowerment transmitted through him to the unhealthy believer. (Clearly all healers possess the ability to empower patients with whom they have established a healing relationship or therapeutic working alliance.) In the seventeenth century, Sydenham recognized and described syndromes that, despite the outward appearance of physical maladies, in reality were related to identifiable, heavily emotionally charged life events and circumstances. He described but did not name *somatization,* which is the experience and expression of psychological stress and conflict in physical rather than in emotional terms. Burton later described the physical (somatic) and hypochondriacal preoccupation that today is a recognized concomitant of mood and anxiety disorders. Almost a half century ago, and long before the popularization of the holistic approach to health and illness, Alexander[2] wrote: "Once again, the patient as a human being with worries, fears, hopes, and despairs, as an indivisible whole and not merely the bearer of organs ... of a diseased liver or stomach ... is becoming the legitimate object of medical interest. In the last two decades increasing attention has been paid to the causative role of emotional factors in disease." Brown and colleagues[3] wrote an insightful landmark paper identifying six striking characteristics appearing repeatedly in a number of patients manifesting obvious functional overlay.

These characteristics include: (1) vague history, confused chronology, or introduction of material ostensibly having nothing to do with the injury and symptoms; (2) expression of open or veiled resentment toward caretakers because of alleged mismanagement and neglect; (3) dramatic descriptions of the symptoms and the patient's reactions to them; (4) difficulty in localization and description of pain and other symptoms ... or a complaint of pain in many areas, obscuring a pain that might originally have had an anatomic focus; (5) failure of the usual forms of treatment to give significant relief of pain; and (6) accompanying neurotic symptoms: acute and chronic anxiety, insomnia, irritability, pressure-like headaches, depression, crying spells, chronic fatigue, acute anxiety attacks or chronic anxiety and peculiar gaits suggesting hysteria. At the same time, these authors underscored the fact that in 12 of 12 patients, the "clinical picture was from both somatogenic and psychogenic causes." The first sentence of this chapter is meant to dispel once and for all the *either or* notion—that chronic pain is of *either* organic *or* psychogenic origin.

DISABILITY AND CHRONIC PAIN

The problem of chronic pain and disability, which is growing at an alarming rate, has reached gargantuan proportions and is associated with astronomical costs for health care, Workers' Compensation, and physical injury. In 1988, Frymoyer and Gordon[4] wrote that low back pain disabled 5.4 million Americans each year and cost at least $16 billion annually. In 1992, Ford[5] reported that at least 10% of all medical-surgical patients have *no objective evidence* of physical disease. (The author's experience suggests that 10% is a low estimate.) Lipowski[6] described an even higher percentage of functional illness, especially depression, among patients presenting to primary care providers with physical, not psychological, complaints. The message is clear: depressed and otherwise psychologically unwell persons frequently do not recognize the psychological nature of their problem. In fact, they usually deny vehemently any psychological or emotional dimension in their clinical picture. Their massive denial, lack of insight, and resistance to accepting and confronting psychological factors involved in their chronic pain makes them particularly difficult to treat.

The fact that *somatizers* often go weeks, months, or even years with an incorrect diagnosis and ongoing disability indicates that something is wrong with our approach to chronic pain. Misdiagnosis of the somatizer is the inevitable precursor to prolonged and ineffective treatment, and frequently to multiple and inappropriate chemical, electrical, and imaging studies; inappropriate medications, including narcotics (which frequently compound the problem); or, worse yet, to invasive procedures, including surgical intervention. After over 40 years of experience caring for back pain, it is clear to this author that *surgery is rarely indicated.* Most "failed backs" are found in unfortunate individuals who should never have had surgery in the first place, or who, needing surgery, did not have the right procedure at the right time and at the right level. Frymoyer[7] states that the "failed surgical back" is usually the result of poor surgical judgment.

The purpose of this chapter is to describe and define the dynamic and psychosocial issues involved with and frequently fueling chronic pain syndromes, to review those presenting signs and symptoms that should alert the astute clinician to the issue of functional overlay, to outline briefly a comprehensive history format, to review the adjunctive use of psychological testing, and to describe management strategies for this frustrating and often passive, resistant, and noncompliant group of patients. Typically, many of these patients simultaneously proclaim ardently how much they want to get better while conveying, with their mixed-message behavior, that they really are going to (and unconsciously wish to) remain disabled. Timely recognition and appropriate treatment of the chronic back pain patient not only is cost effective, but also ultimately benefits the doctor spiritually and materially. In the highly scrutinized health care environment of today, the practitioner must establish a reputation for the kind of comprehensive treatment protocol that *gets patients back to work (and to life in full) and keeps them there.*

TERMS AND CONCEPTS

Several terms and concepts frequently encountered in the chronic pain vocabulary are defined or discussed in the following section.

Alexithymia

Sifneos[8] coined this term to describe those individuals who (literally) have no words for their feelings. *Lex* is the Greek root meaning *word.* The thymus is the gland thought by the ancients to be the seat of the emotions, hence *thymia.* Persons troubled by alexithymia, rather than recognizing their innermost feelings, bury and deny them only to have them surface as physical symptoms that seem to, but do not, have a physical basis.

Compensation and Litigation

If the benefits (or potential benefits in fantasy) derived from staying ill outweigh the benefits of regaining health, the patient will not likely get well. It is generally recognized in the healing professions that some patients seem clearly to thrive on being disabled. One does not need a professional degree to understand that a person suing for an injury-related disability will less likely profit financially if the disability resolves. This situation leads naturally to a consideration of *gain* (see subsequent section).

Compliance

Some patients fail to comply with treatment regimens designed for their benefit. This failure may best be understood as an impediment to or as unconscious resistance to healing. These unfortunate souls, for reasons they themselves rarely understand and of which they usually are unaware, *need* to be in pain, *need* to suffer, *need* to feel like powerless victims, and *need* to be cared for *without losing face.* Others, a smaller subset, are at least partially aware of their motives. They exhibit pain behavior fueled by anger, resentment, or a wish to retaliate.

Denial

Individuals who somatize typically deny that they are experiencing significant emotional or psychological stress, much as an alcoholic denies having a problem with alcohol. Denial blinds an individual to the psychological problem and precludes insight. Denial can and frequently does constitute a tremendous barrier to recovery.

Depression

Many persons who are depressed neither look nor feel depressed. If asked about their mood, they will deny depression. Instead, they exhibit chronic pain (often chronic back pain) or other somatic complaints, as an *initial manifestation* of their depression,[9] often deluding the well-intentioned doctor. Their pain allows them to seek and to receive medical/chiropractic care and attention while simultaneously denying the mood disorder and often the life stress, chaos, and conflict fueling it. Emotional neediness is a hallmark of depression. Unfortunately, the unrecognized depression remains untreated.

Dreams

Dreams have been described as *the royal road to the unconscious.*[10] Certainly, the dreams of patients often reveal (in their symbolism) conflicts, fears, and wishes that lie buried outside of conscious awareness. They may clarify issues constituting barriers to recovery.

Fear

At a conscious level, fear frequently bespeaks a wish at an unconscious level, particularly in the patient whose actions and words signal a double or conflicting message.

Functional Overlay

This venerable term in the medical vernacular is not part of official medical nomenclature. Nonetheless, it is useful in describing those nonphysical (i.e., psychological and emotional) factors that color the way in which patients present themselves. It is also accurate because it does not suggest an either/or dichotomy between physical and psychological symptoms.

Gain

For practical purposes, gain can be thought of as *primary, secondary,* and *tertiary.*

PRIMARY GAIN

Primary gain addresses psychological needs: being taken care of while *feeling* independent. Primary gain is entirely *within* the individual, and involves self image and self esteem. It allows the disabled person to deny passive dependency, because the illness (i.e., the back condition) is forcing the dependency and, but for it, the patient would be an independent and responsible member of society. The person unable to work because of disability can see him- or herself as absolved of responsibility by the illness, which is not their fault.

SECONDARY GAIN

This term describes those material benefits (special attention, care taking, sick leave, relief from some if not all responsibilities to others such as alimony or child support payments, compensation payments, awards, ongoing payments from disability carriers, and the like) derived from outside the individual. The ministrations of others to one who is disabled are secondary gains. Although secondary gain figures prominently in chronic pain syndromes, it is often not as potent a force as primary gain.

TERTIARY GAIN

This relatively new term describes those material and psychological gains enjoyed by those caring for the disabled one. The spouse may have a *need* to be a caretaker, the lawyer may have a *need* to keep the patient disabled and out of work to maximize winnings, a doctor may *need* to keep the patient dependent on ongoing care and manipulation (in more than one sense) rather than to teach the patient self–sufficiency, and the psychiatrist may nurture ongoing passive dependency for considerations that have little to do with the welfare of the patient. Tertiary gain usually involves a conflict of interest, an issue that behooves all health care and legal providers to self-monitor.

Motivation

Virtually all patients state that they want nothing more than to get better. Most of them *do* want to get better and most of them do get better. The remaining few, however, with their ongoing complaints of pain and their problematic behavior, bespeak a conflict of which they have little if any awareness: *consciously,* they want to get better, but *unconsciously,* they

want and need to be cared for—or loved. Thus, the double message that identifies the somatizer. These patients, in their passivity, are often misunderstood as poorly motivated. The clinician should remain mindful that actions speak louder than words, and understand that what appears to be poor motivation may in reality be a powerful (unconscious) conflict.

Parallel History

The parallel history is the record of important psychosocial events and circumstances experienced during and before those typically included in the history of present condition.[11] When viewed against the backdrop of the formative years, the parallel history often makes clear the events and circumstances that may be fueling a chronic pain syndrome in the vulnerable person.

Somatization

Somatization is the expression of unconscious feelings and emotions in physical rather than emotional terms. The somatizing patient, believing with a conviction of delusional proportion that his or her symptoms are solely and totally of physical origin, typically seeks medical rather than psychiatric care.[12] Unfortunately this conviction often leads the unsuspecting doctor to inappropriate and rather far-flung diagnoses and equally inappropriate and unsuccessful treatment.

Somatization Diathesis

Certain individuals, emotionally short-changed or scarred during their formative years, evidence a proclivity to somatize in the face of stressful untoward events or circumstances of adult life, especially ones that awaken feelings buried in the unconscious and rooted in the past. These individuals are said to harbor a *somatization diathesis.*[1]

RECOGNITION

It is proverbially true that if one *thinks* of the right diagnosis, one will likely *make* the right diagnosis. Nowhere is this more apt than in the recognition of back pain complicated and colored by psychological factors. Unfortunately, even today, many textbooks fail to include a discussion of psychological factors as they apply to chronic musculoskeletal symptoms, including neck, shoulder, and back pain. The aim of this section is to spotlight the characteristics of this group of patients, to outline an interview format helpful in identifying them, and to review the use of the Pain Drawing, the Minnesota Multi Phasicz, and other select psychological tests.

Red Flags

The following listing of *red flags*—signs, symptoms, and other clues that alert the clinician to the likelihood that psychological and emotional factors figure significantly in the clinical presentation[1]—are arranged in groups reflecting history, psychosocial issues, disturbances of mood, and examination findings.

RED FLAGS I (HISTORY)

- Vague, inconsistent, and implausible history of injury, often unwitnessed
- Symptoms that proliferate from one body area or system to several, often culminating in total body pain
- Highly emotionally charged pain descriptors: torturing, suffocating, cutting, wretched, blinding, exhausting, searing, scalding, stabbing, wrenching, punishing, grueling, cruel, vicious, penetrating, piercing, terrifying, fearful, crushing, gnawing, pounding, beating, and the like
- Obvious hyperbole in history: "...I couldn't move ... my legs collapsed ... I was numb all over ... I couldn't or can't do anything ..."
- Obvious discrepancies during evaluation: the patient who reports an inability to sit for more than 10 minutes but sits for an hour or more relating the history
- A lengthy history of life-long hard work and responsibility with a professed desire to return to work, which, unfortunately, is now precluded by pain
- Marked passivity, inappropriate activity curtailment, frequently with concomitant weight gain and marked physical deconditioning
- Acceptance of disabled status: "I've just learned to accept my limitations."
- History that only narcotics afford pain relief, with gradually escalating narcotic use

RED FLAGS II (PSYCHOSOCIAL ISSUES)

- Externalizing responsibility or blame for occupational, relationship, mood, or financial problems
- Emotional constriction: keeping feelings inside
- Tearfulness or weeping during interview
- Denial that the manifest somatic problem is in any way related to life events and circumstances, except to blame life failures on the purported physical illness: (e.g., "but for my back pain, everything would be A-okay")
- A verbalized fear of ongoing disability. Such a *fear* frequently represents an unconscious wish to be taken care of, especially in persons emotionally short-changed in their youth.

RED FLAGS III (DISTURBANCES OF MOOD)

- Dissatisfaction or frustration with job or anger at a boss or doctors frequently represents unrecognized (displaced) anger at parenting figures, which may culminate in verbalized resentment at the way the claim is handled, the way a disability is (not) accommodated, or the way treatment is rendered
- Failure of reasonable treatments, in the face of which patients may report worsening symptoms. Such failures may reflect resentment at authority figures displaced from parents or supervisors onto the unsuspecting and often bewildered doctor.
- The doctor begins to sense his or her own anger directed at the patient. This "countertransference" frequently signals the passive-aggressive behavior of a smiling, manifestly compliant, but latently angry or enraged person. The challenge for the doctor is then to recognize his or her feelings to better control behavior. It is a grievous error for the doctor to return in kind the anger of passive-aggressive patients.

- Visiting emergency rooms for narcotics, escalating drug needs, increasing alcohol abuse, or gaining weight may represent a thinly veiled emotional hunger and neediness in concert with a proclivity to address that hunger with drugs or food

RED FLAGS IV (EXAMINATION FINDINGS)

- Theatrical presentation: walking with an obviously unnecessary cane (often carried in the wrong hand), a strange limp, or maintaining a bizarre posture
- Nonanatomic sensory findings, such as glove-stocking or half-body hypesthesia
- Nonanatomic motor findings, such as giveway weakness on muscle testing or on toe or heel walking, or obviously suboptimal grip attempts
- Significant difference between observed and formally tested ranges of motion
- Significant difference between straight-leg raising in sitting versus recumbent postures
- Inappropriate cervical compression test (e.g., causing low back pain or causing legs to give way)
- Inappropriate withdrawal or exaggerated tenderness response on gentle palpation or percussion, especially if the patient grabs the examiner's hand in theatrical fashion

None of this information is really new. In 1940, Fetterman[13] identified symptoms, including dramatic pain descriptors, preoccupation with pain, fear of increasing helplessness, and the utility (i.e., secondary gain) of the symptoms, that have a "neurotic ring." More recently, Waddell[14,15] described physical signs and symptoms that bespeak functional overlay. In essence, when the examiner encounters any of these red flags, he or she should document them and make an attempt to account for them. All too often, they are mentioned in a medical report, only to be ignored in the discussion of findings. *Everything* in a comprehensive evaluation has meaning.

Depression

Eighty percent of persons suffering from depression are evaluated by primary care providers: chiropractors, family physicians, internists.[6] These patients usually do not realize that they are depressed, because their particular kind of depression is manifest by *physical symptoms* rather than by a *mood disturbance*. Back pain frequently is an *initial* manifestation of depression. The patient whose depression progresses to become clinically evident understandably (albeit usually incorrectly) concludes that the depression was caused by the chronic pain. Terms such as *depression without depression, masked depression,* and *pain as a depression equivalent* have been used to describe this particular group of patients. Other common somatic symptoms of depression are headaches, fatigue (including pseudo-*chronic fatigue syndrome*), weakness, shortness of breath, dizziness, palpitations, gastrointestinal complaints such as nausea and diarrhea, paresthesias, blurred vision, temporomandibular joint problems, ringing in the ears, diminished libido and/or sexual dysfunction, and generalized pain (including pseudo-*fibromyalgia* or *fibromyositis*). It is axiomatic that no person should be given a diagnosis of *chronic fatigue syndrome, fibromyalgia,* or *fibromyositis* without an evaluation that includes careful psychodiagnostic assessment by a professional who understands that chronic pain and/or chronic fatigue may be (and not infrequently are) the initial manifestations of an occult and clinically inapparent depression.

Somatizing/depressed individuals (who are usually highly resistant to psychological interpretations of their symptoms) often are so convinced that their problem is physical, and *only* physical, that they persuade their doctors of their delusional misconception. Because these patients have a *mood* (i.e., psychological) disorder, they do not get better in response to treatment directed at a *physical* problem. Typically, they request and receive extension after extension of their disability. One should beware of the patients who state: "The doctors just can't find out what's wrong with me." They frustrate their doctors who, not recognizing or even suspecting that they are depressed, unwittingly collude with them, seeking consultations and diagnostic tests directed at discovering a *physical* explanation for the pain. The astute doctor, however, may recognize early on that these patients will remain disabled. They deliver a double message: mouthing words about their independence, their tolerance of pain, and their frustration with their physical problem, their passive, dependent behavior bespeaks emotional need and dependence, intolerance of and incapacitation by pain, and complacency in accepting the invalid status.

The double message of the somatizer is as follows. Their words say:

- I started working at an early age and I have worked hard all my life.
- I have always been very independent.
- I can take a lot of pain . . . I'm not one to complain (denial).
- I just want to get better so I can have my life back.
- All I want to do is return to work.

while their behaviors say:

- Because I had to fend for myself as a youngster, I want the care *now* I didn't get *then.*
- My pain forces me to be passive and dependent (legitimizing invalidism).
- I am a victim, disabled and helpless in the face of this terrible pain.
- I need to remain disabled because now I am being taken care of.
- I don't want to go back to work . . . (maybe) . . . I want the educational opportunity (vocational rehabilitation) I forfeited when I dropped out of school.

Blumer and Heilbronn[9] described the typical characteristics of the person with a chronic pain syndrome:

- Limited formal education
- Holds overly strenuous routine or otherwise dissatisfying job
- Has had unmet dependency needs since early in life
- Began work at an early age (i.e., had no opportunity to really *be* a child)

- Worked at hard jobs a long time before becoming disabled by pain
- Family role model for pain and/or disability (identification)
- Often school drop-out

These authors explain that, "by virtue of providing for others and not being fully able to depend on their own parents as children . . . they had postponed gratification of such needs until a minor injury provided a rational and socially acceptable means of depending on others for emotional and economic support." Chronic (back) pain, in such instances, is an expression of *emotional* and *psychological* pain, totally outside of the conscious awareness of the patient.

Pain (emotional) begets **Pain** (physical i.e. psychogenic)

Because the pain-prone patient is one who seeks and usually receives endless and costly studies or interminable treatment and *does not get better,* it is important to recognize the diagnosis of somatization early. In 1959, Engel[16] outlined his understanding of psychogenic pain and its relationship to depression: ". . . a common error by the physician is to assume that the patient is depressed because he has pain. Investigation will usually make clear that the experience of pain serves to attenuate the guilt and shame of the depression . . ." Psychogenic (or somatoform or idiopathic) pain, rather than being a *cause* is more frequently a *manifestation* of depression. This is to say that patients whose psychogenic pain represents depression do not feel much, if any, depression. Instead, they experience pain. Engel also recognized that narcotic addiction frequently complicates the management of these patients. Unfortunately, some well-intentioned but ill-informed lawyers will object to psychological examination of the chronic pain patient (in accident-related litigation) on the grounds that the client is making no claim for psychological injury. Whenever chronic pain is a manifestation of an unrecognized (i.e., unconscious) depression or other mood disturbance, the patient does not even know of the mood disturbance. The most effective way to prevent and obfuscate accurate diagnosis and impede optimal treatment is to preclude psychological investigation of chronic pain that has failed to improve in response to treatment directed at a physical disorder.

Substance Abuse

The chronic pain patient frequently demands, and then receives, prescription after prescription for narcotic analgesics, reporting that nothing else relieves the pain. Such patients are at risk for drug dependency and iatrogenic addiction. The addicted patient invariably denies such addiction, asserting, "I only take the narcotic for my pain . . . I only take it when I *really* need it . . . nothing else (but the narcotic) helps . . ." This litany, or its equivalent, indicates that the *sensation* of pain has become a *withdrawal symptom-equivalent,* which requires the narcotic for its relief. The patient neither realizes nor understands this concept, insisting only that the pain is "real." It is. Almost all pain is real, but the sufferer has no way of knowing whether it is *physical* or *psychological* or both. Pain is pain. Pain represents a final common pathway. When pain becomes chronic and incapacitating, decimating lives of workers and their families, it is the task of the specialist to understand the diverse factors causing it, no matter how difficult the challenge.

Somatization Diathesis

Becker[1] identified a *somatization diathesis* in those individuals who, in one significant way or another, were emotionally short-changed during their formative years. Identifying these individuals involves looking for a history of *abandonment, abuse,* or *alcoholism* in a parenting figure. Because these individuals, in their youth, had to fend for themselves when they were ill-prepared to do so, they arrived in adult life lacking the coping and emotional resources to manage the ordinary demands and responsibilities of daily occupational and social functioning, to say nothing of significant additional stress. Should such individuals suffer the loss of a person on whom they depend, they are prone to develop physical symptoms that garner for them some level of caretaking, even if it is not exactly what they need.

ABANDONMENT

Abandonment takes many forms. A parent who, because of illness or occupational demands, must spend weeks or months away from the home may well be abandoning his child emotionally. The parent who, because of chronic illness, infirmity, or chronic pain, curtails activities and time with the child in effect emotionally abandons the child. The parent who leaves because of separation, divorce, or death abandons the child. Loving means *having time for.* No substitute, material or otherwise, can compensate when a parent is unable to be with and to be "there for" the child. A child abandoned during the formative years is ill-prepared for the demands and responsibilities of mature adult life. The process of parenting involves the gradual (not sudden and catastrophic) withdrawal of caretaking and the simultaneous nurture of emerging independence.

ABUSE

Abuse takes several forms. *Emotional* abuse can occur in the form of name-calling or ridiculing or subjecting the child to a constant state of anxiety in the face of parental fighting, yelling, screaming, and inappropriate favoritism. Abuse, however, can also be *physical,* involving inappropriate or frequent corporal punishment, beating, or actual battering. Lastly, abuse can be *sexual,* either as a single episode or on an ongoing basis. Adults who were abused as children commonly harbor both unconscious guilt and unconscious rage, either or both of which can fuel not only abusive and rebellious behavior, but also a chronic pain syndrome.

ALCOHOLISM

The child of an alcoholic parent is, at the very least, emotionally short-changed, not only by the emotional unavailability of the parent (leaving residual neediness within the child), but also by the negative role model that alcoholic behavior presents.

SURGICAL OUTCOME

Schofferman and colleagues[17] observed that patients who had experienced abandonment, abuse, and alcoholism were more likely than those who had not experienced such emotional trauma to have poor results after back surgery. They identified five childhood traumas that are risk factors: physical, sexual, or emotional abuse, abandonment, and alcoholism (or other drug abuse) by or on the part of a primary caregiver, and reported an 85% chance of an unsuccessful surgical outcome in those individuals with three or more of these risk factors. This information has clear implications regarding both history-taking and treatment approaches. Most "failed backs" reflect unwise diagnostic decisions based on incomplete (or ignored) psychosocial histories. Frymoyer and Gordon[4] identify poor patient selection as the reason for poor surgical outcome.

Factors Predicting Disability

Low back pain typically is a self-limiting symptom. Most patients with acute low back pain respond promptly to appropriate treatment and are back at work in short order. In a subset of patients, however, pain becomes chronic. The term chronic back pain was used in the past to describe pain of more than 6 months duration, but Frymoyer[7] redefined chronic back pain as pain of *more than 3 months duration.* Becker[1] commented that, in most cases, chronic back pain can be identified in even less than 12 weeks. Frymoyer identified several factors that are important in predicting prolonged disability after back injury. They include the duration of the current disability; a history of previous disability; psychosocial factors; occupational requirements; job dissatisfaction; and whether or not the patient has retained a lawyer.

Other factors identified with back pain and/or symptomatic disk disease that frequently prolong disability or serve as barriers to recovery include obesity, inactivity, deconditioning, lack of aerobic fitness, smoking and other substance (alcohol, marijuana, cocaine, legal or illegal narcotic) abuse, exposure to vehicular vibration, and a troubled family situation (e.g., children leaving the nest, illness, death, marital discord, divorce, or other losses). A short period of employment before an on-the-job injury often bodes ill in terms of prognosis.

Examination Format

The cornerstone of evaluation of an injured person is an accurate description of the person and of his or her work. Such a description is possible only after medical and other relevant records are reviewed, and the individual is interviewed and examined. At times, it is necessary to interview a spouse or other family member. The process of evaluation takes time and should never be rushed.

The review of records is most revealing if it is arranged and presented chronologically. This process may take the form of handwritten notes, but a more efficient means is through dictation for subsequent word processor input. A chronologic review of the records affords the best opportunity to understand something of the backdrop against which an injured person must be viewed. Record review is the task of a doctor and should not be delegated. Sometimes extremely subtle medical record entries provide vitally important clues to the comprehensive understanding of an illness and disability.

A *comprehensive history* is the foundation on which an understanding of an injured person rests. It is important to establish rapport with the individual being examined as quickly as possible. The good doctor is first and foremost a good listener. The task of eliciting a good history is both a challenge to and an opportunity for the examiner.

Interviewing is a skill. Almost all persons coming for an initial examination after an injury (and virtually all those coming for a medicolegal evaluation) are anxious. A gentle, reassuring, kindly approach helps to calm them. Some injured persons are angry. It is particularly important that the doctor not respond to them in kind. Frequently, if the doctor simply listens quietly, the anger dissipates and patients are better able to talk about their problems. Many patients, particularly chronic pain patients, have gone through life viewing every human being with whom they come in contact as an adversary. These individuals have a way of "setting up" the doctor as an adversary as well. The doctor should communicate in word and deed his or her determination to listen to, to understand, and to work and collaborate with the patient in the process of healing. Occasionally, an individual will become tearful or weep during an interview. At such times, it is best to maintain a brief silence while trying to understand what triggered the tears. Remember, *everything* in such a setting has meaning, which emphasizes the need for the doctor, and not a lay "historian," to obtain the history.

An overall structural framework for the history assures thoroughness and minimizes the likelihood of serious oversight. The following evaluation format, which has undergone many revisions, has proven useful.

HISTORY FORMAT

The history format encompasses material appropriate for both chiropractic as well as medical or psychosocial evaluation. All areas are important for a comprehensive understanding of the individual being examined.

I. *Identifying Data*
- Name of patient, address, marital status, age, occupation, and employer

- Date of evaluation
- Date of injury, if relevant
- Job description, including physical demands
- Employer and date of hire
- History of previous Workers' Compensation claims or personal injury litigation
- Time periods out of work, current income source (ascertain income while working versus income while disabled)
- Note any job or work load changes before injury
- Ask about rumored layoffs or plant closings
- Ask about any suspensions, or censures for unsatisfactory work performance
- Reason for evaluation

II. *Present Condition*
- List all symptoms attributed to injury—their onset, frequency, and severity. Note symptoms present before injury of focus.
- Chronologic history of present condition, including all previous treatment methods and responses.
- If an injury is involved, a detailed history of that injury is needed, with particular attention paid to discovering and understanding the probable mechanism (in terms of biomechanical forces) of injury. Otherwise, as detailed as possible a history of onset of symptoms should be documented.

III. *Past Medical History*
- Describe previous accidents or injuries, operations, medical conditions, hospitalizations, and any pre-existing disability.
- Note current use of medications, appliances, and physical therapy or similar techniques, as well as clinical responses.
- Note previous chiropractic treatment with clinical response.
- Describe current and past use of alcohol, tobacco, caffeine, and other drugs of abuse.
- History of current or past psychological difficulties and treatment. Ask specifically about anxiety, depression, and suicidal thoughts or attempts.

IV. *Review of Systems and Psychological Symptom Inventory*
- Ask about general health and pose appropriately focused questions pertaining to the head, eyes, ears, nose, and throat, as well as the cardiorespiratory, vascular, gastrointestinal, musculoskeletal, neurologic, and urogenital systems. Ask about sexual function. In females, ascertain number of pregnancies, live births, and miscarriages or abortions with dates. Ask about premenstrual syndrome.
- Ask specifically about depression, sleep problems, crying, difficulty with concentration or memory, loss of energy, easy fatigability, irritability, temper outbursts, physical violence, social withdrawal, dreams, self-esteem, sense of guilt, phobias, panic attacks, hyperventilation, fainting, dizziness, tremors, excess sweating, childhood bedwetting, history of shoplifting or stealing or gambling problems, and hallucinations.

V. *Chronologic, Educational, and Work History, Including Military Experience*
- Note schools attended, interests, performance, extracurricular activities, disciplinary problems, diplomas and/or degrees. If school drop-out, ascertain why.

- Note all major jobs, work dates, job satisfaction, and reason for leaving. Ask specifically about extended periods of unemployment.
- Comprehensive description of the work place and duties, as well as quality of relationships with employers, supervisors, and co–workers.
- Ask specifically about job satisfaction.
- Specifically document any work tasks precluded by the physical or psychological condition of the individual, with reasons for such preclusion.

VI. Personal History

- Note composition of household, any recent or impending changes, and recent deaths or serious illness in family or friends.
- Assess changes in and stability of living arrangements.
- Ask about increasing debts, financial problems, and bankruptcy.
- Check interpersonal relationships: marital or spousal; children, especially children by other marriages; parents; in-laws; and siblings.
- Obtain history of investigations and arrests (including driving while intoxicated), and note any periods of incarceration.

VII. Family History

Note significant medical or emotional problems, specifically depression, nervous breakdown, alcoholism, suicide, psychiatric hospitalization, or disability involving family members.

VIII. Biographical Information

- Developmental history, noting quality of bond to parents, siblings, step–parents, or others.
- Ask specifically about harsh or unusual punishment, physical or sexual abuse.
- Ask person to describe *mother . . . father.*
- Assess quality of bond to siblings, parents, and other family members.
- Determine when the individual left home and why.
- Obtain affectional relationship history (including history of abuse) to assess any difficulty in maintaining stable and mature intimate relationships.
- If divorce has been involved, inquire about alimony and/or child-support payments.

IX. Social and Recreational History

- Note range of interests, hobbies, pursuit of sports, recreational activities with friends and family.
- Specifically document any activities that the patient feels are precluded because of physical or psychological conditions and the reasons for such preclusion.
- Specifically ask about and try to determine in detail the patient's physical fitness program, if any. Assess the patient's initiative, motivation, and perseverance in maintaining a comprehensive fitness or physical rehabilitation program.

X. Mental Status Examination:

- Briefly describe the following: appearance during the interview, attitude, attention, eye contact, posture, flow of speech, content of speech, unusual mannerisms, movements or behavior, and observed as well as reported range of mood. Ask about suicidal thoughts or behavior.
- Check specifically: orientation, calculation, digit span, ability to

make reasonable judgments, and recent and remote memory. Many of these functions are particularly important in elderly persons who may, because of memory difficulties, be unable to comply with complicated treatment routines.

XI. Physical Examination

The format for the physical examination is beyond the scope of this chapter. It is clear, however, that the cornerstone of a thorough evaluation of a person with chronic spinal pain is a comprehensive history (which does not neglect the psychosocial arena), and a careful physical and mental status examination.

Psychological Tests

Just as radiography and other imaging studies are diagnostic tools that work in concert with the history and physical examination to refine the doctor's ability to establish accurate diagnoses, so also does psychological testing aid in establishing accurate diagnoses in the psychological arena. Nothing from a physical standpoint is as valuable a diagnostic instrument as a comprehensive history and physical examination. So also nothing from a psychological standpoint is as valuable as a comprehensive *parallel* history and a mental status examination.[11] Imaging, laboratory, electrical, and psychological tests are important and necessary adjuncts to the comprehensive assessment of the patient with chronic pain. The psychologist interpreting the tests serves as a consultant to the chiropractor, much as a radiologist interpreting imaging studies is a consultant to the primary practitioner.

Of the hundreds of psychological tests available, only a few are of general utility by the nonpsychological professional with regard to chronic pain syndromes in general and to chronic back pain in particular. These few tests, however, are immeasurably helpful. They have been described in detail and discussed by Southwick[18] and by Becker and Smith.[19]

The MMPI (currently the MMPI-2) represents the gold standard. Wiltse and Rocchio[20] showed that a certain MMPI profile (plotted on a graph) is associated with a poor result following chemonucleolysis. It is my experience that an MMPI profile characteristic of somatization usually is associated with evidence of a *somatization diathesis* in the history and suggests that a poor result is likely after back surgery for pain, regardless of the underlying pathology. Certainly, an MMPI-2 is imperative in any case of back, neck, or shoulder pain that fails to respond to reasonable treatment in a timely fashion, or one in which "the doctors just cannot find out what is wrong." No patient with a "failed back" should have further operative procedures without first undergoing thorough psychological assessment.

Southwick[18] detailed the evidence supporting appropriate use of the MMPI. The test is used widely and appropriately so. The MMPI-2 (1989) has largely, if not totally, supplanted the MMPI.

In addition to three scales that assess the validity of the individual test protocol, the major MMPI-2 scales include:

- Hypochondriasis (Hs): abnormal concern over bodily health
- Depression (D): dysphoria, worry, discouragement, low self-esteem
- Hysteria (Hy): inappropriate happy acceptance of adverse or stressful events or circumstances in general (denial)
- Psychopathic deviate (Pd): moodiness, resentment, maladjustment, defiance of authority, anger
- Masculinity-femininity (Mf): Aesthetic vocational interests, artistic interests, sexual orientation
- Paranoia (Pa): persecution, being easily hurt, suspiciousness
- Psychasthenia (Pt): narcissism, anxiety, self-concern, self-doubt, feelings of being forced, constitutional inadequacy
- Schizophrenia (Sc): alienation, delusions, influence of external agents
- Hypomania (Ma): expansiveness, irritability, egotism, the other side of depression

These descriptors are simplistic and not intended to encourage the amateur interpretation of MMPI-2 profiles. The interpretation of the MMPI-2 requires an extremely broad understanding of that specific test instrument. Normally, the MMPI-2 and other psychological test measures are interpreted by a clinical psychologist with special training and specific expertise in the area of psychological test administration and interpretation. Validity scales are built into the MMPI. Lees-Haley[21] devised a fake-bad scale for the MMPI-2, which has proven useful in identifying patients who may be consciously misrepresenting fact or even frankly malingering.[21] Full-blown malingering is, in my experience, infrequent. A more common situation is *unconscious* or to some degree *conscious* embellishment of symptoms wherein the hyperbole is part of the patient's theatrical (i.e., hysterical) character style. At the other end of the continuum is pure *somatization,* which is almost as uncommon as pure malingering. Most chronic pain patients represent a mix of somatization plus underlying organic pathology plus some symptomatic embellishment, not necessarily in any conscious attempt to be deceitful.

PAIN DRAWING

A picture is worth a thousand words. Mooney and co-workers[22] described a means of evaluation in which the patient draws, on the front and back of a body outline, the precise location of pain, specifically using symbols to indicate *numbness, burning, pins and needles, and stabbing.* The pain drawing is remarkable in its correlation with the history, especially the parallel history, and the MMPI-2. Brown[23] concluded that the pain drawing (along with magnetic resonance imaging) is especially useful as a diagnostic adjunct in cases of back and lower extremity pain.

CHRONIC PAIN TEST BATTERY

Becker and Smith[19] outline a small psychological test battery useful in chronic pain evaluation, including: (a) an intelligence assessment (it is important to know if a patient is literate and how effectively the patient can reason before administering an MMPI-2); (b) self-report measures, such as the pain drawing; (c) a personality test, such as the MMPI-2; and (d) projective tests, such as the Rotter Incomplete Sentences test, in which the patient completes a full sentence, given only one or two words. Examples from this test include:

- Back home - - -
- What annoys me - - -
- A mother - - -
- My greatest fear - - -
- When I was a child - - -
- The future - - -
- What pains me - - -
- My father - - -

Use of appropriately selected psychological testing derives several benefits, including revealing evidence of depression, factual misrepresentation, and the psychological assets and liabilities of a patient. In terms of the clinical prognosis, these tests demonstrate the ability of the individual to benefit from psychotherapy or counseling and the likelihood of compliance with exercise regimens or of persevering in functional restoration or vocational rehabilitation programs. The marketplace is replete with so-called "self-report" test measures. In general, these are not tests that look beneath the surface, but rather they indicate how the patient *wishes to be perceived.* They have, therefore, limited usefulness.

Becker and Smith[19] point out that although psychological tests can be scored blindly (e.g., by a computer or a psychologist who has not interviewed or even seen the patient), the conclusions are most accurate when the interpreting psychologist has performed a screening interview and a mental status examination to provide a backdrop against which the hard test data are best interpreted. The chiropractor who wishes to use psychological testing for chronic spine pain patients should establish a relationship with a clinical psychologist who is knowledgeable about chronic pain, somatization, depression, symptom embellishment, malingering, and the like and then work with that individual on a regular basis. This working relationship is particularly effective when the chiropractor and the psychologist confer to formulate appropriate management strategies for each patient with chronic pain.

Patients, particularly those who may harbor a somatization diathesis, are frequently resistant to undergoing psychological evaluation. They tend to distort the meaning and value of such testing with interpretations such as "the doctor thinks it's all in my head," "the doctor doesn't believe me," or "the doctor thinks I'm crazy." Explaining to the patient that he or she is to undergo a *chronic pain evaluation* is less threatening to an emotionally fragile and rigidly defended person than is a *psychological evaluation* or, worse yet, a *psychiatric evaluation.* Most patients readily acknowledge chronic pain, and most can accept the reality that chronic pain and mood and behavior are related. It is often helpful to review with the chronic pain patient his or her failure to regain health despite reasonable treatment, and to point out that a chronic pain evaluation may yield findings that suggest additional treatment strategies. Using patience, understanding, and tact, the doctor can usually persuade the resistant person to undergo a comprehensive chronic pain evaluation.

The use of psychological testing as a diagnostic adjunct in the evaluation of chronic pain is accepted as standard practice. Failure to consider psychological evaluation (including testing) in the face of a refractory chronic pain syndrome, particularly before performing invasive procedures, is negligent.

TREATMENT CONSIDERATIONS

The care of many patients with chronic back pain can be satisfactorily managed by the treating chiropractor, either alone, or if medication is indicated, in concert with a physician. Chronic back pain, especially the kind that lingers or smolders, waxing and waning with time, can be extremely frustrating to the doctor. Sometimes "cure" (meaning long–lasting ablation of pain) is not possible. When it is not, the patient should be so advised and assisted in establishing realistic goals. This preparation is best done in a way that enables the patient to understand in a positive light the implications of living with back pain. The doctor may say, "You will just have to learn to live with it. I've done all I can do." The response of the patient, particularly one who is depressed, may be "I'm never going to get better . . . I'll have to go on suffering . . . I'll never be able to do anything . . . I will not get my life back." These sentences reflect what typical chronic pain patients tell themselves, and illustrate considerable *cognitive distortion,* a kind of negative and defeatist thinking that is characteristic of depression. It is essential to enable the patient to understand that he or she should live (with the pain) to the *fullest. Living with* rather than *suffering with* and *being incapacitated by* the pain is the vital concept to instill.

One talk with a patient is rarely, if ever, enough. Patients with chronic pain are, as a group, more needy (i.e., dependent) than most, and they respond best to ongoing and repetitive support that can be diminished in frequency as they get the message and begin to act on it.

The treatment approach to a chronic pain syndrome must be *goal directed* and *time limited.* It is also counterproductive to help the patient "accept" the chronic pain, because "acceptance" is invariably misunderstood by the patient as meaning ongoing passive incapacitation, helplessness, and victimization. The most effective treatment strategy is the sports medicine (no pain—no gain) approach of working through pain to optimal flexibility, strength, stamina, endurance, and aerobic fitness. The role of each and every member of the treatment team must be supportive of such an approach. Physically conditioned and aerobically fit individuals are less susceptible to incapacitating chronic pain syndromes.[4]

Chiropractor as Therapist/Teacher

Psychotherapy is the practice of listening to the patient talk in a supportive, understanding, and appropriately interactive way that leads to a doctor/patient bond within which healing can be facilitated and nurtured. It has been around since recorded time, antedating Sigmund Freud by several millennia. For many pain patients, especially those who remain productive, the doctor may be able to serve effectively in lieu of a therapist. Living with a degree of chronic pain means focusing increasingly on the resumption of as many activities of daily occupational, family, social, and recreational functioning as possible. Simply because an exercise or activity (done by a deconditioned individual) causes an increase in pain is no reason to stop the activity. Indeed, unless the chronic pain patient pushes on with an appropriate functional restoration program, despite some pain, little if any sustained progress will likely follow. Patients must understand this fundamental principle. (Many patients have no understanding of the concepts involved in progressive conditioning or aerobic training, and need ongoing guidance and supervision.)

If a chronic back pain patient can maintain a relatively high level of musculoskeletal function through the ongoing, infrequent (i.e., once a month or with time, only three or four times a year) contact with a trusted chiropractor, the ongoing chiropractic visits require no other justification. Many patients respond positively to ongoing and infrequent supportive *psychotherapy.* The parallel is apt. The chiropractor with a healing touch usually knows how to manage these challenging individuals, teaching them patiently every step of the way. The proof of effectiveness is the resumption of optimal physical function.

In Latin, "doctor" means teacher (hence words like doctrine and indoctrinate). The effective chiropractor understands that he or she must function as a teacher to enable patients to heal themselves. Teaching patients with chronic back pain how to develop and maintain conditioning and fitness, as well as how to become relatively self-sufficient, is a critically important task of the doctor. Motivation, initiative, and perseverance are vitally important ingredients of such a program. The injured worker who stops a comprehensive physical fitness maintenance program after returning to work soon becomes a candidate for reinjury or re-emergence of symptoms.

For the patient, the bottom-line measure of the effectiveness of a treatment protocol is function: at home, at work, with the family, and at play. In more resistant cases, a treatment team can be effective, wherein the chiropractor works collaboratively with the family physician or the psychologist or psychiatrist. These providers should confer regularly to share insights and understanding and to coordinate, unify, and manage care. If psychological evaluation reveals the likelihood of a masked depression or of pain as a depression equivalent, or if the patient complains of insomnia because of pain, a trial of antidepressant medication is warranted. Details of such therapy are beyond the scope of this chapter, but they have been outlined by Becker[1] and others.

Although many patients who somatize can be satisfactorily managed by the chiropractor or by a chiropractor/family practitioner team, some fail to make progress. They should be referred for psychodiagnostic evaluation and, if indicated, for surgical evaluation as well. The criteria for satisfactory management include:

- Progress in the stretching/strengthening/fitness program without recurrent setbacks and endless return-to-work date extensions
- Progress in reaching a permanent and stationary status and satisfactory maintenance of that status
- Either returning to work on a sustained basis or entering and completing a vocational rehabilitation program, finding appropriate gainful employment post-training, and sustaining work performance
- Discontinuation of narcotic analgesics. Only in rare instances are narcotics indicated in chronic back pain management. A small subset of patients function more satisfactorily with a low level of maintenance narcotic than without the narcotic. Identification of such patients requires considerable skill and experience in assessment and management of chronic pain syndromes and is best undertaken by a physician skilled in algology.
- Resumption of family, social, and recreational physical activity appropriate for age and spinal condition. Ongoing passive dependency, bespeaking psychological regression, is unacceptable and, in and of itself, is a reason for referral.
- At the outset, with a chronic back pain patient, *long-range goals* (resumption of most, if not all activities of daily family, social, occupational, and recreational function; maintenance through a home exercise and aerobic fitness program of fitness, stamina, and endurance) and *short-range goals* (progressive learning of a home exercise and fitness program; acquisition of skills to enable a high degree of self-sufficiency with infrequent monitoring; weaning from reliance on narcotic analgesics; treatment of depression or pain as a depression equivalent, if present; progress in general physical activity level without recurrent setbacks, which indicate that more specialized treatment is indicated), should be established with target dates to avoid endless prolongation of disability. About 99% of all back pain patients should recover promptly. When they do not, something may be seriously wrong, and that something may escape definition if the psychological domain is not included among the differential diagnostic considerations.

Psychiatric, Psychological, and Supportive Treatment Methods

An in-depth description of treatment methods is beyond the scope of this chapter; however, several are identified briefly. The actual choice of treatment may vary with the community resources that are available.

ACUPUNCTURE

Acupuncture has been used by Chinese practitioners for centuries. Recent work suggests it may have some value in chronic pain syndromes.[24]

BEHAVIORAL THERAPY

This type of therapy is rooted in the pioneering work of Skinner, who recognized that behavior is shaped by its consequences. Sternbach[25] describes an approach that identifies: (1) undesirable (maladaptive) pain behaviors that interfere with the patient's life and constitute barriers to recovery; (2) desirable (adaptive) behaviors that the patient has but fails to use; (3) working with family, *reinforcers* that encourage the desirable behaviors (2) and strategies to discourage, if not to extinguish, the undesirable behaviors (1).

COGNITIVE THERAPY

This form of therapy is based on the work of Beck and colleagues.[26] Cognitive therapy helps the patient to recognize the *cognitive distortions* characteristic of the thinking of depressed persons, and to acquire the inner resourcefulness to overcome passive dependency and the "victim complex."

RELAXATION THERAPY, BIOFEEDBACK AND HYPNOSIS

Alone or in combination, these methods have shown limited success. Those patients who manifest the cycle illustrated in Figure 19.1, a form of tension myalgia, may respond to a treatment approach that involves the therapist *teaching* and the patient *learning* skills that culminate in a high degree of patient self-sufficiency. Relaxation, accomplished through medication, biofeedback, or self-hypnosis may increase a motivated patient's sense of self–sufficiency and control while

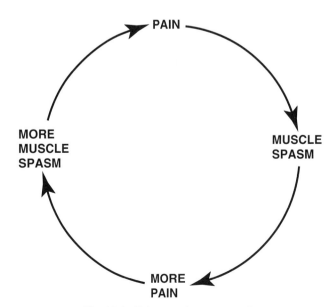

Fig. 19.1. Pain-muscle spasm cycle.

diminishing or extinguishing maladaptive thoughts of helplessness and victimization.

FAMILY THERAPY

Rowat and Jeans[27] state that "learning to live with pain is a family affair." Certainly, when a major wage earner or provider becomes disabled for an extended period of time, the impact on the family may be devastating. In the worst case scenario, the passive/dependent patient can become a virtually helpless invalid. Indeed, some chronic pain patients are as much of a demand on families as is a newborn infant. Additionally, most chronic pain patients manifest depressive spectrum symptoms, including insomnia, irritability, fatigability, lack of motivation, diminished self-esteem, social withdrawal, and diminished libido. It is not unusual for families to collapse and marriages to fail when an overworked spouse cannot shoulder yet another extra burden. Frequently, mounting bills lead to bankruptcy and sometimes homes are lost. Family therapy can sometimes help the family understand the underpinnings of the chronic pain syndrome and to learn strategies that may avert disaster. The family that learns to encourage and reinforce the patient's *active living* and to extinguish the patient's *passive suffering* has a greater chance of survival.

PHARMACOTHERAPY

The chiropractor should discover what medications the patient is taking. *Narcotics,* except under special circumstances, are inappropriate for chronic pain patients and may only diminish energy and motivation. Patients with chronic pain syndromes are at risk for developing iatrogenic substance abuse disorders. They frequently seek narcotic prescriptions from several providers. Appropriate team management of such patients designates only one provider to prescribe and manage pain medications. Ongoing regular use of narcotics diminishes endorphin production, thereby robbing the patient of a biologic mechanism intended to help cope with physical pain. Aspirin is one of the best analgesics in the entire pharmacopoeia. The practice of taking aspirin with a full glass of water effectively minimizes gastric irritation in most individuals.

The use of *anxiolytics* and *sedative-hypnotics* (benzodiazepines, barbiturates) is inappropriate in most cases of chronic pain syndrome. Especially in the presence of dependent and/or somatizing dynamics, these agents tend to diminish energy levels and motivation, thereby effectively sabotaging recovery efforts. Like marijuana, when used regularly, they may be associated with the *amotivational syndrome,* a serious barrier to active recovery.

Antidepressant medications are among the most useful in chronic pain syndromes. Insomnia attributed to pain by the patient often signals an unrecognized depression. Therefore, in this group of patients, antidepressants are more effective than sedative-hypnotic medications. Newer antidepressant agents, including fluoxetine, sertraline, and paroxetine, have not yet been studied extensively in the treatment of chronic pain syndromes, but they may prove effective against pain that is a depression equivalent. These newer medications appear to have a more favorable side effect profile than the traditional tricyclic compounds.

Muscle relaxants may help when identifiable and ongoing muscle spasm is a part of the clinical picture. This class of medication is most appropriate in acute cases and when used regularly, like sedative hypnotics, may diminish energy, motivation, and initiative. The efficacy of these drugs has been questioned. Carisoprodol has acquired a reputation as an aphrodisiac.

Street Drugs, Nutrition, Alcohol, and Tobacco

Marijuana has an effect similar to the benzodiazepines. When used regularly, it is associated with the *amotivational syndrome. Alcohol abuse* signals a self-destructive behavior pattern that may effectively undermine the best-intended efforts of the caregiver.

Many chronic pain patients are overweight. It behooves the chiropractor to teach these individuals something about nutrition, including lowering intake of dietary fat, and increasing intake of fiber, grains, fruits, and vegetables. Telling a patient simply to lose weight is usually ineffective. Teaching a patient the basics of nutrition in the light of current knowledge sometimes helps. Refractory patients may have success with a formal weight reduction program. The role of diet in conjunction with exercise in a weight loss program must be instilled.

Many patients with chronic back pain have never been informed about the relationship between smoking, back pain, and disk degeneration.[4] Part of a comprehensive attack (i.e., educational program) on chronic back pain should *always* involve encouraging the patient to stop smoking. Indeed, the patient's willingness or resistance to do so will serve as an excellent index of motivation. Ultimately, of course, patients do what they want to do and what they are motivated to do.

Functional Restoration

Many persons with chronic pain syndrome are not at all psychologically insightful and their care is best managed with a functional restoration approach as described by Polatin.[28] Such an approach involves careful assessment of the patient's clinical condition, particularly with regard to flexibility, strength, and aerobic conditioning. The injured worker with chronic back pain usually has rested for a long period and has become increasingly out of condition with each day of passivity and rest. The patient must be taught to recognize *deconditioning,* and to address that state, rather than pain, as the focus of concern. A functional restoration program is most effective when led by a team, which includes the primary provider (chiropractor, family physician, or internist), the physical and occupational therapist, and the psychologist. Optimal management presumes ongoing team conferences, at least by telephone.

The important phases of a functional restoration program after initial in-depth evaluation include stretching, progressive resistance exercises, work simulation tasks, and aerobics. The patient learns what to do on his or her own (without fancy or expensive equipment) and is monitored until at least pre-injury (if not optimal) function is restored. A typical functional restoration program for a refractory patient (which can be modified for more active or for well-motivated patients) consists of four phases:

- Phase I. Evaluation and detailed physical assessment, including range of motion and strength measurement.
- Phase II (2 to 6 weeks). Supervised stretching. The focus is on improving any mobility deficits and overcoming apprehension. The patient must understand that hurt does not equal harm and that successful completion of the program cannot occur without "pushing through" pain consequent to remobilization of tired, flabby musculature. The patient must be taught and, through support and encouragement, motivated in an incrementally graduated home program. The patient is best evaluated weekly.
- Phase III (3 weeks with progressive time increases).This exercise and rehabilitation program gradually and incrementally increases until functional restoration (or optimal restoration) is achieved. The patient is repetitively taught the need to maintain gains (strength, stamina, and aerobic fitness) made in the program, so that deconditioning will not sabotage the physical rehabilitation. The person out of work on temporary disability must understand that establishing wellness through functional restoration is the *first and foremost priority*.
- Phase IV. The follow-up phase. Most patients with chronic pain manifest return-to-work apprehension and require firm, directive, but understanding support. At this stage, it may be appropriate to negotiate with the employer if a residual disability requires special accommodation; to pursue job placement if the patient has lost employment; or to pursue a vocational rehabilitation program if the patient has reached a permanent and stationary status with residual disability that would preclude return to the previous employment setting.

Timely identification of those individuals who are vulnerable to develop chronic pain syndromes, and working with them to teach and encourage them about the importance of their active involvement in and responsibility for their recovery, will result in more effective and faster physical rehabilitation. Impediments and stumbling blocks to recovery should be identified early on and addressed. The fundamental importance of emphasizing conditioning (and not focusing on pain) is underscored. The injured worker must learn to work through the pain with a no pain—no gain philosophy. The temporary aggravation of pain when the patient with a chronic pain syndrome embarks on this program should be anticipated and identified as a reason to press on, rather than to slack off. The physically supple, strong, and aerobically fit individual is not likely to develop much less sustain a disabling chronic pain syndrome.

CONCLUSIONS

It is important for the practicing chiropractor to recognize, evaluate, test, and treat patients with chronic back pain in whom psychological and emotional factors are adversely coloring the clinical presentation, thereby constituting barriers to recovery. Prompt recognition and comprehensive supportive and aggressive treatment of these troubled individuals is of signal importance if they are to relinquish passive/dependency and maladaptive pain behaviors and regain a more active lifestyle.

REFERENCES

1. Becker GE: Chronic Pain, Depression, and the Injured Worker. Psychiatr Ann 21:1, 1991.
2. Alexander F: Psychosomatic Medicine. New York, WW Norton, 1950.
3. Brown T, Nemiah JC, Barr JS, et al: Psychological factors in low back pain. N Engl J Med 251:123, 1954.
4. Frymoyer JW, Gordon SL (eds): New Perspectives in Low Back Pain. American Academy of Orthopaedic Surgeons, Workshop, Airlie, VA, 1988.
5. Ford CV: The role of somatization in medical practice. Spine 17:S338, 1992.
6. Lipowski ZJ: Somatization and depression. Psychosomatics 31:13, 1990.
7. Frymoyer JW: Back pain and sciatica. N Engl J Med 318:291, 1988.
8. Sifneos PE: Short Term Psychotherapy and Emotional Crisis. Cambridge, Harvard University Press, 1972.
9. Blumer D, Heilbronn M: Chronic pain as a variant of depressive disease. J Nerv Ment Dis 170:381, 1982.
10. Freud S: Strachey J, Freud A (eds): The Standard Edition of the Complete Psychological Works. London, The Hogarth Press, 1953, p 608.
11. Sandler JL, Becker GE: Addressing the relationship between back pain and distress in your patients. J Musculoskel Med 10:26, 1993.
12. Lipowski ZJ: Somatization: The concept and its clinical application. Am J Psychiatr 145:1358, 1988.
13. Fetterman JL: Vertebral neuroses. Psychosom Med 2:265, 1940.
14. Waddell G, McCulloch GA, Kummel, et al: Nonorganic physical signs in low back pain. Spine 5:117, 1980.
15. Waddell G, Pilowsky J, Bond M: Clinical assessment and interpretation of abnormal illness behavior in low back pain. Pain 39:41, 1989.
16. Engel GL: "Psychogenic" pain and the pain-prone patient. Am J Med 26:899, 1959.
17. Schofferman J, Anderson D, Hines R, et al: Childhood psychological trauma correlates with unsuccessful lumbar spine surgery. Spine 17 (Suppl):S138, 1992.
18. Southwick SM, White AA: The use of psychological tests in the evaluation of low-back pain. J Bone Joint Surg [Am] 65:560, 1983.
19. Becker GE, Smith RB: Psychological factors in back pain. In Kirkaldy–Willis WH, Burton CV (eds): Managing Low Back Pain. New York, Churchill Livingstone, 1992.
20. Wiltse LL, Rocchio PD: Preoperative psychological tests as predictors of success of chemonucleolysis in the treatment of the low-back syndrome. J Bone Joint Surg [Am] 57:479, 1975.
21. Lees-Haley PR: A fake bad scale on the MMPI-2 for personal injury claimants. Psychol Rep 68:203, 1991.
22. Mooney V, Cairns D, Robertson J: A system for evaluating and treating chronic back disability. West J Med 124:370, 1976.
23. Brown M: The Pathophysiology and Diagnosis of Low Back Pain and Sciatica. American Academy of Orthopaedic Surgeons, Instructional Course Lectures XLI, 1992, pp 205-215.

24. Deyo RA: Non-operative treatment of low back disorders. In Frymoyer JW (ed): The Adult Spine: Principles and Practice. New York, Raven Press, 1991.

25. Sternbach R: Behavior therapy. In Wall P, Melzack R (eds): Textbook of Pain. 2nd Ed. Edinburgh, Churchill Livingstone, 1989.

26. Beck AT, Rush AJ, Shaw BF, et al: Cognitive Therapy of Depression. New York, Guilford Press, 1979.

27. Rowat KM, Jeans ME: A collaborative model of care: Patient, family, and health professionals. In Wall P, Melzack R (eds): Textbook of Pain. 2nd Ed. Edinburgh, Churchill Livingstone, 1989.

28. Polatin PB: The functional restoration approach to chronic low back pain. J Musculoskel Med 7:17, 1990.

20 Patient/Doctor Interaction

WILLIAM H. KIRKALDY-WILLIS

SCOPE OF OUR RELATIONSHIPS

The interaction between medical doctor and patient, chiropractor and patient, and medical doctor and chiropractor leads to an integration, a oneness that embraces these three and their environment. The resultant combinations are addressed throughout this chapter. Relationships matter more than any individual factors.

> "In the realm of science, the unbiased observer records facts from the world around us . . . In the field of art, the observer is involved in a personal assessment of the objects studied . . . In the sphere of religion, two or more people are involved in personal interaction."

These words of Macmurry[1,2] define the scope of human relationships. In the work of any health care professional, all three areas of study—science, art, and religion—are important. Chiropractic embraces all three areas, which is why it has so much to offer.

THE INDIVIDUAL

Each person is made of four different, yet interconnected, parts: the physical, the cognitive (logical), the emotional, and the spiritual. This image can be illustrated simply by drawing a circle that represents the individual, dividing it into four quadrants, and imagining a door between each division to illustrate the connection between the parts (Fig. 20.1). A practical application follows:

> Each one of the four parts influences the others. A big difference is noted between a disk herniation in a person who is in good mental, emotional, and spiritual health and one in an individual who has mental or emotional problems. A complete diagnosis includes the other three components as well as the physical findings.

The same approach is required for treatment. It is often easy to treat a woman with a sacroiliac syndrome who is otherwise in good health, but the same treatment is difficult in an individual who is resentful toward her employer.

THE INDIVIDUAL AND THE ENVIRONMENT

The environment also can, for convenience, be considered in four parts (Fig. 20.2): the workplace; home; social gathering, consisting of activities in the club or the church; and hobbies. There is further interaction between the individual and the different parts of the environment. A simple practical application follows:

> The diagnosis must include not only the physical or mental problems within the individual, but also how the patient feels about life at work, at home, and in the external environment. A facet syndrome may be a minor problem in a person who is happy at work and at home. A sacroiliac syndrome may present a difficult problem for a person whose spouse is unsympathetic.

> In prescribing treatment, the answer may be found by introducing a change in the workplace or adjustment to life in the home rather than in chiropractic manipulation or drug, injection, or other therapy. The writer recalls the case of a young man with symptoms suggestive of a cauda equina syndrome who recovered rapidly when plans were made for his mother-in-law to take a long vacation in a distant part of the country.

The wise physician, chiropractor, or physical therapist sees the patient as someone with four parts to their make-up living in a four-part environment. Practitioners cannot help every patient with all possible aspects of their problem, but they may need to approach the problem in greater detail sometimes. Often it is helpful to allow the patient time to tell all he or she wants to say about him- or herself. We should be as prepared to refer a patient to a social worker, industrial adviser, or psychologist as we would to a neurosurgeon or orthopedic surgeon.

LISTENING: A BASIC SURVIVAL SKILL

A study at the University of Minnesota suggests that 60% of misunderstandings in business result from poor listening. Eight percent of all business communications must be repeated. Rarely is more than 20% of what top management says understood five levels below. Sixty percent of customers who stopped buying from a company did so because of poor listening, an attitude of indifference to the client. Eighty percent of the day in business is spent in communication, but time spent in listening is often at only a 25% efficiency level.[3] Poor listening skills are responsible for many of our failures and for much dissatisfaction felt by our patients.

Frank discussion of religion has often been difficult, awkward, and sometimes taboo. It has taken three or four hundred years to recover from the dictum propounded by Descartes, who taught that the Mind and the Body are two separate entities in any individual. For many years, both doctor and patient have felt uncomfortable discussing religious matters.

405

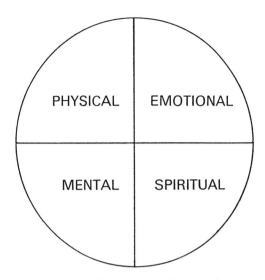

Fig. 20.1. Four aspects of personality.

This attitude is changing, however. Many of us now feel at ease when talking about our world, our universe, and our Creator. The approach of many, particularly younger people, to this subject is often one that differs from tenets once considered orthodox. As physicians, we need to keep open minds with respect to different ideas and beliefs. The good physician sits beside the patient prepared to listen, rather than standing over the patient or sitting behind the desk, prepared to make pronouncements about the individual's health.

MANAGING SEVERAL PROBLEMS AT THE SAME TIME

Although a great deal of our work helping people back to health is quite straightforward, it often can be difficult and tax our capacities to the limit. Ackhoff, an expert adviser and writer on the subject of business and industrial management, commented, as quoted by Dixon,[4] that problems in these areas rarely occur in isolation. In a plant or factory, several problems typically exist at the same time: they are constantly changing and interacting with another. Ackhoff calls this continuing process "mess." In his opinion, a good chief executive

officer is not merely someone who can manage a problem, but one who maintains control when coping with a "mess."

From this discussion of the individual and the environment, it is easy to see the common ground between the business executive and the health care professional. In helping his or her patients, the physician or chiropractor must be prepared to deal with this "mess" frequently. To realize that physician-patient situations often are fraught with this kind of difficulty is to minimize the stress experienced by the therapist. In addition, it enables him or her to understand more easily the thoughts, feelings, and attitudes of the patient.

It is curious that we human beings have two opposing facets within us. On the one hand, we want to be different, stand out among our fellows—brilliant football player, top of the class, early promotion; on the other hand, we want to merge with the crowd—have the same ideas and habits and wear the same clothes. These warring factors make the "mess" more complex.

Of the many ways to deal with this "mess," the most valuable is laughter, *with* and not against someone else, often about something ridiculous. We can sit beside our patients, chatting naturally, getting them to laugh, laughing with them, sometimes when necessary being ourselves the butt of the joke to enhance the interaction.

HAWTHORNE EFFECT[5,6]

Management at the Western Electric Plant at Hawthorne in the western United States was anxious to improve the output of the workers. They employed a team of sociologists who visited the plant, talked to the workers, and inspected the workshops. Among other things, they decided to increase the lighting in several areas. At once, the output from the workers increased dramatically. Everyone was delighted. At this point, one of the visitors suggested a further change. They told the workers that they planned to help them further but were careful not to say what they intended to do. They then decreased the strength of the lighting to a point below the original level. To the surprise of the management, the output of the workers increased still further. In fact, the workers had been influenced not by the strength of the light but by the

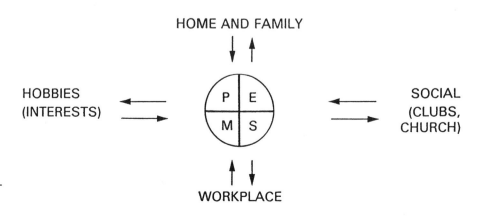

Fig. 20.2. The individual and the environment.

feeling that both management and the team of sociologists were interested in their welfare.

In commenting on the Hawthorne effect, Dixon notes that the scientist, in designing experiments, does his or her best to minimize or eliminate this phenomenon, which is one kind of placebo effect. Dixon thinks that using this effect forms the basis of a good deal of his practice and is a central feature of family medicine. The author concurs in regard to his practice as well.

OBTAINING THE PATIENT'S CONFIDENCE

The effect of putting the preceding principles into practice in our office and clinics is to build up a patient's confidence in him or herself as well as in the physician or chiropractor.

Our interaction with each patient should begin with a friendly greeting, a handshake, walking with him or her from the waiting room to the office, sitting beside him or her and not behind our desk. These things are little but very important, and represent the invaluable combination formed when patient and therapist work together.

Legend has it that in teaching his apprentices, Hippocrates stressed the value of obtaining the patient's confidence. It is reported that he went so far as to say that even in cases of the direst of diseases, the contentment engendered by the patient's conviction of the real concern of the physician could be the main factor responsible for a cure.

Chiropractors have an advantage in that their particular skill requires them to lay hands on their patients. This action itself induces confidence. The rest of us should share this advantage, by touching the patient with our hands during the examination and placing a reassuring hand on his or her shoulder when saying goodbye. In referring to a specialist, one patient said, "He never laid a hand on me to examine me. He came into the room, greeted me briefly and them asked his resident to tell him what he had found. Then he told me I would need a CT scan, a myelogram, and an operation. I was not satisfied. I said I would think it over. I didn't go back to see him again."

HOLISTIC DIMENSION

Obtaining the patient's confidence stems from our regarding him or her as an entire, integrated being, a unity, someone of value—the physical, mental, emotional, and spiritual working in combination. The term draws attention to an important fact, already considered to some extent: as we look on our patients, set out to diagnose their ills, and attempt to treat them, we must think of them, all the time, as a whole man or woman in their own particular environment. In so doing, we try to get alongside the patient, with or almost a part of him or her, to help solve the problem.

HOW SYMBOLS AND METAPHORS WORK

The use of symbols and metaphors has a powerful effect on the patient. They help the patient overcome the feelings of loss of wholeness and oneness, loss of control, vulnerability, and isolation from friends, relatives, and colleagues.

Symbols and metaphors are very personal. Each individual has the ability to make his or her own symbols. Sometimes, external events over which we seem to have no control make symbols for us. Groups of people and nations also have their symbols. A symbol often, perhaps always, carries more weight than logic.

The situation in which we find ourselves is not always friendly. Friends, acquaintances, doctors, nurses, even chiropractors can disturb the working of our symbols and metaphors by their attitude, their thoughts, their words, and their actions. All of us can recall examples of being abrupt, unkind, or unfeeling in treating a patient. Reminding ourselves of such occurrences encourages us to do better in the future.

The following scenario occurred in a major teaching hospital. Cystoscopy was to be performed in a large room with bright lighting in the presence of several doctors, nurses, and orderlies. The patient was taken to the room from the ward without any preoperative medication. He had to get himself across from the stretcher to the operating table. His legs were placed in stirrups, all of him in full view of all persons in the room. The surgeon then injected a local anesthetic per urethram. A few minutes later, the cystoscope was passed, a painful procedure. This experience of both pain and embarrassment affected the patient adversely, leaving a permanent scar, with fear of and dislike for the urologist. A few changes in procedure, a few minutes of explanation by the surgeon the previous evening, and some arrangements for more privacy could have made the whole procedure less traumatic, both physically and symbolically.

RESTORING THE PATIENT'S SELF–RESPECT

Fortunately, it is usually not difficult for the caring physician or chiropractor to help the patient regain his or her feeling of wholeness, belonging, and worth. The physician or chiropractor can listen carefully and with concern to the patient's account of the assault on his or her dignity. Some sample exchanges follow:

- He or she can then say "I agree, this is thoroughly bad, let's see what we can do about it together."
- The patient can be seen as often as is necessary to help him or her feel happy, free from embarrassment, and at ease again.
- The practitioner can put him– or herself in the patient's shoes, saying "Yes, if that happened to me I would be really mad."
- The practitioner can say, "After what you have told me, I would be reluctant to undergo cystoscopy. I can imagine how you felt."
- Another patient said, "Once I had a catheter passed by a rough, inexperienced assistant. It was very painful. In my case, I was told not to be a sissy. I decided not to go to that surgeon ever again unless driven to it." The physician replied, "I'd make the same decision myself."
- A physician said to a patient, "Yes, some years ago, like you, I had on one occasion to take all my clothes off and wait for the doctor

while standing in front of five or six men and women. They seemed to be enjoying my predicament."

All of these situations sound ridiculously simple. The reader may think that they are not helpful. I believe they are extremely important for ensuring a fruitful interaction between patient and physician/chiropractor. Certainly, the patient can do some things for the doctor or chiropractor: having a bath before their appointment; washing the feet thoroughly; and wearing clean underwear.

PREVENTION: PROMOTING HEALTH

The most important measures for the future are in the realm of prevention. Fortunately, individuals now involved in health care are concerned with the promotion of active health and not just with the correction of a disease process. This cogent lesson has been learned mostly in the field of sports medicine. The rest of us owe a debt of gratitude to the pioneers in this field. Our motto should be "health through activity."

The tools and resources needed for disease prevention are well known. We need now to refine and develop them. Chiropractors and medical practitioners learning to work together in harmony is probably the most significant advance in the field of musculoskeletal illness and treatment. These professionals have different yet complementary skills and attitudes. For the last 25 years of practice, my work in increasing cooperation with chiropractors has turned out to be of great benefit to chiropractor, physician, and patient, and was of great assistance in teaching and in research. When chiropractor and physician work together, almost in symbiosis, the result is something of far greater power than the sum of the two working alone. An analogy can be helpful. The power resulting from fusion of interests on the spiritual plane is comparable to that released by the fusion of hydrogen atoms on the physical.

Sometimes the chiropractor takes the lead and sometimes it is the physician. Each should learn from the other. The chiropractor can help the physician by making treatment simpler and more cost effective. Quick, almost immediate intervention by the physician makes things better for both patient and chiropractor if something suddenly goes wrong in the management of a disk herniation or spinal stenosis, or sudden development of cauda equina syndrome.

Back School

The availability of this facility is essential. The physician or chiropractor should be able to send a patient at any time with delay of no more than 2 or 3 days. A back school may be staffed by physical and/or occupational therapists, sometimes with volunteer help, or by two or three chiropractors. It may be in the office of a chiropractor, physical therapist, or physician, or in a gymnasium or hospital outpatient department. In many instances, educational advances from the back school benefit the community. The back school has been discussed extensively elsewhere.

Fitness Center

Even small North American cities have one or two fitness centers, and large cities have many. This type of venture is usually run by a trained therapist or exercise physiologist. They were started for the benefit of those engaged in athletic activities of all kinds, to both promote fitness and help the resolution of minor musculoskeletal injuries. The client attends at his or her own volition, does his or her own work-out, and asks for help and advice as necessary. Many chiropractors and some physicians use the fitness center to supplement what they can do for the patient in their office and what the patient can do at home. They refer the patient to the therapist in charge, being careful to let the latter know by phone or written note the nature of the problem, with perhaps some suggestions as to the type of exercise likely to be useful. The therapist has free rein to direct and advise the patient and to control his or her activity.

While the patient is attending a fitness center, the health care practitioner and therapist can have frequent discussions about the progress made. The chiropractor or physician sees the patient at regular intervals. Sometimes, the professional personally attends the same fitness center, which provides additional valuable contact with both patient and demonstrates that the doctor does the things that he or she advises patients to do. Every chiropractic or medical office should have access to such a supportive program.

Coulehan[7] outlined the dimensions of treatment outcome. The doctor-patient interaction is expressed in three ways: (1) focal, the treatment method; (2) symbolic, resulting from both cognitive and affective influences; and (3) behavioral, again from these two influences. The routine of the fitness center affords all three. It provides the incentive to develop both the physical and the spiritual well-being of the client.

Elastic Bodysuit

The rationale for wearing an elastic bodysuit for the prevention and treatment of low back pain is similar to that put forward by athletes engaged in many different kinds of sporting activities: downhill and cross country skiing: bobsledding; water skiing; and scuba diving, among other things; elastic trunks or suits are often worn by football, tennis, and basketball players and by cyclists; weight lifters wear a similar garment. This type of garment supports trunks and pelvis (focal), gives confidence and endurance (behavioral), and expresses the idea that the athlete is striving for oneness, body, mind and spirit combined and integrated (symbolic).[8]

Physician and chiropractors have been slow to grasp the fact that an elastic bodysuit is not a rigid corset but something that enhances activity exactly as the corresponding garment does for the athlete. We need to rethink this means of making extra provision for prevention and treatment. In the context of doctor/patient interaction, it is the symbolic aspect that is the most cogent.

ASCENT OF THE SPIRITUAL

A series of steps lead upward from what might be considered the purely physical (if such a state existed) to the completely spiritual (something not seen in this world). In our work as health care practitioners, we are concerned with the spectrum that lies between these two extremes.

Religion and Healing

Abdul Baha writes, "Religion and Science are the two wings on which man's intelligence can soar to the heights. It is not possible to fly with one wing alone. With the wing of religion alone an individual would fall into the quagmire of superstition. With the wing of science alone he or she would fall into the despairing slough of materialism."[9]

Edison patented 1093 inventions and turned the inventions of others into a success. In 1879, after many unsuccessful attempts, he made the first electric light bulb. His team produced latex from Golden Rod after examining hundreds of plants. When asked where his ideas came from, he used to smile and point to the sky.

Quite ordinary men and women like ourselves believe in the existence of a God who is all powerful and prepared under certain conditions to intervene in our affairs, provided this intervention does not compromise our free will. We seek this help through what we call "prayer." It is wise to do this more often than we do.

Either/Or: Both/And

Something is lacking in the way we think. Perhaps it has always been that way. In most situations, we think in terms of either/or. The chiropractor or osteopath thinks in terms of manual therapy, the physician in terms of medication or surgery. In Saskatoon, the process of chiropractors and orthopedic surgeons learning to work together was at first painful for both sides. Out of this effort came a "both/and" approach resulting in a synthesis of both disciplines, something new for us, to the benefit of both ourselves and our patients.

Turning to consideration of the physical and the spiritual, we encounter the same difficulty. Many spiritually minded health care professionals see no need for anything other than physical and material methods of treatment. Priests and ministers who have a concern for healing often tend to think in spiritual terms only. The best approach is a synthesis of the two. Intermediate steps on the journey from the Physical to the Spiritual contain elements of both, and are mentioned only briefly.

Other Resources

Back school, already mentioned, deals not only with material facts but also with the interaction of instructors and clients and with the whole group in the class. Discussion of their problems during breaks is as important as any instruction given.

Meditation, relaxation, and imagery can be a part of Back School or they can be taught individually, both with great benefit. An integral part of this process is how to manage stress. This subject is discussed at length by Zahourek.[10]

Use of the imagination should be cultivated. Sanford[11] tells how she was able to help a small boy with a serious heart condition. She discovered that he was fascinated by football. She said, "Let's play a game." He nodded and agreed. "Billy, imagine that you are playing football and that you are getting better and better at it. One day your team is playing against the best team in the league. You play so well that you score more goals than anyone else and win the game for your side. You hear some of the onlookers say 'Just look at Billy, how fast he can run, how well he tackles, how strongly he kicks the ball. We'd like to be like him. He must be so fit and well.' Billy was thrilled." Sanford continues, "Can you make a picture of that in your mind three or four times every day." Once again Billy, nodded vigorously. He did this every day. After a few months, be became perfectly fit and well again, no problem with his heart. He later became a great football player.

The Institute for the Advancement of Human Behavior, another resource, is in Stamford, Connecticut. This organization of psychologists, psychiatrists, and other practitioners plans seminars and meetings dealing with the psychologic and immunologic aspects of both wellness and disease.

Publications

Siegel wrote of lessons learned about self-healing from a surgeon's experience with exceptional patients.[12] His approach combines orthodox medicine with the spiritual. The American Cancer Society has produced a pamphlet entitled *Say it with the Heart* to help those suffering from cancer. It is full of helpful suggestions and emphasizes the importance of the patient's attitude and feelings. Another book by Simonton, Matthews–Simonton, and Creighton appeals equally to health care professionals and patients with cancer.[13] The underlying philosophy is that we are all responsible for our own health and illnesses, and that we participate, consciously or unconsciously, in creating our own physical, emotional, and spiritual health. The knowledge gained from reading this book can also be applied to the management of many other conditions, be they physical, emotional, and spiritual. (*Getting Well Again* is also available in video cassette.

Power of Prayer

Many of us believe that the natural indwelling defenses against foreign invaders and disease, including the immune system, were given to us by God as part of our make-up; that our environment contains many resources for healing, substances like penicillin and digitalis; and that health care professionals and others have their source of training directly from Him—it is no accident that hospitals and clinics had their origin in the monasteries of the Middle Ages.

It is not too great a stretch of the imagination to believe in the existence of an all-powerful being, prepared under certain circumstances to intervene in our affairs. Again, we seek this help through prayer. It is easy to ignore the existence of a power greater than ourselves when the sun is shining. Then our god may well be golf, our savior the computer, our inspiration gained from thoughts of sex. When ill health and disaster loom ahead, we are more inclined to look above and beyond ourselves for help. Fortunate is the man or woman, health care professional or patient, who seeks to take advantage both of the natural provisions for health and wellness and of those from the supernatural realm.

One example makes the point more clear. The people involved were tough sturdy fishermen. The captain and four members of the crew of a small craft lived for 11 days without food in a rubber raft after their 29-meter fishing boat sank. They were eventually rescued. When questioned later, one of the crew said, "We did a lot of praying. I definitely believe that God was watching over us. Every time we made a stupid mistake or something went wrong we would just slump our heads and start praying heavily—and bingo something would happen. We did a lot of soul searching and now I think we're going to enjoy the simpler things in life. Instead of shooting for the stars we're going to sit down and smell the flowers."

The same sort of revelation can occur when someone is suffering from severe low back pain, at a time when both patient and doctor are at wit's end. A priest in the Episcopal Church developed severe back and leg pain of sudden onset. He contacted a friend who in turn called his friend, an orthopedic surgeon. The surgeon examined the man and thought he had an acute L4-5 disk herniation. This suspicion was confirmed by a CT scan. Members of the priest's church prayed for him that night. On his next visit, the surgeon prayed for him as well, with some reluctance (surgeons do not usually pray for priests!). In the middle of that night, the patient woke up and realized all his pain had gone. From that point, he had a rapid and uneventful recovery. The priest later said that he had experienced two miracles: the first, that a surgeon had visited him in his own home, and the second, the healing of his back.

SUMMARY

Interaction between physician, chiropractor, and patient is both fundamental and complex. The resulting relationships are the phenomena of most importance. They depend on something more than science alone. The raw materials of which they are built come from a variety of sources:

- A careful study of science and its branches
- The humanities
- Philosophy
- Myth, the story with a meaning
- Behavior, symbol and metaphor

The combination of these sources with the greatest significance are those with a strong symbolic content. Good relations stem from our seeking the best for one another. The search may involve us in efforts to understand aspects of a person's psyche that range from slight differences in dress to grasping the nature of an individual's reaction to a situation of life and death. At times, it is not difficult for the discerning physician to empathize with the distress felt by a patient, sharing the symbolic content and the behavioral aspects of the situation. The practitioner must shift from time to time from close identity on the stage to standing back in the wings.

In the process of travelling with a client from a state of distress to one of complete well-being, we should be prepared to seek help from other sources. Complete rapport between the physician and the chiropractor is of greatest significance and also is rewarding. The convergence of ideas and beliefs held by students and teachers from two different backgrounds produces within them the stimulation required to conquer new areas in the spectrum of musculoskeletal illness.

Given the large a number of different approaches to spiritual healing, it is essential to respect beliefs that are different from our own. It is good to be aware of the presence and involvement of the Creator in any and every scenario in which client and helper seek health and wholeness. This statement does not imply that we are always talking about such awareness. When we ourselves do not have access to the "throne of grace," we should feel free to refer the client to someone else who has. The One who sits on the throne is able to come "alongside" us just as we are taught to come alongside our clients in their need.

REFERENCES

1. Macmurry J: Reason amd Emotion. London, Faber and Faber, 1935.
2. Macmurry J: Creative Society. London, Faber and Faber, 1935.
3. Blanchard K: Listening: a Basic Business Skill. Inside Guide, Newsletter for Canadian Plus. Toronto, Grant N.R. Geall, June, July and August, 1992.
4. Dixon T: The philosophies of family medicine (editorial) Can Fam Physician 35:743, 1989.
5. Chapman-Smith D: Reflections on the Hawthorne effect. Chiropractic Report (editorial). Vol 4, 1989, p 1.
6. Dixon T: In praise of the Hawthorne Effect (editorial). Can Fam Physician 35:703, 1989.
7. Coulehan L: The treatment act: An analysis of the clinical art in chiropractic. J Manipulative Physiol Ther 14:1, 1990.
8. Kirkaldy-Willis WH: Energy stored for action: The elastic bodysuit. In Kirkaldy-Willis WH, Burton CV (eds): Managing Low Back Pain. New York, Churchill Livingstone, 1992.
9. Abdul Baha: Paris talks. London, Baha'i Public Trust, 1973, p 143.
10. Zahourek R: Relaxation and Imagery. Philadelphia, WB Saunders, 1988.
11. Sanford A: The Healing Light. New York, Ballantine Books, 1983.
12. Siegel BS: Love, Medicine and Miracles. New York, Harper & Row, 1986.
13. Simonton OC, Matthews S, Creighton JL: Getting Well Again. New York, Bantam Books, 1980.

21 Place of Active Care in Disability Prevention

VERT MOONEY

The difficulty of defining and treating a soft tissue injury to the back is well known. Nonetheless, the primary therapeutic focus is now changing from relieving pain to restoring function. The ability to measure functional capacity, especially for the returning worker, becomes increasingly important.

MEASURING FUNCTIONAL CAPACITY

Most back injuries, whether industrial or recreational, occur without a verifiable site of injury. No repeatable, valid test is available to pinpoint the location of the painful soft tissue injury. It must indeed be a soft tissue injury, because radiographic and bone scan changes are consistently absent in what has been classified "motion disorders of the spine," i.e., postinjury back pain. Degenerative changes may be seen radiographically, but these findings are nonspecific. In no study have these changes been correlated with specific back pain.

Without specific nerve root signs, there are no reproducible physical findings. From the chiropractic and physical therapy view, the previous statement is incorrect, but current medical theory holds firm to this tenet. Because of this difference in opinion, the consensus report of the Quebec Task Force on Motion Disorders of the Spine was forced to classify the back ailment strictly on the basis of pain location and its duration of complaint.[1] This document also proposes that no matter what the soft tissue injury, problems typically resolve within 7 weeks. If spontaneous recovery does not occur, the problem should be defined from a multidisciplinary perspective. Intensive investigation of cause should be initiated early, before a long delay allows the burdens of deconditioning to emerge.

Because the specific site of injury is unknown, palliative care was considered appropriate. Until the last decade, rest, physical therapy techniques that reduced pain, muscle relaxant medication, and analgesics were the standard of care. Certainly, manipulative care can speed the rate of healing, but the mechanism is not known.[2] The emerging concepts of sports medicine, however, led us all to realize that soft tissue injuries are not best treated passively. For injuries to extremity joints, gradual progressive exercise programs to enhance the organization of scar repair in the strained connective tissues have become the standard methods of care. A combination of exercise with treatments such as the application of ice to reduce the pain reaction is now recommended for ankle strains and similar injuries. It is therefore reasonable that exercise is equally appropriate for individuals with low back injuries. No matter where the soft tissue injury—disk, facet joints, ligaments, or muscle tendon junction—progressive exercises should be of benefit. Another important concept is that when exercises are used as the major treatment tool, the measurement of functional capacity replaces the patient's assessment of pain as the basis for evaluating progress.

Sports medicine experience also showed that rest produces deconditioning of cardiovascular as well as peripheral musculature. Similar information began to emerge from the space program, in which the reduction in physical stress associated with gravity-reduced space travel produced measurable deficits in function.[3] The space travel model also revealed not only that the absence of physical stress hinders the healing of injured soft tissue, but also deterioration in function of otherwise healthy tissues could be expected to follow prolonged rest. It is rational, therefore, to turn to the measurement of function as a starting point in an appropriate exercise program. We need to establish the current baseline of function. Aerobic testing can supply baseline of performance (Fig. 21.1).

PERFORMANCE LEVELS

Objective measurement of function is accomplished fairly easily in the realm of sports testing. Performance levels in the athlete are measurable, and norms against which to assess performance can be readily established. Athletic performance is a summation of many physical characteristics, including strength, endurance, neuromotor control, and motivation. To make the best use of performance measurement, specific components are identified for testing. Furthermore, no one test can reliably predict total performance.

Range of Motion

Early in the analysis of performance, range of motion was recognized as a measurable entity, and the absence of normal range was used as a possible predictor of deficient performance. Range of motion of the extremities is nicely measured by goniometers and thus became a standard of physical therapy assessment of extremity function; the validity of such measurement can be verified in the opposite limb. For the back, however, range of motion of the hips had to be separated from that of the lumbar spine. Thus, in the late 1960s, specific discrimination of lumbar range was established using inclinometers.[4] This method of evaluating lumbar capacity is

411

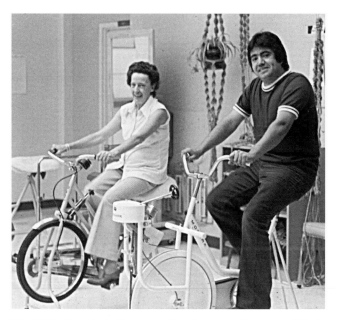

Fig. 21.1. Aerobic testing using bicycle ergometers is a relatively inexpensive measure of performance. Consistency of effort and attitude toward physical function can often be determined by evaluating aerobic performance.

now standard, according to the AMA Guidelines for Impairment.[5] In fact, the delineation of lumbar range is the only objective measurement of function for the assessment of spinal impairment in these guidelines. This measurement does not give a total picture, but no other functional capacity tests for the spine have been judged reliable and valid by consensus. Also, some clinicians believe they can recognize intersegmental variations in motion, but such a finding is not measurable.[6]

Range testing is insufficient to evaluate the functional capacity of the extremities. A significant innovation in the late 1960s was the development of the capacity to control the variable of speed in muscle function.[7] This isokinetic testing allowed an individual to create as much torque as feasible, while allowing force to be measured throughout the range by controlling velocity. This type of measurement proved to be an excellent guide for sports medicine physicians trying to evaluate the relative strength of flexors and extensors and status of rehabilitation after injuries to various joints. The use of isokinetic devices as training/exercise tools has come into question, however, because the incompletely controllable impact forces may cause additional injury.

Not until the early 1980s was the concept of isokinetic testing applied to the back. Using converted extremity equipment and normal subjects, the first study was conducted in Japan in 1980.[8] Although the investigators did not have a method of normalizing the torque curves, and the equipment required that subjects be recumbent for testing, several points emerged that are confirmed by current studies. In normal subjects, the extensors are stronger than the flexors of the back, and the difference is more significant in men than in women.

Age definitely influences the strength of trunk muscles: older subjects are notably weaker than younger individuals. The relative strengths of extensors and flexors, however, remain the same during the aging process.

Smidt et al (also using converted equipment) took measurements while subjects were sitting, a more realistic posture in terms of back performance.[9] The results confirmed that men are significantly stronger in torso musculature than women, and that the extensors in normal individuals are significantly stronger than the flexors. As in most of the early studies, the number of subjects was small. Furthermore, factors such as fitness and patient size were not considered. Nonetheless, the sitting posture could be of use in isolating trunk musculature from hip musculature.

Mayer et al[10] performed the first major study using equipment specifically designed to test back performance isokinetically. This group compared significant numbers of subjects (125 normal and 286 chronic back pain patients). The patients were tested while standing, which probably permits a more realistic evaluation of lifting performance. The investigators also used the weight of the subject as a method of normalizing the data (torque/body weight), making comparison among subjects more valid. Again, extensors were stronger than flexors in normal subjects, but extensor muscles proved significantly weaker than flexors in individuals with chronic back pain. At higher speeds, torque production was significantly less in individuals with back pain than in normal subjects.

The study also demonstrated the extreme variability of initial evaluation in back pain patients. Consistency of performance in spite of pain, however, can be expected when the patients are familiar with the machine. The study showed that pain does not limit consistency when the patients are making maximal efforts. The equipment became available as a method for identifying willful submaximal or misleading performance on the part of the patients. The concept that only maximal effort could provide consistent performance was proposed in this study. This theory assumes no performance feedback to the subject is being tested. It also assumes an accurate measurement tool.

Another variation in the objective of back muscle performance was the assessment of trunk rotatory performance with isokinetic torque measurement equipment.[11] Torque measurement was accomplished with the subject sitting. Rotational torque in normal subjects was about 50% of extensor torque. Torque production was significantly decreased in back pain patients, to about 65% of extensor torque. Patients were not tested until they had achieved normal range, which was easily definable using this equipment. The authors of this study also attempted to compare myoelectric performance with dynamic performance using isokinetic equipment, but they could make few correlations. No study has yet been able to use electromyography as a specific predictor or discriminator of individuals with low back pain.

All of these studies involved the use of equipment from Cybex (Ronkonkoma, NY), the only manufacturer of such devices at that time. Other manufacturers have emerged since

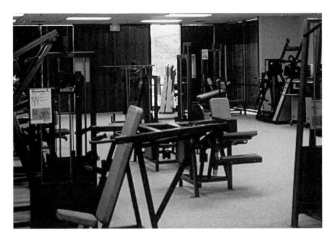

Fig. 21.2. Example of a strengthening circuit manufactured by Cybex. In the far right corner is the lumbar testing machine for evaluating sagittal flexion and extension isokinetic torque.

the lapsing of some Cybex patents, which has led to a virtual explosion in the marketing of functional testing equipment. In addition, many manufacturers supply exercise equipment modeled on the original Nautilus equipment designed 30 years ago (Fig. 21.2).

A limitation of all the early studies was that the individual was constrained to the same position on each occasion of testing in an effort to achieve repeatable data. Each of us has a specific strategy for lifting and lowering that is based on our unique configuration of biomechanical factors. When strapped into a sitting or standing position, we do not lift the way we normally would (Fig. 21.3). Another isokinetic test allows the patient to lift in any posture desired. This simulated lifting task was performed from a standing position. In the initial report of this test, low back pain patients could lift only an average of 67% of the value lifted by normal subjects.[12] Again, at higher speeds, patients performed poorly in comparison with normal subjects. The equipment seemed to be safe, and the results of isokinetic performance testing were more consistent than those of single position isometric testing using the same equipment. Patients tested isometrically in incompletely isolated postures sometimes complained of pain, whereas those individuals tested isokinetically usually did not. Finally, a poor correlation existed between isokinetic performance and isometric performance. Isokinetic testing was therefore advocated as a safer, more reliable means to test lifting performance. It had the potential to provide specific numbers in terms of torque and work production, but with the equipment used in this study, anatomic isolation was poor.

Isodynamic/Isometric Testing

An alternative to isokinetic testing is a computerized system labeled isodynamic. Manufactured by Isotechnologies (Hillsborough, NC), this constant-load device simultaneously measures change in torque and velocity in all three planes of motion (sagittal, frontal, and transverse). With so many variables

operating at the same time, comparison from one day to another and from one individual to another is more difficult than with isokinetic equipment. Nonetheless, normal levels of function have been reported.[13] Once again, women have lower torque and velocity measures than men. One of the most important contributions from studies using this equipment is that speed of performance is a major discriminator between individuals with back pain.[14] Investigators using this equipment have also observed that with increasing fatigue, muscle substitution and greater deviation in the arc of motion occur.

Such evaluation of lateral bending and rotation simultaneously with flexion and extension is a unique property of this equipment.[15] The point is that different systems of measurement can provide alternative perspectives on human performance. It also underscores the emerging awareness that one specific measure cannot totally summarize or diagnose with certainty the incapacity resulting from soft tissue injury in the back.

Various other methods can be used to evaluate free lifting. The subjects are tested in such a way that they can lift or lower any weight that the computerized equipment defines. They can lift straight or in a twisting mode to various heights. Numeric representation of performance, graphic feedback, and a printout of performance are available.

Simpler methods of evaluating free lifting involve having the individual lift graduated weights. Performance is then measured in terms of increasing amounts of weight lifted over

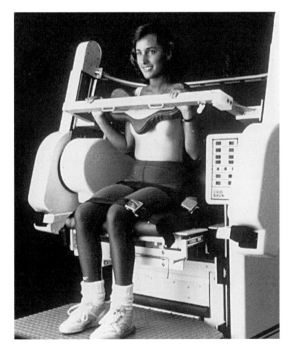

Fig. 21.3. Device manufactured by the Lordan Company with an adjustable platform allows testing while sitting or standing. Unfortunately, stabilization of the pelvis cannot be fully achieved. Also, intense, variable resistance concentric and eccentric exercise is not available.

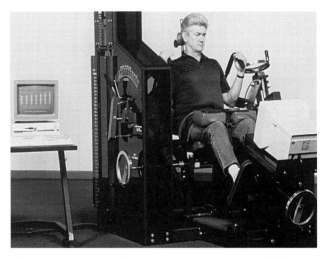

Fig. 21.4. Design of this equipment completely stabilizes the pelvis so that testing accurately documents lumbar extensor muscular strength. Also, variable resistance concentric and eccentric strength training is provided to the lumbar extensor muscles. This equipment provides the most significant amount of isolation, and thus, specific training of any device currently available.

time. For safety and to avoid overexertion, limits on performance can be identified. For instance, in the Pile test, 5- or 10-lb weights are added in 30-second intervals, and the subject lifts and lowers the weights four times in 30 seconds.[16] This type of test provides an alternative to methods requiring expensive equipment. Normal standards and comparisons of the performance of back pain patients against such standards for these tests have been recorded. An improved weights in a box test, known as Epic, has been developed that defines deficit relative to normal ability.[17]

Although isometric testing was the first functional test method with which to assess lumbar performance and then compare it with the expected performance of worker, this single-dimension method has not maintained its primacy in lumbar assessment.[18] In simple, unconstrained isometric testing, the posture of the test subject is difficult to control. In addition, the significant weak link cannot be easily identified—unconstrained isometric testing depends on arm strength, trunk strength, and leg strength, but standard test methods cannot readily separate the contribution of each of these factors.

Another isometric lumbar test, the Sorenson test, requires the subject to hold the trunk parallel to the floor while the torso is unsupported. In industrial populations in Denmark, the inability to hold such a posture for a minute or more correlated with an increased incidence of back injury.[19] This finding implies that strength has something to do with back pain.

New equipment has been developed, however, that specifically segregates lumbar isometric performance from that of the arms and legs. This equipment, made by MedX (Ocala, FL), identifies isometric performance at specific equidistant points in lumbar range from full flexion to full extension. The thoracolumbar spine is totally isolated from all other anatomy.

With these design characteristics, the equipment has proven to be extremely reliable and repeatable in testing lumbar strength (Fig. 21.4).[20] This equipment can also be used for exercise training. Because of the intensity of the variable resistance exercise, full potential for strengthening can be reached with only one or two sessions per week. In addition, strengthening correlates significantly with diminished pain complaint.[21]

PAIN TREATMENT

Given our improved ability to measure strength, we must recognize our inability to locate specifically the soft tissue site of injury in back pain. Quantitative assessment of function seems to be the only way to obtain objective data. This concept is not totally accepted. Hasson and Wise criticized earlier investigators for not dividing patient groups into diagnostic categories; however, the diagnostic categories they suggested are nonverifiable, i.e., sacroiliac strain versus facet syndrome versus disk pathology.[22] This problem is identical to that which plagues the treatment of chronic back pain: most of the sources of pain are nonverifiable. Pain in the back usually is without representation of specific nerve root dysfunction. The role of deconditioning—the impairment of physical capacity that may result from prolonged pain-limited behavior—cannot easily be evaluated with a simple physical examination. Such barriers to understanding have led to the development of pain clinics with a focus on the perception of pain rather than on the sources of pain. Behavioral control of pain has been the project in these centers, but restoration of functional capacity and return to work have not been measured goals.

The focus on treating the pain alone has led to a general suspicion, particularly among third-party payers, that rehabilitation for chronic pain may be ineffective and in fact many be no better than a placebo in attaining specific societal goals, such as return to work.[23] Fordyce and colleagues noted that pain clinics tend to treat the experience of pain but not the disability associated with pain behavior. Pain often is associated with the deconditioning syndrome, and technology now allows us to measure this extent of deconditioning. In the case of the back, objective lumbar function testing has been of great value in the treatment and rehabilitation of individuals with chronic back pain.[24]

It is a great improvement to base evaluation on functional and strength testing rather than on simple alteration in the patient's report of pain function. With this more objective methodology, the focus is on returning the patient to work and normal life activities. But how can we use this improved ability to measure to enhance active care?

REHABILITATION

One of the most important areas of community knowledge has emerged from the availability of widespread observation of sporting events. With television coverage, many more people witness injuries sustained during various professional sports. They also observe the rapid return of this athlete to action within several days or weeks after significant injury. Thus, the reality of effective care in sports medicine is readily evident to the public at large.

What are the principles of sports medicine? Put simply, progress in treatment is based on measured changes in function. The athlete views discomfort as irrelevant in terms of return of function. Moreover, the easily understood principles of soft tissue repair are applied to these athletes. Gradual progressive exercises that challenge the soft tissues consistently and progressively constitute a reliable therapeutic maneuver. This process is the way we all learned to treat a sprained ankle. Transferring these principles to other joints, including the back, is simple. Are these principles applicable to industrial injuries as well?

A reasonable approach to the injured worker is to consider that individual an industrial athlete. The project is to convince that individual that the principles are just as applicable to his or her injury as they were to the injured athlete they saw on television. Outcome in the treatment of any joint, including the back, can be measured by using various tests of function. As described previously, excellent equipment is available for measuring strength and endurance in a reproducible, objective sense. It is also possible to identify levels of consistent performance and effort on the part of the injured individual.

The injured worker must want to get better for the treatment program to be of benefit. Certainly, most people truly do want to get better and to avoid pain and disability. Their desires for recovery are usually enthusiastic if the treatment is initiated early. With prolonged delay in rational treatment, however, factors of deconditioning of the soft tissues, as well as of the psyche, emerge. Habituation to pain develops. Perhaps some pleasure with absence from work may occur. Under these circumstances, significant social disruption also can occur. Litigation perhaps can develop wherein the successful litigation depends on proof of severity and level of pain and disability. Once these psychosocial problems are involved with the repair process, chances for success are considerably limited.

Even under these circumstances, however, modern techniques offer a tool to urge the deconditioned worker back to healthy behavior. The programs are generically known as *work hardening centers.* Hereto, the earlier the disabled worker participates, the more successful the approach. What are these principles?

QUEBEC TASK FORCE: PRINCIPLES FOR EVALUATION AND TREATMENT

Certainly, the back injury problem is one that has been addressed by many experienced clinicians and scientists. A wide array of concepts and various areas of emphasis have been reported. As mentioned previously, a consensus of these concepts is now available. In 1987, a document was published stating those principles deemed most appropriate for the evaluation and treatment of back injuries. The project was initi-

ated by the Canadian Institute for Workers Health and Safety. Thus, the Quebec Task Force on Spinal Disorders was convened. Included in this task force were a wide array of experts in medicine, law, and therapy.[25]

This extensive consensus report identified various factors that would increase costs, e.g., excessive, unnecessary diagnostic testing, such as magnetic resonance imaging, CT, and electromyography without clinical justification. Surgical intervention with little clinical justification also was noted. One of the most important factors in increasing costs was the use of ineffective physical therapy techniques, such as ultrasound. The use of the therapies was "hit or miss" in large part because few objective data were used to support the benefits of any type of treatment program. Finally, the report noted that employers often are reluctant to allow an employee who is still having pain to return to work. This situation led to prolonged treatment and, of course, enhanced legal costs. Delay in receiving effective care was also noted as a factor in driving up costs. What is effective care?

This report revealed that most complaints were nonspecific in that no anatomic cause could be identified to explain the patient's complaint. Even though the source of the problem was unexplained, however, bed rest turned out to be an inappropriate form of treatment. This study also reported that surgery alone is not predictably effective in treating back pain. Associated with this concept is that the decision to use surgical care should be made only after the patient has participated in an *active* rehabilitation program and has demonstrated lack of improvement. It was also noted that residual chronic pain was not a contraindication for return to work. This concept was further reinforced by an excellent prospective study that documented a greater than 80% rate in the ability to return to work for chronically disabled people even though they had some residual back pain.[26]

The task force also found that the majority of costs associated with back disorders are incurred by 10 to 15% of the patients with symptoms that have lasted longer than 7 weeks. Thus, the concept proposed from this consensus report is that seven weeks is the time at which a problem is considered chronic. Chronicity may be defined as the time at which a soft tissue problem no longer can be expected to heal spontaneously. This document also identified the milestone of acute injury as 1 week, and subacute injury from 1 week to 7 weeks. This differentiation is valuable in that if one expects spontaneous resolution of a problem in the acute and subacute phase, developing a more vigorous and expensive treatment plan during that phase is inappropriate in most cases.

There is some support for the concept put forth by McKenzie that a method to prevent the back injury from deteriorating into a more significant problem can be implemented by a specific exercise program that evaluates physical maneuvers by which the pain is changed. Studies have shown that if this program is initiated within the first 4 weeks, excellent or good results can be expected in 98% of cases; if, however, the program is initiated after 4 weeks, the percentage of success drops to about 80%.[27]

A relatively simple exercise program was documented by Choler et al.[28] At this acute and subacute phase, some methods in the form of heat or cold likely are useful; however, the literature includes no justification, as supported by the Quebec Task Force Study, that other techniques such as diathermy, massage, and repeated hot packs offer any benefit to enhance the rate of recovery. It must be emphasized that treatment is to a nonspecific problem, and the only definition of improvement in the McKenzie concept is centralization of the pain to the mid-low back. If the pain progresses further in a peripheral manner, the therapist must recognize that the exercise program proposed is inappropriate. The exercise may be extension, flexion, or side-shifting based on what happens to the pain. At least, this type of program has the benefit of some relatively objective measurement of progress. *Indeed, a method to measure progress should be at the core of all efficient, effective treatment plans.*

PROVIDING CARE IN TODAY'S HEALTH CARE ENVIRONMENT

The reason for interest in the sports medicine approach, i.e., measurement of progress by some objective maneuver, is the matter of reimbursement. As the health care system begins to look for greater efficiencies, it is apparent that more documentation as to the level of dysfunction is the basis on which reimbursement is more likely to be provided. The system responds more specifically to payment for medical care that is focused on documenting how the patient is functioning better, rather than how they might be feeling better. It is apparent to the providers that even though the patient may feel better briefly, no benefit has been served in terms of reimbursement for medical care without long-term change in function. Documentation of progress is the essence on which billings are reimbursed. Lack of measurable progress is the documentation on which useful medical care for soft tissue injuries has ceased. This is essentially a sports medicine approach. It is unlikely that the future health care dollar will pay for maintenance level care for benign, nondestructive disease.

A plan of care that reflects this attitude is noted in Table 21.1. This treatment guideline has been accepted by several preferred provider organizations in the Southern California area. It speaks specifically toward documentation of function.

In industrial back injuries, experience shows that the patient seldom arrives at an appropriately oriented treatment program within the first several weeks. In those patients for whom treatment is delayed, some deconditioning occurs. In this group of patients, and those that have not improved in the McKenzie type of program, one may expect a relative loss of range and strength. The reality of this phenomenon is documented by the fact that an ICD-9 Code 728.2 makes available a definition of deconditioning by the diagnosis of muscular wasting and disuse atrophy. This diagnosis can be objectively demonstrated by specific testing. Therefore, a treatment plan that strengthens the soft tissues and can document the benefit

Table 21.1. Treatment of Medical Back Problems

- A program of progressive exercise should be initiated after no more than 2 to 3 days of bed rest. Passive methods (either ice or hot packs) are only useful as an adjunct to exercise. Other techniques are not appropriate.
- An objective, reproducible functional assessment should occur if more than 2 weeks of treatment are required.
- Most patients need instruction on appropriate exercise but do not need a formal program of physical therapy. When physical therapy is indicated, duration should not exceed 6 weeks and frequency should not exceed three treatments weekly.
- Diagnostic radiographs are seldom appropriate initially and, with rare exceptions, are not appropriate at intervals during treatment.
- Unless neurologic function has deteriorated or progressive exercise has failed, specific diagnostic techniques (e.g., CT scan, magnetic resonance imaging, bone scan, EMG, nerve conduction studies) are not appropriate.
- More than 75% of employed patients with medical back problems return to work within 4 weeks of onset. Careful re-evaluation of the treatment plan is warranted if the patient has not progressed significantly in 4 weeks.
- If treatment lasts 6 weeks, the patient should be evaluated by an appropriate medical specialist. The evaluation should include objective measurement of functional status, reassessment of treatment goals, and confirmation of appropriateness of treatment.
- If the patient has not returned to work within 3 months, the patient should be referred to a specialized center for computerized re-assessment and care planning.

of treatment by objective testing is justified. These tools were described previously.

SUMMARY

Active exercise programs are effective in disability prevention. It is important to separate the concepts of impairment and disability. Impairment is the physical weak link(s) that limit function. If we can isolate anatomy sufficiently, we should be able to test the deficit and evaluate progress and treatment by further testing.

Disability, on the other hand, refers to the limits that prevent return to the previous level of function. In addition to the "weak link" is an array of personal and human factors that create disability, including age, sex, education, secondary gain, and overall attitude. Some factors of disability may involve acquiring bad habits such as substance abuse, obesity, marital and family upheaval, and anxiety and depression. All of these factors seem to be enhanced by diminishing physical activity. Physical activity that is focused on improving healthy behavior is the anecdote to these disabling problems. Frequently, coaching in positive health habits is necessary. This coaching does not necessarily fall into the patient care realm of any specific clinician; all practitioners who come in contact with disabled patients need to focus on these positive factors. Active exercise, not preaching, seems to have the greatest opportunity to effect a significant change.

REFERENCES

1. Spitzer WO, LeBlanc FE, Dupuis M: Scientific approach to the assessment and management of activity–related spinal disorders. Spine 12:S1, 1987.

2. Haldeman S, Phillips RB: The spinal manipulative theory in the management of low back pain. In Frymoyer JW (ed): The Adult Spine: Principles and Practice. New York, Raven Press, 1991, pp 1581–1605.

3. Lamb L, Johnson RL, St. Jens PM: Cardiovascular conditioning during chair rest. Aerospace Med 35:646, 1964.

4. Loebl W: Measurements of spinal posture and range in spinal movements. Am J Phys Med Rehabil 9:103, 1967.

5. Engelberg AL (ed): Guides to the Evaluation of Permanent Impairment. 3rd Ed. Chicago, American Medical Association, 1988.

6. Gitelman R: A chiropractic approach in biomedical disorders of the lumbar spine and pelvis. In Haldeman S (ed): Modern Developments in the Principles and Practice of Chiropractic. New York, Appleton Century Crofts, 1980.

7. Thistoe H, Hislop HJ, Mofford M, et al: Isokinetic contraction: A new concept of resistive exercise. Arch Phys Med Rehabil 48:279, 1967.

8. Hasue M, Fujiwara M, Kikuchi S: A new method of quantitative measurement of abdominal and back muscle strength. Spine 5:143, 1980.

9. Smidt G, et al: Muscle strength at the trunk. J Orthop Sports Phys Ther 1:165, 1980.

10. Mayer T, Smith S, Keeley J, et al: Quantification of lumbar function. Part 2: Sagittal plane trunk strength in chronic low-back pain patients. Spine 10:765, 1985.

11. Mayer T, Smith SS, Kondraske G, et al: Quantification of lumbar function. Part 3: Preliminary data on isokinetic torso rotation testing with myoelectric spectral analysis in normal and low-back pain subjects. Spine 10:912, 1985.

12. Kishino N: Quantification of lumbar function. Part 4: Isometric and isokinetic lifting simulation in normal subjects and low back pain dysfunction patients. Spine 10:921, 1985.

13. Seeds R, Levine J, Goldberg HM: Normative data for isostation B-100. J Orthop Sports Phys Ther 9:141, 1987.

14. Seeds R, Levine JA, Goldberg HM: Abnormal patient data for the isosation B-100. J Orthop Sports Phys Ther 10:121, 1988.

15. Parnianpour M, Nordin M, Frankel VH, et al: Triaxial coupled isometric trunk measurements. Presented at Orthopedic Research Society Meeting, Atlanta, January 1988, p 379.

16. Mayer T, Kishing ND, Nichols G, et al: Progressive isoinertial lifting evaluation. I. A standardized protocol and normative database. Spine 13:993, 1988.

17. Alpert J, Matheson L, Beam W, et al: The reliability and validity of two new tests of maximum lifting capacity. J Occup Rehabil 1:13, 1991.

18. Chaffin DB, Parek KS: A longitudinal study of low back pain as associated with occupational weight lifting factors. J Am Ind Hyg Assoc 10:513, 1973.

19. Biering-Sorenson F: Physical measurements as risk indicators for low back trouble over a one year period. Spine 9:45, 1984.

20. Graves JE, Pollock ML, Carpenter DM, et al: Quantitative assessment of full range of motion isometric lumbar extension strength. Spine 15:289, 1990.

21. Graves JE, Pollock ML, Foster D, et al: Effect of training frequency and specificity on isometric lumbar extension strength. Spine 15:504, 1990.

22. Hasson SM, Wise DD: Instrumented testing of the back. Surg Rounds Orthop 10:28, 1989.

23. Fordyce W, Roberts A, Sternbach R: The behavioral management of chronic pain: A response to critics. Pain 22:113, 1985.

24. Mayer T, Gatchell RJ, Kishino N, et al: A prospective short-term study on chronic low back pain patients utilizing novel objective functional measurement. Pain 25:53, 1986.

25. Spitzer UO: The scientific approach to the assessment and management of activity related to spinal disorders. Spine 12:1, 1987.

26. Mayer TT, Gatchel R, Mayer H, et al: A prospective two year study of functional restoration in industrial low back injury. JAMA 250:450, 1987.

27. Donelson RG, Silva G, Murphy K: The centralization phenomenon: Its usefulness in evaluating and treating sciatica. Spine 15:211, 1990.

28. Choler U, Larsson R. Nachemson A: Back pain attempt at a structural treatment program for patients with low back pain. SPRI Report 188, Social Planerings–och Rationaliseringsintsitut Rapport, Stockholm, 1985.

Index